GAZMEN]

MW01092353

HERBAL
VADE MECUM

800 Herbs, Spices, Essential Oils, Lipids, Etc.

Constituents, Properties, Uses, and Caution

HERBACY PRESS
Rutherford, New Jersey

Published March 2003
Reprinted with corrections, November 2003, January 2004, May 2004, December 2004, July 2005, May, 2006, December 2006, June 2008, July 2009, January 2019

Disclaimer
The intent of this book is solely informational and educational. The information and suggestions in this book are not intended to replace the advice or treatments given by health professionals. Only they, based on individual disorders, can recommend the appropriate botanicals. Although the need of consulting health professionals in the book is not emphasized for all the botanicals, it doesn't mean that the rest can be used without their advice. The author has made every effort to present accurate information. However, neither he nor the publisher shall be responsible or liable for any problem arising from the information in this book.

ISBN-13: 978-0-9713209-2-5
ISBN-10: 0-9713209-2-6
Library of Congress Control Number: 2001093998

Printed in the United States of America

Cover and text design by
The Author

Published by
Herbacy Press
144 Wheaton Place
Rutherford, NJ 07070

To Silva, Juna, Lira, Marin, and Gres

CONTENTS

PREFACE

The purpose of this book is to provide concise information on constituents, properties, uses, and caution for a selected list out of the vast number of worldwide botanicals (herbs, spices, essential oils, resins, balsams, fixed oils, fats, gums, etc.) chiefly used in food, pharmaceutical and cosmetic industries, and family practice. Included are some bioactive substances such as beta glucans (lentinan, schizophyllan) obtained from medicinal mushrooms (shiitake, etc.; see Beta Glucans), bromelain (see Pineapple), camphor (q. v.), and soy lecithin (see Soy). Some monographs such as Ayahuasca, Khat and Syrian Rue are included mainly for toxicological purposes.

The approximately 800 botanicals are grouped in 657 short monographs listed alphabetically according to the common names of the plants from which they are derived.

Each botanical includes a description of its main constituents (suggestions for possible constituents are often included), properties (often detailed for important active constituents such as ephedrine, caffeine, and many others), uses (separated by internal and external uses), and caution (contraindications, side effects, some known or possible interactions with drugs).

The reader can go directly to the monographs or select them from the therapeutic checklist at the end of the book, where monographs are classified according to the organ systems and disorders, and from the list of various effects and uses. The reader can check uses and caution, which are clearly separate, and connect the two with the given properties, because they are mostly harmonious. The glossary of medical terms explains the terminology used under properties. Others, with broader interests, will find for each botanical, a concise and classified description about those most important active constituents, which justify properties, uses, and reasons for caution. The glossary of chemical terms explains the most important constituents of botanicals.

I have tried to keep a certain style throughout the book and done my best to avoid or at least minimize errors. Realizing that no book can be free from errors, I will be very grateful for any comments and suggestions that will improve the book for later revisions.

Gazmend Skenderi

Note: Unless otherwise specified, the described herbs and most of the spices are used dry.
h. p. is used as an abbreviation for herbal product.

ACEROLA

Other Common Name(s): Barbados cherry, West Indian cherry
Botanical Name(s): *Malpighia emarginata* DC. = *Malpighia glabra* L. = *Malpighia punicifolia* L. [Fam.: Malpighiaceae]
Fruit (cherry)
Constituents: Vitamin C (very rich; the unripe fruits are almost two times richer than the ripe ones), β-carotene (= provitamin A), flavonoids (anthocyanins: cyaniding and pelargonidin glycosides; flavonols: quercetin glycosides), minerals (calcium, iron, phosphor), organic acids (malic acid, etc.), sugars (glucose, fructose, sucrose), a heat resistant enzyme, etc.
Properties: Acidulous, refrigerant, mild astringent, antioxidant. Acerola exerts all the effects attributed to vitamin C.
Uses: Internally it is used (as a tea, h. p., jam, preserve) for feverish and thirsty states, minor diarrhea, as a vitamin C supplement, beneficial due also to its antioxidant effect. Externally it is used (as a gargle) for sore throat.
Caution: There are no contraindications or side effects when used properly.

References: (3) Vol. 5, p. 672; (8) p. 351; (9) p. 6; (52) p. 471; (57) p. 511.

ACHYRANTHES

Other Common Name(s): pigs' knee, twotooth achyranthes
Botanical Name(s): *Achyranthes bidentata* Blume [Fam.: Amaranthaceae]
Root
Constituents: Triterpenoid saponins (achyranthes saponins; with aglycone: oleanolic acid), phytosterols (phytoecdysteroids: ecdysterone, inokosterone, etc.), etc. It possibly contains high concentrations of potassium nitrate and calcium oxalate.
Properties: Anti-inflammatory and analgesic, diuretic, antispasmodic, vasodilatory, antihypertensive, emmenagogue, mild uterotonic. Its main active constituents are considered saponins and phytoecdysteroids. Phytoecdysteroids have been shown to increase protein biosynthesis (esp. in the liver). If present, potassium nitrate (chiefly unchanged KNO_3, partly may be reduced to potassium nitrite, KNO_2) may contribute to the diuretic and antihypertensive effects and may account for the dilatory effect on the neck of uterus after topical applications of achyranthes root.
Uses: Internally it is used (as a tea, h. p.) for rheumatic complaints (incl. rheumatoid arthritis), inflammatory and spastic conditions of the genitourinary, gastrointestinal and hepatobiliary tracts, secondary amenorrhea and oligomenorrhea (= ceased / infrequent / scanty menstruation without pathology) and a hypotonic uterus. In traditional gynecologic practice it is also used (by topical application) to induce dilation of the neck of uterus (= cervix uteri) and then apply curettage. Externally it is used (as a mouthwash) for inflammations of the mouth and (as a wet compress, poultice) for minor

1

wounds.

Caution: Unless advised by a health professional, achyranthes should not be taken during pregnancy. Before using it for gynecologic disorders, the problem should be judged by a health professional. Manufacturers should evaluate calcium oxalate content. If it results to be in high concentrations, achyranthes should be avoided in cases of a known history of oxalate kidney stones. Otherwise, there are no reports of contraindications or side effects when used properly.

References: (1) Vol. 4, p. 56; (3) Vol. 2, p. 895; (12a) p. 624; (18) p. 140; (31) p. 714; (36) p. 508; (41) Vols. 1-7; (42) Vol. 3, pp. 86, 88; (45) p. 157; (53) p. 287; (65) pp. 445, 842.

ACONITE

Other Common Name(s): friar's cap, monkshood, wolf's bane
Botanical Name(s): *Aconitum napellus* L. [Fam.: Ranunculaceae]
Root (tuber)
Constituents: Alkaloids (diterpenoid compounds: aconitine, its decomposition products, etc.), organic acids (aconitic acid, etc.), starch, resin, etc.
Properties: Analgesic, antipyretic, local anesthetic.
Uses: Internally and externally it is still used (only in a combination product) for neuralgic pains (incl. trigeminal neuralgia) and rheumatic pains (incl. myalgias = muscular pains). Combined with autumn crocus (= colchicum) it is used for gouty and arthritic conditions.
Caution: Aconite is very toxic and is not for self-treatment. Ingestion of even 0.2-0.5 grams of the root that contains 1 % aconitine may cause death to an adult.

References: (1) Vol. 4, p. 72; (3) Vol. 2, p. 1066; (5) Vol. 1, p. 17; (9) p. 7; (12) p. 1077; (13) p. 280; (23) p. 323; (36) p. 405; (46) p. 4; (47) p. 388; (48) p. 1052.

ADONIS, SPRING

Other Common Name(s): false hellebore, pheasant's eye
Botanical Name(s): *Adonis vernalis* L. [Fam.: Ranunculaceae]
Aerial part
Constituents: Cardiac glycosides (chiefly adonitoxol = adonitoxigenol-rhamnoside, also cymarin = k-strophanthin-α = k-strophanthidin-cymaroside), flavonoids (chiefly flavone-C-glycosides), etc.
Properties: Spring adonis exerts strophanthus-like cardiotonic effect, but milder. It has also shown diuretic, coronary dilatory and sedative effects. It is less cumulative than digitalis. See DIGITALIS; STROPHANTHUS.
Uses: Internally it is used (as a standardized product) for early stages of heart failure (stages I and II, according to NYHA) and it is beneficial for cases associated with nervous cardiovascular problems.

2

Caution: Spring adonis is toxic and not for self-treatment. It is used only as directed by a health professional. Spring adonis products should be standardized to the cardiac glycosides content. See DIGITALIS.

References: (1) Vol. 4, p. 93; (3) Vol. 2, p. 1103; (6) pp. 37, 38; (7) p. 109; (8) p. 25; (11) p. 119; (13) p. 190; (16) p. 97; (19) p. 23; (23) p. 169; (28) p. 133; (36) p. 319; (37) p. 22; (46) p. 16; (48) p. 747.

AERVA

Other Common Name(s): 1) Aerva lanata 2) Javanese aerva, Javanese wool plant

Botanical Name(s): 1) *Aerva lanata* (L.) Juss. ex Schult. 2) *Aerva javanica* (Burm. f.) Juss. ex Schult. = *Aerva persica* (Burm. f.) Merrill = *Aerva tomentosa* Forssk. [Fam.: Amaranthaceae]

Aerial part

Constituents: Triterpenoid saponins, flavonoids (flavonols, methoxy-flavones, flavanones; chiefly as glycosides), phytosterols (5-sterols: β-sitosterol, etc.), water-soluble polysaccharides, etc.

Properties: Diuretic, anti-inflammatory, expectorant, demulcent, emollient, antimicrobial, antioxidant, antihyperglycemic, immunomodulant, antitumoral. Saponins and flavonoids account for the diuretic, anti-inflammatory and expectorant effects. β-Sitosterol has been shown to inhibit the biosynthesis of prostaglandins and leukotrienes and may account at least in part for the anti-inflammatory effect. Its immunomodulant and antitumoral effects are due at least in part to water-soluble polysaccharides and flavonoids.

Uses: Internally it is used as a flushing-out treatment (= herbal tea or product + liquids: more than 2 liters per day; sometimes combined with a medication) for inflammations of the genitourinary tract (cystitis, urethritis, etc.), urinary gravel and nonobstructive stones, to prevent relapsing urinary infections / gravel / stones, for inflammations of the upper respiratory tract (bronchitis, pharyngitis, etc.; coughs due to thickened bronchial secretion) and gastrointestinal tract (diarrhea, etc.), and as an adjuvant for diabetes. Externally it is used for minor skin inflammations and hemorrhoids.

Caution: There are no reports of contraindications or side effects when used properly. Nevertheless, a flushing-out treatment is contraindicated in cases of obstructive urinary stones, edema due to impaired heart or kidney function and kidney inflammations (here can be used on health professional's advice to enhance the effects of an antimicrobial therapy).

References: (1) Vol. 4, p. 101; (3) Vol. 2, p. 1110; (41) Vols. 1-7; (52) p. 19; (57) p. 15.

AGAR

Other Common Name(s): agar agar

Agar is a dried mucilaginous substance, extracted from red algae (Class:

Rhodophyceae), mainly *Gelidium* spp.: *Gelidium capense* (S.G. Gmelin) P.C. Silva = *Gelidium cartilagineum* (L.) Gaillon; *Gelidium amansii* (Lamouroux) Lamouroux; *Gelidium pacificum* Okamura; etc.; *Gracilaria* spp.: *Gracilaria confervoides* (L.) Grev.; *Gelidiella acerosa* (Forssk.) Feldman et Hamel; etc.

Constituents: Polysaccharides, namely agarose (ca. 2/3) and agaropectin (ca. 1/3), which are polymers of galactose and sulfated galacturonic acid. Depending on sources, to the sulfate rests are attached metallic elements (calcium, etc.)

Properties: Bulk laxative, demulcent, suspending and emulsifying, gelling.

Uses: Internally (at higher doses) it is used for chronic constipation and (at lower doses: in a combination product) as a gastrointestinal demulcent. Agar is extensively used in the production of suspensions, emulsions, suppositories, tablets, among others.

Caution: As a laxative it should not be taken in cases of bowel obstruction. Agar may impair the absorption of some drugs. In view of this, when taking a vital oral medication, drugs should be taken about one hour apart from agar products. Otherwise, there are no reports of contraindications and side effects when used properly.

References: (2) Vol. 2, p. 778; (3) Vol. 2, p. 1141; (7) p. 226; (8) p. 278; (9) p. 9; (11) p. 44; (13) p. 361; (48) p. 57.

AGARIC

Other Common Name(s): white agaric, larch agaric
Botanical Name(s): *Polyporus officinalis* Vill. = *Fomes officinalis* Faull. [Fam.: Polyporaceae]
Agaric (cap of the fungus, deprived of the outer coat), **agaricin**

Constituents: Agaric contains a resin (with agaricin = agaricic acid = α-cetylcitric acid), phytosterols (eburicoic and dehydroeburicoic acids), polyacetylenes, bitter principles, etc.

Properties: Agaricin has shown antihidrotic (= sweat-inhibiting) effect, which is due to its partial atropine-like action. It needs several hours to exert its effect.

Uses: Internally are still used (agaric or agaricin: in a combination product) to alleviate excessive sweating (in pulmonary tuberculosis, etc.). It has also been used for bronchial asthma and spastic constipation. Due to its bitter taste agaric is still an ingredient in some bitter liqueurs.

Caution: Both agaric and agaricin should be used only as directed by an experienced practitioner. At higher doses than recommended they may cause paralysis of smooth muscles and at toxic doses they cause respiratory arrest and death.

References: (3) Vol. 4, p. 1034; (5) Vol. 2, p. 126; (8) p. 454; (28) p. 158; (37) pp. 31, 552; (41) Vols. 1-7; (46) p. 19.

AGARWOOD, CHINESE

Other Common Name(s): Chinese eaglewood
Botanical Name(s): *Aquilaria sinensis* (Lour.) Gilg [Fam.: Thymeleaceae]
Resinous heartwood
Constituents: Volatile oil (with sesquiterpenes: baimuxinol, isobaimuxinol, etc.), chromones, especially derivatives of 2-(2-phenylethyl) chromone, etc.
Properties: Aromatic, antispasmodic, diuretic, analgesic, antipyretic, tonic, and it is claimed to be aphrodisiac.
Uses: Internally it is chiefly used (as an h. p.) for spastic and inflammatory conditions of the gastrointestinal tract (nausea, vomiting, cramps, irritable bowel syndrome), upper respiratory tract (bronchial asthma, spastic bronchitis, the common cold) and genitourinary tract (with urinary gravel and non-obstructive stones), and for rheumatic complaints (incl. arthritic pains).
Caution: There are no reports of contraindications or side effects when used properly.

References: (1) Vol. 4, p. 309; (3) Vol. 3, p. 165; (31) p. 347; (41) Vols. 1-7; (52) p. 63; (57) p. 57.

AGRIMONY

Other Common Name(s): 1) church steeple, agrimony 2) fragrant agrimony, agrimony
Botanical Name(s): 1) *Agrimonia eupatoria* L. 2) *Agrimonia procera* Wallr. [Fam.: Rosaceae]
Aerial part
Constituents: Tannins (chiefly condensed t.), flavonoids (flavones: luteolin, etc.; flavonols: quercetin, etc.), phenolic acids (ferulic and vanillic acids, etc.), triterpenes (ursolic acid, etc.), etc.
Properties: Astringent, antibacterial, anti-inflammatory, mild choleretic. The astringent and antibacterial (against *Shigella* spp.: *S. dysenteriae*, etc.; *Staphylococcus* spp.: *S. aureus*, etc.) effects are due in large part to tannins, potentiated by flavonoids and ferulic acid. Ferulic acid has also shown mild choleretic and liver protective effects. Ursolic acid tastes bitter.
Uses: Internally it is used (as a tea, h. p.) for inflammations of the gastrointestinal tract (gastritis, diarrhea, etc.) and genitourinary tract (cystitis, urinary incontinence), and as an adjuvant (only combined with other herbs) for chronic hepatobiliary disorders. Externally it is used (as a mouthwash, gargle) for inflammations of the mouth and throat, and (as a wash, wet compress, poultice) for minor skin inflammations, wounds and eczemas.
Caution: There are no reports of contraindications or side effects when used properly.

References: (2) Vol. 2, p. 45; (3) Vol. 2, p. 1151; (6) p. 146; (8) p. 30; (16) p. 26; (17) p. 39; (19) p. 164; (27) p. 24; (28) pp. 71, 94; (46) p. 37; (47) p. 447; (51) p. 100.

AJUGA

Other Common Name(s): bugle, blue bugle, common bugle
Botanical Name(s): *Ajuga reptans* L. [Fam.: Lamiaceae (Labiatae)]
Aerial part
Constituents: Bitter principles (iridoids: ajugol and ajugoside, both closely related to harpagoside of devil's claw), phytosterols (phytoecdysteroids: ajugalactone, cyasterone), Lamiaceae tannins (rosmarinic acid and other caffeic acid derivatives), flavonoids (anthocyanins), etc.
Properties: Bitter tonic, astringent, anti-inflammatory, vulnerary, mild laxative. Cyasterone has been shown to increase protein synthesis in liver cells. Iridoids have shown bitter tonic, choleretic, liver protective, laxative, diuretic, anti-inflammatory, antibacterial, antiviral, antifungal and immunomodulant effects, among others. Based on constituents, ajuga may exert artichoke-like effects (incl. choleretic, cholagogic, liver protective).
Uses: Internally it is used (as a tea, h. p.) for loss of appetite and nonulcer dyspepsia (with flatulence, minor constipation) associated with minor hepatobiliary disorders (impaired bile secretion and flow). It is also used as an antidyscratic (= blood purifier; tea, h. p.) for atopic eczema (= chronic eczema of internal origin) and chronic rheumatic complaints. Externally it is used (as a mouthwash, gargle) for inflammations of the mouth and throat, and (as a wash, wet compress, poultice) for minor wounds.
Caution: There are no reports of contraindications or side effects when used properly.

References: (1) Vol. 4, p. 154; (3) Vol. 2, p. 1157; (10) p. 47; (31) pp. 714, 715; (35) p. 139; (41) Vols. 1-7; (51) p. 158.

AKEBIA

Other Common Name(s): five-leaf akebia
Botanical Name(s): *Akebia quinata* (Houtt.) Decne. [Fam.: Lardizabalaceae]
Stem
Constituents: Triterpenoid saponins (akebiasaponins, etc.), flavonoids (flavonols), minerals (potassium), phytosterols (5-sterols: stigmasterol, etc.), a triterpene (betulin), sugars (sucrose, etc.), a cyclitol (myo-inositol), etc.
Properties: Diuretic, anti-inflammatory, "vitamin P"-like, mild laxative. It is diuretic due in large part to potassium and saponins and mild laxative due at least in part to saponins. The anti-inflammatory effect may be due to saponins, enhanced by phytosterols and flavonols. The "vitamin P"-like (= helps in normalizing an increased microvascular permeability and fragility) effect is due to flavonols (see BUCKWHEAT).
Uses: Internally it is used as a flushing-out treatment (= herbal tea or product + liquids: more than 2 liters per day; sometimes combined with a medi-

6

cation) for inflammations of the genitourinary tract (cystitis, etc.), urinary gravel and nonobstructive stones, to prevent relapsing urinary infections / gravel / stones, (as a tea, h. p.) for sluggish bowels, inflammations of the upper respiratory tract (also as a diaphoretic hot tea), and as an antidyscratic (= blood purifier) and anti-inflammatory (tea, h. p.) for chronic rheumatic complaints (incl. rheumatoid arthritis) and atopic eczema (= chronic eczema of internal origin).

Caution: Akebia should not be taken during pregnancy, as there are reports of emmenagogic effect. At higher doses than recommended akebia may cause gastrointestinal irritations (with nausea, vomiting, diarrhea). A flushing-out treatment is contraindicated in cases of obstructive urinary stones, edema due to impaired heart or kidney function and kidney inflammations (here can be used on health professional's advice to enhance the effects of an antimicrobial therapy).

References: (1) Vol. 4, p. 157; (3) Vol. 2, p. 1158; (12a) p. 206; (41) Vols. 1-7; (42) Vol. 4, pp. 348, 349; (52) p. 26.

ALDER

Other Common Name(s): black alder, common alder, European alder
Botanical Name(s): *Alnus glutinosa* (L.) Gaertn. [Fam.: Betulaceae]
Bark
Constituents: Tannins (possibly of condensed type), flavonoids (flavonols: hyperin, etc.), triterpenes (δ-amyrenone, etc.), phytosterols (β-sitosterol, etc.), etc.
Properties: Astringent.
Uses: Externally it is used (as a gargle, mouthwash) for inflammations of the mouth and throat, (as an enema) for hemorrhoids, (as a wash) for minor skin inflammations, wounds and ulcers, and (as a vaginal irrigation / sitz bath / wash) for leukorrhea.
Caution: There are no reports of contraindications or side effects when used properly. At higher doses than recommended alder causes gastrointestinal irritations and constipation.
Leaf
Constituents: Tannins (possibly of condensed type), flavonoids (flavonols: hyperin, etc.), phytosterols, resinous acids, wax, etc.
Properties: Astringent.
Uses: Externally it is used (as a gargle, mouthwash) for inflammations of the mouth and throat, and (as an enema) for hemorrhoids. Internally it is used (as a tea, h. p.) for minor diarrhea.
Caution: See Bark.
Note: Among other alders, which in traditional medicine are used for almost the same indications are white alder or European alder: *Alnus incana* (L.) Moench.; and American alder or speckled alder: *Alnus incana* (L.) Moench.

ssp. *rugosa* (Du Roi) R.T. Clausen = *Alnus rugosa* (Du Roy) Spreng.

References: (1) Vol. 4, p. 207; (3) Vol. 2, p. 1218; (5) Vol. 1, p. 55; (10) p. 6; (18) p. 155; (27) p. 242; (35) p. 17; (41) Vols. 1-7; (52) p. 34.

ALETRIS

Other Common Name(s): blazing star, colic root, star grass, true unicorn
Botanical Name(s): *Aletris farinosa* L. [Fam.: Liliaceae (Melanthiaceae)]
Root
Constituents: Bitter principles, steroidal saponins (with aglycone: diosgenin, as in wild yam), volatile oil, resin and starch, but no tannins. The bitter taste is possibly due to alkaloids, or at least aletris may contain them.
Properties: Bitter tonic, antispasmodic (esp. uterine active), estrogenic, diuretic, mild sedative.
Uses: Internally it is used (as a tea, h. p.) for loss of appetite and nonulcer dyspepsia (with flatulence, minor cramps, etc.) and primary dysmenorrhea (= painful menstruation without pathology). It is also used as an antidyscratic (= blood purifier; tea, h. p.) for chronic rheumatic complaints.
Caution: Aletris should not be taken during pregnancy and lactation, in cases of peptic ulcers and before using it for gynecologic disorders, the problem should be judged by a health professional. At higher doses than recommended aletris causes gastrointestinal irritations (with nausea, vomiting, diarrhea). Manufacturers should evaluate alkaloids.

References: (1) Vol. 4, p. 173; (3) Vol. 2, p. 1176; (9) p. 11; (15) p. 19; (18) p. 305; (27) p. 25; (35) p. 824; (36) pp. 51, 474; (41) Vols. 1-7; (42) Vol. 2, p. 345; (44) p. 55; (46) p. 41; (52) p. 29; (55) p. 246; (66) p. 111.

ALFALFA

Other Common Name(s): lucerne
Botanical Name(s): *Medicago sativa* L. [Fam.: Fabaceae (Leguminosae)]
Leaf
Constituents: Proteins, crude fiber, triterpenoid saponins (soyasapogenol A-E), phytosterols (5-sterols: β-sitosterol, etc.), flavonoids (isoflavones: daidzein, formononetin, etc.), coumestans (= coumarono-coumarins: coumestrol, etc.), amino acids, chlorophyll, carotenoids, vitamins, minerals, organic acids, etc.
Properties and Uses: Internally it is used as a supplement of vitamins, chlorophyll, minerals and phytoestrogens (coumestrol, daidzein, formononetin, etc.). Coumestrol exerts a much stronger estrogen-like effect than daidzein and formononetin (see: KUDZU; RED CLOVER; SOY).
Caution: There are no reports of contraindications or side effects when used properly. As with other herbs with estrogen-like effects, alfalfa should not be taken in cases of estrogen receptor-positive (ER+) tumors. During preg-

nancy and lactation it can be used on health professional's advice.

References: (3) Vol. 5, p. 732; (9) p. 13; (21) p. 23; (41) Vols. 1-7; (47) p. 1858.

ALKANET

Other Common Name(s): Spanish bugloss
Botanical Name(s): *Alkanna tinctoria* (L.) Tausch [Fam.: Boraginaceae]
Root
Constituents: Naphthoquinones (collectively referred to as alkanna red: esters of alkannin), tannins, unsaturated pyrrolizidine alkaloids (= UPAs), etc.
Properties, Uses, and Caution: For its antibacterial, astringent and wound-healing effects, it has been used internally for diarrhea and externally for wounds, varicose ulcers and other dermatologic disorders. UPAs have been shown to be toxic (hepatotoxic, carcinogenic!) therefore alkanna is no longer used for medicinal purposes. Alkanna is still used as a red coloring ingredient in the production of lipsticks, hair dyes and oils, among others. For dosage limits of UPAs see COLTSFOOT.

References: (1) Vol. 4, p. 176; (3) Vol. 2, p. 1192; (9) p. 19; (17) p. 45; (36) p. 248; (37) p. 43; (41) Vols. 1-7.

ALLSPICE

Other Common Name(s): Jamaica pepper, myrtle pepper, pimenta
Botanical Name(s): *Pimenta dioica* (L.) Merr. = *Pimenta officinalis* Lindl. = *Eugenia pimenta* DC [Fam.: Myrtaceae]
Fruit (unripe)
Constituents: Volatile oil (with eugenol, etc.), resin, fixed oil, starch, organic acids, flavonoids (flavonols, flavan-3-ols = catechins), tannins (proanthocyanidins, etc.), vitamins, minerals, etc.
Properties: Aromatic, stomachic, carminative, antibacterial, antifungal, antiviral, due to volatile oil (cf. CLOVE), and antioxidant is due in large part to flavonoids and proanthocyanidins.
Uses: Allspice is chiefly used as a spice, and as a cheap substitute of clove (see CLOVE). Consumption in moderate amounts is also beneficial due to its antioxidant effect. Internally it is used (as a tea, h. p.) for nonulcer dyspepsia (with fullness, flatulence, nausea, etc.) and minor inflammations of the gastrointestinal tract (diarrhea) and upper respiratory tract (the common cold). Externally it can be used much like clove (see CLOVE).
Caution: There are no reports of contraindications or side effects when used properly.
Note: Volatile oil obtained by steam distillation from the fruit or leaf is very rich in eugenol and is often used as a substitute for clove oil.

References: (3) Vol. 6a, p. 663; (9) p. 20; (24) p. 457; (45) p. 246; (52) p. 598.

ALMOND

Botanical Name(s): *Prunus dulcis* (Miller) D. A. Webb [Fam.: Rosaceae]

Almond oil

It is the fixed oil (not the volatile oil!), obtained by cold expression from the seeds of bitter or sweet variety.

Constituents: Chiefly glycerides (fatty acids component: chiefly oleic and linoleic acids, also palmitic and stearic acids), etc.

Properties: Emollient, demulcent, mild laxative.

Uses: Externally it is used as an ingredient in creams, ointments and lipsticks, and (unmixed) for chapped hands and skin irritations. Internally it is used for minor constipation. The refined oil is used in pharmaceutical practice in the production of oily solutions (eyedrops, eardrops, injections).

Caution: Almond oil should not be taken in cases of bowel obstruction. Otherwise, there are no reports of contraindications or side effects when used properly. Almond oil is not to be confused with the essential / volatile oil of bitter almond. When unprocessed, the essential oil of bitter almond contains hydrocyanic acid (toxic!).

References: (3) Vol. 6a, p. 938; (5) Vol. 1, p. 876; (9) p. 22; (10) p. 7; (11) p. 72; (12) p. 254; (13) p. 386; (48) p. 138.

ALOE

Other Common Name(s): 1) Aloe vera, Barbados aloe, Curaçao aloe, aloe 2) Cape aloe

Botanical Name(s): 1) *Aloe vera* (L.) Burm.f. = *Aloe barbadensis* Mill. 2) *Aloe ferox* Mill. [Fam.: Liliaceae (Asphodelaceae)]

Aloe

It is the dried juice of the leaf and has a dark brown color.

Constituents: Anthranoids (C-glycosides: barbaloin = aloin, etc.; free anthraquinones), resin, bitter principles, chromone-C-glycosides (A. vera: aloeresin B = aloesin, etc., no aloeresin A; Cape a.: aloeresins B and A), etc.

Properties: Laxative (large intestine stimulant laxative), bitter, choleretic. See SENNA.

Uses: Internally it is used (usually as a combination product) for constipation (atonic, non-spastic). See SENNA.

Caution: See SENNA.

Aloe vera gel

It is the colorless mucilaginous gel that exudes from the fresh leaf after eliminating the outer layer.

Constituents: Chiefly water and mucilage (mucilaginous polysaccharides: glucomannans), also glycoproteins, amino acids, enzymes, minerals, lipids, tannins, small amounts of anthranoids, etc.

Properties: Emollient, demulcent, anti-inflammatory, antibacterial, antifun-

10

gal, wound-healing, immunomodulant, antihyperglycemic. The effects are due in large part to mucilages, also glycoproteins, tannins, anthranoids, etc.

Uses: <u>Externally</u> it is used (as a lotion, cream, spray, lip balm, etc.) for skin inflammations, minor burns (incl. sunburns) and wounds, chaps, and common acne, among others. <u>Internally</u> it may be beneficial for diabetes and inflammatory conditions of the gastrointestinal tract.

Caution: Aloe vera gel should not be applied to severe wounds and burns.

References: (1) Vol. 4, pp. 213, 222; (3) Vol. 2, p. 1219; (6) p. 336; (8) p. 41; (9) p. 25; (11) p. 53; (12) p. 914; (13) p. 297; (14) p. 19; (17) pp. 49, 53; (20) p. 25; (23) p. 103; (46) p. 43; (47) p. 484; (48) p. 434; (59) pp. 33, 43.

AMBRETTE

Other Common Name(s): musk mallow
Botanical Name(s): *Abelmoschus moschatus* Medic. = *Hibiscus abelmoscus* L. [Fam.: Malvaceae]
<u>Seed</u> (musk seed)
Constituents: Volatile oil (see Oil of ambrette), fixed oil, mucilaginous polysaccharides, phytosterols (5-sterols: β-sitosterol, etc.), phosphatides (incl. phosphatidyl-choline = lecithin), an alkaloid (α-cephaelin), resin, etc.
Properties: Aromatic, bitter tonic, carminative, antispasmodic, insecticidal.
Uses: Musk seed is chiefly used in liqueur industry, in the production of some bitters. <u>Internally</u> it is used (as a tea, h. p.) for loss of appetite and nonulcer dyspepsia (with flatulence, minor cramps) and as an adjuvant for minor fatigue and headaches. <u>Externally</u> it is used as an insecticide.
Caution: There are no reports of contraindications or side effects when used properly.
<u>Oil of ambrette</u>
It is the volatile oil obtained by steam distillation from the musk seed.
Constituents: Farnesyl acetate, ambrettolide, etc.
Properties and Uses: Due to its musk-like aroma it is chiefly used as a fragrance ingredient in cosmetics and perfumery. It is also used as a flavor ingredient in some bitters.
Caution: In seldom cases it may cause skin allergic reactions.

References: (1) Vol. 4, p. 3; (3) Vol. 5, p. 79; (9) p. 30; (37) p. 1; (41) Vols. 1-7; (52) p. 1.

AMMONIAC

Other Common Name(s): ammoniac-plant
Botanical Name(s): *Dorema ammoniacum* D. Don [Fam.: Apiaceae (Umbelliferae)]
<u>Ammoniac</u> (ammoniac gum, ammoniacum)
It is a gum-oleoresin, the dried exudate of the flowering and fruiting stems.

Constituents: Volatile oil (with linalool, citronellol, etc.), resin (with a coumarin derivative: ammoresinol), soluble gum, salicylic acid and its derivatives.

Properties: Rubefacient, counterirritant, antispasmodic, expectorant, emmenagogue.

Uses: Externally it is used (as a plaster, poultice) for rheumatic pains (incl. arthritic pains) and neuralgic pains (incl. sciatica), and (as an ointment) for skin infections (incl. boils). Internally it is used (usually as a combination product) for chronic inflammatory and spastic conditions of the upper respiratory tract (spastic bronchitis, etc., bronchial asthma; coughs due to thickened bronchial secretion).

Caution: Ammoniac should not be taken during pregnancy. Possibly, ammoniac acts through the autonomic nervous system. In view of this, doses higher than recommended should be avoided. Due to its rubefacient and counterirritant effects, it should be used with caution in cases of peptic ulcers. Otherwise, there are no reports of contraindications or side effects when used properly.

References: (2) Vol. 2, p. 530; (3) Vol. 4, p. 712; (4) Vol. 1, p. 382; (15) p. 24; (36) pp. 290, 474; (37) p. 431; (41) Vols. 1-7; (49) Vol. 2, p. 479; (52) p. 262.

ANDROGRAPHIS

Other Common Name(s): creat, green chiretta, Indian chiretta
Botanical Name(s): *Andrographis paniculata* (Burm. f.) Nees [Fam.: Acanthaceae]
Aerial part
Constituents: Bitter principles (a diterpenoid lactone: andrographolide; etc.), flavonoids (methoxy-flavones), minerals (potassium, etc.), etc.

Properties: Bitter tonic, anti-inflammatory, antipyretic, antibacterial, choleretic, liver protective, mild immunomodulant. Andrographolide is thought to be the main active constituent, with its bitter tonic and liver protective effects. Many methoxy-flavones have shown anti-inflammatory, antioxidant, antiviral, antibacterial and antifungal effects.

Uses: Internally it is used (as a tea, h. p.) for loss of appetite and nonulcer dyspepsia (with flatulence, minor constipation), inflammations of the liver (chronic hepatitis, liver damage), upper respiratory tract (the common cold, bronchitis), gastrointestinal tract (diarrhea), and genitourinary tract. Andrographis is also used for feverish states, minor fatigue and convalescence.

Caution: There are no reports of contraindications or side effects when used properly. Nevertheless, it is best to avoid it during pregnancy and lactation. At higher doses than recommended andrographis may cause gastrointestinal irritations (with nausea, vomiting, diarrhea).

References: (3) Vol. 3, p. 81; (5) Vol. 1, p. 79; (13) p. 426; (31) p. 388; (36) pp. 437, 491; (37) p. 83; (41) Vols. 1-7; (52) p. 49; (57) p. 44.

ANEMARRHENA

Botanical Name(s): *Anemarrhena asphodeloides* Bunge [Fam.: Liliaceae (Anthericaceae)]
<u>Root</u> (rhizome)
Constituents: Steroidal saponins (timosaponins; with aglycone: sarsapogenin), xanthones (mangiferin, etc.), lignans (hinokiresinol and related compounds), tannins, polysaccharides (anemaranes), etc.
Properties: Anti-inflammatory (cortisone-like effect), antipyretic, platelet aggregation inhibitory, expectorant, laxative, diuretic. Saponins may account for most of the effects. Mangiferin has shown anti-inflammatory, liver protective and antiviral effects. Lignans have shown anti-inflammatory, liver protective, immunomodulant, antibacterial, antiviral, and other effects.
Uses: <u>Internally</u> it is used (as a tea, h. p.) for inflammations of the upper respiratory tract (the common cold, bronchitis, etc.; coughs due to thickened bronchial secretion), gastrointestinal tract (with constipation), and genitourinary tract, for feverish states, and as an adjuvant for bronchial asthma.
Caution: Anemarrhena should not be taken in cases of diarrhea. Otherwise, there are no reports of contraindications or side effects when used properly.

References: (1) Vol. 4, p. 277; (3) Vol. 3, p. 82; (18) p. 310; (31) pp. 435, 536; (36) p. 507; (41) Vols. 1-7; (48) p. 279.

ANGELICA

Other Common Name(s): archangel, European angelica
Botanical Name(s): *Angelica archangelica* L. = *Angelica officinalis* Moench = *Archangelica officinalis* (Moench) Hoffm. [Fam.: Apiaceae (Umbelliferae)]
<u>Root</u> (rhizome)
Constituents: Volatile oil (with β- and α- phellandrene, etc.), coumarins (umbelliferone, etc.), furanocoumarins (xanthotoxin, imperatorin, etc.), phenolic acids (caffeic acid derivatives), etc.
Properties: Aromatic, bitter tonic, antispasmodic, choleretic, cholagogue, carminative, antibacterial, diuretic.
Uses: <u>Internally</u> it is used (as a tea, h. p.) for loss of appetite and nonulcer dyspepsia (with fullness, flatulence, burping, heartburn, aerophagia = swallowing of air, minor cramps, nausea, etc.) associated with impaired bile secretion and flow, and for inflammation of the upper respiratory tract (bronchitis, etc.). Angelica is a flavor ingredient in some bitters. <u>Externally</u> it is used (as a partial bath, liniment) for rheumatic pains, (as a mouthwash, gargle) for inflammations of the mouth and throat, and (as a wet compress) for bruises.
Caution: Angelica should not be taken during pregnancy and lactation. When handling angelica avoid contact with skin and when taking its prod-

ucts avoid exposure to strong sunrays as it may cause phototoxic skin irritations.

References: (2) Vol. 2, p. 95; (6) pp. 128, 183; (8) p. 59; (9) p. 32; (13) p. 328; (15) p. 26; (16) p. 124; (17) p. 62; (19) p. 28; (20) p. 28; (23) p. 62; (28) pp. 101, 107; (46) p. 83; (48) p. 272; (51) p. 136.

ANGOSTURA

Other Common Name(s): angustura, cusparia
Botanical Name(s): *Angostura trifoliata* (Willd.) T.S. Elias = *Cusparia febrifuga* Humb. ex DC. = *Galipea officinalis* Hancock [Fam.: Rutaceae]
Bark
Constituents: Volatile oil (with sesquiterpenes: galipol, etc.), bitter principles (angosturin, etc.), quinoline alkaloids (galipine, cusparine, etc.), vitamin B_1, etc.
Properties: Aromatic, bitter tonic, antipyretic, antispasmodic, antidiarrheal. Galipine and cusparine have shown antispasmodic effect.
Uses: Internally it is used (as a tea, h. p.) for loss of appetite and nonulcer dyspepsia (with fullness, flatulence, minor cramps), diarrhea, feverish states and minor fatigue. It is a flavor ingredient in some bitters, but not the one known as Angostura Bitters.
Caution: There are no reports of contraindications or side effects when used properly. As with other bitter herbs, higher doses cause gastrointestinal irritations (with nausea, vomiting).

References: (2) Vol. 2, p. 747; (3) Vol. 4, p. 391; (8) p. 209; (9) p. 35; (27) p. 33; (31) pp. 272, 274; (37) p. 570; (41) Vols. 1-7; (45) p. 212; (46) p. 86; (47) p. 534; (49) Vol. 2, p. 304.

ANGURATÉ

Botanical Name(s): *Mentzelia cordifolia* Dombey ex Urb. et Gilg [Fam.: Loasaceae]
Aerial part (stems and branches)
Constituents: Flavonoids (flavonols: quercetin, kaempferol), bitter principles (iridoids: decaloside, its derivatives), phenolic acids (caffeic acid, etc.), coumarins (scopoletin, etc.), mucilaginous polysaccharides, β-sitosterol, etc.
Properties: Bitter tonic, anti-inflammatory, antispasmodic, antiulcer (= prevents or helps in healing peptic ulcers). Iridoids have shown bitter tonic, choleretic, liver protective, laxative, diuretic, anti-inflammatory, antibacterial, antiviral, antifungal and immunomodulant effects, among others. Caffeic acid has shown antiulcer, liver protective and anti-inflammatory effects, among others. Scopoletin has shown anti-inflammatory, antispasmodic, antibacterial and antifungal effects.
Uses: Internally it is used (as a tea, h. p.) for loss of appetite and dyspeptic disorders (with minor cramps, etc.), convalescence and minor fatigue, and it may prevent and heal peptic ulcers.

Caution: There are no reports of contraindications or side effects when used properly.

References: (3) Vol. 5, p. 781; (8) p. 373; (12) p. 438; (37) p. 880; (31) pp. 364, 474, 569; (41) Vols. 1-7; (42) Vol. 4, p. 403.

ANISE

Botanical Name(s): *Pimpinella anisum* L. = *Anisum vulgare* Gaertn. [Fam.: Apiaceae (Umbelliferae)]

Fruit (commonly called seed)

Constituents: Volatile oil (see Anise oil), coumarins, flavonoids, phenolic acids (caffeic and chlorogenic acids), fixed oil, proteins, minerals, phytosterols, etc.

Properties: Aromatic, sialagogue (= increases the flow of saliva), expectorant (chiefly bronchial secretagogue effect), stomachic, antispasmodic (gastrointestinal active), carminative, antibacterial. Most of the effects are due to the volatile oil. Phenolic acids, coumarins and flavonoids contribute to the effects in the gastrointestinal tract.

Uses: Internally it is used (as a tea, h. p.) for inflammatory and spastic conditions of the upper respiratory tract (bronchitis, tracheitis, laryngitis; coughs due to thickened bronchial secretion), nonulcer dyspepsia (with flatulence, minor cramps, irritable bowel syndrome) and to prevent griping effects of the anthranoid laxatives (senna, cascara, aloe, etc.). In traditional medicine it is used as a galactagogue to promote the secretion of milk. Anise is widely used as a flavor ingredient in food industry.

Caution: Anise should be avoided during pregnancy. In rare cases, if hypersensitive to anethole, it may cause allergic reactions. Otherwise, there are no reports of contraindications or side effects when used properly.

Anise oil

It is the volatile oil obtained by steam distillation from freshly crushed fruits.

Constituents: Chiefly trans-anethole.

Uses: Internally it is used (usually as a combination product or a few drops in a glass of water) very much like anise fruit.

Caution: See ANISE, STAR.

References: (1) Vol. 6, p. 137; (3) Vol. 6a, p. 671; (6) pp. 95, 128; (7) p. 172; (8) p. 427; (12) p. 692; (13) p. 125; (15) p. 160; (16) p. 70; (17) p. 66; (19) p. 29; (20) p. 30; (23) p. 83, 216; (27) p. 33; (46) p. 92; (47) p. 544; (48) p. 513.

ANISE, STAR

Other Common Name(s): Chinese star anise

Botanical Name(s): *Illicium verum* Hook. f. [Fam.: Illiciaceae (Magnoliaceae)]

Fruit

Constituents: Volatile oil (see Star anise oil), fixed oil, phospholipids and glycolipids, phytosterols, vitamin E, flavonoids, phenolic acids, etc.

Properties: Aromatic, sialagogue (= increases the flow of saliva), expectorant (chiefly bronchial secretagogue effect), antispasmodic (bronchial active), stomachic, carminative, antibacterial.

Uses: Internally it is used (as a tea, h. p.) for inflammations of the upper respiratory tract and nonulcer dyspepsia (with flatulence, cramps, etc.). It is an important spice used in Chinese cookery.

Caution: Star anise should be avoided during pregnancy. In rare cases, if hypersensitive to anethole, it may cause allergic reactions. Otherwise, there are no reports of contraindications or side effects when used properly.

Star anise oil

It is the volatile oil obtained by steam distillation from freshly crushed fruits.

Constituents: Chiefly trans-anethole.

Uses: Internally it is used (usually in a combination product) very much like star anise fruit.

Caution: Star anise oil should not contain cis-anethole (toxic!). Cis-anethole is found in oils that are stored unprotected from light and particularly when they are produced artificially. See also caution, under fruit.

References: (1) Vol. 5, p. 515; (3) Vol. 5, p. 228; (9) p. 36; (12) p. 693; (17) p. 66; (36) p. 495; (46) p. 89; (48) p. 569; (49) Vol. 2, p. 157.

ANNATTO

Other Common Name(s): achiote, lipstick tree
Botanical Name(s): *Bixa orellana* L. [Fam.: Bixaceae]
Seed (anotto, orléana)
Constituents: Carotenoids (chiefly bixin, also norbixin). Bixin is very closely related to crocin of saffron (q. v.).

Properties: Although bixin and norbixin are carotenoids, they do not exert vitamin A effects.

Uses: Annatto is used as a yellow coloring ingredient in food, pharmaceutical and cosmetic industries. There are available liposoluble extracts (rich in bixin) and water-soluble extracts (rich in norbixin salts).

Caution: There are no reports of contraindications or side effects in the amounts used in foods and drugs.

References: (3) Vol. 3, p. 479; (5) Vol. 1, p. 169; (9) p. 39; (12) p. 614; (36) p. 459; (48) p. 776; (49) Vol. 2, p. 230.

APPLE

Other Common Name(s): cultivated apple

Botanical Name(s): *Malus pumila* Mill. = *Malus domestica* (Borkh.) Borkh. [Fam.: Rosaceae]

Fruit (dried slices); **Pectin**

Constituents: (Fruit): Pectin, sugars (fructose, etc.), organic acids (malic acid, etc.), tannins, phenolic acids, minerals, flavonoids, amino acids (asparagine, etc.), vitamins, volatile oil (pleasant odor).

Properties: Astringent, adsorbent, antibacterial, antidiarrheal, and it helps in normalizing intestinal flora. The mentioned effects are due in large part to pectin, but to the overall beneficial effects contribute also other constituents (organic acids, tannins, minerals, etc.).

Uses: Internally it is used (as a tea, h. p.) for minor diarrhea and is recommended for children and the elderly. Apple, particularly its residue from the production of juices, is used in the production of pectin. Pectin is used (usually in a combination product) for diarrhea and gastroenteritis, as an adjuvant for peptic ulcers and for complaints due to irritating effects of antibiotics and other agents. As with mucilaginous polysaccharides (see PSYLLIUM), pectin may bind dietary cholesterol in the intestinal tract and increase its fecal excretion. Therefore, pectin and pectin-rich products may be beneficial for high cholesterol. In food industry pectin is used as a gelling ingredient. Dried apple peel is incorporated in herbal teas.

Caution: Apple products (incl. pectin) should not be taken in cases of bowel obstruction. Pectin may impair the absorption of some drugs. In view of this, when taking a vital oral medication, drugs should be taken about one hour apart from pectin / pectin-rich products. Otherwise, there are no reports of contraindications or side effects when used properly.

References: (1) Vol. 5, p. 751; (3) Vol. 5, p. 678; (6) p. 62; (8) p. 352; (37) p. 1035; (48) p. 118; (49) Vol. 2, p. 424.

ARJUNA

Botanical Name(s): *Terminalia arjuna* (Roxb. ex DC.) Wight et Arn. [Fam.: Combretaceae]

Bark (stem bark)

Constituents: Triterpenoid saponins (with aglycones: arjunolic acid, etc.), minerals (very rich in calcium), flavonoids (methoxy-flavones, -flavanones, -chalcones), tannins (rich), phytosterols (5-sterols: β-sitosterol, etc.), etc.

Properties: Cardiotonic (increases the contractility of the heart muscle), mild antihypertensive, diuretic, sedative, astringent, antioxidant.

Uses: Internally it is chiefly used (as a tea, h. p.) for minor cases of heart failure, hypertension and nervous cardiac disorders, and for inflammations of the gastrointestinal tract (diarrhea, etc.) and genitourinary tract (cystitis, etc.). Externally it is used (as a wet compress, poultice) for minor skin inflammations and wounds.

Caution: Arjuna is best used on health professional's advice. A combination with cardioactive glycosides or herbs (digoxin, lily-of-the-valley, etc.) should be avoided or made only by a health professional. To arjuna apply all contraindications for calcium (e. g. hypercalciuria, calcic urinary stones, hypercalcemia, etc.). Tetracyclines should be taken about 2 hours apart from arjuna as it may impair their absorption.

References: (1) Vol. 6, p. 913; (3) Vol. 6c, p. 43; (36) p. 493; (41) Vols. 1-7; (42) Vol. 3, pp. 438, 439, 443, 446; (45) p. 141; (52) p. 788.

ARNICA

Other Common Name(s): European arnica
Botanical Name(s): *Arnica montana* L. [Fam.: Asteraceae (Compositae)]
Flower
Constituents: Sesquiterpene lactones (helenalin, etc., their esters), flavonoids, coumarins, volatile oil, water-soluble polysaccharides, phenolic acids, polyacetylenes, carotenoids, etc.
Properties: Anti-inflammatory, rubefacient, counterirritant, analgesic, antibacterial, antifungal. Most of the effects are attributed to sesquiterpene lactones.
Uses: Externally it is used (as a solution, ointment: on unbroken skin parts) for bruises, sprains, minor skin inflammations (incl. those after insect bites), fungal skin infections, boils, minor rheumatic pains, and (as a mouth-wash, gargle) for inflammations of the mouth and throat.
Caution: Arnica is no longer recommended for internal use. Externally it should not be applied to open wounds or ulcers. Arnica may cause allergic contact dermatitis to persons hypersensitive to other Asteraceae plants (e. g. chamomile, feverfew, ragweed, tansy, yarrow) that contain sesquiterpene lactones. Follow carefully the manufacturer's instructions as it may cause blisters if left on the painful site longer than advised, and even necrosis if used concentrated products.

References: (1) Vol. 4, p. 345; (3) Vol. 3, p. 214; (6) p. 339; (7) p. 290; (8) p. 73; (12) p. 488; (13) p. 312; (16) p. 39; (17) p. 78; (19) p. 30; (20) p. 34; (22) p. 219; (28) p. 196; (46) p. 103; (47) p. 585; (48) p. 627.

ARNICA, FALSE

Other Common Name(s): Mexican arnica
Botanical Name(s): *Heterotheca inuloides* Cass. [Fam.: Asteraceae (Compositae)]
Flower
Constituents: Volatile oil (with 1- and 2-naphthol derivatives, sesquiterpenes), flavonoids (flavonols: rutin, etc.), phenolic acids (chlorogenic acid, etc.), tannins, coumarins (umbelliferone, etc.), bitter principles, etc. Possibly, the reported bitter principles are sesquiterpene lactones.

18

Properties: Anti-inflammatory, astringent, wound-healing, bitter tonic, mild antispasmodic, laxative and diuretic.

Uses: Externally it is used (as a wash, wet compress, paint) for minor wounds, and (as a poultice, ointment) for bruises and sprains. Internally it is chiefly used in traditional medicine as a diaphoretic hot tea for feverish states and inflammations of the upper respiratory tract, and as a mild laxative and diuretic.

Caution: At higher doses than recommended false arnica causes gastrointestinal irritations (with nausea, vomiting, diarrhea). False arnica may cause allergic contact dermatitis to persons hypersensitive to other Asteraceae plants (e. g. chamomile, feverfew, ragweed, tansy, yarrow) that contain sesquiterpene lactones. Otherwise, there are no reports of contraindications or side effects when used properly.

References: (1) Vol. 5, p. 440; (5) Vol. 3, p. 277; (37) p. 659; (41) Vols. 1-7; (52) p. 372.

ARROWROOT

Other Common Name(s): arrowroot, St. Vincent arrowroot, West Indian arrowroot

Botanical Name(s): *Maranta arundinacea* L. [Fam.: Marantaceae]

Starch (arrowroot starch)

It is prepared from fresh tubers. Fresh tubers contain starch, proteins (with amino acids: tryptophan, etc.), a bitter principle and a protease inhibitor.

Properties: Nutrient, demulcent.

Uses: Internally it is used (as a tea, jelly) for inflammations of the gastrointestinal tract (including diarrhea), and is recommended for children and the elderly. In pharmaceutical industry it is used the same as other starches.

Caution: Arrowroot should be used as a prepared starch only and not the unprocessed underground organ.

Note: Arrowroot starch is also produced from other sources, including African arrowroot: *Canna edulis* Ker-Gawl. [Fam.: Cannaceae]; Indian cane, flowering reed root: *Canna indica* L. [Fam.: Cannaceae]; Brazilian arrowroot, cassava: *Manihot esculenta* Crantz [Fam.: Euphorbiaceae]; sweet potato: *Ipomoea batatas* (L.) Lam. [Fam.: Convolvulaceae]; East arrowroot: *Curcuma angustifolia* Roxb.; *Curcuma rubescens* Roxb., *Curcuma leucorrhiza* Roxb.; Indian arrowroot, Zedoary (q. v.): *Curcuma zedoaria* (Christm.) Roscoe [Fam.: Zingiberaceae]

References: (1) Vol. 5, p. 772; (2) Vol. 2, p. 282; (5) Vol. 1, pp. 215, 372, 608, 689; (36) p. 498.

ARTICHOKE

Other Common Name(s): cynara, garden artichoke, globe artichoke

Botanical Name(s): *Cynara scolymus* L. [Fam.: Asteraceae (Compositae)]

Leaf

Constituents: Phenolic acid derivatives (fresh leaves and alcoholic extracts: chiefly 1,5-dicaffeoyl-quinic acid and 5-caffeoyl-quinic acid = chlorogenic acid; extracts prepared with hot water: chiefly cynarin = 1,3-dicaffeoyl-quinic acid), bitter principles (sesquiterpene lactones: cynaropicrin, etc.), flavonoids (flavones as luteolin glycosides: cynaroside, scolymoside), etc.

Properties: Bitter tonic, choleretic, cholagogue, liver protective, promotes regeneration of liver cells, increases secretion of pancreatic juice (= external secretion of pancreas that passes into duodenum), antioxidant, cholesterol and triglyceride reducing, mild diuretic. The effects in the hepatobiliary tract, including cholesterol and triglyceride reducing effects, are due in large part to cynarin and its related compounds. To these effects contribute also cynaropicrin (esp. as bitter tonic, also choleretic) and luteolin (esp. as cholesterol and triglyceride reducer, also anti-inflammatory).

Uses: Internally it is used (as a tea, h. p.) for loss of appetite and nonulcer dyspepsia (with fullness, flatulence, bloating, nausea, sluggish bowels), especially when they are associated with hepatobiliary disorders (impaired bile secretion and flow, chronic cholecystitis, nonobstructive gallstones) and insufficient external secretion of pancreas, and for high cholesterol and triglycerides. For its bitter tonic effects artichoke is also recommended for convalescents and the elderly.

Caution: Artichoke should not be taken in cases of biliary obstruction. In cases of nonobstructive gallstones it can be used but only on health professional's advice. Artichoke may cause allergic contact dermatitis to persons hypersensitive to other Asteraceae plants (e. g. arnica, chamomile, feverfew, ragweed, tansy, yarrow) that contain sesquiterpene lactones. Otherwise, there are no reports of contraindications or side effects when used properly.

References: (1) Vol. 4, p. 1117; (3) Vol. 4, p. 415; (6) p. 144; (7) p. 191; (8) p. 213; (9) p. 42; (12) p. 782; (16) p. 134; (19) p. 32; (20) p. 36; (23) p. 122; (27) p. 74; (28) p. 106; (31) p. 404; (41) Vols. 1-7; (46) p. 248; (48) p. 247; (74) p. 282.

ARTICHOKE, JERUSALEM

Other Common Name(s): sunchoke, topinambur
Botanical Name(s): *Helianthus tuberosus* L. [Fam.: Asteraceae (Compositae)]
Root (tuber-like rhizome)
Constituents: Chiefly inulin (a polymer of almost only fructose; very rich in autumn), also proteins, minerals (rich in potassium), tannins, diterpenes, etc., but no starch.
Properties: Nutrient, mild laxative, mild diuretic. Inulin reaches large intestine almost unchanged, where enzymes split it. The produced fructose acts as an osmotic laxative.
Uses: Internally it is used as a dietetic aid to diabetics and for minor consti-

pation. Through acidic hydrolysis are produced syrupy or dried hydroly-sates, which consist chiefly of fructose. They are used as sugar substitutes for diabetics and as mild laxatives and diuretics.

Caution: Jerusalem artichoke should be avoided in cases of impaired renal function. Consumption of amounts larger than recommended may cause bloating and diarrhea. Otherwise, there are no reports of contraindications or side effects when used properly.

References: (1) Vol. 5, p. 416; (3) Vol. 5, p. 33; (12) p. 339; (23) p. 142; (36) p. 207; (37) p. 648; (48) p. 85.

ASAFETIDA

Other Common Name(s): giant fennel
Botanical Name(s): *Ferula assa-foetida* L.; *Ferula foetida* (Bunge) Regel [Fam.: Apiaceae (Umbelliferae)]
<u>Asafetida</u> (gum asafetida, devil's dung)
It is the gum-oleoresin obtained by incisions made to the rhizome and root.
Constituents: Resin (with coumarin derivatives, etc.), volatile oil (with di-sulphides; unpleasant smelling) and gum.
Properties: Carminative, antispasmodic, intestinal antiseptic, expectorant (bronchial secretagogue effect), sedative, aromatic.
Uses: <u>Internally</u> it is used (as an h. p., usually combined with other herbs) for inflammatory and spastic conditions of the gastrointestinal tract (flatu-lence, bloating, cramps, irritable bowel syndrome, etc.) and upper respira-tory tract (spastic bronchitis, bronchial asthma). It has also been used for hysterical neurosis and similar nervous disorders. It is still used as a flavor ingredient in food industry.
Caution: Asafetida should not be used during pregnancy and lactation and in infants. At doses higher than recommended it may cause diarrhea and headache, among others. Otherwise, there are no reports of contraindications or side effects when used properly.

References: (2) Vol. 2, p. 697; (3) Vol. 4, p. 980; (8) p. 260; (14) p. 24; (15) p. 34; (36) p. 289; (37) p. 523; (46) p. 115; (47) p. 614; (48) p. 582; (49) Vol. 2, p. 479; (65) p. 143.

ASARABACCA

Other Common Name(s): European wild ginger
Botanical Name(s): *Asarum europaeum* L. [Fam.: Aristolochiaceae]
<u>Root and aerial part</u>
Constituents: Volatile oil (chiefly with trans-isoasarone = α-asarone, trans-isoeugenol, or trans-isoelemicin; depending on chemotype; contained almost only in root), tannins (condensed t.), phenolic acids, mucilaginous polysac-charides, invert sugar, etc.

21

Properties: Expectorant (bronchial secretagogue effect), antispasmodic (bronchial active), diuretic, emmenagogue.

Uses: Internally it is still used (the chemotype with trans-isoasarone, in a standardized combination product) for inflammatory and spastic conditions of the upper respiratory tract (spastic bronchitis, tracheitis, laryngitis, etc., bronchial asthma; coughs due to thickened bronchial secretion). In traditional practice the root is still used as a sniffing powder.

Caution: Asarabacca should not be taken during pregnancy and lactation. At higher doses than recommended it causes gastrointestinal irritations (with heartburn, nausea, vomiting, diarrhea).

References: (1) Vol. 4, p. 379; (3) Vol. 3, p. 281; (8) p. 83; (13) p. 146; (27) p. 47; (37) p. 147; (46) p. 107; (47) p. 620; (51) p. 65; (73) p. 433.

ASH, EUROPEAN

Other Common Name(s): common ash
Botanical Name(s): *Fraxinus excelsior* L. [Fam.: Oleaceae]
Bark (from young twigs)
Constituents: Coumarins (fraxinol, isofraxidin, scopoletin, etc.), bitter principles (iridoids), tannins, phytosterols (5-sterols: stigmasterol, etc.), sugars (mannitol, glucose, galacturonic acid), etc.
Properties: Bitter tonic, antipyretic, antirheumatic.
Uses: Internally it is used (as a tea, h. p.) for rheumatic complaints (incl. rheumatoid arthritis) and feverish states.
Caution: There are no reports of contraindications or side effects when used properly.
Leaf
Constituents: Flavonoids (flavonols: quercetin, kaempferol, etc.), bitter principles (iridoids), coumarins, sugars (mannitol, etc.), triterpenes (ursolic acid, etc.), phenolic acids, tannins, etc.
Properties: Diuretic, antipyretic, antirheumatic, laxative.
Uses: Internally it is used (as a tea, h. p.) for rheumatic complaints (incl. rheumatoid arthritis), feverish states and minor constipation.
Caution: There are no reports of contraindications or side effects when used properly.

References: (1) Vol. 5, p. 191; (3) Vol. 4, p. 1050; (8) p. 268; (10) p. 19; (27) p. 140; (28) p. 184; (37) p. 557; (41) Vols. 1-7; (46) p. 618; (47) p. 1381.

ASH WEED

Other Common Name(s): bishop's weed, goutweed, ground elder
Botanical Name(s): *Aegopodium podagraria* L. [Fam.: Apiaceae (Umbelliferae)]
Aerial part

22

Constituents: Volatile oil, coumarins, phenolic acids (caffeic and chloro-genic acids), flavonoids (flavonols), polyacetylenes, phytosterols (5-sterols: β-sitosterol, etc.), etc. It possibly contains small amounts of furanocou-marins.

Properties: Based on its constituents, it possibly exerts stomachic, chol-eretic, antioxidant, anti-inflammatory, diuretic, mild antispasmodic and an-tibacterial effects.

Uses: Fresh ash weed is still added to salads with beneficial effects on the gastrointestinal, hepatobiliary and genitourinary tracts. Internally it is used as an antidyscratic (= blood purifier; tea, h. p.) for chronic rheumatic com-plaints. Externally it is used (as partial bath, poultice) for rheumatic pains.

Caution: There are no reports of contraindications or side effects when used properly. Nevertheless, ash weed is best avoided during pregnancy and lac-tation. Due to the possible presence of furanocoumarins, when handling the herb avoid contact with skin and when taking its products, avoid exposure to strong sunrays as it may cause phototoxic skin irritations.

References: (1) Vol. 4, p. 99; (3) Vol. 2, p. 1109; (10) p. 133; (35) p. 368; (42) Vol. 6, pp. 569, 574; (47) p. 413; (49) Vol. 2, p. 486; (51) p. 135; (52) p. 18.

ASHWAGANDHA

Other Common Name(s): withania
Botanical Name(s): *Withania somnifera* (L.) Dunal [Fam.: Solanaceae]
Root

Constituents: Steroidal lactones (withanolides: withaferin A, withanolides D, E, etc.), alkaloids (piperidine type: anaferine, etc.; pyrazole type: withasomnine, etc.; pyrrolidine type: cuskohygrine, etc.), phytosterols, etc.

Properties: Adaptogenic, sedative, mild hypnotic (by elevating levels of GABA = GABA-mimetic effect), antispasmodic, anti-inflammatory, anti-tumoral, antibacterial, antifungal, immunomodulant, antioxidant, aphrodisi-ac. Some withanolides have shown anti-inflammatory, antibacterial, im-munomodulant and antitumoral effects, among others. Alkaloids may ac-count at least in part for the sedative and antispasmodic effects.

Uses: Internally it is used (as a tea, h. p.) for minor nervousness, anxiety, impaired concentration and insomnia associated with stress, minor spastic conditions of the gastrointestinal tract (it may be helpful for irritable bowel syndrome, especially when associated with stress), genitourinary tract (due to inflammations, non-obstructive urinary stones), and upper respiratory tract (spastic coughs), and for rheumatic complaints (incl. rheumatoid arthri-tis). It may be beneficial for male low sexual drive, especially when associ-ated with stress. Externally it is used (as a poultice) for boils and swellings.

Caution: Ashwagandha should not be taken during pregnancy and lactation. Alcoholic drinks may interact with ashwagandha. A possible combination of ashwagandha with sedative, hypnotic and antidepressant drugs should be made only by a health professional. Otherwise, there are no reports of contraindications or side effects when used properly.

References: (3) Vol. 6c, p. 513; (6) p. 239; (12) p. 515; (18) p. 241; (22) p. 243; (29) p. 124; (31) p. 721; (36) pp. 92, 320; (41) Vols. 1-7; (45) p. 150; (52) p. 868; (68) p. 230.

ASPARAGUS

Botanical Name(s): *Asparagus officinalis* L. [Fam.: Liliaceae]
Root
Constituents: Steroidal saponins (asparagosides), polysaccharides (fructans), minerals (rich in potassium), a phenol glycoside (coniferin), amino acids (asparagine, etc.), etc.
Properties: Diuretic. The diuretic effect is due in large part to saponins and potassium salts.
Uses: Internally it is used (as a tea, h. p.; usually combined with other herbs) as a flushing-out treatment (= herbal tea or product + liquids: more than 2 liters per day; sometimes combined with a medication) for inflammations of the genitourinary tract (cystitis, etc.), urinary gravel and nonobstructive stones, to prevent relapsing urinary infections / gravel / stones, and as an antidyscratic (= blood purifier; tea, h. p.) for chronic rheumatic complaints and atopic eczema (= chronic eczema of internal origin).
Caution: There are no reports of contraindications or side effects when used properly. Nevertheless, a flushing-out treatment is contraindicated in cases of obstructive urinary stones, edema due to impaired heart or kidney function and kidney inflammations (here can be used on health professional's advice to enhance the effects of an antimicrobial therapy).

References: (1) Vol. 4, p. 397; (3) Vol. 3, p. 289; (6) p. 185; (8) p. 85; (9) p. 47; (16) p. 166; (19) p. 215; (24) p. 311; (27) p. 44; (28) p. 163; (37) p. 149; (46) p. 113; (47) p. 631; (48) p. 86; (49) Vol. 2, p. 53.

ASTRAGALUS

Other Common Name(s): 1) membranous milkvetch, astragalus 2) Mongolian milkvetch, astragalus
Botanical Name(s): 1) *Astragalus membranaceus* (Fisch. ex Link) Bunge 2) *Astragalus mongholicus* Bunge = *Astragalus membranaceus* (L.) (Fisch. ex Link) Bunge var. *mongholicus* (Bunge) P.K. Hsiao [Fam.: Fabaceae (Papilionaceae)]
Root (huang qi)
Constituents: Polysaccharides (incl. water-soluble p.), triterpenoid saponins (astragalosides I-X, etc.), amino acids (incl. GABA = gamma aminobutyrric acid), flavonoids (isoflavones: formononetin, calycosin, etc.), lignans (lariciresinol, syringaresinol, etc.), phytosterols (5-sterols: β-sitosterol, etc.), etc.

Properties: Immunomodulant (by stimulating the activity of T-lymphocytes and macrophages and the interferon production), liver protective, anti-inflammatory, diuretic, antibacterial, antiviral, antihyperglycemic, antioxidant. It is also reported to exert mild cardiotonic effect (= positive inotropic effects = increases the contractility of the heart muscle), thought to be due in large part to saponins. The immunomodulating effect is due in large part to water-soluble polysaccharides. Lignans have shown liver protective, immunomodulant, anti-inflammatory, antibacterial, and antiviral effects, among others.

Uses: Internally it is used (as a tea, h. p.; usually combined with a medication) to ease and shorten the duration of the common cold and flu and other viral or bacterial infections (often of relapsing nature) of the upper respiratory tract (bronchitis, etc.), genitourinary tract (chronic nephritis, etc.), gastrointestinal tract (diarrhea, etc.) and the liver (chronic hepatitis, etc.). Astragalus is also used to enhance the effects of a cancer therapy, for minor fatigue and feeling of weakness and it may be beneficial for minor cardiac insufficiencies associated with infective conditions. As an anti-inflammatory and antidyscratic (= blood purifier; tea, h. p.) it is used for atopic eczema (= chronic eczema of internal origin) and other chronic skin disorders.

Caution: Astragalus should not be taken during pregnancy and lactation. For minor cardiac insufficiencies it should be used only on health professional's advice. Unless advised by a health professional, it should not be taken for more than 8 weeks. Before a possible resuming, a break for 2-3 weeks is required. See ECHINACEA; BETA GLUCANS.

References: (1) Vol. 4, pp. 409, 415; (9) p. 50; (31) p. 435; (41) Vols. 1-7; (53) p. 27; (59) p. 50.

ATRACTYLODES, BAI-ZHU

Botanical Name(s): *Atractylodes macrocephala* Koidz. = *Atractylis macrocephala* (Koidz.) Hand.-Mazz. [Fam.: Asteraceae (Compositae)]
Root (rhizome) (bai zhu)
Constituents: Furano-sesquiterpenes (chiefly atractylone, also atractylenolides I-III, etc.; chiefly steam distilling), polyacetylenes (atractylentrioles), polysaccharides (β-D-mannans, β-D-fructans), volatile oil (with atractylone, etc.), a coumarin (scopoletin), phytosterols, etc.
Properties: Diuretic, stomachic, carminative, anti-inflammatory, antioxidant, liver protective, immunomodulant, antibacterial, antiviral, anticoagulant, antihyperglycemic. The diuretic effect may be due at least in part to the steam distilling compounds and the disintegration products of polysaccharides. Furano-sesquiterpenes account for the anti-inflammatory, antioxidant and liver protective effects, and possibly the anticoagulant effect. The immunomodulant effect is due to polysaccharides. Many polyacetylenes are considered natural antibiotics. Scopoletin has shown anti-inflammatory, antispasmodic, antibacterial and antifungal effects.

Uses: <u>Internally</u> it is used as a flushing-out treatment (= herbal tea or product + liquids: more than 2 liters per day; sometimes combined with a medication) for inflammations of the genitourinary tract (cystitis, etc.), urinary gravel and nonobstructive stones, to prevent relapsing urinary infections / gravel / stones, and (as a tea, h. p.) for inflammations of the gastrointestinal tract (loss of appetite, nonulcer dyspepsia, diarrhea) and liver (chronic hepatitis).

Caution: There are no reports of contraindications or side effects when used properly and if not adulterated with the toxic root of *Atractylis gummifera* L. Nevertheless, a flushing-out treatment is contraindicated in cases of obstructive urinary stones, edema due to impaired heart or kidney function and kidney inflammations (here can be used on health professional's advice to enhance the effects of an antimicrobial therapy).

References: (2) Vol. 2, p. 224; (9) p. 529; (13) p. 428; (29) p. 18; (31) pp. 46, 364; (36) p. 509; (41) Vols. 1-7; (45) p. 172; (52) p. 87.

AUTUMN CROCUS

Other Common Name(s): colchicum, meadow saffron
Botanical Name(s): *Colchicum autumnale* L. [Fam.: Colchicaceae (Liliaceae)]
<u>Seed</u>, <u>root</u> (tuber)
Constituents: Tropolone alkaloids (chiefly colchicine, also colchicoside, demecolcine, etc.), etc.
Properties: Anti-inflammatory and anti-gout, antimitotic (= inhibits or disrupts a type of cell division). Colchicine exerts anti-inflammatory and anti-gout effects by decreasing the migration of polymorphonuclear leukocytes and by indirectly stopping the deposition of uric acid to the inflamed area.
Uses: <u>Internally</u> it is used (as a standardized product, pure colchicine) for the treatment of acute attacks of gout and for the prophylaxis and treatment of familial paroxysmal peritonitis (= familial Mediterranean fever = FMF).
Caution: Colchicine and colchicum are highly toxic. Only colchicum standardized products or pure colchicine are used, as directed by a health professional. They should not be taken during pregnancy and lactation. Among the reported side effects are gastrointestinal irritations (with nausea, abdominal pains, vomiting, diarrhea) and possible liver and kidney damage. These occur particularly in subjects with preexisting gastrointestinal, liver and kidney disorders.

References: (1) Vol. 4, p. 946; (3) Vol. 4, p. 235; (6) p. 247; (8) p. 181; (11) p. 181; (12) p. 1011; (13) p. 279; (19) p. 103; (23) p. 282; (37) p. 353; (46) p. 342; (48) p. 949; (49) Vol. 2, p. 71; (50) p. 197; (72) nr. 43001; (74) p. 320.

AVENS

Other Common Name(s): geum, herb bennet, wood avens

Botanical Name(s): *Geum urbanum* L. [Fam.: Rosaceae]
<u>Root</u> (rhizome)
Constituents: Tannins (condensed and hydrolyzable t.), volatile oil (with eugenol, etc.), a phenol glycoside (gein = eugenol-vicianoside), phenolic acids (caffeic and chlorogenic acids), etc.
Properties: Astringent, anti-inflammatory, antibacterial. The astringent and anti-inflammatory effects are attributed to its high tannins content.
Uses: <u>Internally</u> it is used (as a tea) for diarrhea, inflammations of the gastrointestinal tract (gastritis, ulcerative colitis, etc.) and hemorrhoids. <u>Externally</u> it is used (as a mouthwash, gargle) for inflammations of the mouth and throat, (as a paint) for gingivitis (= inflammations of the gums), denture and canker sores, (as a wet compress, enema) for hemorrhoids, and (as a wash, wet compress) for minor skin inflammations and wounds.
Caution: At higher doses than recommended avens causes gastrointestinal irritations (with nausea, vomiting) and constipation. Otherwise, there are no reports of contraindications or side effects when used properly.

References: (1) Vol. 5, p. 263; (3) Vol. 4, p. 1130; (8) p. 283; (15) p. 102; (17) p. 249; (20) p. 40; (27) p. 77; (35) p. 73; (41) Vols. 1-7; (47) p. 1449; (49) Vol. 2, p. 422; (51) p. 98; (87) Vol. 1, p. 196.

AVOCADO

Other Common Name(s): alligator pear
Botanical Name(s): *Persea americana* Mill. = *Laurus persea* L. = *Persea gratissima* Gaertn. [Fam.: Lauraceae]
<u>Avocado oil</u>
It is the fixed oil produced by expressing the dried pulp of the fruit. The refined oil is more preferred.
Constituents: Glycerides (fatty acids component: oleic acid, etc.), fat-soluble vitamins (rich in vit. E), sterols (5-sterols: cholesterol, campesterol, β-sitosterol), triterpenes, carotenoids, etc.
Properties: Emollient.
Uses: <u>Externally</u> it is used (as an ointment, cream, body oil) in the practice of natural cosmetics for skin care and beneficial massages.
Caution: There are no reports of contraindications or side effects when used properly.
<u>Note</u>: Avocado is a valuable potassium supplement.

References: (1) Vol. 6, p. 70; (3) Vol. 6a, p. 533; (8) p. 414; (9) p. 54; (41) Vols. 1-7; (45) p. 118; (52) p. 580.

AYAHUASCA

Ayahuasca is a brewed beverage that the Amazonian tribes make using chiefly the stems of caapi or ayahuasca: *Banisteriopsis caapi* (Spruce ex

Griseb.) Morton = *Banisteriopsis inebrians* Morton [Fam.: Malpighiaceae]. They incorporate other herbs, particularly *Diplopterys cabrerana* (Cuatr.) Gates [Fam.: Malpighiaceae], *Psychotria viridis* Ruiz et Pavon, and *Psychotria carthaginensis* Jacq. [Fam.: Rubiaceae].

Constituents: Ayahuasca beverage contains indole alkaloids of β-carboline group (harman alkaloids: harmine = banisterine, harmaline, tetrahydroharmine = THH) and a tryptamine derivative (N, N-dimethyltryptamine = DMT) as its chief constituents. While caapi contains the mentioned β-carboline alkaloids, the three added herbs contain DMT, but no alkaloids.

Properties and Caution: Ayahuasca beverage is hallucinogenic. The chief constituent responsible for its hallucinogenic effect is considered DMT and to a lesser extent β-carboline alkaloids. These alkaloids are also monoamine oxidase (= MAO) inhibitors and thought to protect DMT from the oxidative deamination. This leads to a synergistic effect.

References: (1) Vol. 4, p. 458; (13) p. 287; (49) Vol. 2, p. 291; (61) p. 274; (62) p. 155; (81) p. 351.

BACCHARIS TRIMERA

Other Common Name(s): carqueja
Botanical Name(s): *Baccharis trimera* (Less.) DC. = *Baccharis genistelloides* (Lam.) Pers. var. *trimera* (Less.) Baker [Fam.: Asteraceae (Compositae)]
<u>Aerial part</u>
Constituents: Volatile oil (with monoterpenes: carquejol, etc.), bitter principles (diterpenoid lactones), flavonoids (chiefly flavones), and possibly triterpenoid saponins.
Properties: Aromatic, bitter tonic, choleretic, antipyretic, antibacterial.
Uses: <u>Internally</u> it is used (as a tea, h. p.) for loss of appetite and nonulcer dyspepsia (with flatulence, change of bowel habits, etc.) associated with minor hepatobiliary disorders. Baccharis is also used for minor fatigue, feverish states and convalescence. <u>Externally</u> it is used (as a wash, wet compress, poultice) for minor skin inflammations and wounds.
Caution: Baccharis should not be taken during pregnancy and lactation. Otherwise, there are no reports of contraindications or side effects when used properly.

References: (1) Vol. 4, p. 448; (3) Vol. 3, p. 346; (41) Vols. 1-7; (42) Vol. 3, pp. 487, 541; (52) p. 93.

BACOPA

Other Common Name(s): herb-of-grace, Indian pennywort, water hyssop
Botanical Name(s): *Bacopa monnieri* (L.) Pennell = *Herpestis monniera* (L.) Kunth [Fam.: Scrophulariaceae].

Aerial part
Constituents: Triterpenoid saponins (bacosides A, B), minerals (rich in potassium), a sugar alcohol (rich in mannitol), flavonoids (flavones: luteolin, etc.), triterpenes (betulinic acid, etc.), phytosterols (5-sterols: stigmasterol), alkaloids (nicotine, etc.), a pseudoalkaloid (3-formyl-4-hydroxy α-pyran), hydrocarbons (octacosane, etc.), etc.
Properties: Bacopa exerts nootropic effect (= increases cognitive function), which is attributed to bacosides, but the presence of potassium and small concentrations of nicotine and 3-formyl-4-hydroxy α-pyran may play an important role. It has also sedative, diuretic, anti-inflammatory, antioxidant, demulcent, emollient, stomachic, laxative, and cardiotonic properties. The effects are mild. The diuretic effect is due in large part to potassium.
Uses: Internally it is chiefly used as an adjuvant (tea, h. p.) for impaired mental performance (incl. cognitive function). It is also used (usually combined with other herbs) for chronic rheumatic complaints, as a flushing-out treatment (= herbal tea or product + liquids: more than 2 liters per day; sometimes combined with a medication) for inflammations of the genitourinary tract (cystitis, etc.), urinary gravel and nonobstructive stones, to prevent relapsing urinary infections / gravel / stones, and (as a tea, h. p.) for inflammations of the upper respiratory tract (bronchitis, laryngitis with hoarseness, etc.; coughs) and gastrointestinal tract (gastritis, impaired digestion, sluggish bowels, minor constipation). Bacopa extract may be used as a potassium supplement in a therapy with potassium depleting diuretics (e. g. hydrochlorthiazide). Externally it is used (expressed juice from leaves: as a wet compress) for rheumatic pains.
Caution: There are no reports of contraindications or side effects when used properly. Nevertheless, bacopa is best used as directed by an experienced practitioner. As a potassium supplement it should be used only on health professional's advice. In some regions of India bacopa is called brahmi, a name used in some other regions for gotu kola: *Centella asiatica* (L.) Urb.

References: (3) Vol. 3, p. 347; (5) Vol. 1, p. 150, Vol. 3, p. 275; (36) p. 502; (41) Vols. 1-7; (42) Vol. 6, pp. 366, 746; (45) p. 173; (52) p. 94; (57) p. 106; (69) p. 27.

BAILAHUÉN

Botanical Name(s): *Haplopappus baylahuen* Remy [Fam.: Asteraceae (Compositae)]
Leaf, aerial part
Constituents: Volatile oil, resin, flavonoids (flavanones, flavonols), coumarins, anthranoids, tannins, etc. It possibly contains bitter principles (diterpenoid lactones), phenolic acids and polyacetylenes.
Properties: Aromatic, bitter tonic, choleretic, anti-inflammatory, antibacterial, mild laxative, mild astringent. Its bitter tonic and hepatobiliary effects may be attributed to bitter diterpenoid lactones and phenolic acids. Flavon-

oids contribute to anti-inflammatory, polyacetylenes to antimicrobial, anthranoids to laxative and tannins to astringent effects, respectively.

Uses: Internally it is used (as a tea, h. p.) for loss of appetite and nonulcer dyspepsia (with fullness, flatulence, change of bowel habits, etc.) associated with minor disorders of the hepatobiliary tract (chronic cholecystitis, nonobstructive gallstones, chronic hepatitis) and for inflammations of the upper respiratory tract (also as a diaphoretic hot tea for the common cold and feverish states) and genitourinary tract (cystitis, urethritis, prostatitis, etc.). To enhance the effects in problems of the genitourinary tract, the fluid intake (incl. herbal teas) should be more than 2 liters per day. Externally it is used (as a wet compress, poultice) for minor skin inflammations and wounds.

Caution: Bailahuén should not be taken during pregnancy and lactation, biliary obstruction and severe liver disorders. Otherwise, there are no reports of contraindications or side effects when used properly.

References: (2) Vol. 2, p. 834; (3) Vol. 5, p. 14; (12) pp. 445, 778; (18) p. 284; (31) pp. 46, 388, 645; (35) p. 427; (37) p. 639; (41) Vols. 1-7; (52) p. 361.

BALLOON VINE

Other Common Name(s): heart pea, winter cherry
Botanical Name(s): *Cardiospermum halicacabum* L. [Fam.: Sapindaceae]
Leaf
Constituents: Tannins (rich in condensed and hydrolyzable t.), triterpenoid saponins, triterpenes, phytosterols (5-sterols: β-sitosterol, etc.), flavonoids (flavones: luteolin, etc.), a cyclitol (quebrachitol), alkaloids (?), etc.

Properties: Astringent, anti-inflammatory, analgesic, antipruritic, sedative, diuretic. It is also reported to exert emmenagogic and oxytocic effects. β-Sitosterol and related phytosterols have been shown to inhibit the biosynthesis of prostaglandins and leukotrienes and may account in large part for the anti-inflammatory and antipruritic effects.

Uses: Externally it is used (as a wet compress, poultice, liniment, ointment) for eczemas and other skin inflammatory conditions (with itching or pruritus), and rheumatic pains (incl. arthritic pains). Internally it is used (as a tea, h. p.) for inflammations of the gastrointestinal tract (diarrhea, etc., incl. hemorrhoids; also when minor hemorrhages are present, but on professional's advice), genitourinary tract (cystitis, etc.) and upper respiratory tract (bronchitis, etc.), and for rheumatic complaints (incl. rheumatoid arthritis).

Caution: Unless advised by a health professional, it should not be taken during pregnancy and lactation. Manufacturers should evaluate the reported alkaloids. *Cardiospermum* spp. is reported to contain cyanogenic glycosides, hence manufacturers should run tests and evaluate them. Otherwise, there are no reports of contraindications or side effects when used properly.

References: (1) Vol. 4, p. 681; (18) p. 188; (19) p. 37; (23) p. 330; (36) p. 42; (37) p. 279; (41) Vols. 1-7; (45) p. 181; (52) p. 154.

BALM, LEMON

Other Common Name(s): balm, bee balm, melissa, melissa balm
Botanical Name(s): *Melissa officinalis* L. [Fam.: Lamiaceae (Labiatae)]
Leaf
Constituents: Volatile oil (with citral a = geranial, citral b = neral, citron-ellal, etc.), Lamiaceae tannins (rosmarinic acid and other caffeic acid de-rivatives), bitter principles (triterpenes: ursolic and oleanolic acids), flavo-noids (flavones: luteolin and its glycosides), etc. The amount and constitu-ents of the volatile oil depend on origin, climate, year and cut, among oth-ers.

Properties: Sedative, antispasmodic, carminative, mild choleretic, antibac-terial, antiviral (against *Herpes simplex* type 2), mild astringent. Volatile oil, though in small amounts, plays an important role in the sedative, antispas-modic and carminative effects. The choleretic, antibacterial, antiviral and astringent effects are due in large part to rosmarinic acid and other related caffeic acid derivatives, which have also been shown to inhibit the biosyn-thesis of leukotrienes and prostaglandins.

Uses: Internally it is used (as a tea, h. p.) for insomnia and minor headaches (associated with stress), nervousness, anxiety, nervous heart complaints (e. g. cardiac arrhythmias), nonulcer dyspepsia (with flatulence, minor cramps, nausea), primary dysmenorrhea (= painful menstruation without pathology), and as a diaphoretic hot tea for the common cold and feverish states. Exter-nally it is used (as a cream with a standardized extract) for cold sores (= herpes simplex), and (as a mouthwash) for inflammations of the mouth.

Caution: There are no reports of contraindications or side effects when used properly. For best results it should be used leaves derived from *Melissa of-ficinalis* ssp. *officinalis*, which are relatively much richer in volatile oil.

Reference: (1) Vol. 5, p. 811; (3) Vol. 5, p. 759; (8) p. 366; (9) p. 57; (12) pp. 708, 782; (13) p. 103; (16) p. 181; (17) p. 383; (19) p. 157; (23) pp. 51, 296; (27) p. 216; (47) p. 1866; (48) p. 510; (51) p. 168.

BALMONY

Botanical Name(s): *Chelone glabra* L. [Fam.: Scrophulariaceae]
Aerial part
Constituents: It is reported to contain bitter principles and resins. It possi-bly contains iridoids and a phenol glycoside (syringin = glucoside of sinapyl alcohol, based on positive results from Ehrlich- and Syringin-Tests).
Properties: Bitter tonic, antispasmodic, choleretic, laxative. Many iridoids, besides their bitter tonic effect, have shown choleretic, liver protective, laxative, diuretic, anti-inflammatory, antibacterial, antiviral, antifungal and immunomodulant effects, among others. Possibly, through hydrolysis (in the intestinal tract) and oxidation (chiefly in the liver), syringin (if present) is converted to sinapic acid (as with the conversion of salicin of willow bark to

salicylic acid). Sinapic acid has shown liver protective, antibacterial and antifungal effects.

Uses: <u>Internally</u> it is used (as a tea, h. p.) for loss of appetite and nonulcer dyspepsia (with fullness, minor cramps, minor constipation, etc.) associated with minor hepatobiliary disorders (impaired bile secretion and flow, chronic cholecystitis, nonobstructive gallstones). In traditional medicine it is also used as an antidyscratic (= blood purifier; tea, h. p.) for atopic eczema (= chronic eczema of internal origin) and chronic rheumatic complaints.

Caution: There are no reports of contraindications or side effects when used properly.

References: (3) Vol. 3, p. 841; (10) p. 24; (15) p. 62; (17) p. 519; (18) p. 255; (22) p. 200; (31) p. 487; (32) Vol. 3, p. 1768; (35) p. 77; (36) p. 220.

BARBERRY

Other Common Name(s): European barberry
Botanical Name(s): *Berberis vulgaris* L. [Fam.: Berberidaceae]
<u>**Root bark**</u>, <u>**bark**</u>
Constituents: Isoquinoline alkaloids (root bark is richer), chiefly of protoberberine type (berberine, jatrorrhizine, etc.), also benzophenanthridine type (palmatine, etc.) and bisbenzyl-isoquinoline type (berbamine, etc.), tannins, etc.

Properties: Bitter tonic, cholagogue, antibacterial (against *Bacillus dysenteriae*, etc.), antifungal (against *Candida*), antiprotozoal (against *Entamoeba, Giardia, Leishmania, Trichomonas*), diuretic. The effects are due in large part to the high berberine content.

Uses: <u>Internally</u> it is used (as a tea, h. p.) for bacterial / fungal / protozoal infections of the gastrointestinal tract (chronic diarrhea, amebic dysentery), loss of appetite and nonulcer dyspepsia, and hepatobiliary disorders (impaired bile secretion and flow, nonobstructive gallstones, possibly hepatic amebiasis) often associated with them. <u>Externally</u> it is used (as an ointment that contains its tincture) for psoriasis and common acne (= acne vulgaris), (as a vaginal irrigation / sitz bath / wash, suppository) for vulvovaginitis, and (as a mouthwash, paint) for canker sores. See also COPTIS.

Caution: Barberry bark should not be taken during pregnancy and lactation and is best avoided in infants. At higher doses than recommended barberry causes gastrointestinal irritations (with nausea, vomiting, diarrhea).

<u>**Berry**</u> (ripe)
Constituents: Organic acids (malic acid, etc.), vitamin C (fresh berries are richer), phenolic acids (chlorogenic acid, etc.), anthocyanins, pectin, sugars, triterpenes (ursolic acid, etc.), etc.

Properties: Acidulous, refrigerant, mild laxative, mild bitter tonic.
Uses: <u>Internally</u> it is used (as a tea) for feverish and thirsty states, minor constipation and loss of appetite, and as a vitamin C supplement (jams pro-

duced with fresh berries, etc.). Externally it is used (as a mouthwash, gargle) for inflammations of the mouth and throat.

Caution: Only ripe berries should be used, as they normally are alkaloid-free. Nevertheless, the alkaloids content should be known before processing. There are no reports of contraindications or side effects when used properly.

References: (1) Vol. 4, p. 488; (3) Vol. 3, p. 415; (6) pp. 148, 190, 193; (8) p. 97; (9) p. 66; (13) p. 234; (15) p. 39; (29) p. 19; (37) p. 197; (41) Vols. 1-7; (44) p. 121; (46) p. 406; (47) p. 701; (51) p. 249; (66) p. 177; (71) p. 282.

BARLEY

Botanical Name(s): *Hordeum vulgare* L. [Fam.: Poaceae (Gramineae)]
Decorticated grain (peeled barley)
Constituents: Starch, sugars (sucrose, maltose, fructose, etc.), proteins (hordeine: rich in glutamic acid), minerals (phosphor, magnesium), fixed oil, vitamins (vit. E, niacin, pantothenic acid, vit. B_6, B_2, B_1, folic acid), etc.
Properties: Nutrient, demulcent.
Uses: Internally it is used (as a tea) for inflammations of the gastrointestinal tract (gastritis, diarrhea). Roasted barley is also used as a coffee substitute.
Caution: There are no reports of contraindications or side effects when used properly. Germinated barley should be avoided as it contains hordenine (= N, N-dimethyltyramine), a biogenic amine with sympathomimetic activity, much like tyramine (see CEREUS, NIGHT-BLOOMING).

References: (3) Vol. 5, p. 98; (27) p. 246; (28) p. 30; (35) p. 84; (37) pp. 671, 1123; (49) Vol. 2, p. 19.

BASIL

Other Common Name(s): sweet basil, garden basil
Botanical Name(s): *Ocimum basilicum* L. [Fam.: Lamiaceae (Labiatae)]
Aerial part
Constituents: Volatile oil (see Sweet basil oil), tannins, flavonoids (flavonols), Lamiaceae tannins (rosmarinic acid and other caffeic acid derivatives), phytosterols, triterpenes, etc.
Properties: Aromatic, stomachic, antispasmodic, carminative, anti-inflammatory, diuretic, antimicrobial. Rosmarinic acid and other related phenolic acid derivatives have been shown to inhibit the biosynthesis of leukotrienes and prostaglandins, and to exert choleretic, antibacterial and antiviral effects. Flavonoids and coumarins may contribute to the antispasmodic effect.
Uses: Basil is chiefly used as a spice. Internally it is used (as a tea) for loss of appetite and nonulcer dyspepsia (with flatulence, minor cramps, nausea, etc.), and for minor inflammations of the gastrointestinal tract (diarrhea, etc.), genitourinary tract (cystitis, urethritis, epididymitis, leukorrhea, pyelitis, etc.) and upper respiratory tract (the common cold, bronchitis, etc.). To enhance the effects in problems of the genitourinary tract, the fluid intake

33

(incl. herbal teas) should be more than 2 liters per day. Externally it is used (as a mouthwash, gargle) for inflammation of the mouth and throat, (as a mouthwash, chewing) for bad breath, (as a wet compress, poultice, ointment) for wounds, and (as a hair rinse) for hair loss.

Caution: Basil should not be taken during pregnancy and lactation. Otherwise, there are no reports of contraindications or side effects when used properly.

Sweet basil oil
It is the volatile oil obtained by steam distillation from the fresh aerial part.

Constituents: Linalool, methylchavicol (= estragole), eugenol, etc.; depending on the origin, etc.

Properties: Aromatic.

Uses: It is chiefly used as a fragrance ingredient in cosmetics and perfumery and to improve the aroma of tobacco. It can also be tried as insect-repellent.

Caution: There are no reports of irritating or toxic effects when used properly (in small amounts) as a fragrance ingredient.

References: (3) Vol. 6a, p. 288; (8) p. 385; (9) p. 68; (10) p. 26; (17) p. 104; (27) p. 49; (35) p. 87; (47) p. 669; (51) p. 174.

BAY

Other Common Name(s): bay laurel, sweet bay, true bay

Botanical Name(s): *Laurus nobilis* L. [Fam.: Lauraceae]

Leaf
Constituents: Volatile oil (see Bayleaf oil), bitter principles (sesquiterpene lactones: costunolide, etc.), tannins (condensed t.), aporphine alkaloids, flavonoids (flavonols), lignans, phenolic acids, etc.

Properties: Aromatic, stomachic, carminative, antimicrobial, expectorant.

Uses: Bayleaf is chiefly used as a spice. Internally it is used (as a tea) for loss of appetite and nonulcer dyspepsia (with flatulence, minor cramps), and for inflammations of the upper respiratory tract (bronchitis, etc.; coughs due to thickened bronchial secretion) and genitourinary tract (cystitis, urethritis, leukorrhea, etc.). To enhance the effects in problems of the genitourinary tract, the fluid intake (incl. herbal teas) should be more than 2 liters per day. Externally it is used (as a wash, wet compress) for minor wounds, (as a partial bath) for sweating feet, and (as a mouthwash, chewing) for bad breath.

Caution: Due to costunolide, which is closely related to sesquiterpene lactones found in Asteraceae plants (e. g. arnica, chamomile, feverfew, ragweed, tansy, yarrow), bayleaf may cause allergic contact dermatitis to persons hypersensitive to them. Otherwise, there are no reports of contraindications or side effects when used properly.

Bayleaf oil
It is the volatile oil obtained by steam distillation from the leaves.

Constituents: Chiefly 1,8-cineole (= eucalyptol), and depending on the origin, also varying amounts of pinenes, linalool, eugenol, bisabolol, etc.
Properties: Aromatic, antimicrobial.
Uses: Bayleaf oil is used as a flavor ingredient in food industry and as a fragrance ingredient in cosmetics and perfumery.
Caution: In rare cases it may cause allergic reactions. Otherwise, there are no reports of contraindications or side effects when used properly.

References: (2) Vol. 3, p. 50; (3) Vol. 5, p. 460; (5) Vol. 1, p. 636; (8) p. 336; (9) p. 69; (10) p. 167; (27) p. 25; (37) p. 811; (49) Vol. 2, p. 168; (51) p. 174.

BAY-RUM-TREE

Other Common Name(s): West Indian bay, myrcia
Botanical Name(s): *Pimenta racemosa* (Miller) J.W. Moore = *Pimenta acris* Kostel [Fam.: Myrtaceae]
Bay oil (= oil of bay, myrcia oil)
It is the volatile oil obtained by steam distillation from the leaves.
Constituents: There are several chemotypes available. Clove type, i. e. phenolic type, contains chiefly eugenol and chavicol. There is an anise type, i. e. non-phenolic type, which contains chiefly methyleugenol and estragole, and a lemon type, i. e. aldehydic type, which contains chiefly citrals (citral a = geranial, citral b = neral).
Properties: Rubefacient, analgesic, antimicrobial.
Uses: Externally it is used (as a liniment) for inflammations of the upper respiratory tract. Bay oil is chiefly used as a fragrance ingredient in cosmetics (e. g. bay rum), adding antiseptic effect to the products. Some insect-repellents contain it. In food industry bay oil is used as a flavor ingredient.
Caution: The application of the pure oil may cause skin irritation. In the production of bay rum, the phenolic type is preferred.

References: (3) Vol. 6a, p. 665; (5) Vol. 1, p. 834; (8) p. 426; (9) p. 71; (12) p. 759; (37) p. 1080; (48) p. 494.

BAYBERRY

Other Common Name(s): 1) southern bayberry, candle berry, wax myrtle 2) northern bayberry
Botanical Name(s): 1) *Morella cerifera* (L.) Sm. = *Myrica cerifera* L. 2) *Morella pensylvanica* (Mirb.) Kartesz = *Myrica pensylvanica* Mirb. [Fam.: Myricaceae]
Root bark
Constituents: Tannins (condensed t.), flavonoids (flavonols: myricitrin, etc.), triterpenes (myricadiol, taraxerol, etc.), gum, starch, an acrid resin, etc.
Properties: Astringent, antimicrobial, wound-healing.

Uses: <u>Internally</u> it is chiefly used (as a tea) for inflammations of the gastro-intestinal tract (diarrhea, ulcerative colitis) and for hemorrhoids. <u>Externally</u> it is used (as a mouthwash, gargle) for inflammations of the mouth and throat, (as a vaginal irrigation / sitz bath / wash) for leukorrhea and vulvovaginitis, and (as a poultice) for minor skin inflammations and ulcers.

Caution: The constituents of the reported acrid resin are not known. In view of this, bayberry should be avoided during pregnancy and lactation. At higher doses than recommended bayberry may cause gastrointestinal irritations (with nausea, vomiting). Otherwise, there are no reports of contraindications or side effects when used properly.

References: (3) Vol. 5, p. 917; (9) p. 72; (10) p. 26; (15) p. 146; (20) p. 41; (35) p. 87; (37) p. 934; (42) Vol. 5, p. 138; (47) p. 1937.

BEAN, COMMON

Botanical Name(s): *Phaseolus vulgaris* L. [Fam.: Fabaceae (Leguminosae)]
Pod
Constituents: Minerals (silicic acid, potassium, chromium), flavonoids, trigonelline, amino acids (arginine, etc.), allantoin, sugars, vitamin C, etc.
Properties: Mild diuretic (due to potassium, silicic acid, flavonoids). Due to its chromium content it may exert mild antihyperglycemic effect.
Uses: <u>Internally</u> it is used (combined with other herbs) as a flushing-out treatment (= herbal tea or product + liquids: more than 2 liters per day; sometimes combined with a medication) for inflammations of the genitourinary tract (cystitis, etc.), urinary gravel and nonobstructive stones, to prevent relapsing urinary infections / gravel / stones, and as an antidyscratic (= blood purifier; tea, h. p.) for chronic rheumatic complaints and skin disorders. It is also incorporated in herbal teas used as adjuvant for diabetes.
Caution: There are no reports of contraindications or side effects when used properly. Nevertheless, a flushing-out treatment is contraindicated in cases of obstructive urinary stones, edema due to impaired heart or kidney function and kidney inflammations (here can be used on health professional's advice to enhance the effects of an antimicrobial therapy).

References: (3) Vol. 6a, p. 559; (5) Vol. 1, p. 821; (6) pp. 185, 186; (8) p. 421; (16) p. 153; (17) p. 438; (19) p. 88; (23) p. 277; (24) p. 92; (47) p. 2097; (51) p. 106.

BEAR'S BREECH

Botanical Name(s): *Acanthus mollis* L. [Fam.: Acanthaceae]
Root
Constituents: Not well known. It is reported to contain mucilaginous polysaccharides and tannins. It possibly contains saponins, iridoids and a storage sugar (stachyose).
Properties: Emollient, astringent, wound-healing, demulcent, diuretic.

Uses: <u>Externally</u> it is used (as a wash, wet compress, poultice) for minor skin inflammations, burns and wounds, and (as a mouthwash, gargle) for inflammations of the mouth and throat. <u>Internally</u> it is used (as a tea) for inflammations of the gastrointestinal tract (diarrhea, etc.), genitourinary tract (cystitis, prostatitis, etc.), and upper respiratory tract (bronchitis, etc.; coughs).

Caution: There are no reports of contraindications or side effects when used properly.

References: (3) Vol. 2, p. 878; (5) Vol. 1, p. 10; (18) p. 256; (27) p. 16; (36) p. 49; (42) Vol. 6, p. 386; (45) p. 157; (47) p. 384; (52) p. 8.

BEAR'S FOOT

Other Common Name(s): 1) yellow leafcup 2) whiteflower leafcup
Botanical Name(s): 1) *Polymnia uvedalia* L. 2) *Polymnia canadensis* L. [Fam.: Asteraceae (Compositae)]

Root

Constituents and Properties: It is reported to contain tannins, a resin and sugars. Bear's foot belongs to the Heliantheae tribe. Among constituents found in this tribe are sesquiterpene lactones (they have shown anti-inflammatory, antibacterial, antitumoral effects), diterpenes (they have shown bitter tonic, anti-inflammatory effects), acetophenones (they have shown inhibitory effect on platelet aggregation and biosynthesis of prostaglandins and leukotrienes), benzofurans (they have shown antibacterial and antifungal effects), phenolic acids (they have shown liver protective, choleretic, antibacterial, antifungal, antiviral, antioxidant, anti-inflammatory effects), polyacetylenes (they have shown antifungal and antibacterial effects, etc.).

Uses: <u>Internally</u> it has been used as a tonic, laxative and analgesic, for the enlargement of spleen and liver and for dyspeptic disorders. <u>Externally</u> it has been used for painful swellings, minor skin inflammations, and as a hair tonic. There are plants of genus *Polymnia* that accumulate boron. If it is present, it could be a natural supplement of boron, which is recently recommended for the prevention of osteoporosis.

Caution: Bear's foot is best avoided during pregnancy and lactation. At doses higher than recommended it causes gastrointestinal irritations (with nausea, vomiting, diarrhea). If sesquiterpene lactones are present, bear's foot may cause allergic contact dermatitis to persons hypersensitive to other Asteraceae plants (e. g. arnica, chamomile, feverfew, ragweed, tansy, yarrow) that contain them. The toxic unsaturated pyrrolizidine alkaloids (= UPAs) are found only in a few species of Heliantheae tribe. Nevertheless, manufacturers should evaluate them and consider their limits. For dosage limits of UPAs see COLTSFOOT.

References: (5) Vol. 3, p. 482; (10) p. 27; (18) pp. 278, 283; (31) pp. 338, 466, 472, 645; (32) Vol. 1, p. 479; (35) p. 91; (36) p. 50; (41) Vols. 1-7; (44) p. 424; (52) p. 620; (64) pp. 1466, 1474; (91) p. 161.

BEAR'S GARLIC

Other Common Name(s): wild garlic
Botanical Name(s): *Allium ursinum* L. [Fam.: Liliaceae (Alliaceae)]
Aerial part (fresh)

Constituents: Its active constituents are chiefly the disintegration products of alliin (allicin, ajoenes), free amino acids (arginine, asparaginic acid, glutamic acid, etc.), etc. See also GARLIC.

Properties: Cholesterol and triglyceride reducing, platelet aggregation inhibitory, antihypertensive, antibacterial, antifungal, anthelmintic. It acts similar to garlic, but milder. See also GARLIC.

Uses: Bear's garlic is chiefly used as a spice and it is beneficial due to the mentioned effects. Internally it is consumed fresh or taken as a tea for inflammations of the gastrointestinal tract (impaired digestion, flatulence, diarrhea) and upper respiratory tract (bronchitis, tracheitis, laryngitis, colds), worm infestations (as an enema, or taken as a tea), and as an adjuvant for hypertension and preventive for arteriosclerosis. Externally it is used (as a wash, wet compress, poultice) for minor skin inflammations.

Caution: At higher doses than recommended bear's garlic may cause gastrointestinal discomfort (nausea, vomiting). Otherwise, there are no contraindications or side effects when used properly.

References: (1) Vol. 4, p. 202; (3) Vol. 2, p. 1215; (8) p. 40; (13a) p. 111; (23) pp. 116, 177; (37) p. 47; (47) p. 479.

BEDSTRAW

Other Common Name(s): 1) bedstraw, cleavers, clivers, goosegrass, stickywilly 2) lady's bedstraw, yellow bedstraw
Botanical Name(s): 1) *Galium aparine* L. 2) *Galium verum* L. [Fam.: Rubiaceae]
Aerial part

Constituents: Flavonoids (flavonols: quercetin, rutin, etc.; etc.), iridoids (asperuloside, etc.), tannins (possibly condensed t.), phenolic acids (caffeic acid derivatives), etc.

Properties: Diuretic, astringent, anti-inflammatory. Flavonoids may account at least in part for its diuretic effect. Iridoids have shown bitter tonic, choleretic, liver protective, anti-inflammatory, laxative, diuretic, antibacterial, antiviral, antifungal and immunomodulant effects, among others. Caffeic acid derivatives and tannins may account for the anti-inflammatory and astringent effects.

Uses: Internally it is used (as a tea, h. p.; usually combined with other herbs) as a flushing-out treatment (= herbal tea or product + liquids: more than 2 liters per day; sometimes combined with a medication) for inflammations of the genitourinary tract (cystitis, etc.), urinary gravel and non obstructive stones, to prevent relapsing urinary infections / gravel / stones, and as an antidyscratic (= blood purifier) and anti-inflammatory (tea, h. p.) for atopic eczema (= chronic eczema of internal origin) and chronic rheumatic complaints. It is also used for inflammations of the gastrointestinal tract (minor diarrhea, etc.). Externally it is used (as a wash, wet compress, poultice) for minor skin inflammations, wounds, ulcers, poison ivy dermatitis, bruises and sprains, and (as a vaginal irrigation / sitz bath / wash) for leukorrhea and vulvovaginitis.

Caution: There are no reports of contraindications or side effects when used properly. Nevertheless, bedstraw should not be taken in cases of edemas due to impaired heart or kidney function, obstructive urinary stones and kidney inflammations (here can be used on health professional's advice to enhance the effects of an antimicrobial therapy).

References: (1) Vol. 5, pp. 220, 225; (3) Vol. 4, pp. 1086, 1087; (10) p. 165; (12) p. 438; (14) p. 61; (15) p. 96; (17) p. 246; (20) p. 78; (31) p. 569; (35) p. 91; (41) Vols. 1-7; (44) p. 241; (45) p. 212; (51) p. 192.

BEEBALM

Other Common Name(s): 1) lemon beebalm, prairie bergamot 2) spotted beebalm, plains beebalm, pony beebalm 3) beebalm, white bergamot, wild bergamot 4) horsemint, American horsemint, monarda, origanum, spotted beebalm 5) wild bergamot beebalm, beebalm, Oswego tea

Botanical Name(s): 1) *Monarda citriodora* Cerv. ex Lag. 2) *Monarda pectinata* Nutt. 3) *Monarda clinopodia* L. 4) *Monarda punctata* L. 5) *Monarda fistulosa* L. [Fam.: Lamiaceae (Labiatae)]

Aerial part

Constituents: Volatile oil (with phenols: thymol, thymohydroquinone, etc.; also quinones: thymoquinone; etc.), flavonoids, Lamiaceae tannins (rosmarinic acid and other caffeic acid derivatives), triterpenes (ursolic acid, etc.), bitter principles (ursolic acid, possibly diterpenoid lactones), etc.

Properties: Aromatic, bitter tonic, sedative, antispasmodic, carminative, antimicrobial, anti-inflammatory, diuretic, expectorant, counterirritant.

Uses: Internally it is used (as a tea, h. p.) for minor inflammatory and spastic conditions of the gastrointestinal tract (impaired digestion, flatulence, nausea, intestinal cramps, chronic diarrhea) and upper respiratory tract (bronchitis, laryngitis, etc.; minor coughs due to thickened bronchial secretion; also as a diaphoretic hot tea for the common cold and feverish states). Externally it is used (as a mouthwash, gargle) for inflammations of the mouth and throat and (as a poultice, liniment) for rheumatic pains.

Caution: There are no reports of contraindications or side effects when used properly. Nevertheless, beebalms are best avoided during pregnancy and lactation.

References: (3) Vol. 5, pp. 880, 881, 882; (29) p. 76; (35) p. 546; (37) p. 918; (44) pp. 346, 347; (45) p. 234; (52) p. 505; (57) p. 539.

BEET, RED

Botanical Name(s): *Beta vulgaris* L. ssp. *vulgaris* var. *conditiva* Alef [Fam.: Chenopodiaceae]
Root
Constituents: Minerals (rich in iron and copper), betalain pigments* (chiefly the red-violet betacyanins: betanin = betanidin-glucoside, etc.; also some yellow betaxanthins: vulgaxanthin, etc.), allantoin, amino acids, etc. *) Betalain pigments are not to be confused with anthocyanins, which are flavonoids found in bilberry, elderberry, cornflower and many other fruits and flowers, or with betaine, which is a biogenic amine.
Properties: Antianemic, tonic, "detoxifying". The antianemic and tonic effects are due to the iron and copper content. The hepatorenal "detoxifying" effect may be attributed to betalain pigments, allantoin and amino acids.
Uses: Internally it is used (as an h. p., juice, consumed fresh) for anemia, chronic liver and kidney ailments, and to enhance the effects of a tumor therapy. Red beet is claimed to be valuable for any condition that we need to cleanse our body from toxins.
Caution: To enhance the effects of a tumor therapy the unprocessed red beet juice should be used as directed by a health professional. In some individuals red beet pigments are not completely transformed, due to which urine results colored (beeturia). This is not a sign to be concerned about.

References: (3) Vol. 3, p. 430; (8) p. 100; (23) p. 240; (36) p. 339; (37) p. 202.

BEET, SUGAR

Botanical Name(s): *Beta vulgaris* L. ssp. *vulgaris* var. *altissima* Doell [Fam.: Chenopodiaceae]
Juice
Constituents: Sugars (sucrose, etc.), biogenic amines (betaine, etc.), galactinol (= myo-inositol-glucoside), a phenol glycoside (coniferin = glucoside of coniferyl alcohol), triterpenoid saponins (aglycone: oleanolic acid), phytosterols, amides (glutamine, etc.), purine bases, amino acids, organic acids.
Properties: Liver protective, promotes regeneration of liver cells, triglyceride and cholesterol reducing. Its main active constituents are considered betaine and myo-inositol.
Uses: Internally it is used for chronic liver disorders (chronic hepatitis, fatty liver, etc.).
Caution: There are no reports of contraindications or side effects when used properly.

References: (3) Vol. 3, p. 430; (8) p. 99; (23) p. 125; (37) p. 202; (49) Vol. 2, p. 133.

BELLADONNA

Other Common Name(s): deadly nightshade
Botanical Name(s): *Atropa belladonna* L. [Fam.: Solanaceae]
Leaf, **root**
Constituents: Both contain tropane alkaloids. Fresh leaf contains chiefly (−)-hyosciamine, while dried leaf and extracts contain chiefly atropine = (±)-hyosciamine, and (fresh, dried) also belladonnine, scopolamine, among other alkaloids. Root contains almost the same alkaloids (more belladonnine, plus cuskohygrine), but no flavonols. Among other constituents found in the leaf are flavonols, coumarins, tannins, and organic acids.
Properties: Due to the parasympatholytic (= anticholinergic = antimuscarinic) activity of hyosciamine / atropine, belladonna exerts antispasmodic and antisecretory effects, among others.
Uses: Internally it is used (usually in a standardized combination product) for spastic conditions of the gastrointestinal tract (irritable bowel syndrome, spastic constipation, peptic ulcers, vomiting), biliary tract (gallstones, cholecystitis), genitourinary tract (urinary stones, urinary incontinence) and upper respiratory tract (spastic bronchitis).
Caution: Belladonna is toxic. Today the extracts standardized to hyosciamine / atropine are used and especially the isolated alkaloids, which are given by prescription only. Belladonna should not be taken in cases of tachycardia, glaucoma, retention of urine due to prostatic hyperplasia, bowel obstruction and during pregnancy, among others.

References: (1) Vol. 4, p. 423; (3) Vol. 3, p. 309; (5) Vol. 1, p. 143; (11) p. 149; (12) p. 970; (13) p. 239; (14) p. 31; (19) p. 228; (37) p. 154; (46) p. 133; (48) p. 811; (74) p. 320.

BENZOIN TREE

Other Common Name(s): 1) Siam benzoin, Siam styrax 2) Sumatra benzoin
Botanical Name(s): 1) *Styrax tonkinensis* (Pierre) Craib ex Hartwich 2) *Styrax benzoin* Dryand.; *Styrax paralleloneurus* Perk. [Fam.: Styracaceae]
Benzoin (benzoe)
Is a balsamic resin, the dried exudate obtained by wounds made to the bark.
Constituents: Siam benzoin contains benzoic acid (free, as coniferyl-benzoate and other esters), triterpenoid acids (siaresinolic acid, etc.) and vanillin. Sumatra benzoin contains very much the same constituents, but benzoic acid is partly replaced by cinnamic acid.
Properties: Antimicrobial, anti-inflammatory, wound-healing, expectorant.
Uses: Externally it is used (Benzoin Tincture, Compound Benzoin Tincture) mainly for small cuts, also for eczema and fungal skin infections (= derma-

tomycosis), and (as a mouthwash: diluted tincture) for inflammations of the mouth. Internally it is used (as an inhalation) for inflammations of the upper respiratory tract. Benzoin is chiefly used in cosmetics and perfumery. Siam benzoin is also used as an antioxidant for some ointment bases.

Caution: In rare cases benzoin may cause allergic reactions.

References: (1) Vol. 6, p. 847; (3) Vol. 6b, p. 617; (8) p. 539; (9) p. 81; (11) p. 105; (12) p. 748; (13) p. 137; (37) p. 192; (46) p. 138; (48) p. 257.

BERGENIA

Other Common Name(s): leather bergenia
Botanical Name(s): *Bergenia crassifolia* (L.) Fritsch [Fam.: Saxifragaceae]
Leaf (= Siberian tea, Tschager tea)
Constituents: Phenol glycosides (arbutin = hydroquinone-glucoside), some free hydroquinone, tannins (chiefly gallotanins), a bitter principle (an aromatic alcohol glycoside: rhododendrin), flavonoids, an isocoumarin (bergenin = cuscutin), etc.
Properties: Urinary antiseptic, astringent, anti-inflammatory. Due to its high arbutin content it acts much like uva-ursi (see UVA-URSI). Bergenin has shown anti-inflammatory effect.
Uses: Internally it is used (as a tea, h. p.) chiefly for inflammations of the genitourinary tract (cystitis, urethritis, prostatitis, pyelonephritis), and also gastrointestinal tract (diarrhea, etc.; also when minor hemorrhages are present, but on professional's advice). To enhance the effects, urine should be slightly alkaline (this can be done by consuming a diet rich in vegetables and / or taking about a teaspoonful / day of baking soda) and the fluid intake (incl. herbal teas) should be more than 2 liters per day.
Caution: See UVA-URSI.

References: (1) Vol. 4, p. 497; (3) Vol. 3, p. 424; (5) Vol. 1, p. 162; (13) p. 304; (19) p. 43; (31) p. 541; (48) p. 246.

BETA GLUCANS

Lentinan
Lentinan is a high molecular weight D-glucan (= D-glucose polymer), which consists of a long main chain made of β-(1→3) linked D-glucose units and side chains made of β-(1→3) and β-(1→6) linked D-glucose units. Side chains are linked to every 5th D-glucose unit of the main chain. Lentinan occurs in **shiitake** or Chinese black mushroom: *Lentinula edodes* (Berk.) Pegler. = *Lentinus edodes* (Berk.) Sing. [Fam.: Tricholomataceae]

Schizophyllan
Schizophyllan is a D-glucan very similar to lentinan. Its main chain is the same as lentinan. The small difference is in the structure of side chains and

the fact that side chains are linked to every 3rd D-glucose unit of the main chain. It occurs in **suehirotake** or split-gill: *Schizophyllum commune* Fries [Fam.: Schizophyllaceae].

Properties: β-(1→3)-D-glucans, prepared from the mentioned mushrooms or some other species (see Note), have shown immunomodulant, antitumoral and antibacterial effects. The effects are mainly attributed to their role in stimulating T-lymphocytes and macrophages.

Uses: Standardized β-(1→3)-D-glucan products (known as Beta 1,3 / 1,6 D-glucan; Beta 1,3 D-glucan; Beta 1,3 Glucan; Beta Glucan) are chiefly used to enhance the effects of cancer and infection therapies. Even when used alone, they have been shown to increase the survival rate of cancer patients and to decrease the intensity and the relapse of bacterial, viral or fungal infections.

The mentioned mushrooms, besides β-D-glucans, contain other constituents (triterpenes, phytosterols, biogenic amines, polyacetylenes, thiophenes, trace minerals, etc.). These mushrooms, as well as those mentioned below (see Note), are considered adaptogens. They have been shown to improve mental and physical performance, immune response and blood levels of cholesterol and glucose, among others.

Caution: As with Echinacea and other immunomodulants, β-(1→3)-D-glucan products should not be taken in cases of chronic debilitating illnesses such as multiple sclerosis, tuberculosis, diffuse connective tissue diseases (rheumatoid arthritis, scleroderma, systemic lupus erythematosus, Behçet's syndrome, etc.), AIDS, etc. Only a health professional should decide and monitor a combination therapy with β-D-glucan products and anticancer drugs. For other cases, unless advised by a health professional, they should not be taken for more than 8 weeks. Before a possible resuming, a break for 2-3 weeks is required. See ECHINACEA.

Note: Other mushrooms rich in β-D-glucans, similar to lentinan and schizophyllan, are: **kawaratake** or turkey tail: *Trametes versicolor* (L. ex Fr.) Pilat = *Coriolus versicolor* (L. ex Fr.) Quel. [Fam.: Polyporaceae]; **maitake**: *Grifola frondosa* (Dicks ex Fr.) S.F. Gray [Fam.: Polyporaceae]; **poria**: *Wolfiporia cocos* (F.A. Wolf) Ryvarden & Gilb. = *Poria cocos* F.A. Wolf [Fam.: Polyporaceae]; **reishi**: *Ganoderma lucidum* (Curt. ex Fr.) Karst.; *Ganoderma japonicum* (Fr.) Lloyd; **artist's conk**: *Ganoderma applanatum* (Pers.) Pat. [Fam.: Ganodermataceae]; etc.

References: (2) Vol. 2, p. 752; Vol. 3, pp. 61, 528; (9) p. 425; (12) p. 375; (13) p. 550; (37) pp. 820, 1235; (48) p. 42; (77) p. 25.

BETELNUT PALM

Other Common Name(s): areca
Botanical Name(s): *Areca catechu* L. [Fam.: Arecaceae (Palmae)]
<u>Seed</u> (betel nut, areca nut)

Constituents: Piperidine alkaloids (chiefly arecoline, also arecaidine, etc.), tannins (condensed t.), phlobaphenes (areca red), sugars, fixed oil, etc.

Properties: Taeniafuge. Due to the parasympathomimetic activity of arecoline, areca promotes secretion of saliva and sweat, and increases peristalsis.

Uses: <u>Internally</u> it is used (as an h. p.) in veterinary practice for tapeworm infestations.

Caution: Betel nut is toxic. Even eight grams of betel nut can be fatal to an adult. Chewing betel-mastic is not advisable as arecoline causes bronchial spasms, bradycardia (= slow heart beat) and other side effects. Chronic abuse leads to neurologic problems of the oral cavity and throat.

References: (3) Vol. 3, p. 184; (5) Vol. 1, p. 105; (8) p. 69; (10) p. 15; (11) p. 147; (13) p. 273; (37) p. 126; (48) p. 871; (49) Vol. 2, p. 4.

BETHROOT

Other Common Name(s): birth root, purple trillium, red trillium, wakerobin

Botanical Name(s): *Trillium erectum* L. = *Trillium pendulum* Willd. [Fam.: Liliaceae]

<u>Root</u> (rhizome)

Constituents: Steroidal saponins (trillin, trillarin, etc.; with aglycone: diosgenin, chlorogenin, cryptogenin, etc.), tannins, flavonoids (a kaempferol glycoside, etc.), resin, etc. It has been reported to contain an alkaloid.

Properties: Uterotonic, mild oxytocic, astringent, hemostatic, mild expectorant.

Uses: <u>Internally</u> it is chiefly used (as a tea, h. p.) for menorrhagia / hypermenorrhea (= prolonged / heavy menstruation), postpartum hemorrhage (= h. following childbirth), as an adjuvant for metrorrhagia (= nonmenstrual uterine bleeding), also for hemorrhages of the urinary tract associated with gravel or nonobstructive stones, and more seldom for coughs (incl. coughing of blood). <u>Externally</u> it is used (as a vaginal irrigation / sitz bath / wash) for leukorrhea, and (as a poultice, ointment) for minor skin inflammations, wounds and ulcers.

Caution: It should not be taken during pregnancy and lactation. Before taking it for any kind of bleeding, the problem should be judged by a health professional. Manufacturers should evaluate the reported alkaloids.

References: (3) Vol. 6c, p. 277; (10) p. 30; (15) p. 217; (29) p. 117; (36) p. 478; (37) p. 1402; (41) Vols. 1-7; (44) p. 568; (47) p. 2730; (52) p. 817; (71) p. 9.

BETONY, MARSH

Other Common Name(s): woundwort, marsh woundwort

Botanical Name(s): *Stachys palustris* L. [Fam.: Lamiaceae (Labiatae)]

44

Aerial part
Constituents: Volatile oil, bitter principles (iridoids: harpagide, acetyl-harpagide), flavonoids (flavones: palustrinoside, isoscutellarein, etc.), Lamiaceae tannins (rosmarinic acid and other caffeic acid derivatives), proline-betaines (betonicine, stachydrine), etc.
Properties: Aromatic, bitter tonic, astringent, anti-inflammatory, antioxidant, wound-healing, mild antispasmodic. See also BETONY, WOOD.
Uses: Internally it is used (as a tea, h. p.) for loss of appetite and nonulcer dyspepsia (with flatulence, minor cramps, change of bowel habits, etc.) and minor cases of primary dysmenorrhea (= painful menstruation without pathology). Externally it is used (as a poultice) for wounds.
Caution: There are no reports of contraindications or side effects when used properly.

References: (3) Vol. 6b, p. 510; (10) p. 289; (12) p. 438; (16) p. 131; (28) p. 173; (31) p. 569; (35) p. 862; (41) Vols. 1-7; (44) p. 543.

BETONY, WOOD

Botanical Name(s): *Stachys officinalis* (L.) Trev. = *Betonica officinalis* L. = *Stachys betonica* Benth. nom. illeg. [Fam.: Lamiaceae (Labiatae)]
Aerial part
Constituents: Volatile oil, bitter principles (a diterpenoid lactone: betolide; iridoids), Lamiaceae tannins (rosmarinic acid and other caffeic acid derivatives), proline-betaines (betonicine, stachydrine), flavonoids, a biogenic amine (choline), etc.
Properties: Aromatic, bitter tonic, astringent, anti-inflammatory, wound-healing, mild antispasmodic. Iridoids have shown bitter tonic, choleretic, liver protective, anti-inflammatory, laxative, antibacterial, antiviral, antifungal and immunomodulant effects, among others. The effects are mild. Proline-betaines have shown cholagogic effect. Betonicine has also shown anti-inflammatory effect. Rosmarinic acid and other related caffeic acid derivatives have been shown to inhibit the biosynthesis of leukotrienes and prostaglandins and to exert choleretic, antibacterial and antiviral effects.
Uses: Internally it is used (as a tea, h. p.) for loss of appetite and nonulcer dyspepsia (with fullness, flatulence, minor cramps, change of bowel habits, etc.), inflammations of the upper respiratory tract (bronchitis, etc.; also as a diaphoretic hot tea for the common cold and feverish states), and for minor fatigue with headache. Externally it is used (as a wash, poultice) for minor wounds and ulcers, and (as a mouthwash, gargle) for inflammations of the mouth and throat.
Caution: There are no reports of contraindications or side effects when used properly.

References: (3) Vol. 6b, p. 506; (12) p. 782; (15) p. 41; (24) p. 83; (27) p. 53; (28) p. 201; (31) p. 247; (35) p. 97; (37) p. 1300; (41) Vols. 1-7; (47) p. 2598.

BILBERRY

Other Common Name(s): European blueberry, huckleberry, whortleberry
Botanical Name(s): *Vaccinium myrtillus* L. [Fam.: Ericaceae]
Berries
Constituents: Tannins (oligomeric and polymeric proanthocyanidins), flavonoids (anthocyanins: glycosides of cyanidin, delphinidin, etc.; flavonols; catechins), sugars, organic acids (citric and malic acids, etc.), pectin, etc.
Properties: Astringent, intestinal antiseptic, antidiarrheal, antioxidant, anti-inflammatory. Bilberry anthocyanins have shown antioxidant and "vitamin P"-like (= help in normalizing an increased microvascular permeability and fragility) effects. Bilberry has been shown to improve night vision, which is due to its anthocyanins.
Uses: Internally it is used (as a tea, h. p.) for inflammations of the gastrointestinal tract (diarrhea, ulcerative colitis) and for hemorrhoids. For minor cases of nonspecific diarrhea it is also recommended for children and the elderly. Bilberry extracts standardized to the anthocyanins content and the isolated and purified bilberry anthocyanins are used for age-related macular degeneration (= AMD). Externally it is used (as a mouthwash, gargle) for inflammations of the mouth and throat and (as a wash, wet compress) for minor skin inflammations and eczemas.
Caution: There are no reports of contraindications or side effects when used properly.
Leaf
Constituents: Tannins (proanthocyanidins), flavonoids (flavonols, catechins), iridoids, phenolic acids, triterpenes, minerals (chromium, manganese), quinolizidine alkaloids (in traces), etc.
Properties: Astringent, anti-inflammatory, claimed antihyperglycemic.
Uses: Internally it is used (as a tea, h. p.; usually combined with other herbs) for minor inflammations of the gastrointestinal and genitourinary tracts. In traditional medicine it is used as an adjuvant for diabetes. Externally it is used (as a mouthwash, gargle) for inflammations of the mouth and throat, and (as a wash, poultice) for minor skin inflammations and burns.
Caution: There are no reports of contraindications or side effects when used properly.

References: (1) Vol. 6, p. 1052; (3) Vol. 6c, p. 369; (6) pp. 155, 328; (7) p. 212; (8) p. 573; (9) p. 84; (16) p. 83; (17) pp. 403, 406; (19) p. 102; (22) p. 64; (23) p. 93; (26) p. 55; (27) p. 227; (35) p. 99; (46) p. 951; (47) p. 1949; (48) p. 361.

BIRCH

Other Common Name(s): 1) European white birch, silver birch, weeping birch 2) white birch, downy birch
Botanical Name(s): 1) *Betula pendula* Roth = *Betula verrucosa* Ehrh
2) *Betula pubescens* Ehrh. = *Betula alba* L. [Fam.: Betulaceae]

Leaf

Constituents: Flavonoids (flavonols: hyperin and other quercetin glycosides, etc.), saponin-like triterpenes, tannins (condensed t.), minerals (potassium, etc.), phenolic acids (caffeic acid, etc.), volatile oil (small amounts; with methyl salicylate, etc.), etc.

Properties: Diuretic, mild antimicrobial. The diuretic effect is due in large part to flavonoids, potassium and saponin-like triterpenes.

Uses: Internally it is used as a flushing-out treatment (= herbal tea or product + liquids: more than 2 liters per day; sometimes combined with a medication) for inflammations of the genitourinary tract (cystitis, etc.), urinary gravel and nonobstructive stones, to prevent relapsing urinary infections / gravel / stones, and as an antidyscratic (= blood purifier; tea, h. p.) for chronic rheumatic complaints and atopic eczema (= chronic eczema of internal origin). Externally it is used (as a poultice) for boils and (as a wash, wet compress) for milk crust and hair loss (due to fungal infections).

Caution: There are no reports of contraindications or side effects when used properly. Nevertheless, a flushing-out treatment is contraindicated in cases of obstructive urinary stones, edema due to impaired heart or kidney function and kidney inflammations (here can be used on health professional's advice to enhance the effects of an antimicrobial therapy).

Sprout

Constituents: Flavonoids (methoxy-flavonols), volatile oil (very rich; with β-betulenol, abscisic acid, etc.), triterpenoid saponins, bitter principles, etc.

Properties: Aromatic, choleretic, diuretic.

Uses: Externally it is used (as a wash: mainly combined with other herbs) for skin diseases and as an ingredient in some hair wash products. Internally it is used (usually combined with other herbs) for inflammations of the genitourinary and hepatobiliary tracts.

Caution: There are no reports of contraindications or side effects when used properly.

Bark

Constituents: Triterpenes (rich in betulin), tannins (condensed t.), phenolic acids (salicylic and vanillic acids), benzoic acid, a bitter glycoside (betuloside), resin, volatile oil, etc.

Properties: Astringent, mild antimicrobial. The effects are due in large part to tannins. To the antimicrobial effect may contribute phenolic acids and benzoic acid. Betulinic acid, which is produced by converting the isolated betulin, has been shown to inhibit certain tumors and HIVs.

Uses: Externally it is used (as a wash, partial bath) for skin inflammatory conditions and sweating feet, and (as a poultice) for boils.

Caution: There are no reports of contraindications or side effects when used properly.

References: (1) Vol. 4, p. 501; (3) Vol. 3, p. 434; (8) p. 100; (12) p. 853; (13) p. 318; (16) p. 159; (17) p. 107; (19) p. 46; (23) p. 276; (27) p. 54; (28) p. 183; (37) p. 203; (46) p. 141; (47) p. 710; (48) p. 760; (51) p. 244.

BIRTHWORT

Other Common Name(s): European aristolochia
Botanical Name(s): *Aristolochia clematitis* L. [Fam.: Aristolochiaceae]
Aerial part
Constituents: Aromatic nitro-compounds (aristolochic acids), alkaloids, choline, trimethylamine, phenolic acids, volatile oil, flavonoids, methyl inositol, phytosterols, etc.
Properties, Uses, and Caution: In traditional medicine birthwort has been used internally for menstrual disorders and externally for infected wounds, among others. Due to its high toxicity birthwort is no longer used. Some of aristolochic acids have shown nephrotoxic and carcinogenic effects (cf. GINGER, CANADIAN WILD; SNAKEROOT, VIRGINIA).

References: (2) Vol. 2, p. 171; (3) Vol. 3, p. 205; (8) p. 70; (10) p. 32; (13a) p. 330; (29) p. 13; (37) p. 128; (46) p. 101; (47) p. 577.

BISTORT

Other Common Name(s): snakeweed
Botanical Name(s): *Polygonum bistorta* L. [Fam.: Polygonaceae]
Root
Constituents: Tannins (hydrolyzable and condensed t.), starch (rich), phenolic acids (sinapic acid, etc.), sugars (glucose, etc.), proteins, etc.
Properties: Astringent, demulcent, anti-inflammatory.
Uses: Internally it is used (as a tea, h. p.) for inflammations of the gastrointestinal tract (diarrhea, ulcerative colitis, incl. hemorrhoids; also when minor hemorrhages are present, but on professional's advice). Externally it is used (as a mouthwash, gargle, paint) for inflammations of the mouth and throat (incl. canker sore), (as a vaginal irrigation / sitz bath / wash) for leukorrhea, (as a wet compress, ointment) for hemorrhoids and anal fissure, and (as a wet compress) for minor cuts, wounds and ulcers (incl. sore nipples). It is also used as a substitute of rhatany.
Caution: There are no reports of contraindications or side effects when used properly. Nevertheless, at higher doses than recommended bistort causes gastrointestinal irritations (with constipation, nausea, vomiting).

References: (1) Vol. 6, p. 76; (3) Vol. 6a, p. 815; (5) Vol. 1, p. 864; (10) p. 32; (15) p. 167; (24) p. 289; (27) p. 57; (28) pp. 94, 124, 175; (35) p. 105; (37) p. 1103.

BITTER CANDYTUFT

Other Common Name(s): clown's mustard
Botanical Name(s): *Iberis amara* L. [Fam.: Brassicaceae (Cruciferae)]
Aerial part (fresh)

Constituents: Bitter principles (cucurbitacins: cucurbitacin E, etc.), glucosinolates (glucoiberin, etc.), flavonoids (flavonols: kaempferol and quercetin glycosides), bitter principles (cucurbitacins; in traces), etc. Under the action of enzymes (when the fresh material is crushed; partly with drying) glucoiberin liberates 3-methylsulphinyl-propyl isothiocyanate, responsible for the pungent flavor, and then is partly further transformed to a biogenic amine (3-methylsulphinyl-propylamine).

Properties: Relieves gastrointestinal inflammations and cramps, decreases gastric acid secretion, mild antimicrobial.

Uses: <u>Internally</u> it is used (combined with other herbs) mainly for inflammatory and spastic conditions of the gastrointestinal tract (gastritis, gastroenteritis, heartburn, irritable bowel syndrome). <u>Externally</u> it is used (as a poultice) for rheumatic pains.

Caution: Unless advised by a health professional, it should not be taken during pregnancy as it may induce uterine contractions.

Seed

Constituents: Bitter principles (cucurbitacins: cucurbitacins E, I, etc., much richer than the aerial part), glucosinolates (glucoiberin = 3-methylsulfinyl-propyl-glucosinolate, etc.; much richer than the aerial part), fixed oil, etc.

Properties: Bitter tonic, choleretic, antimicrobial, rubefacient, counterirritant. The bitter tonic and choleretic effects are due in large part to cucurbitacins. Under the action of enzymes (when the seed is crushed and comes into contact with moisture and lukewarm temperature) glucoiberin liberates the volatile and pungent 3-methylsulfinyl-propyl isothiocyanate (in higher concentrations than the aerial part), responsible for most of the the effects.

Uses: <u>Externally</u> it is used (as a poultice) for rheumatic and neuralgic pains and inflammations of the upper respiratory tract. <u>Internally</u> it is used (as a tea, h. p.; combined with other herbs) for nonulcer dyspepsia (with fullness, flatulence, bloating, cramps, etc.) associated with impaired bile secretion.

Caution: Bitter candytuft is toxic and should be used with caution and only as directed by an experienced practitioner. It should not be taken during pregnancy and lactation.

References: (1) Vol. 5, p. 502; (3) Vol. 5, p. 221; (8) p. 320; (12) p. 516; (19) p. 39; (23) p. 65; (24) p. 461; (31) p. 96; (37) p. 695; (41) Vols. 1-7; (45) p. 220; (47) p. 1600; (67) p. 807; (72) nr. 59164.

BITTERSWEET

Other Common Name(s): bitter nightshade, climbing nightshade, dulcamara, woody nightshade

Botanical Name(s): *Solanum dulcamara* L. [Fam.: Solanaceae]

Twigs (2-3 year old)

Constituents: Glycoalkaloids (= glycosidic steroidal alkaloids; their aglycones are free alkaloids: solasodine, etc.), steroidal saponins (dulcamaric acid, etc.), tannins, bitter principles (glycosides: dulcamarin, etc.), etc.

Properties: Anti-inflammatory, diuretic, immunomodulant, astringent, anti-fungal, expectorant, antispasmodic. Glycoalkaloids and saponins account for most of the effects. Solasodine has shown cortisone-like anti-inflammatory effect. As with potato, its glycoalkaloids have shown parasympatholytic activity (belladonna-like or atropine-like effect; see BELLADONNA). Tannins are astringent and contribute to the anti-inflammatory effect.

Uses: Internally it is used (as a tea, h. p.) chiefly as an anti-inflammatory and antidyscratic (= blood purifier) for atopic eczema (= chronic eczema of internal origin) and chronic rheumatic complaints, and for inflammatory and spastic conditions of the upper respiratory tract (spastic bronchitis, bronchial asthma, etc.; coughs due to thickened bronchial secretion). Externally it is used (as a wash, poultice) for eczema and other skin inflammatory conditions.

Caution: Bittersweet should not be taken during pregnancy and lactation. At higher doses than recommended bittersweet causes gastrointestinal irritations (with nausea, vomiting), due in large part to saponins. Otherwise, there are no reports of contraindications or side effects when used properly (esp. as a standardized product).

References: (1) Vol. 6, p. 737; (3) Vol. 6b, p. 437; (6) pp. 239, 356; (8) p. 524; (12a) p. 221; (19) p. 49; (23) pp. 278, 332; (24) p. 90; (27) p. 108; (28) p. 157; (41) Vols. 1-7; (46) p. 490; (47) p. 1242; (48) p. 1063.

BLACK CHERRY

Other Common Name(s): wild black cherry, Virginian prune
Botanical Name(s): *Prunus serotina* Ehrh. [Fam.: Rosaceae]
Bark (inner bark)
Constituents: A cyanogenic glycoside (prunasin), an enzyme (prunase), organic acids (trimethoxy-benzoic acid, etc.), tannins (condensed t.), coumarins (scopoletin, etc.), etc. When bark is ground and mixed with luke-warm water, prunasin is hydrolyzed (under the action of the enzyme) liberating hydrocyanic acid (toxic!), benzaldehyde and glucose.

Properties: Aromatic, cough suppressant, antispasmodic, astringent.

Uses: Internally it is used (as a tea, h. p.) for inflammatory and spastic conditions of the upper respiratory tract (bronchitis, tracheitis, etc.; irritating dry coughs) and gastrointestinal tract (diarrhea, cramps). It is also used in flavoring syrupy medicines (incl. cough medicines). Externally it is used (as a poultice) for minor skin inflammations, (as a poultice, powder) for cuts, ulcers and wounds, and (as a gargle) for inflammations of the throat.

Caution: Black cherry should not be taken during pregnancy and lactation. Black cherry bark products should be standardized to the cyanogenic glycosides content, expressed as hydrocyanic acid. Maximum dose of hydrocyanic acid for adults is considered 0.002 gram (= 2 mg), as a single dose, and 0.006 gram (= 6 mg), as a daily dose.

References: (3) Vol. 6a, p. 950; (5) Vol. 1, p. 881; (9) p. 155; (10) p. 281; (11) p. 57; (15) p. 171; (36) p. 335; (37) pp. 218, 1136; (44) p. 443; (46) p. 1152.

BLACK COHOSH

Other Common Name(s): black bugbane, black snakeroot, rheumatism weed

Botanical Name(s): *Actaea racemosa* L. = *Cimicifuga racemosa* (L.) Nutt. [Fam.: Ranunculaceae]

Root (rhizome)

Constituents: Saponin-like triterpenoid glycosides (actein, cimicifugoside) and their free aglycones (acetylacteol, cimigenol), phenolic acids (derivatives of caffeic and hydroxycinnamic acids), quinolizidine alkaloids (cytisine, N-methylcytisine), flavonoids (an isoflavone: formononetin; etc.), resins, etc. Formononetin is not found in alcoholic extracts.

Properties: LH (= luteinizing hormone) inhibitory, anti-inflammatory, antispasmodic, peripheral vasodilatory, antihypertensive. Most of the effects are attributed to saponin-like triterpenoid glycosides. Its extracts have been shown to inhibit the production of luteinizing hormone without changing levels of FSH (= follicle-stimulating hormone). It is also claimed to exert estrogen-like effect thought to be due to formononetin. Formononetin, compared especially to coumestrol, a coumestan derivative (see: ALFALFA; KUDZU; RED CLOVER; SOY) but also genistein, an isoflavone (see: RED CLOVER; SOY), exerts a very weak estrogen-like effect, and it doesn't influence serum levels of luteinizing hormone. Cytisine and N-methylcytisine, with their nicotine-like action, are possibly involved in the effects (cf. BLUE COHOSH).

Uses: Internally it is used (as an h. p.) for menopausal syndrome (with hot flashes, sweating, tachycardia, insomnia, emotional instability, depressive mood, fatigue, decreased vaginal lubrication, etc.), premenstrual syndrome = PMS (with breast pain = mastodynia, nervousness, insomnia, emotional instability, depressive mood, fatigue, headache, pelvic discomfort, nausea, loss of appetite, dyspepsia, constipation, edema, etc.) and primary dysmenorrhea (= painful menstruation without pathology; incl. juvenile dysmenorrhea), and as an adjuvant for the prevention of postmenopausal problems (osteoporosis, high cholesterol and triglycerides, breast and uterine cancer, etc.) and prostate cancer.

Caution: Black cohosh should be used on health professional's advice (esp. in cases with breast pain = mastodynia). It should not be used during pregnancy and lactation, in children under 12 years, and in cases of estrogen receptor-positive (ER+) tumors. It should not be taken for more than 6 months. In rare cases it may cause mild stomach upset. At higher doses than recommended it causes nausea, dizziness and headache.

References: (2) Vol. 2, p. 374; (3) Vol. 4, p. 10; (6) p. 311; (7) p. 271; (8) p. 157; (9) p. 88; (12) p. 518; (13) p. 405; (14) p. 34; (16) p. 170; (19) p. 64; (20) p. 80; (22) p. 190; (23) p. 369; (31) p. 420; (41) Vols. 1-7; (46) p. 310; (47) p. 983; (48) p. 761; (59a) p. 55.

BLACK HAW

Other Common Name(s): nannybush
Botanical Name(s): *Viburnum prunifolium* L. [Fam.: Caprifoliaceae]
Bark
Constituents: Coumarins (aesculetin, scopoletin), flavonoids (a biflavone: amentoflavone), triterpenes (oleanolic and ursolic acids), tannins, phenolic acids (chlorogenic acid, etc.), phytosterols (5-sterols: β-sitosterol), bitter principles (see triterpenes), etc.
Properties: Antispasmodic (uterine active), sedative. The effects are mild. Scopoletin has shown antispasmodic and anti-inflammatory effects, among others.
Uses: Internally it is used (as a tea, h. p.) for minor uterine spastic conditions such as primary dysmenorrhea (= painful menstruation without pathology) and spastic pregnancy.
Caution: There are no reports of contraindications or side effects when used properly. Nevertheless, before using black haw, the gynecologic problem should be judged by a health professional.

References: (2) Vol. 3, p. 774; (3) Vol. 6c, p. 435; (6) p. 306; (8) p. 585; (9) p. 89; (10) p. 36; (13) p. 304; (15) p. 230; (17) p. 616; (31) p. 364; (44) p. 595; (46) p. 1761; (71) p. 240.

BLACKBERRY

Other Common Name(s): 1) blackberry; 2) dewberry
Botanical Name(s): 1) *Rubus fruticosus* L. 2) *Rubus caesius* L. [Fam.: Rosaceae]
Leaf
Constituents: Tannins (hydrolyzable t.), flavonoids (flavonols), organic acids (citric and isocitric acids), triterpenes (ursolic acid, etc.), mucilaginous polysaccharides, volatile oil (traces), etc.
Properties: Astringent, antidiarrheal.
Uses: Internally it is used (as a tea, prepared by decoction) for diarrhea and (as a tea, prepared by infusion) for minor inflammations of the gastrointestinal tract. Externally it is used (as a mouthwash, gargle) for inflammations of the mouth and throat, (as a vaginal irrigation / sitz bath / wash) for leukorrhea, (as a wash, wet compress) for skin inflammations and hemorrhoids, and (as a partial bath) for sweating feet. When fermented and then dried the leaf gains a black tea-like flavor, for which it is used as a caffeine-free substitute (prepared by infusion).
Caution: There are no reports of contraindications or side effects when used properly.
Root
Constituents: Tannins (hydrolyzable t.), organic acids, a triterpenoid saponin (villosine), etc.

Properties: Astringent, antidiarrheal.
Uses: Root is used much like leaf, but not as a black tea substitute.
Caution: See Leaf.
Note: For almost the same indications (esp. diarrhea) in traditional medicine is also used the root or root bark derived from other blackberry (*Rubus*) species such as Allegheny blackberry: *Rubus allegheniensis* Porter; smooth blackberry: *Rubus canadensis* L.; blackberry: *Rubus corchorifolius* L. f. = *R. villosus* Thunb.; cut-leaf blackberry, blackberry: *Rubus laciniatus* Willd.; etc.

References: (3) Vol. 6b, p. 188; (8) p. 494; (16) pp. 80, 148; (17) p. 509; (19) p. 56; (24) p. 101; (27) p. 295; (35) p. 108; (44) p. 486; (46) p. 964; (47) p. 2358; (52) p. 679; (57) p. 720.

BLADDERWRACK

Other Common Name(s): 1) bladderwrack, dyer's fucus, red fucus, rockwrack 2) knotted wrack, kelp
Botanical Name(s): 1) *Fucus vesiculosus* L. = *Fucus quercus marina* Gmel. 2) *Ascophyllum nodosum* Le Jol. = *Fucus scorphioides* O. F. Müller [Fam.: Fucaceae]
Bladderwrack and knotted wrack (= kelp) are rockweeds, brown algae (Class Phaeophyceae).
Constituents: Iodine (bound to proteins, in variable amounts), bromine, and other minerals (copper, zinc, arsenic, etc.), carotenoids, polysaccharides (fucoidin = a glucose polymer; alginic acid, etc.), etc.
Properties and Uses: Internally it is still used as an adjuvant for minor cases of endemic goiter (= enlargement of thyroid gland due to iodine deficiency), to control overweight, and for arteriosclerosis, among others.
Caution: Bladderwrack products should be standardized to the iodine content and used based on advice and monitored by a health professional, considering the same contraindications that apply to iodine.

References: (1) Vol. 4, p. 393, Vol. 5, p. 201; (5) Vol. 2, p. 22; (13) p. 409; (17) p. 232; (48) p. 48; (49) Vol. 1, p. 351.

BLESSED THISTLE

Other Common Name(s): holy thistle
Botanical Name(s): *Cnicus benedictus* L. = *Centaurea benedicta* (L.) L. [Fam.: Asteraceae (Compositae)]
Aerial part
Constituents: Bitter principles (sesquiterpene lactones: cnicin, etc.) and lactonic lignans, polyacetylenes, flavonoids (flavones: luteolin, etc.), volatile oil, triterpenes (oleanolic acid, etc.), etc.
Properties: Aromatic, bitter tonic, antipyretic, antimicrobial. Besides its very bitter taste, cnicin has shown antibacterial effect.

Uses: <u>Internally</u> it is used (as a tea, h. p.) for loss of appetite and nonulcer dyspepsia (with fullness, flatulence, bloating, minor cramps, change of bowel habits) and as an adjuvant for feverish states, minor fatigue, convalescence and decreased resistance to infections. Blessed thistle is also incorporated in herbal products used for chronic hepatobiliary disorders. It is also used as a flavor ingredient in some bitters. <u>Externally</u> it is used (as a wash, wet compress) for ulcers and wounds.

Caution: There are no reports of contraindications or side effects when used properly. Nevertheless, blessed thistle is best avoided during pregnancy and lactation. As with other bitter herbs, at higher doses than recommended it causes gastrointestinal irritations (with nausea, vomiting). It may cause allergic contact dermatitis to persons hypersensitive to other Asteraceae plants (e. g. arnica, chamomile, feverfew, ragweed, tansy, yarrow) that contain sesquiterpene lactones.

References: (2) Vol. 2, p. 387; (3) Vol. 4, p. 166; (6) pp. 133, 147, 150; (8) p. 175; (13) p. 165; (14) p. 126; (15) p. 70; (16) p. 135; (17) p. 158; (19) p. 42; (20) p. 160; (23) p. 63; (31) p. 608; (46) p. 253; (47) p. 824; (48) p. 621.

BLOODROOT

Other Common Name(s): red puccoon, red root
Botanical Name(s): *Sanguinaria canadensis* L. [Fam.: Papaveraceae]
Root (rhizome)
Constituents: Isoquinoline alkaloids (chiefly of benzophenanthridine type: sanguinarine, chelerythrine; also protoberberine type: berberine), etc.
Properties: Antibacterial, antifungal, anti-inflammatory, local anesthetic. The effects are due in large part to sanguinarine, but also berberine and chelerythrine contribute to the overall effect.
Uses: <u>Externally</u> it is used (as a mouthwash, toothpaste, paint) for the prevention of dental caries, for inflammations of the mouth (gingivitis, stomatitis, etc.), (as a gargle) for inflammations of the throat, (as a wash, wet compress) for wounds, and (as a paint: fresh juice) for warts (common w., plantar w.) and corns.
Caution: There are no reports of contraindications or side effects when used properly. Bloodroot should not be used internally, especially during pregnancy and lactation and in infants.

References: (2) Vol. 3, p. 497; (3) Vol. 6b, p. 265; (8) p. 508; (9) p. 92; (11) p. 161; (15) p. 187; (22) p. 230; (29) p. 103; (31) p. 218; (35) p. 115; (44) p. 515; (46) p. 1425; (47) p. 2424; (48) p. 917; (52) p. 694; (66) p. 429.

BLUE COHOSH

Botanical Name(s): *Caulophyllum thalictroides* (L.) Michx. [Fam.: Berberidaceae (Leonticaceae)]

Rhizome (with roots, papoose root)

Constituents: Quinolizidine alkaloids (N-methylcytisine = caulophylline, etc.), triterpenoid saponins (caulosaponin, etc.), resins, volatile oil (traces), etc.

Properties: Uterotonic, mild oxytocic, diuretic. Caulosaponin has shown oxytocic effect, i. e. stimulates contractions of the uterine smooth musculature and promotes rapid childbirth. Cytisine and N-methylcytisine, both present also in black cohosh (q.v.), exert nicotine-like effects (by binding to nicotinic acetylcholine receptors) and, in small amounts, may potentiate the effects of caulosaponin.

Uses: Internally (at lower doses) it is used for a hypotonic uterus and to support a pregnancy, and (at higher doses) it is used to induce labor and check postpartum hemorrhage (= hemorrhage following childbirth).

Caution: Blue cohosh should be used only as directed by a health professional. Normally, it should not be used during lactation and in cases of cardiovascular diseases and peptic ulcers.

References: (1) Vol. 4, p. 741; (3) Vol. 3, p. 776; (8) p. 129; (9) p. 93; (15) p. 54; (20) p. 82; (25) p. 206; (29) p. 24; (44) p. 144; (45) p. 73; (47) p. 863; (65) p. 406; (66) p. 212; (68) p. 32; (71) pp. 10, 22; (75) p. 139.

BLUE FLAG

Other Common Name(s): 1) larger blue flag; 2) southern blue flag

Botanical Name(s): 1) *Iris versicolor* L. 2) *Iris virginica* L. = *Iris caroliniana* Watson [Fam.: Iridaceae]

Root (rhizome)

Constituents: Volatile oil (with furfurol, etc.), a lipoid resin (containing esters of saturated alcohols with saturated fatty acids), phytosterols, polysaccharides (fructans), sucrose, tannins, etc.

Properties: Bitter tonic, cholagogue, laxative, diuretic, and (esp. when fresh) rubefacient, counterirritant.

Uses: Internally it is used (as a tea, h. p.) for inflammatory conditions of the biliary tract (chronic cholecystitis, nonobstructive gallstones) and complaints associated with them (impaired digestion, sluggish bowels, constipation, headache, nausea). It is also used as an antidyscratic (= blood purifier; tea, h. p.) for atopic eczema (= chronic eczema of internal origin) and chronic rheumatic complaints. Externally it is used (as a poultice, ointment) for rheumatic pains, bruises and sprains, and (as a wet compress, ointment) for chronic skin disorders (eczema, psoriasis), wounds and ulcers.

Caution: Blue flag should not be taken in cases of biliary obstruction. During pregnancy and in cases of nonobstructive gallstones it can be used but only on health professional's advice. At higher doses than recommended and when using the fresh root, blue flag causes gastrointestinal irritations (with nausea, vomiting, diarrhea).

References: (2) Vol. 2, p. 883; (3) Vol. 5, p. 279; (14) p. 40; (15) p. 120; (20) p. 44; (41) Vols. 1-7; (44) p. 278; (46) p. 778; (47) p. 1636; (66) p. 324.

BOG BEAN

Other Common Name(s): buck bean, marsh trefoil
Botanical Name(s): *Menyanthes trifoliata* L. [Fam.: Menyanthaceae (Gentianaceae)]
Leaf
Constituents: Bitter principles (seco-iridoids: menthiafolin, etc.), seco-iridoid alkaloids (gentialutine, etc.), flavonoids (hyperin, etc.), coumarins (scopoletin, etc.), phenolic acids (caffeic acid, etc.), triterpenes (betulinic acid, etc.), tannins, etc.
Properties: Bitter tonic, mild choleretic, liver protective, mild laxative. Iridoids have shown bitter tonic, choleretic, liver protective, laxative, diuretic, anti-inflammatory, antibacterial, antiviral, antifungal and immunomodulant effects, among others. To its hepatobiliary effects contribute also phenolic acids.
Uses: Internally it is used (as a tea, h. p.) for loss of appetite and nonulcer dyspepsia (with fullness, belching, heartburn, flatulence, minor cramps, sluggish bowels, minor constipation). It is also used for feverish states, convalescence, minor fatigue and decreased resistance to infections.
Caution: Unless advised by a health professional, bog bean should not be taken during pregnancy and lactation. At higher doses than recommended it causes gastrointestinal irritations (with nausea, vomiting, diarrhea). Otherwise, there are no reports of contraindications or side effects when used properly.

References: (2) Vol. 3, p. 211; (3) Vol. 5, p. 781; (8) p. 374; (13) p. 162; (14) p. 41; (15) p. 144; (16) p. 136; (17) p. 587; (19) p. 48; (20) p. 45; (23) p. 60; (24) p. 88; (29) p. 76; (35) p. 117; (46) p. 1635; (47) p. 1885.

BOLDO

Botanical Name(s): *Peumus boldus* Molina [Fam.: Monimiaceae]
Leaf
Constituents: Aporphine alkaloids (boldine, etc.), volatile oil (with ascaridol, p-cymene, cineole), coumarins, flavonoids (flavonols), tannins, resin, etc.
Properties: Choleretic, cholagogue, stomachic, antispasmodic, antioxidant, antimicrobial, anti-inflammatory, diuretic, anthelmintic. Its main active constituent is considered boldine, but also volatile oil and flavonoids contribute to the overall effect.
Uses: Internally it is used (as a tea, h. p.; usually combined with other herbs) for nonulcer dyspepsia (with minor cramps) associated with minor hepatobiliary disorders (impaired bile secretion and flow, nonobstructive gall

56

stones, chronic cholecystitis) and for inflammations of the lower urinary tract (cystitis).

Caution: Boldo should not be taken in cases of biliary obstruction, severe liver disorders and during pregnancy and lactation. In cases of nonobstructive gallstones, boldo can be used but only on health professional's advice. Boldo should not be taken for a prolonged period as it may lead to neurotoxic effect, due to ascaridol.

References: (3) Vol. 6a, p. 554; (6) pp. 148, 149; (7) p. 191; (9) p. 95; (12) p. 683; (13) p. 278; (15) p. 155; (16) p. 119; (17) p. 110; (19) p. 51; (20) p. 46; (22) p. 74; (23) p. 134; (28) p. 106; (46) p. 159; (47) p. 725; (48) p. 910.

BONDUC

Botanical Name(s): *Caesalpinia bonduc* (L.) Roxb. = *Caesalpinia bonducella* (L.) Fleming [Fam.: Fabaceae (Leguminosae)]
<u>Seed</u> (nikkar nut, nicker bean / seed)
Constituents: Bitter principles (diterpenoid lactones: α-, β-caesalpins, etc.), a benzopyran derivative or homoisoflavone (bonducellin), tannins, saponins, resin, phytosterols, fixed oil (unpleasant smelling), possibly alkaloids, etc.
Properties: Bitter tonic, antipyretic, antispasmodic, diuretic, and it is claimed to be aphrodisiac.
Uses: Bonduc is chiefly used in traditional medicine. <u>Internally</u> it is used (as a tea) for feverish states, spastic conditions of the upper respiratory tract (bronchial asthma) and gastrointestinal tract (colics) and for minor edemas. Roasted seed is used as an adjuvant for diabetes.
Caution: Bonduc should not be taken during pregnancy and lactation. Otherwise, there are no reports of contraindications or side effects when used properly.

References: (3) Vol. 3, p. 560; (5) Vol. 1, p. 196; (10) p. 201; (41) Vols. 1-7; (45) p. 178; (52) p. 137; (57) p. 135.

BONESET

Other Common Name(s): thoroughwort
Botanical Name(s): *Eupatorium perfoliatum* L. [Fam.: Asteraceae (Compositae)]
<u>Aerial part</u> (leaf and flowering top)
Constituents: Bitter principles (sesquiterpene lactones: euperfolide, etc.), water-soluble polysaccharides, flavonoids (eupatorin, astragalin, etc.), hydrocarbons (dotriacontane, etc.), diterpenes, triterpenes, phytosterols, etc.
Properties: Bitter tonic, antipyretic, choleretic, cholagogue, laxative, immunomodulant. The effects are mild. The immunomodulant effect is due to water-soluble polysaccharides and is possibly enhanced by bitter principles (sesquiterpene lactones, diterpenes).

Uses: Internally it is used (as a tea, h. p.) for loss of appetite and nonulcer dyspepsia (with sluggish bowels), inflammations of the upper respiratory tract (bronchitis, etc.; also as a diaphoretic hot tea for the common cold and feverish states) and to enhance resistance to viral and bacterial infections.

Caution: Boneset should not be taken during pregnancy and lactation. At higher doses than recommended it causes gastrointestinal irritations (with nausea, vomiting, diarrhea). It may cause allergic contact dermatitis to persons hypersensitive to other Asteraceae plants (e. g. arnica, chamomile, feverfew, ragweed, tansy, yarrow) that contain sesquiterpene lactones. There are no reports that it contains unsaturated pyrrolizidine alkaloids (= UPAs). Nevertheless, as there are reports on their presence in Heliantheae tribe (boneset is included here), manufacturers should evaluate them. For dosage limits of UPAs see COLTSFOOT.

References: (6) p. 262; (8) p. 257; (9) p. 96; (10) p. 40; (13) p. 554; (15) p. 86; (20) p. 48; (46) p. 568; (47) p. 1315; (66) p. 277.

BORAGE

Botanical Name(s): *Borago officinalis* L. [Fam.: Boraginaceae]
Borage oil
It is the fixed oil obtained from the seeds.

Constituents: Chiefly glycerides, with fatty acids component high proportions of linoleic acid and gamma-linolenic acid (= GLA), which are omega-6 fatty acids, and oleic acid.

Properties and Uses: See EVENING PRIMROSE

Caution: See EVENING PRIMROSE. Normally, the UPAs are found in far below the accepted limits. As in rare cases they have been found in concentrations enough to be toxic, manufacturers should evaluate them. For dosage limits of UPAs see COLTSFOOT.

Aerial part
Constituents: Mucilaginous polysaccharides (rich), tannins, minerals (silicic acid, etc.), unsaturated pyrrolizidine alkaloids (= UPAs: amabiline, etc.; hepatotoxic and carcinogenic!), saturated pyrrolizidine alkaloids (thesinine, etc.; non-toxic), saponins, etc.

Properties: Emollient, anti-inflammatory, astringent. The emollient effect is due to mucilaginous polysaccharides. The anti-inflammatory and astringent effects are due in large part to tannins.

Uses: Externally it is used (as a wet compress, poultice, h. p.) for skin inflammations.

Caution: Due to its serious side effects (hepatotoxic, carcinogenic) internal use is no longer recommended. In borage products, the UPAs content should be within limits. For dosage limits of UPAs see COLTSFOOT.

References: (1) Vol. 4, p. 528; (3) Vol. 3, p. 489; (5) Vol. 1, p. 173; (8) p. 102; (9) p. 98; (19) p. 52; (20) p. 49; (22) p. 194; (24) p. 97; (27) p. 57; (29) p. 20; (35) p. 119; (48) p. 157.

BROOKLIME

Other Common Name(s): European brooklime
Botanical Name(s): *Veronica beccabunga* L. [Fam.: Scrophulariaceae]
Aerial part
Constituents: Bitter principles (iridoids: aucubin, etc.), phenolic acids (caffeic acid, etc.), phytosterols (5-sterols: β-sitosterol, etc.), hydrocarbons (n-triacontane, etc.), tannins, etc.
Properties: Bitter tonic, diuretic, laxative. The effects are mild and due in large part to iridoids and phenolic acids.
Uses: <u>Internally</u> it is used (as a tea, h. p.; usually combined with other herbs) for loss of appetite and nonulcer dyspepsia (with sluggish bowels, minor constipation), inflammations of the upper respiratory and genitourinary tracts, and as an antidyscratic (= blood purifier; salad, fresh juice, tea, h. p.) for atopic eczema (= chronic eczema of internal origin). Dried herb is an ingredient in herbal tea blends.
Caution: There are no reports of contraindications or side effects when used properly.

References: (1) Vol. 6, p. 1117; (3) Vol. 6c, p. 431; (5) Vol. 1, p. 1125; (10) p. 42; (35) p. 123; (37) p. 1446; (47) p. 2805.

BRYONY

Other Common Name(s): 1) white bryony; 2) red bryony
Botanical Name(s): 1) *Bryonia alba* L. 2) *Bryonia cretica* L. ssp. *dioica* (Jacq.) Tutin = *Bryonia dioica* Jacq. [Fam.: Cucurbitaceae]
Root
Constituents: Bitter principles (triterpenes: cucurbitacins and derivatives), phytosterols, fatty acids, resin (bryoresin), a triterpene (bryonolic acid), etc. Red bryony is much richer in cucurbitacins than white bryony.
Properties: Strong purgative, diuretic, counterirritant.
Uses: <u>Internally</u> it is used (as a tea, h. p.; only combined with other herbs) mainly for constipation, also as an antidyscratic (= blood purifier) for chronic rheumatic complaints. <u>Externally</u> it is used (as an ointment, etc.: mainly combined with other herbs) for bruises and rheumatic pains.
Caution: Bryony is toxic due in large part to cucurbitacins. It should not be taken during pregnancy and lactation. At higher doses than recommended it causes gastrointestinal irritations (with nausea, vomiting, heavy diarrhea) and genitourinary tract (with kidney damage), among others.

References: (1) Vol. 4, p. 568; (3) Vol. 3, p. 523; (8) p. 108; (13) p. 403; (24) p. 364; (27) p. 60; (28) p. 120; (37) p. 240; (46) p. 165; (47) p. 733; (48) p. 760.

BUCHU

Other Common Name(s): short buchu, round buchu
Botanical Name(s): *Agathosma betulina* (P.J. Bergius) Pillans = *Barosma betulina* (Bergius) Bartl. et H.L. Wendl. [Fam.: Rutaceae]
Leaf
Constituents: Volatile oil (with diosphenol, pseudo-diosphenol, some terpinen-4-ol, pulegone, etc.), flavonoids (diosmin, rutin), mucilaginous polysaccharides, resin, etc.
Properties: Antimicrobial, diuretic. Diosphenol has shown urinary antiseptic effect, while terpinen-4-ol is a strong diuretic. Both diosmin and rutin exert "vitamin P"-like effect (= help in normalizing an increased microvascular permeability and fragility).
Uses: Internally it is used (as a tea, h. p.) for inflammations of the genitourinary tract (cystitis, cystopyelitis, urethritis, prostatitis). To enhance the effects in problems of the genitourinary tract, the fluid intake (incl. herbal teas) should be more than 2 liters per day.
Caution: There are no reports of contraindications or side effects when used properly. Nevertheless, buchu is best avoided during pregnancy and lactation. At higher doses than recommended it may cause gastrointestinal and renal irritations.
Note: Oval buchu: *Agathosma crenulata* (L.) Pillans = *Barosma crenulata* (L.) Hook, and long buchu: *Agathosma serratifolia* (Curtis) Spreeth = *Barosma serratifolia* (Curtis) Willd. contain much smaller amounts of diosphenol or do not contain it at all.

References: (1) Vol. 4, p. 467; (1) Vol. 3, p. 369; (8) p. 96; (9) p. 104; (13) p. 402; (14) p. 43; (15) p. 15; (17) p. 101; (19) p. 58; (20) p. 51; (36) p. 272; (37) p. 181; (46) p. 167; (47) p. 741; (48) p. 562.

BUCKTHORN

Other Common Name(s): purging buckthorn
Botanical Name(s): *Rhamnus cathartica* L. [Fam.: Rhamnaceae]
Fruit (ripe berry)
Constituents: Anthranoids (glycosides: glucofrangulins, frangulins; free anthraquinones: frangula-emodin, etc.), flavonoids (flavonols: rhamnetin, rhamnetin glycosides, etc.), pectin, tannins, etc.
Properties: Laxative (large intestine stimulant laxative). See SENNA.
Uses: Internally it is used (as a tea, h. p.) for constipation (atonic, non-spastic) and when softer stools or easier defecation is sought such as in cases of hemorrhoids and after surgeries (anorectal, abdominal region in general).
Caution: See SENNA.

References: (1) Vol. 6, p. 393; (3) Vol. 6b, p. 89; (12) p. 909; (13) p. 297; (19) p. 133; (23) p. 106; (36) p. 242; (37) p. 1182; (46) p. 1522; (47) p. 2295; (48) p. 439.

BUCKWHEAT

Botanical Name(s): *Fagopyrum esculentum* Moench = *Polygonum fagopyrum* L. [Fam.: Polygonaceae]

Aerial part

Constituents: Flavonoids (flavonols: chiefly rutin = quercetin-3-rutinoside; chiefly in leaves and flowers), phenolic acids, small amounts of naphthodianthrones (fagopyrin, etc.; chiefly in flowers, esp. when young).

Properties: Rutin exerts "vitamin P"-like effect (= helps in normalizing an increased microvascular permeability and fragility; P = permeability). As with many other flavonoids, rutin and quercetin are antioxidants.

Uses: Buckwheat is chiefly used as a natural source in the production of rutin. Internally it is used (as a standardized product to rutin content, isolated rutin) for the prevention and treatment of capillary hemorrhages, vascular retinopathy, as an adjuvant for allergic and infectious conditions, and as an antioxidant. Buckwheat is often combined with vitamin C and / or rose hips.

Caution: There are no reports of contraindications or side effects for rutin. When using ground buckwheat, it should be considered that it may contain fagopyrin, particularly if the flowering plant (esp. with young flowers) and not only the leaves have been ground. Fagopyrin is a photosensitizer, like hypericin found in St. John's wort (q. v.).

References: (1) Vol. 5, p. 137; (3) Vol. 4, p. 915; (6) p. 376; (9) p. 453; (12) p. 843; (13) p. 319; (19) p. 59; (37) p. 513; (48) p. 328.

BUGLEWEED

Other Common Name(s): 1) Virginia bugleweed 2) European bugleweed, gipsywort, water horehound

Botanical Name(s): 1) *Lycopus virginicus* L. 2) *Lycopus europaeus* L. [Fam.: Lamiaceae (Labiatae)]

Aerial part

Constituents: Phenolic acids (ester-like derivatives of caffeic and hydroxycinnamic acids: lithospermic acid, etc.), flavonoids (flavones, methoxyflavones, flavonols), minerals (Zn, Mn, F), coumarins, phytosterols, etc.

Properties: Antithyrotropic. It also lowers prolactin level, when this is elevated. The effects are chiefly attributed to lithospermic acid.

Uses: Internally it is used (as a standardized product) chiefly for minor cases of hyperthyroidism (= Basedow's disease) and complaints associated with it (nervousness, insomnia, tachycardia, weakness, hyperhidrosis, etc.) and for mastodynia (= breast pain).

Caution: It should be used only standardized products and as directed by a health professional. It should not be taken in cases of hypothyroidism and should not be combined with sedative-hypnotic drugs. A possible combination with herbal sedatives should be made only by a health professsional. At higher doses and when taken for a prolonged period, it may lead to goiter, and a prompt discontinuation of this medication may worsen the condition.

References: (2) Vol. 3, pp. 132, 141; (3) Vol. 5, p. 608; (6) p. 214; (8) p. 348; (13) p. 418; (19) p. 247; (22) p. 196; (23) pp. 150, 368; (37) p. 846; (47) p. 1807.

BUPLEURUM

Other Common Name(s): Chinese thoroughwax
Botanical Name(s): *Bupleurum chinense* DC.; *Bupleurum scorzonerifolium* Willd. = *Bupleurum falcatum* L. var. *scorzonerifolium* (Willd.) Ledeb. [Fam.: Apiaceae (Umbelliferae)]

<u>Root</u>
Constituents: Triterpenoid saponins (saikosaponins A, D, etc.), lignans, polyacetylenes (saikodiynes), polysaccharides (bupleurans), chromones (saikochromone, etc.), phytosterols (7-sterols: α-spinasterol; 5-sterols: stigmasterol), volatile oil, etc.
Properties: Anti-inflammatory (corticosteroid-like effect, much like licorice; cf. LICORICE), analgesic, antipyretic, immunomodulant, liver protective, cholesterol reducing, antiulcer (= prevents or helps in healing peptic ulcers), sedative, antiepileptic. Bupleurum has been shown to increase levels of cAMP (= cyclic adenosine monophosphate) and to help in normalizing plasma levels of transaminases (GOT and GPT). Saikosaponins have shown anti-inflammatory, antiviral, liver protective, sedative and antitumoral effects, among others. Bupleurans have shown immunomodulant and antiulcer effects. Many lignans have shown liver protective, immunomodulant, anti-inflammatory and antiviral effects, while many polyacetylenes have shown antibacterial effect.
Uses: <u>Internally</u> it is used (as a tea, h. p.) for inflammations of the liver (chronic hepatitis), kidneys (chronic nephritis) and upper respiratory tract (influenza, the common cold, bronchitis, etc.), PMS (= premenstrual syndrome), primary dysmenorrhea (= painful menstruation without pathology), secondary amenorrhea and oligomenorrhea (= ceased / infrequent / scanty menstruation without pathology), a hypotonic uterus, auditory disorders (impaired hearing, vertigo = a type of dizziness) and for minor cases of nervous tension and decreased concentration associated with fatigue.
Caution: Unless advised by a health professional, bupleurum should not be taken during pregnancy and lactation. Before using it for dysmenorrhea or other gynecologic disorders, the problem should be judged by a health professional. At higher doses than recommended it may cause drowsiness and gastrointestinal discomfort. Alcoholic drinks may interact with bupleurum. A possible combination of bupleurum with sedative, hypnotic and antidepressant drugs should be made only by a health professional. Otherwise, there are no reports of contraindications or side effects when used properly.

References: (1) Vol. 4, p. 580; (3) Vol. 3, p. 534; (12) p. 535; (13) pp. 217, 428; (29) p. 22; (31) pp. 46, 435; (36) p. 437; (41) Vols. 1-7; (48) p. 682; (59) p. 67; (71) p. 262; (77) p. 159.

BURDOCK

Other Common Name(s): 1) great burdock 2) lesser burdock, common burdock
Botanical Name(s): 1) *Arctium lappa* L. 2) *Arctium minus* Bernh. [Fam.: Asteraceae (Compositae)]
Root
Constituents: Volatile oil, polyacetylenes, thiophenes, phenolic acids (caffeic and chlorogenic acids, etc.), lignans, sesquiterpene lactones, triterpenes, phytosterols, inulin, mucilaginous polysaccharides, etc.
Properties: Diuretic, mild choleretic, antimicrobial, wound-healing.
Uses: Internally it is used (as a tea, h. p.; usually combined with other herbs) as an antidyscratic (= blood purifier) for atopic eczema (= chronic eczema of internal origin) and chronic rheumatic complaints, and for minor inflammations of the genitourinary, gastrointestinal and hepatobiliary tracts. Externally it is used (as a wash, wet compress) for chronic skin disorders (eczema, psoriasis, dandruff), and (as a poultice) for boils.
Caution: Burdock may contain allergenic sesquiterpene lactones (e. g. dehydrocostuslactone, with a methylene group in the lactone ring) therefore it may cause allergic contact dermatitis to persons hypersensitive to other Asteraceae plants (e. g. arnica, chamomile, feverfew, ragweed, tansy, yarrow) that contain them. Otherwise, there are no reports of contraindications or side effects when used properly.

References: (2) Vol. 2, p. 141; (3) Vol. 3, p. 173; (8) p. 65; (9) p. 107; (14) p. 48; (17) p. 98; (20) p. 52; (23) p. 276; (24) p. 193; (27) p. 48; (28) p. 160; (35) p. 143; (46) p. 129; (47) p. 570; (48) p. 172.

BURNET

Other Common Name(s): 1) great burnet, sanguisorba 2) salad burnet, garden burnet
Botanical Name(s): 1) *Sanguisorba officinalis* L. 2) *Sanguisorba minor* Scop. = *Poterium sanguisorba* L. [Fam.: Rosaceae]
Aerial part, root
Constituents: Tannins (hydrolyzable and condensed t.; root is richer), triterpenes (ursolic acid, etc.), triterpenoid saponins, phenolic acids (aerial part: caffeic acid derivatives), flavonoids (aerial part: flavonols), etc.
Properties: Astringent, anti-inflammatory, antimicrobial.
Uses: Internally it is used (as a tea, h. p.) for inflammation of the gastrointestinal tract (diarrhea, ulcerative colitis, incl. hemorrhoids; also when minor hemorrhages are present, but on professional's advice). Externally it is used (as a mouthwash, gargle) for inflammations of the mouth and throat, and (as

a wash, wet compress) for minor skin inflammations, eczemas, local bleedings, wounds, burns and hemorrhoids.

Caution: At higher doses than recommended and when taking strong teas, it may cause gastrointestinal irritations (with nausea, vomiting). Otherwise, there are no reports of contraindications or side effects when used properly.

References: (1) Vol. 6, pp. 587, 589; (3) Vol. 6b, p. 270; (5) Vol. 1, p. 966; (9) p. 535; (10) p. 50; (15) p. 188; (20) p. 54; (24) p. 353; (47) p. 2428.

BURNET, THORN

Botanical Name(s): *Poterium spinosum* L. = *Sarcopoterium spinosum* (L.) Spach [Fam.: Rosaceae]
Root bark
Constituents: Triterpenoid pseudosapogenins (tormentillic acid, etc.) and pseudosaponins (tormentoside = diglucoside of tormentillic acid, etc.), tannins (OPCs = oligomeric proanthocyanidins; hydrolyzable tannins), etc.
Properties: Mild antihyperglycemic (chiefly due to triterpenoids), astringent (due to tannins).
Uses: Internally it is used as an adjuvant (tea, h. p.) for diabetes. Externally it is used (as a mouthwash) for inflammations of the mouth.
Caution: There are no reports of contraindications or side effects when used properly.

References: (1) Vol. 6, p. 607; (3) Vol. 6a, p. 848; (8) p. 460; (18) p. 170; (23) p. 142.

BUTCHER'S BROOM

Other Common Name(s): box holly
Botanical Name(s): *Ruscus aculeatus* L. [Fam.: Liliaceae]
Root (rhizome)
Constituents: Steroidal saponins (ruscin, ruscoside, etc., with aglycones ruscogenin and neo-ruscogenin), glycolic acid, sucrose, resin, etc.
Properties: Vasotonic (esp. venotonic), antiexudative, anti-inflammatory, topical vasoconstrictor, diuretic. The mentioned effects are due in large part to steroidal saponins.
Uses: Internally it is used (as a standardized product to steroidal saponins expressed as ruscogenins: capsule, tablet, suppository) for peripheral venous disorders (varicose veins in the legs, hemorrhoids, etc.), postthrombotic syndrome, and (as a tea, h. p.) for minor inflammations of the genitourinary tract. To enhance the effects in problems of the genitourinary tract, the fluid intake (incl. herbal teas) should be more than 2 liters per day. Externally it is used (as an ointment, applied mainly in combination with suppositories) for hemorrhoids.
Caution: In rare cases it may cause gastrointestinal irritations (with nausea,

etc.). Otherwise, there are no reports of contraindications or side effects when used properly.

References: (3) Vol. 6b, p. 200; (5) Vol. 1, p. 257; (6) p. 77; (8) p. 497; (10) p. 52; (12a) p. 688; (16) p. 114; (19) p. 146; (22) p. 149; (23) p. 111; (27) p. 274; (35) p. 128; (37) p. 1205; (48) p. 697.

BUTTERBUR, PURPLE

Other Common Name(s): petasites, sweet coltsfoot
Botanical Name(s): *Petasites hybridus* (L.) P. Gaertn. et al. = *Petasites officinalis* Moench [Fam.: Asteraceae (Compositae)]
Leaf, **root** (rhizome)
Constituents: Sesquiterpenes (petasins: petasin, neopetasin, isopetasin, etc.; root is much richer), mucilaginous polysaccharides, flavonoids (leaf), unsaturated pyrrolizidine alkaloids (= UPAs; leaf: in traces or absent; root: in different amounts, depending on origin), volatile oil, minerals, etc.
Properties: Antispasmodic and antiallergic (by inhibiting the biosynthesis of leukotrienes), demulcent, emollient, mild antihypertensive. The antispasmodic, anti-inflammatory and antihypertensive effects are due in large part to petasins. The demulcent and emollient effects are due to mucilage.
Uses: Internally it is used (as a standardized extract) for spastic, allergic and inflammatory conditions of the upper respiratory tract (spastic bronchitis, bronchial asthma, allergic rhinitis, laryngitis with hoarseness; spastic dry coughs), spastic conditions of the genitourinary tract (gravel, nonobstructive urinary stones), primary dysmenorrhea (= painful menstruation without pathology), biliary tract (nonobstructive gallstones) and gastrointestinal tract (peptic ulcers, etc.; it may be helpful for irritable bowel syndrome), and minor hypertension and headaches especially when they are associated with nervous tension. Externally it is used (leaf: as a poultice, wet compress) for minor wounds and ulcers.
Caution: Purple butterbur should not be taken during pregnancy and lactation and before using it for dysmenorrhea the gynecologic problem should be judged by a health professional. Its products should be standardized to petasins and the content of UPAs (hepatotoxic and carcinogenic!) should be within limits. For dosage limits of UPAs see COLTSFOOT.

References: (1) Vol. 6, p. 83; (3) Vol. 6a, p. 535; (6) p. 190; (7) p. 248; (8) p. 415; (12) p. 477; (13) p. 420; (17) p. 428; (19) p. 174; (23) p. 224; (27) p. 126; (46) p. 1091; (47) p. 2084; (48) p. 845.

BUTTERNUT

Other Common Name(s): white walnut
Botanical Name(s): *Juglans cinerea* L. [Fam.: Juglandaceae]
Bark (inner bark)
Constituents: Naphthoquinones (juglone, etc.), fixed oil, volatile oil, tannins (hydrolyzable t.), resin, etc.

Properties: (At low doses): Bitter tonic, cholagogue, antimicrobial, anti-fungal. (At high doses): Pungent bitter, laxative, anthelmintic. Applied externally it is rubefacient. Juglone is considered its main active constituent but also tannins contribute to the overall effect.

Uses: Internally it is used (as a tea, h. p.; at low doses) for nonulcer dyspepsia associated with minor hepatobiliary disorders (impaired bile secretion and flow), for diarrhea, and (as a tea, h. p.; at high doses) for constipation and intestinal worms. Externally it is used (as a wash, wet compress) for minor skin inflammations, eczema, wounds, ulcers and hemorrhoids, and (as a poultice) for bruises, sprains, and rheumatic pains (incl. arthritic pains).

Caution: Unless advised by a health professional, laxative doses should be avoided during pregnancy. At higher doses than recommended it may cause gastrointestinal irritations (with nausea, vomiting, diarrhea).

References: (3) Vol. 5, p. 330; (5) Vol. 1, p. 620; (10) p. 53; (29) p. 65; (35) p. 150; (36) pp. 436, 476; (37) p. 740; (42) Vol. 4, pp. 281, 283; (44) p. 279; (47) p. 1659; (52) p. 409; (58) pp. 50, 147, 171; (65) p. 180; (66) p. 325.

BUTTERWORT

Other Common Name(s): bog violet
Botanical Name(s): *Pinguicula vulgaris* L. [Fam.: Lentibulariaceae]
Aerial part
Constituents: A phenylpropanoid acid (*trans*-cinnamic acid), bitter principles (iridoids: globularin, etc.), flavonoids (isoscutellarein glycosides, etc.), minerals, volatile oil (traces), etc.

Properties: Antispasmodic (esp. bronchial active). Trans-cinnamic acid has shown antispasmodic effect. Iridoids have shown bitter tonic, choleretic, liver protective, anti-inflammatory, antimicrobial and immunomodulant effects, among others.

Uses: Internally it is used (as a tea, h. p.) for minor inflammatory and spastic conditions of the upper respiratory tract (spastic bronchitis, laryngitis with hoarseness, coughs: spastic dry cough, whooping cough), similarly to sundew with which is also combined in herbal products. See SUNDEW.

Caution: There are no reports of contraindications or side effects when used properly.

References: (1) Vol. 6, p. 157; (3) Vol. 6a, p. 676; (5) Vol. 1, p. 838; (6) p. 107; (12) p. 438; (24) p. 136; (31) pp. 476, 569.

CABBAGE

Other Common Name(s): white cabbage
Botanical Name(s): *Brassica oleracea* L. var. *capitata* f. alba [Fam.: Brassicaceae (Cruciferae)]
Leaf (fresh)

Constituents: Glucosinolates (glucobrassicin = 3-indolylmethyl-glucosinolate etc.; mainly in the intact fresh material), non-protein amino acids (methyl-methionine, etc.), vitamins (A, B complex, C), enzymes, etc.

Properties: Fresh cabbage juice has been shown to shorten the healing time of ulcers. Methyl-methionine is considered an antiulcer factor (vitamin U). Fresh cabbage is also mild rubefacient, antibacterial, and antioxidant. When the fresh material is crushed or processed, glucobrassicin (under the action of enzymes) liberates isothiocyanates (chiefly the non-volatile 3-indolylmethyl-isothiocyanate), which are responsible for the mild pungent flavor and the mentioned effects. See CRESS, GARDEN; MUSTARD.

Uses: Internally it is used (fresh cabbage juice) for inflammatory and ulcerative conditions of the gastrointestinal tract and inflammations of the upper respiratory tract. Externally it is used (as a poultice) for minor infected wounds, ulcers (incl. varicose ulcers), boils, common acne (= acne vulgaris), minor muscular pains.

Caution: Fresh cabbage juice should not be taken in cases of renal failure. Isothiocyanates have been shown to cause goiter. In view of this, a consumption of raw cabbage in excessive amounts and for prolonged periods without breaks should be avoided.

References: (1) Vol. 4, p. 551; (3) Vol. 3, p. 505; (8) p. 106; (13a) p. 107; (27) p. 83; (37) p. 232.

CACAO

Other Common Name(s): cocoa, chocolate tree
Botanical Name(s): *Theobroma cacao* L. [Fam.: Sterculiaceae]
Cacao butter (cocoa butter, theobroma oil)
It is the fixed oil obtained by expressing the roasted seeds.
Constituents: Chiefly glycerides (fatty acids component: oleic, stearic and palmitic acids), small amounts of free fatty acids, phytosterols, etc.
Properties: Emollient.
Uses: Externally it is used as an ingredient in ointments, creams, liniments, lipsticks, soaps, and other skin care and cosmetic products. It has been used as a fatty excipient of suppositories but today it is replaced by semisynthetic equivalents. Cacao butter is an important ingredient in chocolate.
Caution: There are no reports of contraindications or side effects even when taken internally (orally, rectally) if the products are prepared with well-stored cocoa butter.
Prepared cacao (= breakfast cocoa)
It is the powdered residue after expressing cacao butter from the cured, dried, then roasted seeds.
Constituents: Fixed oil (cacao butter), phytosterols, purine alkaloids (chiefly theobromine, also caffeine), starch, sugars, proteins, tannins (oligomeric and polymeric proanthocyanidins), flavonoids (catechins, flavonols), etc.
Properties: Nutrient due in large part to lipids, diuretic due in large part to

theobromine, mild stimulant of the cardiovascular and central nervous systems due in large part to caffeine, and antioxidant due to catechins and proanthocyanidins. Theobromine is a mild diuretic and smooth muscle relaxant, and a weak CNS stimulant. See also COFFEE.

Uses: Breakfast cocoa is consumed (as a beverage, chocolate, etc.) for its nutrient and mild stimulant effects, and it is beneficial also due to its antioxidant effect.

Caution: In rare cases it may cause allergic reactions.

References: (1) Vol. 6, p. 943; (3) Vol. 6c, p. 89; (9) p. 181; (11) p. 74; (12) pp. 251, 1073; (13) pp. 268, 390; (36) p. 402; (37) p. 1364; (48) p. 1080; (49) Vol. 2, p. 259.

CADE JUNIPER

Other Common Name(s): cade, prickly juniper, red juniper
Botanical Name(s): *Juniperus oxycedrus* L. [Fam.: Cupressaceae]
Cade oil (= juniper tar)
It is obtained by destructive distillation (without access of air) from woody portions and branches of cade.

Constituents: Chiefly sesquiterpenes (high boiling point bicyclic hydrocarbons: δ-cadinene, etc.), also phenols (guaiacol = 2-methoxyphenol, ethyl guaiacol, cresol = 4-methylphenol).

Properties: Antimicrobial, keratolytic, antipruritic, anti-eczematous, antiparasitic (against *Sarcoptes scabiei*).

Uses: Externally it is used (as an ointment, liniment, medicinal soap, shampoo) for eczema, psoriasis, lichen planus (= a skin itching condition) and scabies (= the itch), also in veterinary practice.

Caution: There are reports that cade oil has caused contact dermatitis. Some constituents of cade oil have shown carcinogenic effect therefore it should be used only for short periods.

References: (1) Vol. 5, p. 579; (3) Vol. 5, p. 340; (4) Vol. 1, p. 1572; (5) Vol. 2, p. 203; (9) p. 109; (36) p. 270; (37) p. 741; (48) p. 585; (49) Vol. 1, p. 386.

CAJUPUT

Other Common Name(s): cajeput, river tea tree, weeping tea tree
Botanical Name(s): *Melaleuca cajuputi* Powell; *Melaleuca leucadendra* L.; and some other *Melaleuca* spp. [Fam.: Myrtaceae]
Cajeput oil (oil of cajuput)
It is distilled from fresh leaves and twigs, then rectified for medicinal purposes.

Constituents: Chiefly 1,8-cineole (= eucalyptol = cajeputol), also pinene, terpineol, etc.

Properties: Antimicrobial, rubefacient and analgesic, expectorant, anthelmintic, insect-repellent.

68

Uses: Externally it is used (as an ointment, liniment) for inflammations of the upper respiratory tract (bronchitis, tracheitis, etc.; coughs due to thickened bronchial secretion), rheumatic pains, neuralgic pains, headaches, abdominal pains, minor skin inflammations, itching, common acne (= acne vulgaris), (as a cotton swab) for toothache, and (as eardrops) for earache. Internally it is used (as an inhalation, in capsules: the rectified oil) for inflammations of the upper respiratory tract (bronchitis, tracheitis, etc.; coughs due to thickened bronchial secretion). In traditional medicine it is also used for intestinal worms and as an insect-repellent.

Caution: See EUCALYPTUS. Internally should be used only the rectified oil.

References: (2) Vol. 3, p. 187; (3) Vol. 5, p. 749; (5) Vol. 1, p. 698; (8) p. 361; (36) p. 278; (37) p. 874; (48) p. 560; (49) Vol. 2, p. 446; (66) p. 192.

CALAMINT

Other Common Name(s): lesser calamint
Botanical Name(s): *Calamintha nepeta* (L.) Savi = *Calamintha officinalis* Moench = *Satureja calamintha* (L.) Scheele [Fam.: Lamiaceae (Labiatae)]
Aerial part
Constituents: Volatile oil (with aryl-ketones: piperitone epoxide, pulegone, etc.; depending on chemotype), bitter principles (a flavanone: poncirin; ursolic acid), triterpenes (calaminthadiol, ursolic acid, etc.), etc.
Properties: Aromatic, bitter tonic, carminative, antispasmodic, diuretic.
Uses: Internally it is used (as a tea, h. p.) for loss of appetite and nonulcer dyspepsia (with bloating, flatulence, minor cramps) and as a diaphoretic hot tea for the common cold and feverish states. It is sometimes used as a spice.
Caution: There are no reports of contraindications or side effects when used properly. Nevertheless, manufacturers should evaluate pulegone content in its volatile oil as it has shown hepatotoxic effect.

References: (1) Vol. 4, p. 595; (3) Vol. 3, p. 563; (35) p. 152; (48) p. 527.

CALAMUS

Other Common Name(s): acorus, sweet calamus, sweetflag
Botanical Name(s): *Acorus calamus* L. [Fam.: Acoraceae (Araceae)]
Root (rhizome)
Constituents: Volatile oil, mucilaginous polysaccharides, starch, tannins, sugars, a biogenic amine (choline), etc. Depending on chemotype, volatile oil contains as its chief constituent a phenylpropanoid, namely β-asarone = cis-isoasarone (higher concentration in the South Asian variety, lower in the European variety, almost not present in the American variety). Volatile oil of the American variety contains sesquiterpenes (acorone, etc.) as its main

69

constituents, instead of β-asarone.

Properties: Aromatic, bitter tonic, demulcent, antispasmodic, carminative, astringent, mild neurocirculatory stimulant. The bitter tonic, antispasmodic and carminative effects are attributed to the essential oil. Calamus is demulcent due to mucilaginous polysaccharides and astringent due to tannins.

Uses: Internally it is used (as a tea, h. p.) for inflammatory and spastic conditions of the gastrointestinal tract (loss of appetite, gastritis, impaired digestion, stomachache, flatulence, intestinal cramps, minor diarrhea) and upper respiratory tract (laryngitis, spastic bronchitis, the common cold, feverish states, etc.; spastic dry coughs). Calamus is also used for minor cases of hypotension (= low blood pressure), fatigue and convalescence. Externally it is used (as a mouthwash, gargle) for inflammations of the mouth and throat, (as a cotton swab or pasty mass applied to the tooth, or by chewing the herb) for toothache, and (as a liniment) for neuralgic and rheumatic pains and neurocirculatory (= nervous and circulatory systems) weakness.

Caution: β-Asarone has shown mutagenic and carcinogenic effects, but only in animal tests. This risk, if it exists for humans, doesn't apply to the American variety: *Acorus calamus* L. var. *americanus* (Raf.) Wulff. = *Acorus calamus* Raf. Calamus root can be used only if it contains less than 0.3 % β-asarone, and therefore the American variety should be preferred. Nevertheless, manufacturers should evaluate the β-asarone content. Calamus is best avoided during pregnancy.

References: (2) Vol. 2, p. 18; (3) Vol. 2, p. 1082; (6) pp. 128, 290; (8) p. 23; (12) p. 66; (13) p. 145; (15) p. 13; (17) p. 116; (19) p. 119; (23) p. 324; (36) p. 275; (37) p. 17; (44) p. 46; (47) p. 770; (48) p. 571; (66) p. 192.

CALENDULA

Other Common Name(s): marigold, pot marigold
Botanical Name(s): *Calendula officinalis* L. [Fam.: Asteraceae (Compositae)]
Flower (ligulate florets)
Constituents: Triterpenes (saponins, alcohols and their esters), carotenoids (rich), water-soluble polysaccharides, flavonoids, coumarins, phytosterols, volatile oil, etc.

Properties: Anti-inflammatory, antiedematous, antibacterial, antifungal, wound-healing, immunomodulant. Its anti-inflammatory and antiedematous effects are due in large part to triterpenes and flavonoids. The wound-healing effect is due in large part to carotenoids and flavonoids. The immunomodulant effect is due to water-soluble polysaccharides.

Uses: Externally it is used (as a lotion, ointment, wet compress, wash) for skin inflammations (incl. eczema), boils, wounds, ulcers (incl. varicose ulcers = ulcus cruris, decubitus ulcers), bruises, sprains, and hemorrhoids, and (as a mouthwash, gargle) for inflammations of the mouth and throat. Calendula is an ingredient in a number of cosmetic products. Internally it is used (usually as a combination h. p.) for inflammations of the gastrointestinal tract.

Caution: There are no reports of contraindications or side effects when used properly. Calendula doesn't seem to contain the allergenic sesquiterpene lactones (see Constituents).

References: (1) Vol. 4, p. 601; (3) Vol. 3, p. 603; (6) pp. 270, 336, 339; (7) p. 288; (8) p. 109; (9) p. 113; (16) p. 34; (17) p. 119; (19) p. 189; (20) p. 58; (22) p. 219; (23) p. 348; (28) pp. 172, 200; (46) p. 185; (47) p. 778; (48) p. 705; (74) p. 353.

CALUMBA

Other Common Name(s): colombo
Botanical Name(s): *Jateorhiza palmata* (Lam.) Miers [Fam.: Menispermaceae]
Root
Constituents: Benzyl-isoquinoline alkaloids (jatrorrhizine, palmatine, columbamine), bitter diterpenes (columbin, etc.), mucilaginous polysaccharides, starch, etc., but no tannins.
Properties: Bitter tonic. The isolated alkaloids have also shown analgesic, antibacterial, antifungal and antiprotozoal effects.
Uses: Internally it is used (as a tea, h. p.) for loss of appetite and nonulcer dyspepsia (with fullness, flatulence, minor cramps, change of bowel habits) and has been recommended for chronic diarrhea and dysentery.
Caution: Calumba should not be taken during pregnancy and lactation. At higher doses than recommended it causes gastrointestinal irritations (with nausea, vomiting) and overdoses have shown narcotic effect. Otherwise, there are no reports of contraindications or side effects when used properly.

References: (1) Vol. 5, p. 557; (3) Vol. 5, p. 315; (8) p. 326; (13) p. 234; (14) p. 50; (15) p. 121; (31) pp. 210, 772; (37) p. 739; (46) p. 371; (48) p. 920.

CAMPHOR

Other Common Name(s): camphor laurel, camphor tree
Botanical Name(s): *Cinnamomum camphora* (L.) J. Presl. = *Camphora officinalis* Nees = *Laurus camphora* L. [Fam.: Lauraceae]
Camphor
Natural camphor or (+)-camphor is separated from the volatile oil of the stems, twigs and roots of camphor tree, while racemic camphor or (±)-camphor is prepared semisynthetically from pinenes. Both are crystalline substances.
Properties: Rubefacient, local anesthetic, analgesic, antipruritic, antimicrobial.

Uses: Camphor is chiefly incorporated in combination products. <u>Externally</u> it is used (as an ointment, lotion) for neuralgic and rheumatic pains, (as an ointment, cream: rub / inhalation) for inflammations of the upper respiratory tract (the common cold, bronchitis, etc.; irritating coughs), and (as a mouthwash) for the oral hygiene or inflammations of the mouth. Racemic camphor has been also used <u>internally</u> as an analeptic (= CNS stimulant), but today is seldom incorporated in some products to be taken by drops.

Caution: Camphor should not be used in infants and the recommended amounts should not to be exceeded.

References: (1) Vol. 4, p. 896; (3) Vol. 4, p. 62; (8) p. 164; (11) p. 82; (12a) p. 353; (13) p. 111; (36) p. 278; (37) p. 262; (48) p. 551; (49) Vol. 2, p. 167; (55) p. 144.

CANADIAN HEMP

Other Common Name(s): black Indian hemp, hemp dogbane
Botanical Name(s): *Apocynum cannabinum* L. [Fam.: Ranunculaceae]
Root
Constituents: Cardiac glycosides (chiefly cymarin = apocymarin = k-strophanthin-α = k-strophanthidin cymaroside; etc.), free strophanthidin, etc.

Properties: Canadian hemp exerts strophanthus-like cardiotonic effect, but milder. It is less cumulative than digitalis. It exerts strong diuretic effect therefore is recommended for edemas. See DIGITALIS.

Uses: <u>Internally</u> it is used (only as a combination h. p.) for early stages of heart failure.

Caution: Canadian hemp is toxic and not for self-treatment. It is used only as directed by a health professional. Its products should be standardized to the cardiac glycosides content. See DIGITALIS.

References: (1) Vol. 4, p. 303; (3) Vol. 3, p. 124; (6) pp. 37, 38; (8) p. 62; (13) p. 192; (37) p. 112; (46) p. 216; (47) p. 557.

CANCHALAGUA

Botanical Name(s): *Centaurium chilensis* (Willd.) Druce = *Erythraea chilensis* Pres. [Fam.: Gentianaceae]
Aerial part
Constituents: Bitter principles (seco-iridoids: sweroside, etc.), xanthones (swerchirin, etc.), triterpenes (oleanolic acid, etc.), tannins, etc.

Properties: Bitter tonic, antipyretic. It possibly exerts mild immunomodulant (due to bitter iridoids) and antidepressive (due to xanthones) effects. Many xanthones (incl. swerchirin) have shown antimicrobial, anti-inflammatory, antiedematous, liver protective and monoamine oxidase (= MAO) inhibiting effects.

Uses: <u>Internally</u> it is used (as a tea, h. p.) for loss of appetite and nonulcer dyspepsia (with fullness, bloating, flatulence, sluggish bowels), feverish

72

states, minor fatigue and convalescence.

Caution: Canchalagua should not be taken during pregnancy and lactation. At higher doses than recommended it causes gastrointestinal irritations (with nausea, vomiting, diarrhea). Otherwise, there are no reports of contraindications or side effects when used properly.

References: (1) Vol. 4, p. 758; (3) Vol. 3, p. 791; (5) Vol. 1, p. 256; (37) p. 295; (52) p. 168.

CAPER BUSH

Botanical Name(s): *Capparis spinosa* L. [Fam.: Capparaceae (Capparidaceae)]
Flower bud (caper)
Constituents: Glucosinolates (glucocapparin = methyl-glucosinolate; mainly in the intact fresh material; cf. CAPER, THREE-LEAF), flavonoids (rich in rutin), triterpenoid saponins, etc.
Properties: Mild stomachic, antioxidant. Under the action of myrosinase (when the fresh material is crushed, partly with processing) glucocapparin liberates methyl isothiocyanate, responsible for the horseradish-like flavor and the mentioned effects.
Uses: For its mustard-like flavor it is used as a spice (usually as caper pickles) and is helpful for mild cases of loss of appetite and nonulcer dyspepsia.
Caution: There are no reports of contraindications or side effects when consumed properly (occasionally, in moderate amounts).

References: (3) Vol. 3, p. 665; (5) Vol. 1, p. 220; (37) p. 266.

CAPER, THREE-LEAF

Other Common Name(s): varuna
Botanical Name(s): *Crataeva nurvala* Buch.-Ham. [Fam.: Capparaceae (Capparidaceae)]
Bark
Constituents: Volatile oil (with methyl-isothiocyanate, etc.; mainly in the processed / dried material), glucosinolates (glucocapparin = methyl-glucosinolate; mainly in the intact fresh material; cf. CAPER BUSH), triterpenoid saponins, phytosterols (5-sterols: β-sitosterol, etc.), proline-betaines (stachydrine, etc.), phenolics (catechins, possibly sinapic acid, etc).
Properties: Diuretic, stomachic, laxative, rubefacient, antimicrobial.
Uses: <u>Internally</u> it is used as a flushing-out treatment (= herbal tea or product + liquids: more than 2 liters per day; sometimes combined with a medication) for inflammations of the genitourinary tract (cystitis, urethritis, prostatitis), urinary gravel and nonobstructive stones, to prevent relapsing urinary infections / gravel / stones, as an antidyscratic (= blood purifier; tea, h. p.) for atopic eczema (= chronic eczema of internal origin), and (as a tea,

h. p.) for inflammations of the upper respiratory tract (bronchitis, etc.) and nonulcer dyspepsia (with impaired digestion, sluggish bowels, constipation, etc.). Externally it is used (as a poultice) for inflammations of the upper respiratory tract and for rheumatic pains.
Caution: See CRESS, GARDEN.

References: (5) Vol. 3, p. 145; (12a) p. 470; (18) p. 208; (31) p. 95; (41) Vols. 1-7; (42) Vol. 3, p. 362; (45) p. 87; (52) p. 225; (57) p. 237.

CAPSICUM

Other Common Name(s): 1) cayenne, cayenne pepper, chili, chili pepper 2) habañero pepper
Botanical Name(s): 1) *Capsicum annuum* L. and its varieties 2) *Capsicum chinense* Jacq. [Fam.: Solanaceae]
Fruit
For external applications, the varieties and hybrids rich in pungent principles are used, while internally are used those with a very low content of these principles.
Constituents: Pungent principles (amides: capsaicin, dihydrocapsaicin, other capsaicinoids), carotenoids (capsanthin, etc.), vitamin C (rich), flavonoids (flavones), volatile oil, etc.
Properties: (Externally): Rubefacient, counterirritant, analgesic, anti-inflammatory. The mentioned effects are due in large part to capsaicin.
Uses: Externally it is used (as a cream, ointment, lotion, gel, plaster) for neuralgic and rheumatic pains (articular, muscular), generally by applying the recommended amount 3-4 times daily, for 4-8 weeks. It is also used (as a gargle) for chronic laryngitis.
Caution: Capsicum products should not be applied on injured or inflamed skin and any contact with the eyes or other mucous membranes should be avoided. It may cause blisters and ulcerations if left on the painful site longer than advised. Products with a very high content in capsaicin (esp. plasters) should be limited to a few days.
Note: Paprika (mild pungent variety of *Capsicum annuum* L.) contains vitamin C (rich), carotenoids (capsanthin, etc.), flavonoids (flavones), pungent principles (very low concentration), volatile oil, etc. It is used internally for nonulcer dyspepsia (with flatulence, sluggish bowels), impaired peripheral circulation and as a vitamin C-rich supplement.

References: (1) Vol. 4, p. 661; (3) Vol. 3, p. 669; (8) p. 113; (9) p. 115; (11) p. 134; (12) pp. 71, 1099; (13) p. 146; (15) p. 47; (16) p. 51; (19) p. 62; (20) p. 60; (29) p. 23; (46) p. 230; (47) p. 814; (48) p. 775.

CARAWAY

Botanical Name(s): *Carum carvi* L. [Fam.: Apiaceae (Umbelliferae)]
Fruit (commonly called seed)

Constituents: Volatile oil (see Caraway oil), phenolic acids (caffeic acid, etc.), coumarins (umbelliferone, etc.), fixed oil, carbohydrates, proteins, etc.
Properties: Aromatic, stomachic, antispasmodic, carminative, choleretic, galactagogue, antimicrobial.
Uses: Caraway is extensively used as a flavor ingredient in culinary practice and in food and liqueur / liquor industries. Internally it is used (as a tea, h. p.) for nonulcer dyspepsia (with fullness, flatulence, bloating, cramps, irritable bowel syndrome), to promote the secretion of milk in nursing mothers, and is added to mixtures of anthranoid laxatives (senna, cascara, etc.) to prevent griping effect.
Caution: There are no reports of contraindications or side effects when used properly.

Caraway oil

It is the volatile oil obtained by steam distillation from the freshly crushed fruits.
Constituents: Chiefly carvone and limonene.
Properties: Aromatic, etc., much like fruit.
Uses: Caraway oil is chiefly used as a fragrance ingredient in cosmetic, perfume and liqueur / liquor industries. Internally it can be used (a few drops in a glass of water; in capsule / dragée) much like caraway seed. Externally it has been used (as a liniment) for skin parasites (scabies = the itch, etc.) and for inflammations of the upper respiratory tract.
Caution: There are no reports of contraindications or side effects when used properly. When taken internally, its dose should be limited to a few drops (on sugar / water).

References: (1) Vol. 4, p. 694; (3) Vol. 3, p. 727; (6) p. 128; (7) p. 198; (8) p. 119; (9) p. 119; (12) p. 706; (13) p. 124; (15) p. 48; (16) p. 126; (17) p. 134; (19) p. 134; (23) p. 81; (45) p. 182; (47) p. 848; (48) p. 518; (51) p. 130.

CARAWAY, BLACK

Other Common Name(s): great pignut
Botanical Name(s): *Bunium bulbocastanum* L. = *Carum bulbocastanum* (L.) W.D.J. Koch [Fam.: Apiaceae (Umbelliferae)]
Fruit (black caraway)
Constituents: Volatile oil (with cuminaldehyde and p-cymene, also farnesol, etc.), fixed oil, sugars, etc.
Properties: Aromatic, carminative, antispasmodic.
Uses: Internally it is used (as a tea, h. p.) for nonulcer dyspepsia (with flatulence, cramps, nausea). In Asia, black caraway is used as a substitute for caraway. Cuminaldehyde is used in perfumery.
Caution: There are no reports of contraindications or side effects when used properly. **This is not about Black Cumin (Nigella sativa L.).**

References: (1) Vol. 4, p. 577; (3) Vol. 3, p. 733; (5) Vol. 1, p. 232; (31) p. 560; (52) p. 132.

CARDAMOM

Other Common Name(s): Mysore cardamom
Botanical Name(s): *Elettaria cardamomum* (L.) Maton var. *cardamomum* [Fam.: Zingiberaceae]
Seed
In trade it is available as a whole fruit (capsule). Seeds are kept in the fruit until required for use.
Constituents: Volatile oil (with 1,8-cineole, α-terpinyl acetate, α-terpineol, etc.), minerals (rich in manganese and iron), carbohydrates, fixed oil, proteins, etc.
Properties: Aromatic, stomachic, cholagogue, carminative, antibacterial, antifungal, antiviral, expectorant, and it is claimed to be aphrodisiac.
Uses: Cardamom is chiefly used as a flavor ingredient in culinary practice and in food and liqueur / liquor industries. Internally it is used (as a tea, h. p.; usually combined with other herbs) for loss of appetite and nonulcer dyspepsia (with flatulence, minor cramps, etc.) and inflammations of the upper respiratory tract (bronchitis, etc.; coughs due to thickened bronchial secretion). In pharmaceutical industry it is used as a flavor ingredient in bitter tasting mixtures and to correct griping effect of anthranoids laxatives. Externally it can be tried (as a liniment, paint) for fungal skin infections.
Caution: Cardamom should not be taken in cases of biliary obstruction, severe liver disorders and during pregnancy. In cases of nonobstructive gallstones it can be used but only on health professional's advice.

References: (1) Vol. 5, p. 38; (3) Vol. 4, p. 767; (6) p. 128; (8) p. 237; (9) p. 121; (12) p. 705; (13) p. 108; (15) p. 81; (16) p. 125; (19) p. 124; (37) p. 462; (46) p. 251.

CARDAMOM, AMOMUM

Other Common Name(s): 1) round cardamom, Chinese / Java / Siam cardamom 2) Chinese cardamom, white-fruit amomum 3) Indian cardamom, Bengal / Nepal / greater cardamom 4) wringed cardamom, tsao-ko cardamom
Botanical Name(s): 1) *Amomum compactum* Sol. ex Maton 2) *Amomum kravanh* Pierre ex Gagnep. 3) *Amomum subulatum* Roxb. 4) *Amomum tsao-ko* Crevost et Lemarié = *Amomum aromaticum* Roxb. [Fam.: Zingiberaceae]
Seed
As with cardamom (q. v.), in trade it is available as a whole fruit (capsule). Seeds are kept in the fruit until required for use.
Constituents: The mentioned species are grouped together as the volatile oils of their seeds besides other monoterpenes (depending on species) contain 1,8-cineole as their chief constituent.
Properties: Aromatic, stomachic, carminative, antimicrobial, antispasmodic. See also CARDAMOM.

Uses: <u>Internally</u> it is used (as a tea, h. p.) for loss of appetite and nonulcer dyspepsia (with flatulence, minor cramps, nausea, vomiting) and inflammations of the upper respiratory tract (spastic bronchitis, etc.; coughs due to thickened bronchial secretion). It is widely used as a spice and in liqueur / liquor industry, much like cardamom. See also CARDAMOM.
Caution: See CARDAMOM.

References: (1) Vol. 4, p. 243; (3) Vol. 3, p. 46; (5) Vol. 1, p. 69; (41) Vols. 1-7; (42) Vol. 2, p. 458.

CAREX, SAND

Other Common Name(s): sand sedge, sea sedge
Botanical Name(s): *Carex arenaria* L. [Fam.: Cyperaceae]
<u>Root</u> (rhizome)
Constituents: Triterpenoid saponins, silicic acid, tannins (proanthocyanidins), volatile oil (with methyl salicylate, cineole, etc.), carbohydrates (mucilaginous polysaccharides, starch, sugars), bitter principles, etc.
Properties: Diuretic, expectorant, anti-inflammatory, mild laxative, mild astringent. It has been designated as German sarsaparilla.
Uses: <u>Internally</u> it is used (as a tea, h. p.; usually combined with other herbs) as an antidyscratic (= blood purifier) and anti-inflammatory for chronic rheumatic complaints and atopic eczema (= chronic eczema of internal origin), and (as a tea, h. p.) for inflammations of the upper respiratory tract (bronchitis, etc.; minor coughs due to thickened bronchial secretion; also as a diaphoretic hot tea for colds) and gastrointestinal tract (gastritis, minor constipation, etc.). <u>Externally</u> it is used (as a wash, wet compress) for minor skin inflammations.
Caution: There are no reports of contraindications or side effects when used properly.

References: (1) Vol. 4, p. 685; (3) Vol. 3, p. 708; (18) p. 326; (23) p. 277; (24) p. 277; (27) p. 76; (37) p. 279; (47) p. 837; (51) p. 48; (52) p. 154.

CARLINE THISTLE

Botanical Name(s): *Carlina acaulis* L. [Fam.: Asteraceae (Compositae)]
<u>Root</u>
Constituents: Volatile oil (with polyacetylenes: carlina oxide, carlilene), resin, inulin, tannins, flavonoids, etc.
Properties: Bitter tonic, aromatic, diuretic, antispasmodic, antimicrobial. Like many other polyacetylenes, carlina oxide has shown antibacterial and antifungal effects.
Uses: <u>Internally</u> it is used (as a tea, h. p.; usually combined with other herbs) for loss of appetite and nonulcer dyspepsia (with minor cramps and constipation, etc.), inflammations of the genitourinary tract (cystitis, etc.) and

upper respiratory tract (bronchitis, the common cold, etc.), and for feverish states. To enhance the effects in problems of the genitourinary tract, the fluid intake (incl. herbal teas) should be more than 2 liters per day. Carline thistle is a component of the Swedish bitter. Externally it is used (as a wash) for minor skin inflammations (due to bacterial / fungal infections), ulcers and wounds, and (as a mouthwash, gargle) for inflammations of the mouth and throat.

Caution: There are no reports of contraindications or side effects when used properly. At higher doses than recommended it causes gastrointestinal irritations (with nausea, vomiting, diarrhea).

References: (1) Vol. 4, p. 691; (3) Vol. 3, p. 717; (5) Vol. 1, p. 228; (8) p. 117; (17) p. 132; (18) p. 283; (24) p. 110; (27) p. 77; (28) pp. 30, 71; (31) p. 48; (37) p. 280; (41) Vols. 1-7; (51) p. 218; (87) Vol. 2, p. 230.

CARNAUBA WAX PALM

Botanical Name(s): *Copernicia prunifera* (Mill.) H.E. Moore = *Copernicia cerifera* (Arruda) Mart. [Fam.: Arecaceae (Palmae)]
Carnauba wax (purified leaf wax)
Constituents: Esters of cerotic acid with myricyl alcohol, free monohydric alcohols, free fatty acids, and hydrocarbons of alkanes series.
Uses: Carnauba wax is used in pharmaceutical and food industries in the production of coated tablets, in dental practice for plasters, in cosmetics for lipsticks and nail polishes and it is an ingredient in products used for polishing leather and furniture, among others.
Caution: Carnauba wax has resulted to be non-toxic.

References: (1) Vol. 4, p. 993; (8) p. 191; (11) p. 76; (12) p. 291; (13) p. 396; (36) p. 190; (48) p. 168; (49) Vol. 2, p. 9.

CAROB

Other Common Name(s): locust bean, St. John's bread
Botanical Name(s): *Ceratonia siliqua* L. [Fam.: Fabaceae (Caesalpiniaceae)]
Carob (bean) gum (locust bean gum)
It is the flour obtained by grinding seeds after they are freed from their coat and germ.
Constituents: Carob bean gum is richer in mucilaginous polysaccharides (carubin) than the whole seed. Seed contains carubin, proteins, lipids, etc. Fruit (pod with seeds) contains cellulose, fat, tannins (condensed t.), proteins, starch, sugars (fructose, glucose, sucrose), etc.
Properties: Demulcent, antidiarrheal.
Uses: Internally it is used (as an h. p.) for minor diarrhea (recommended for infants and children), vomiting (in infants, during pregnancy) and other in-

flammatory conditions of the gastrointestinal tract (gluten intolerance, gastroenteritis), and as an aid to a weight-loss diet. In food industry carob bean gum is extensively used as a thickening ingredient.

Caution: Carob should be taken with sufficient amount of water. It should not be taken in cases of bowel obstruction. Carob may impair the absorption of some drugs. In view of this, when taking a vital oral medication, drugs should be taken about one hour apart from carob products.

References: (2) Vol. 2, p. 323; (3) Vol. 3, p. 811; (8) p. 138; (9) pp. 123, 355; (12) p. 369; (13) p. 373; (37) p. 297; (46) p. 255; (48) p. 100; (49) Vol. 2, p. 356.

CARRAGEEN ALGAE

Carrageen

Carrageen (native carrageen, NC) is the bleached and dried thallus of *Chondrus crispus* Stackh. (= **Irish moss**); *Mastocarpus stellatus* (Stackh.) Guiry = *Gigartina stellata* (Stackh.) Batters = *Gigartina mamillosa* (Gooden. et Woodw.) J. Agardh; and some other red algae (Class: Rhodophyceae, Fam.: Gigartinaceae).

Constituents: Chiefly carrageenan (q. v.), also minerals (rich in chlorides, iodides, bromides; comparatively high concentrations of arsenic), proteins and lipids.

Properties: Demulcent, bulk laxative.

Uses: Internally it is used (as an h. p.; usually combined with other herbs) for chronic constipation and irritating dry coughs.

Caution: Its quality should comply with pharmacopoeial parameters (arsenic content, etc.). As a laxative it should not be taken in cases of bowel obstruction. Otherwise, there are no reports of contraindications or side effects when used properly.

Carrageenan

It is a gum-like (hydrocolloid) obtained by extraction and purification from the mentioned species, but is also obtained from other red algae (genera: *Gigartina, Eucheuma, Iridaea, Hypnea*).

Constituents: It is a straight-chain highly sulfated galactan (galactose polymer), composed of two major fractions (gel-forming and non gel-forming).

Properties: (the food-grade, with molecular weight 200,000-800,000): Suspending, emulsifying, gelling, demulcent, bulk laxative.

Uses: The food-grade (with molecular weight 200,000-800,000) is used in pharmaceutical and food industries in the production of gels, suspensions, emulsions, tablets, creams, toothpastes, ice creams and puddings, among others. It is also used (usually combined with other herbs) as a demulcent and bulk laxative and is incorporated in various weight-loss formulations.

Caution: Carrageenans of lower molecular weight than 50,000 have been shown to be highly toxic. As a laxative it should not be taken in cases of bowel obstruction. Otherwise, there are no reports of contraindications or side effects when used properly.

References: (1) Vol. 4, p. 860; Vol. 5, p. 268; (3) Vol. 3, p. 721; (8) p. 149; (9) p. 124; (11) p. 44; (12) pp. 379, 389; (13) p. 360; (36) p. 209; (37) p. 282; (48) p. 53.

CARROT

Other Common Name(s): 1) wild carrot 2) cultivated carrot
Botanical Name(s): 1) *Daucus carota* L. ssp. *carota* 2) *Daucus carota* L. ssp. *sativa* [Fam.: Apiaceae (Umbelliferae)]
Fruit (commonly called seed; wild carrot)
Constituents: Volatile oil (with pinenes, geraniol, terpinen-4-ol, carotol, etc.), furanocoumarins (psoralene derivatives), flavonoids, fixed oil, etc.
Properties: Diuretic, carminative, antispasmodic, emmenagogue. As with juniper berry, terpinen-4-ol is considered responsible for the diuretic properties. The rest of the effects may be due at least in part to flavonoids and furanocoumarins.
Uses: Internally it is used as a flushing-out treatment (= herbal tea or product + liquids: more than 2 liters per day; sometimes combined with a medication) for inflammations of the genitourinary tract (cystitis, etc.), urinary gravel and nonobstructive stones, to prevent relapsing urinary infections / gravel / stones, and for secondary amenorrhea and oligomenorrhea (= ceased / infrequent / scanty menstruation without pathology).
Caution: Carrot fruit should not be taken during pregnancy. A flushing-out treatment is contraindicated in cases of obstructive urinary stones, edema due to impaired heart or kidney function and kidney inflammations (here can be used on health professional's advice to enhance the effects of an antimicrobial therapy). Otherwise, there are no reports of contraindications or side effects when used properly.
Root (the fresh root of the cultivated carrot)
Constituents: Pectin (rich), sugars (sucrose, glucose), carotenoids (carotenes: very rich in β-carotene), vitamins (C, B_1, B_2, β-carotene = a provitamin A), volatile oil (with mono- and sesquiterpenes), organic acids (malic and citric acids, etc.), polyacetylenes, etc.
Properties and Uses: Carrot is a rich natural supplement of β-carotene, a provitamin A. In the intestinal tract and the liver, β-carotene is converted to vitamin A (1 molecule β-carotene yields 2 molecules vitamin A), which is then stored as such in the liver. Carrot juice has shown mild diuretic and anthelmintic (against pinworms = *Oxyuris* spp.) effects. Due to pectin it is a valuable antidiarrheal, for which carrot root is ground, mixed with water and boiled down to a purée and taken as such by adults or mixed with broth and made a soup-like drink for infants. Pectin and pectin-rich fruits and vegetables are beneficial for high cholesterol. For the effects of pectin see APPLE.
Caution: Carrot (raw, purée) should not be taken in cases of bowel obstruc-

80

tion. Pectin may impair the absorption of some drugs. In view of this, when taking a vital oral medication, drugs should be taken about one hour apart from pectin / pectin-rich products. Otherwise, there are no reports of contra-indications or side effects when used properly.

References: (3) Vol. 4, p. 471; (6) p. 62; (9) p. 127; (10) p. 281; (14) p. 221; (15) p. 77; (19) p. 596; (20) p. 264; (23) p. 117; (27) p. 78; (37) p. 388.

CASCARA AMARGA

Botanical Name(s): *Acosmium panamense* (Benth.) Yakovlev = *Sweetia panamensis* Benth. [Fam.: Fabaceae (Leguminosae)]
Bark (Honduras bark)
Constituents: It is not well studied. It is reported to contain quinolizidine alkaloids (4-α-hydroxysparteine, 5,6-didehydro-α-isosparteine, etc.) and triterpenes (lupeol, etc.).
Properties: Bitter tonic, antipyretic, diuretic, antihyperglycemic.
Uses: Cascara amarga is chiefly used in traditional medicine. Internally it is used (as a tea, h. p.) for loss of appetite and dyspeptic disorders associated with impaired bile secretion, and for feverish states. It is also used for chronic skin diseases especially of syphilitic origin and atopic eczema (= chronic eczema of internal origin), and it may be beneficial for diabetes.
Caution: Due to the potential quinolizidine alkaloids, cascara amarga should be used with caution and only as directed by an experienced practitioner.
Note: Other sources of cascara amarga are bitter bush (*Picramnia pentandra* Sw.) and West Indian snakewood (*Picramnia antidesma* Sw.) [Fam.: Simaroubaceae]. Their barks is reported to contain alkaloids, triterpenes (epibetulin, epibetulinic acid), bitter principles, anthranoids, etc. In traditional medicine their bark is used as a bitter tonic (substitute of cinchona bark).

References: (3) Vol. 6a, p. 652; Vol. 6b, p. 700; (5) Vol. 1, p. 852; (10) p. 61; (41) Vols. 1-7; (52) pp. 595, 770; (66) p. 210.

CASCARA SAGRADA

Botanical Name(s): *Frangula purshiana* (DC.) J.G. Cooper = *Rhamnus purshiana* DC. [Fam.: Rhamnaceae]
Bark
Constituents: Anthranoids (C-glycosides: cascarosides A - D, aloin, chrysaloin; O-glycosides: glycosides of emodin, aloe-emodin, and chrysophanol), etc.
Properties: Laxative (large intestine stimulant laxative). See SENNA. Cascara sagrada has been shown to cause less griping or dependence effects, compared to other anthranoid laxatives (senna, frangula, aloe).

81

Uses: Internally it is used (as an h. p.) for constipation (atonic, non-spastic). See also SENNA.
Caution: See SENNA.

References: (1) Vol. 6, p. 404; (3) Vol. 6b, p. 83; (7) p. 230; (11) p. 52; (12) p. 919; (13) p. 296; (14) p. 52; (17) p. 48; (19) p. 25; (22) p. 59; (23) p. 106; (46) p. 260; (48) p. 433.

CASCARILLA

Other Common Name(s): sweetwood
Botanical Name(s): *Croton eluteria* (L.) Sw. [Fam.: Euphorbiaceae]
Bark
Constituents: Volatile oil (with p-cymene, α-thujone, linalool, eugenol, etc.), bitter principles (diterpenes: cascarillin A, etc.), resin (rich), an organic acid (cascarilic acid), tannins, etc.
Properties: Aromatic, bitter tonic, mild astringent, antimicrobial. Based on its constituents, the strong aromatic volatile oil may account for the antimicrobial effect.
Uses: Internally it is used (as a tea, h. p.) for loss of appetite and nonulcer dyspepsia (with flatulence, atonic diarrhea) and feverish states. It is also used for convalescence, minor fatigue and decreased resistance to infections (esp. in the upper respiratory tract). Externally it is used (as a gargle, mouthwash) for inflammations of the mouth and throat. Cascarilla is used as a flavor ingredient in tobacco and liqueur / liquor industries. Its volatile oil is used in cosmetics and perfumery.
Caution: Cascarilla should not be taken during pregnancy and lactation. At higher doses than recommended it causes gastrointestinal irritations (with nausea, vomiting), headache and insomnia. Otherwise, there are no reports of contraindications or side effects when used properly.

References: (2) Vol. 2, p. 454; (3) Vol. 4, p. 347; (9) p. 130; (10) p. 62; (12a) p. 291; (27) p. 112; (35) p. 166; (37) p. 370; (46) p. 268; (52) p. 228; (66) p. 211.

CASHEW

Other Common Name(s): caju
Botanical Name(s): *Anacardium occidentale* L. [Fam.: Anacardiaceae]
Nut (cashew nut)
Constituents: Fixed oil (see Cashew oil), glycolipids, phospholipids, proteins, starch, etc.
Properties: Mild astringent, antimicrobial (due to trace amounts of anacardic acid and related compounds).
Uses: The roasted nuts are enjoyed as a delicious nutrient and in traditional medicine are used for gastrointestinal problems.

Caution: Only roasted nuts should be used. When roasting, avoid contact with skin as anacardic acid is a strong irritant and may lead to severe eczema.

Cashew oil (= cashew nut shell oil)
It is isolated from the nutshell and consists chiefly of anacardic acid (= an alkyl derivative of salicylic acid) and cardol, both closely related to urushiol, the skin irritant of Poison Ivy.
Properties: Rubefacient, counterirritant, antimicrobial, antifungal.
Uses: Cashew oil is chiefly used in traditional medicine. Externally it is used (as a paint) for warts (common w., plantar w.) and corns, fungal skin infections and psoriasis, among others.
Caution: Cashew oil should not be taken internally. When used externally, besides the normal irritation (see Nut) it may cause allergic reactions, for which a test is recommended. In view of this, cashew oil should be applied under the supervision of an experienced practitioner.

References: (1) Vol. 4, p. 254; (3) Vol. 3, p. 66; (8) p. 51; (10) p. 63; (31) pp. 455, 456; (35) p. 167; (37) p. 80; (45) p. 164; (52) p. 47.

CASTOR

Other Common Name(s): palma christi
Botanical Name(s): *Ricinus communis* L. [Fam.: Euphorbiaceae]
Castor oil
It is the fixed oil obtained by cold expression from the seeds.
Constituents: Chiefly glycerides (fatty acids component: chiefly ricinoleic acid, also oleic and linoleic acids, etc.), etc.
Properties: (At low doses): Laxative, demulcent. (At high doses): Purgative. The active component is ricinoleic acid, a small intestine stimulant laxative / purgative, which is liberated from castor oil after this is attacked by the enzymes there. It is also emollient, when applied externally.
Uses: Internally it is used (at purgative doses) for acute constipation and (at mild laxative doses) for bowel inflammations. It is also used as a solvent for fat-soluble drugs and as an ingredient in lotions, ointments and cosmetic products (soaps, hair-grooming products, etc.), etc. To make its taste more acceptable, it is mixed with lemon juice, milk, or coffee (any of them, in cool temperature).
Caution: Castor oil should be taken on an empty stomach. It should not be taken in chronic constipation and in cases of biliary obstruction and other biliary disorders. During pregnancy it can be used but only on health professional's advice. Castor oil is contraindicated in poisonings caused by fat-soluble agents or after taking fat-soluble drugs that must pass unabsorbed through the digestive system (e. g. male fern extract).

References: (1) Vol. 6, p. 475; (3) Vol. 6b, p. 143; (6) pp. 166, 167; (7) p. 231; (8) p. 487; (9) p. 132; (11) p. 70; (12) p. 256; (13) p. 392; (36) p. 186; (48) p. 144; (49) Vol. 2, p. 270.

CAT'S CLAW

Other Common Name(s): uña-de-gato
Botanical Name(s): *Uncaria tomentosa* (Willd.) DC. [Fam.: Rubiaceae]
Root bark
Constituents: Oxindole alkaloids (either pentacyclic: pteropodine, etc.; or, tetracyclic: rhynchophylline, etc.; depending on chemotype), triterpenes (oleanolic and ursolic acids, etc.), triterpenoid saponins (quinovic acid glycosides), flavonoids (epicatechin), tannins (proanthocyanidins), etc.
Properties: Anti-inflammatory and antirheumatic, (due to esp. the pentacyclic alcaloids), astringent, immunomodulant. The tetracyclic chemotype is of toxicologic importance, not for therapeutic use.
Uses: Internally it is used (as an h. p.) for rheumatic complaints (incl. rheumatoid arthritis), inflammatory and ulcerative conditions of the gastrointestinal tract (gastritis, peptic ulcers, colitis, diverticulitis, hemorrhoids, minor diarrhea), inflammatory conditions (due to allergies, bacterial / viral infections) of the upper respiratory tract. Due to its immunomodulant effect it is also used to enhance the effects of cancer therapies.
Caution: Cat's claw should not be taken during pregnancy and lactation. It is best used on health professional's advice. Manufacturers should not mix two chemotypes. For further caution concerning immunomodulants see ECHINACEA; BETA GLUCANS.

References: (2) Vol. 3, p. 706; (21) p. 97; (22) p. 257; (41) Vols. 1-7; (68) p. 43; (75) p. 154.

CATALPA, SOUTHERN

Other Common Name(s): catawba, cataroba tree, Indian bean tree
Botanical Name(s): *Catalpa bignonioides* Walter = *Bignonia catalpa* L. [Fam.: Bignoniaceae]
Fruit, bark
Constituents: Iridoids (catalpol, very bitter; catalposide, not bitter), phenolic acids (*p*-hydroxybenzoic and *p*-coumaric acids, etc.), fixed oil (in seeds; with glycerides chiefly of linoleic acid), etc.
Properties: Due to iridoids (catalpol, catalposide) it possibly exerts anti-inflammatory, antimicrobial, immunomodulant, choleretic, liver protective, laxative and diuretic effects, among others. *p*-Hydroxybenzoic acid has been shown to stimulate the biosynthesis of specific prostaglandins (possibly PGE_1). PGE_1 has shown anti-inflammatory, bronchodilatory, and immunomodulant effects, among others. This might explain benefits of using catalpa for bronchial asthma and other spastic conditions of the upper respiratory tract.
Uses: Internally it is used (as a tea, h. p.) for inflammatory and spastic conditions of the upper respiratory tract (spastic bronchitis, bronchial asthma, etc.; whooping cough).

Caution: There are no reports of contraindications or side effects when used properly.

References: (2) Vol. 2, p. 308; (3) Vol. 3, p. 767; (12) p. 438; (31) pp. 459, 569, 572; (41) Vols. 1-7; (46) p. 158.

CATECHU

Black catechu (cutch)
It is the dried aqueous extract prepared from the heartwood of *Acacia catechu* Willd. [Fam.: Fabaceae (Mimosaceae)];
Pale catechu (brown cutch, gambir, gambir catechu, white cutch)
It is the dried aqueous extract prepared from the leaf and twig of *Uncaria gambir* (W. Hunter) Roxb. [Fam.: Rubiaceae]
Constituents: (Black c.; Pale c.): Tannins (very rich in condensed t.), also phlobaphenes, flavonoids, gum, and is reported to contain indole alkaloids.
Properties: Astringent, antimicrobial, hemostatic.
Uses: Externally it is used (as a mouthwash, paint) for inflammations of the mouth (incl. bleeding gums), and (as a gargle) for sore throat. Internally it is still used (as an h. p.; only combined with other herbs) for inflammations of the gastrointestinal tract (diarrhea, ulcerative colitis, etc.).
Caution: There are no contraindications or side effects when used properly (in moderate amounts / concentrations and for a short period). At higher doses than recommended it causes gastrointestinal irritations (with nausea, constipation, etc.).

References: (1) Vol. 4, p. 30; (2) Vol. 3, p. 693; (3) Vol. 3, p. 768; Vol. 6c, p. 342; (8) p. 16; (9) p. 135; (14) p. 55; (15) p. 53; (36) p. 229; (37) p. 1419; (48) p. 400; (49) Vol. 2, p. 379.

CATNIP

Other Common Name(s): catmint
Botanical Name(s): *Nepeta cataria* L. [Fam.: Lamiaceae (Labiatae)]
Aerial part
Constituents: Volatile oil (with citral, citronellol, β-caryophyllene, limonene, etc.), bitter principles (iridoids: nepetalactone, etc.), tannins, etc.
Properties: Aromatic, bitter tonic, antispasmodic, sedative, astringent. Its bitter tonic effect is due to iridoids. Volatile oil is responsible for its antispasmodic and sedative effects. Catnip attracts cats, for which nepetalactone is considered responsible.
Uses: Internally it is used as a diaphoretic hot tea for feverish states and the common cold, (as a tea, h. p.) for minor inflammatory and spastic conditions of the gastrointestinal tract (diarrhea, cramps) and minor cases of primary dysmenorrhea (= painful menstruation without pathology) and headaches.
Caution: Catnip is best avoided during pregnancy and lactation. Before using catnip for dysmenorrhea, the gynecologic problem should be judged by

a health professional. Otherwise, there are no reports of contraindications or side effects when used properly.

References: (3) Vol. 6a, p. 176; (9) p. 137; (10) p. 66; (27) p. 117; (29) p. 79; (35) p. 173; (37) p. 962; (46) p. 272; (52) p. 526.

CEDAR, EASTERN RED

Other Common Name(s): pencil cedar, Virginia red cedar
Botanical Name(s): *Juniperus virginiana* L. [Fam.: Cupressaceae]
Cedarwood oil
It is the volatile oil obtained by steam distillation from the wood (sawdust, chips, etc.).
Constituents: Chiefly sesquiterpenes (chiefly α- and β-cedrene, some thujopsene, cedrol, etc.), also monoterpenes.
Properties: Aromatic, antimicrobial, insecticidal, rubefacient, counterirritant, emmenagogue.
Uses: Cedarwood oil is chiefly used as a fragrance ingredient or fixative in cosmetics and perfumery and as an insect-repellent (esp. against clothes moths). Externally it is used (as an ointment, liniment combination product) for neuralgic and rheumatic pains.
Caution: Cedarwood oil is best limited to a fragrance ingredient and insect-repellent and not used internally.
Cedarwood (chips)
Constituents: Volatile oil (see Cedarwood oil), flavonoids (biflavones: amentoflavone, etc.; flavonols; etc.), resin, lignans (podophyllotoxin), etc.
Properties: Aromatic, antibacterial, antiviral, expectorant, diuretic, emmenagogue, insecticidal. The effects are due in large part to the volatile oil. The antiviral effect (incl. papillomaviruses) is due to podophyllotoxin.
Uses: Cedarwood is used only in traditional medicine. Internally it is used (as a tea, h. p.) for inflammations of the upper respiratory tract (the common cold, bronchitis, etc.; coughs due to thickened bronchial secretion; also as a diaphoretic hot tea or inhalation) and genitourinary tract (cystitis, urethritis, etc.), and as an antidyscratic (= blood purifier; tea, h. p.; combined with other herbs) for chronic rheumatic complaints. It is also used for primary dysmenorrhea (= painful menstruation without pathology) and secondary amenorrhea and oligomenorrhea (= ceased / infrequent / scanty menstruation without pathology). To enhance the effects in problems of the genitourinary tract, the fluid intake (incl. herbal teas) should be more than 2 liters per day. Externally it is used (as an ointment: in different concentrations) for minor skin inflammations, scabies (= the itch) and genital warts. It is also used as an insect-repellent, especially against clothes moths.
Caution: Cedarwood should not be taken during pregnancy and lactation.
Note: Cedarwood bark contains a flavanonol, namely taxifolin, which is the

86

structural basis of flavanolignans (silybin, etc.), the active constituents of milk thistle (q. v.).

References: (1) Vol. 5, p. 589; (3) Vol. 5, p. 339; (5) Vol. 2, p. 204; (9) p. 139; (29) p. 66; (44) p. 290; (49) Vol. 1, p. 389; (52) p. 412; (55) pp. 604, 646; (65) p. 146.

CEDRON

Botanical Name(s): *Simaba cedron* Planch. = *Simarouba cedron* Planch. [Fam.: Simaroubaceae]
Seed
Constituents: Bitter principles, including nortriterpenes (quassinoids: cedronin, cedronyline, quassin) and sesquiterpene lactones (cedrin* = valvidin, etc.). It also contains starch, fixed oil, etc. *) Cedrin (= valvidin) is not to be confused with cedrin, which is a flavone found in *Cedrus* spp.
Properties: Bitter tonic, antipyretic, antimalarial, anthelmintic. Nortriterpenes of quassinoid type have shown antiprotozoal (esp. against *Entamoeba* spp., but also *Plasmodium* spp.), antiviral, antibacterial and anthelmintic effects. Cedrin is very closely related to santonin and artemisin, which are known for their anthelmintic effects.
Uses: Internally it is used (as a tea, h. p.) for feverish states, malaria, nonulcer dyspepsia, amebic dysentery, and as a tonic. Externally it is used (as a wash, wet compress, poultice) for wounds, ulcers, and boils.
Caution: Cedron seed should not be taken during pregnancy and lactation. At higher doses than recommended it causes gastrointestinal irritations (with nausea, vomiting).

References: (3) Vol. 6b, p. 405; (10) p. 67; (31) p. 728; (31) p. 728; (35) p. 178; (37) p. 1271; (47) p. 871; (49) Vol. 2, p. 306; (52) p. 725.

CELANDINE

Other Common Name(s): greater celandine
Botanical Name(s): *Chelidonium majus* L. [Fam.: Papaveraceae]
Aerial part
Constituents: Alkaloids (chiefly protoberbcrine type: chiefly coptisine, also berberine, etc.; also benzophenanthridine type: chelidonine, chelerythrine, sanguinarine, etc.), phenolic acids, flavonoids, etc.
Properties: Antispasmodic (biliary and upper gastrointestinal active), cholagogue, choleretic, analgesic, anti-inflammatory, mild sedative. Chelidonine and coptisine account for the antispasmodic, analgesic and sedative effects. The cholagogic and choleretic effects are due in large part to berberine and sanguinarine.
Uses: Internally it is used (as a tea, h. p.) for inflammatory and spastic conditions of the biliary tract (nonobstructive gallstones, cholecystitis) and gastrointestinal tract (gastrointestinal colics, diarrhea, minor spastic constipa-

87

tion). Celandine (combined with other herbs: turmeric, peppermint, etc.) is also used to alleviate complaints following a cholecystectomy. <u>Externally</u> it is used (as a paint: fresh juice) for warts (common w., plantar w.) and corns.

Caution: Celandine should not be taken in cases of severe liver disorders, during pregnancy and lactation, and it should be avoided in infants and children under 12. For any condition with gallstones, it should be used on health professional's advice. Celandine products should be standardized to the alkaloids content. At higher doses than recommended it causes gastrointestinal irritations (with nausea, vomiting, diarrhea). Otherwise, there are no reports of contraindications or side effects when used properly.

<u>**Root**</u> (rhizome)
It is richer in alkaloids (chiefly chelidonine, etc.) than the aerial part and is used for the same purposes.

Caution: See Aerial part.

References: (1) Vol. 4, p. 836; (3) Vol. 3, p. 835; (6) pp. 148, 149; (7) p. 192; (8) p. 143; (13) p. 233; (15) p. 61; (16) p. 122; (17) p. 147; (19) p. 203; (23) p. 131; (37) p. 302; (46) p. 276; (47) p. 916; (51) p. 82; (72) nr. 76006.

CELERY

Botanical Name(s): *Apium graveolens* L. [Fam.: Apiaceae (Umbelliferae)]
<u>**Fruit**</u> (commonly called seed)
Constituents: Volatile oil (with limonene, β-selinene, butylphthalide, etc.), alkyl-phthalides (in volatile oil: butylphthalide, etc.), furanocoumarins, flavonoids (flavones: luteolin; etc.), fixed oil, etc.
Properties: Aromatic, stomachic, carminative, diuretic, antibacterial, antifungal, antispasmodic, sedative, emmenagogue.
Uses: Celery fruit is chiefly used as a spice and it is beneficial for nonulcer dyspepsia (with flatulence, minor cramps). <u>Internally</u> it is used (as a tea, h. p.) for minor inflammatory and spastic conditions of the genitourinary tract (cystitis, urethritis, leukorrhea, gravel, nonobstructive urinary stones), primary dysmenorrhea (= painful menstruation without pathology), and as an antidyscratic (= blood purifier) and mild sedative (tea, h. p.) for chronic rheumatic complaints and minor nervousness. To enhance the effects in problems of the genitourinary tract, the fluid intake (incl. herbal teas) should be more than 2 liters per day.
Caution: Celery fruit should not be taken during pregnancy and lactation, in cases of impaired renal function, and before using it for dysmenorrhea, the gynecologic problem should be judged by a health professional. When handling the herb avoid contact with skin and when taking its products, avoid exposure to strong sunrays as it may cause phototoxic skin irritations. Otherwise, there are no reports of contraindications or side effects when used properly.

Root

Constituents: Volatile oil, a sugar alcohol (mannitol), polysaccharides, phenolic acids, furanocoumarins, amino acids, a biogenic amine (choline), polyacetylenes, etc.

Properties: Stomachic, carminative, diuretic.

Uses: Celery root is chiefly used as a spice and it is beneficial for nonulcer dyspepsia (with flatulence, minor cramps). Internally it is used as a flushing-out treatment (= herbal tea or product + liquids: more than 2 liters per day; sometimes combined with a medication) for inflammations of the genitourinary tract (cystitis, etc.), urinary gravel and nonobstructive stones, to prevent relapsing urinary infections / gravel / stones, and as an antidyscratic (= blood purifier; tea, h. p.) for chronic rheumatic complaints.

Caution: See Fruit.

Aerial part

Constituents: Volatile oil (with limonene, etc.), furanocoumarins, flavonoids, phenolic acids, etc.

Properties: Aromatic, stomachic, carminative, diuretic.

Uses: Fresh celery is chiefly used as a spice and it is beneficial for loss of appetite, nonulcer dyspepsia and minor complaints of the genitourinary tract. Dried celery is used as a diuretic.

Caution: Avoid consumption of excessive amounts during pregnancy and lactation. It may cause phototoxic skin irritations (see Fruit).

References: (1) Vol. 4, p. 292; (3) Vol. 3, p. 122; (6) p. 183; (8) p. 61; (9) p. 141; (13) p. 129; (15) p. 28; (17) p. 75; (24) p. 301; (26) p. 67; (27) p. 311; (46) p. 1451; (47) p. 551; (51) p. 128.

CENTAURY

Other Common Name(s): common centaury, lesser centaury

Botanical Name(s): *Centaurium erythraea* Rafn = *Erythraea centaurium* Borkh. [Fam.: Gentianaceae]

Aerial part

Constituents: Bitter principles (seco-iridoids: chiefly swertiamarin, also sweroside, centapicrin, etc.), seco-iridoid alkaloids (gentianine, etc.), xanthones, triterpenes, phenolic acids, flavonoids, etc.

Properties: Digestive secretagogue (increases secretions of the mouth, stomach, liver and pancreas), anti-inflammatory, antipyretic. It acts much like gentian, but milder. See GENTIAN.

Uses: Internally it is used (as a tea, h. p.) for loss of appetite and nonulcer dyspepsia (with fullness, burping, heartburn, flatulence, minor cramps, sluggish bowels, minor constipation), particularly recommended for children and the elderly. It is also used for convalescence, minor fatigue, decreased resistance to infections and for feverish states.

Caution: Unless advised by a health professional, centaury should not be taken during pregnancy and lactation. At higher doses than recommended it causes gastrointestinal irritations (with nausea, vomiting, diarrhea). Otherwise, there are no reports of contraindications or side effects when used properly.

References: (1) Vol. 4, p. 759; (3) Vol. 3, p. 788; (6) pp. 133, 134, 290; (8) p. 131; (12) p. 454; (13) p. 163; (16) p. 138; (17) p. 141; (19) p. 224; (20) p. 67; (23) p. 58; (27) P. 84; (28) pp. 96, 97; 104; (46) p. 274; (47) p. 873.

CERBERA

Other Common Name(s): Madagascar ordeal bean, gray milkwood
Botanical Name(s): *Cerbera manghas* L. = *Cerbera odollam* Gaertn. = *Tanghinia venenifera* Poir. [Fam.: Apocynaceae]
Seed
Constituents: Cardiac glycosides such as cerberin (= acetylneriifolin), neriifolin, cerberoside, etc., which are closely related to digitalis glycosides. It also contains lignans (cerberalignans).
Properties: Digitalis-like cardioactive. It is reported to have an onset of action shorter than digitoxin. See DIGITALIS.
Uses: Much like digitalis. See DIGITALIS.
Caution: Cerbera is very toxic and not for self-treatment. It is used only as directed by a health professional. Cerbera products should be standardized to the cardiac glycosides content. See DIGITALIS.

References: (1) Vol. 4, p. 788; (3) Vol. 3, p. 815; (41) Vols. 1-7; (42) p. 636; (52) p. 171.

CEREUS, NIGHT-BLOOMING

Other Common Name(s): queen-of-the-night
Botanical Name(s): *Selenicereus grandiflorus* (L.) Britton et Rose = *Cactus grandiflorus* L. = *Cereus grandiflorus* (L.) Mill. [Fam.: Cactaceae]
Flower (flower buds), **aerial part** (flowers and attached stems)
Constituents: Biogenic amines (tyramine, hordenine = N, N-dimethyltyramine, etc.), flavonoids (flavonols: rutin, etc.), etc.
Properties: Cardiotonic, "vitamin P"-like. At recommended doses, due in large part to tyramine, night-blooming cereus increases the contractility of the heart muscle. Tyramine is indirect-acting sympathomimetic, which when taken orally is mainly inactivated by monoamine oxidase (= MAO). When found unchanged in the bloodstream, in small concentrations it increases the contractility of the heart muscle (= positive inotropic effect), among other effects. Flavonols, with their "vitamin P"-like effect (see BUCKWHEAT), contribute positively to the overall effect on the cardiovascular system.
Uses: Internally it is used (as an h. p.; usually combined with other herbs) for minor cardiac insufficiency (with fatigability and difficulty in breathing) and minor cases of hypotension (= low blood pressure) often associated with nervous exhaustion, infectious diseases, anemia and abuse with alcohol,

nicotine and caffeine, and as an adjuvant for menorrhagia / hypermenorrhea (= prolonged / heavy menstruation).

Caution: Night-blooming cereus is best used on health professional's advice. A possible combination with cardioactive herbs (hawthorn, lily-of-the-valley, etc.) should be made only by a health professional. Doses higher than recommended should be avoided because the possible unchanged tyramine may increase blood pressure, among other effects. A concomitant use with MAOI antidepressant drugs (e. g. phenelzine) or herbs (e. g. St. John's wort) as well as certain antihypertensive drugs (reserpine, guanethidine) should be avoided as it may lead to synergistic effects.

References: (1) Vol. 6, p. 658; (3) Vol. 6b, p. 352; (6) p. 43; (12a) p. 449; (13) p. 423; (16) p. 99; (20) p. 68; (24) p. 377; (37) p. 1254; (46) p. 173; (47) p. 752; (49) Vol. 1, p. 154; (67) p. 492.

CHAMOMILE, GERMAN

Other Common Name(s): true chamomile
Botanical Name(s): *Matricaria recutita* L. = *Chamomilla recutita* (L.) Rauschert = *Matricaria chamomilla* L. = *Matricaria suaveolens* L. [Fam.: Asteraceae (Compositae)]

Flower

Constituents: Volatile oil (with sesquiterpenes: α-bisabolol, chamazulene, etc.; a polyacetylene: *cis*-en-in-dicycloether; etc.), flavonoids (flavones: apigenin glycosides, etc.), coumarins (umbelliferone, etc.), mucilaginous polysaccharides, a bitter principle (a sesquiterpene lactone, namely matricin: precursor of chamazulene), etc.

Properties: Mild edative, anti-inflammatory, antispasmodic and mild carminative, antiulcer (= prevents or helps in healing peptic ulcers), wound-healing, antibacterial, antifungal, mild immunomodulant. The mild sedative effect is due at least in part to apigenin. The anti-inflammatory effect is due to chamazulene, α-bisabolol, cis-en-in-dicycloether, matricin and flavonoids. The antispasmodic, antibacterial and antifungal effects are due to α-bisabolol, chamazulene, en-in-dicycloether, flavonoids and coumarins. α-Bisabolol has shown antiulcer effects. The immunostimulant effect is attributed to the mucilaginous polysaccharides.

Uses: Internally it is used (as a tea, h. p.) for minor inflammatory, ulcerative and spastic conditions of the gastrointestinal tract (gastritis, peptic ulcers, flatulence, nausea, irritable bowel syndrome, etc.), primary dysmenorrhea (= painful menstruation without pathology), and (as an inhalation, lozenge) for inflammations of the upper respiratory tract. Chamomile is also recommended to enhance the effects of antimicrobial therapies. Externally it is used (as a mouthwash, gargle, paint, gel) for inflammations of the mouth and throat, (as eardrops) for otitis media, (wet compress, poultice) for sore nipples, hemorrhoids and varicose ulcers, and (as a sitz bath) for anal and genital inflammations and primary dysmenorrhea. It is an ingredient in numerous hair wash, hair dye and skin-care products.

Caution: In very rare cases it may cause allergic contact dermatitis to persons hypersensitive to other Asteraceae plants (e. g. arnica, feverfew, ragweed, tansy, yarrow) that contain sesquiterpene lactones. Before using chamomile for gynecologic disorders, the problem should be judged by a health professional. Otherwise, there are no reports of contraindications or side effects when used properly.

References: (1) Vol. 4, p. 817; (3) Vol. 5, p. 710; (6) pp. 112, 115, 137; (8) p. 358; (12) p. 699; (13) pp. 119, 316; (14) p. 154; (15) p. 139; (16) pp. 29, 89, 142; (17) p. 375; (19) p. 120; (20) p. 69; (46) p. 190; (47) p. 894; (48) p. 520; (59) p. 86; (63): Vol. 1, p. 235.

CHAMOMILE, ROMAN

Other Common Name(s): English chamomile, dog fennel
Botanical Name(s): *Chamaemelum nobile* (L.) All. = *Anthemis nobilis* L. [Fam.: Asteraceae (Compositae)]
Flower
Constituents: Volatile oil (with esters of angelic acid, etc. with butyl, isoamyl alcohols, etc.; pinocarvone, chamazulene, bisabolol, etc.), bitter principles (sesquiterpene lactones: nobilin, etc.), flavonoids, coumarins, polyacetylenes (dehydromatricariaesters), mucilaginous polysaccharides, etc.
Properties: Aromatic, mild bitter tonic, anti-inflammatory and antispasmodic, diuretic, and it is claimed to be mild emmenagogic. Compared to German chamomile its bitter taste is stronger, while it exerts weaker effects as anti-inflammatory and antispasmodic.
Uses: Internally it is used (as a tea, h. p.; usually combined with other herbs) for minor digestive disorders (impaired appetite and digestion, with burping, bloating, sluggish bowels) and primary dysmenorrhea (= painful menstruation without pathology). Externally it is chiefly used as an ingredient in numerous hair wash and hair dye products.
Caution: Roman chamomile is more likely than German chamomile to cause allergic contact dermatitis to persons hypersensitive to other Asteraceae plants (e. g. arnica, feverfew, ragweed, tansy, yarrow) that contain sesquiterpene lactones. Before using it for dysmenorrhea, the gynecologic problem should be judged by a health professional. Otherwise, there are no reports of contraindications or side effects when used properly.

References: (1) Vol. 4, p. 808; (3) Vol. 3, p. 108; (8) p. 141; (12) p. 679; (14) p. 191; (17) p. 144; (20) p. 72; (23) p. 48; (46) p. 187; (47) p. 300.

CHANG SHAN

Botanical Name(s): *Dichroa febrifuga* Lour. [Fam.: Hydrangeaceae]
Root (chang shan), **leaf** (shu chi, chunine)

Constituents: Quinazoline alkaloids, including febrifugine (= β- and γ-di-chroine), isofebrifugine (= α-dichroine) and 4-quinazolone. It contains cou-marins (umbelliferone, etc.), among others.

Properties: Antimalarial, antipyretic. Both febrifugine and isofebrifugine have shown antiprotozoal effect, namely against *Plasmodium* spp. including to some extent *P. falciparum* and *P. vivax*, causatives of malign and benign tertian malarias. Compared to quinine, febrifugine is reported to be about 100 times stronger and isofebrifugine to be as active as quinine.

Uses: Internally it is used (as an h. p. or the isolated febrifugine) for malaria and feverish states.

Caution: Chang Shan can be used during pregnancy, but only as directed by a health professional. At higher doses than recommended it causes gastro-intestinal irritations (with nausea, vomiting, diarrhea) and may lower blood pressure. Even at normal doses it may cause nausea and vomiting.

References: (3) Vol. 4, p. 539; (9) p. 67; (12) p. 949; (13) p. 430; (31) p. 274; (37) p. 405; (48) p. 1043; (49) Vol. 2, p. 427; (80) p. 819.

CHAPARRAL

Other Common Name(s): creosote bush
Botanical Name(s): *Larrea tridentata* (Sessé et Moç. ex DC.) Coville = *Larrea mexicana* Moric. [Fam.: Zygophyllaceae]
Leaf and stem
Constituents: Resin (with lignans: chiefly NDGA = nordihydroguaiaretic acid; phenols: guaiacol derivatives; cf. GUAIACUM), mucilaginous poly-saccharides, flavonoids, triterpenes, phytosterols, wax, etc.

Properties: Antimicrobial, anti-inflammatory, diuretic. NDGA is an antiox-idant and has shown antitumoral, antimicrobial and antifungal effects. Cf. GUAIACUM

Uses: Chaparral is chiefly used for the extraction of NDGA, which is still used in some countries as an antioxidant to preserve animal fats. In tradi-tional medicine the herb has been used internally for inflammations of the upper respiratory tract (bronchitis, the common cold, etc.), gastrointestinal tract (diarrhea, etc.) and genitourinary tract (cystitis, etc.). Externally it is used (as a lotion, wet compress) for minor skin inflammations and wounds, and (as a poultice) for rheumatic pains, among others.

Caution: Internally, chaparral should be used only on health professional's advice. It should not be taken in severe liver and kidney disorders. When applied externally (herbal products, ointments, etc. that contain NDGA as an antioxidant) it may cause skin irritations to hypersensitive persons.

References: (2) Vol. 3, p. 44; (3) Vol. 5, p. 450; (9) p. 148; (11a) p. 467; (12) p. 817; (29) p. 67; (48) p. 291; (49) Vol. 2, p. 292; (52) p. 431; (55) p. 30.

CHAPARRO

Other Common Name(s): chaparro amargoso
Botanical Name(s): *Castela erecta* Turp. ssp. *erecta* = *Castelaria nichol-sonii* (Hook.) Small; *Castela erecta* Turp. ssp. *texana* (Torr. et Gray) Cronq. = *Castela texana* (Torr. et Gray) Rose [Fam.: Simaroubaceae]
Aerial part
Constituents: Bitter principles, as nortriterpenes of quassinoid type (chap-arrin, glaucarubolone, chaparrolide, glaucarubol, etc.), etc.
Properties: Bitter tonic, antipyretic, antiprotozoal. Nortriterpenes of quas-sinoid type have shown antiprotozoal (esp. against *Entamoeba* spp.,), antivi-ral, antibacterial and anthelmintic effects.
Uses: Internally it is used (as a tea, h. p.) for amebic dysentery (incl. possi-bly hepatic amebiasis), and loss of appetite and nonulcer dyspepsia (with fullness, flatulence, etc.).
Caution: Chaparro should not be taken during pregnancy and lactation. At higher doses than recommended it causes gastrointestinal irritations (with nausea, vomiting).

References: (3) Vol. 3, p. 762; (20) p. 223; (31) p. 728; (41) Vols. 1-7; (52) p. 162; (65) p. 884.

CHASTE TREE

Other Common Name(s): monk's pepper tree
Botanical Name(s): *Vitex agnus-castus* L. [Fam.: Verbenaceae]
Fruit (chasteberry, monk's pepper)
Constituents: Iridoids (agnuside = p-hydroxybenzoyl-aucubin, aucubin), flavonoids (chiefly methoxy flavones: casticin, etc.), volatile oil (with cine-ole, etc.), fixed oil, etc.
Properties: Lowers prolactin level, when this is elevated. This is thought to be due to a dopamine-mimetic effect at D-2 receptors in the pituitary (= do-pamine-D2-agonistic effect). The responsible constituents are not yet known. Rational treatments with chaste tree standardized products have re-sulted in an improvement of imbalances of female sex hormones (when se-rum level of estrogens is higher and progesterone is lower than required) and a normalized menstrual cycle.
Uses: Internally it is used (as an h. p.) for premenstrual syndrome = PMS (with breast pain = mastodynia, nervousness, irritability, insomnia, emo-tional instability, depressive mood, fatigue, headache, pelvic discomfort, nausea, loss of appetite, dyspepsia, constipation, edema, etc.), amenorrhea (= absence of menstruation), oligomenorrhea (= infrequent / scanty men-struation) and metrorrhagia (= nonmenstrual uterine bleeding).
Caution: Before using chasteberry for gynecologic disorders, the problem should be judged by a health professional. It should not be taken during pregnancy and lactation, pituitary tumors and breast cancer. Chasteberry

should not be combined with some antipsychotic drugs (those antagonists of dopamine-2 receptors, e. g. haloperidol) as it counteracts them. In rare cases it may cause allergic reaction (skin rash).

References: (1) Vol. 6, p. 1184; (3) Vol. 6c, p. 497; (6) p. 309; (7) p. 268; (9) p. 151; (12) p. 441; (13) p. 425; (16) p. 171; (19) p. 127; (20) p. 19; (22) p. 191; (23) p. 367; (48) p. 755; (50) p. 23; 206; (67) p. 449.

CHAULMOOGRA

Botanical Name(s): *Hydnocarpus kurzii* (King.) Warb. = *Taraktogenos kurzii* King. [Fam.: Flacourtiaceae]
Chaulmoogra oil
It is the fixed oil prepared by cold expression from the ripe seeds.
Constituents: Chiefly glycerides (fatty acids component: hydnocarpic, chaulmoogric and gorlic acids, also stearic, palmitic and oleic acids), phytosterols, etc.
Properties: Antibacterial (esp. against *Mycobacterium leprae*), rubefacient, counterirritant.
Uses: Internally it is used (orally, I.M. injection: Chaulmoogra oil, ethyl hydnocarpate / chaulmoograte) for leprosy. Externally it is used (as an ointment) for leprotic lesions and chronic skin diseases (psoriasis, etc.).
Caution: Due to its toxicity, unsure results and as there are available other drug alternatives, chaulmoogra oil is seldom used today.

References: (2) Vol. 2, p. 863; (3) Vol. 5, p. 110; (10) p. 72; (13) p. 393; (36) p. 187; (37) p. 680; (49) Vol. 2, p. 230; (65) p. 99.

CHEQUÉN

Other Common Name(s): cheken, chekan
Botanical Name(s): *Luma chequen* (Molina) A. Gray = Eugenia *chequen* Molina [Fam.: Myrtaceae]
Leaf
Constituents: Volatile oil (with α-pinene, cineole, etc.), tannins, flavonoids (flavonols), phenolic acids, bitter principles (chekenone, etc. of unknown structure), etc.
Properties: Antimicrobial, expectorant, astringent, diuretic. Volatile oil with its constituents accounts at least in part for the antimicrobial, expectorant and diuretic effects. Flavonols may contribute to the diuretic effect.
Uses: Internally it is used (as a tea, h. p.) for inflammations of the upper respiratory tract (bronchitis, etc.; coughs due to thickened bronchial secretion), gastrointestinal tract (diarrhea, etc.) and genitourinary tract (cystitis, etc.). To enhance the effects in problems of the genitourinary tract, the fluid

intake (incl. herbal teas) should be more than 2 liters per day. Externally it is used (as a wash, wet compress) for minor skin inflammations and wounds.

Caution: There are no reports of contraindications or side effects when used properly. Nevertheless, chequén is best avoided during pregnancy and in severe liver disorders.

References: (1) Vol. 5, p. 133; (3) Vol. 4, p. 861; (10) p. 72; (35) p. 189; (52) p. 294; (57) p. 332.

CHERRY LAUREL

Botanical Name(s): *Prunus laurocerasus* L. = *Laurocerasus officinalis* M. Roem. [Fam.: Rosaceae]
Cherry-laurel water
Constituents: Fresh leaves contain a cyanogenic glycoside (prunasin), a mixture of enzymes (emulsin), etc. When fresh leaves are crushed and mixed with water, under the action of an enzyme (prunase) prunasin is hydrolyzed to release hydrocyanic acid (toxic!), benzaldehyde and glucose. If distilled, the mixture yields cherry-laurel water (Aqua Laurocerasi) and a volatile oil (Oleum Laurocerasi aetheroleum).
Properties: Aromatic, antitussive (cough suppressant effect), antispasmodic.
Uses: Internally it is still used (as a combination product) for coughs (irritating dry coughs) and as a flavoring vehicle especially for cough remedies.
Caution: Cherry-laurel water should not be taken during pregnancy and lactation. Cherry-laurel water contains hydrocyanic acid (toxic!) and should be standardized to 0.1 %. For such a standardized product the maximal single dose is 2 ml., equal to 2-mg (0.002 g) hydrocyanic acid.

References: (3) Vol. 6a, p. 945; (10) p. 72; (37) pp. 122, 218; (47) p. 1716; (48) p. 193.

CHERVIL

Other Common Name(s): garden chervil
Botanical Name(s): *Anthriscus cerefolium* (L.) Hoffm. [Fam.: Apiaceae (Umbelliferae)]
Aerial part
Constituents: Volatile oil (with estragole = methylchavicol, etc.), bitter principles, flavonoids (apiin, etc.), minerals (rich in potassium), etc.
Properties: Aromatic, mild bitter tonic, diuretic, antispasmodic, wound-healing, and possibly emmenagogue. Chervil is reported to decrease or stop the secretion of milk in nursing mothers.
Uses: Chervil is chiefly used fresh as a spice in culinary practice and it is beneficial for loss of appetite and nonulcer dyspepsia (with minor intestinal cramps). Internally it is used (as a tea, h. p.; combined with other herbs) as a diuretic and antidyscratic (= blood purifier) and as a natural supplement of

potassium. Externally it is used (as a poultice) for skin inflammations, eczemas, and wounds.

Caution: Chervil should not be taken during pregnancy. Unless advised by an experienced practitioner, it should not be taken during lactation. As a potassium supplement it should be used on health professional's advice.

References: (3) Vol. 3, p. 114; (9) p. 157; (27) p. 86; (29) p. 11; (37) p. 91; (45) p. 167.

CHESTNUT, SPANISH

Other Common Name(s): European chestnut
Botanical Name(s): *Castanea sativa* Mill. = *Castanea vesca* Gaertn. [Fam.: Fagaceae]
Leaf
Constituents: Tannins (chiefly ellagitannins), flavonoids (flavonols: quercetin, its glycosides, etc.), triterpenes (ursolic acid, etc.), phenolic acids (p-coumaroylquinic acid, etc.), phytosterols, etc.
Properties: Astringent, mild antitussive.
Uses: Internally it is used (as a tea, h. p.) for minor inflammations of the gastrointestinal tract (diarrhea, etc.) and upper respiratory tract (tracheitis, bronchitis, etc.; coughs: irritating cough, whooping cough). Externally it is used (as a mouthwash, gargle) for inflammations of the mouth and throat.
Caution: There are no reports of contraindications or side effects when used properly.

References: (1) Vol. 4, p. 726; (3) Vol. 3, p. 759; (6) p. 102; (8) p. 125; (9) p. 158; (15) p. 52; (17) p. 139; (23) p. 219; (27) p. 80; (35) p. 193; (46) p. 270; (47) p. 857; (51) p. 244.

CHICKWEED

Other Common Name(s): starweed, starwort
Botanical Name(s): *Stellaria media* (L.) Vill. [Fam.: Caryophyllaceae]
Aerial part
Constituents: Triterpenoid saponins, flavonoids (flavonols, etc.), coumarins, phytosterols, etc.
Properties: Expectorant, demulcent, diuretic, emollient, wound-healing, antipruritic.
Uses: Internally it is used (as a tea, h. p.) for inflammations of the upper respiratory tract (bronchitis, etc.; coughs due to thickened bronchial secretion) and as an antidyscratic (= blood purifier; tea, h. p.) for chronic rheumatic complaints and atopic eczema (= chronic eczema of internal origin). Externally it is used (as a poultice) for minor skin inflammations, wounds and ulcers, and (as an ointment) for eczemas and psoriasis.
Caution: There are no reports of contraindications or side effects when used properly.

References: (3) Vol. 6b, p. 526; (9) p. 159; (10) p. 74; (15) p. 198; (24) p. 339; (47) p. 2609; (51) p. 68; (52) p. 543.

CHICORY

Other Common Name(s): common chicory
Botanical Name(s): *Cichorium intybus* L. [Fam.: Asteraceae (Compositae)]
Leaf and root, root
Constituents: Bitter principles (sesquiterpene lactones: lactucin, lactu-copicrin; cf. LETTUCE, WILD), phenolic acids (caffeic, isochlorogenic, cichoric = 2,3-dicaffeoyl-tartaric acid, etc.), flavonoids (leaf: hyperin, etc.), inulin (root), etc.
Properties: Bitter tonic, mild choleretic, laxative, diuretic.
Uses: Internally it is used (as a tea, h. p.) chiefly for loss of appetite and nonulcer dyspepsia (with fullness, heartburn, burping, flatulence, bloating, sluggish bowels, minor constipation) associated with impaired bile secretion. Coffee substitutes are mainly produced from roots of cultivated chicory: *Cichorium intybus* L. var. *sativum* DC. (with over 50% inulin).
Caution: Chicory should not be taken in cases of biliary obstruction. In cases of nonobstructive gallstones it can be used but only on health professional's advice. Chicory may cause allergic contact dermatitis to persons hypersensitive to other Asteraceae plants (e. g. arnica, chamomile, feverfew, ragweed, tansy, yarrow) that contain sesquiterpene lactones. Otherwise, there are no reports of contraindications or side effects when used properly.

References: (1) Vol. 4, p. 867; (3) Vol. 4, p. 3; (8) p. 156; (9) p. 161; (19) p. 240; (27) p. 90; (35) p. 197; (46) p. 305; (47) p. 969; (48) p. 85; (51) p. 222.

CHIRATA

Other Common Name(s): chiretta, East Indian balmony
Botanical Name(s): *Swertia chirayita* (Roxb. ex Fleming) H. Karst. = *Swertia chirata* (Wall.) C.B. Clarke [Fam.: Gentianaceae]
Aerial part
Constituents: Bitter principles (seco-iridoids: swertiamarin, sweroside, etc.), xanthones (swerchirin, mangiferin, chiratol, etc.), xanthones (mangiferin, etc.), flavonoids, triterpenes, etc.
Properties: Bitter tonic, digestive secretagogue (increases secretions of the mouth, stomach, liver and pancreas), mild immunomodulant. Seco-iridoids and xanthones account for most of the effects. Mangiferin, like many other xanthones, has also shown monoamino oxidase (= MAO) inhibitory effects.
Uses: Internally it is used (as a tea, h. p.) for loss of appetite and nonulcer dyspepsia (with fullness, heartburn, flatulence, minor constipation, etc.) associated with chronic liver disorders. It is also used for convalescence, minor fatigue, decreased resistance to infections, and feverish states.

98

Caution: Chirata should not be taken during pregnancy and lactation. It should not be combined with MAOI antidepressant drugs (e. g. phenelzine) or herbs (e. g. St. John's wort) as it may potentiate their effect. At higher doses than recommended it may cause gastrointestinal irritations (with nausea, vomiting, diarrhea).

References: (2) Vol. 3, p. 584; (3) Vol. 6b, p. 701; (8) p. 540; (9) p. 163; (10) p. 75; (31) p. 532; (36) p. 478; (41) Vols. 1-7.

CHIVE

Other Common Name(s): chives
Botanical Name(s): *Allium schoenoprasum* L. [Fam.: Liliaceae (Alliaceae)]
Leaf
Constituents: Chief active constituents are non-volatile sulfur compounds (gamma-glutamyl peptides). It is reported to contain also vitamin C and saponins and it possibly contains free amino acids.
Properties: Much like bear's garlic, but milder. See BEAR'S GARLIC.
Uses: Chive is chiefly used as a spice in salads, soups, etc. A regular consumption of chives may be beneficial like bear's garlic (see BEAR'S GARLIC). Internally it is used in traditional medicine as an anthelmintic for intestinal worms.
Caution: Consumption of chives in excessive amounts may cause gastrointestinal discomfort (nausea, vomiting). Otherwise, there are no reports of contraindications or side effects when used properly.

References: (1) Vol. 4, p. 201; (3) Vol. 2, p. 1216; (52) p. 33.

CHLORELLA

Botanical Name(s): *Chlorella vulgaris* Beij.; *Chlorella pyrenoidosa* Chick.; *Chlorella ellipsoides* Gerneck [Fam.: Oocystaceae]; Class Chlorophyceae (green algae)
They are tiny single-celled green algae (diameter several microns) that grow in fresh waters.
Constituents: Chlorophylls (very rich), proteins (with amino acids: arginine, histidine, cysteine, glutamic acid, alanine, tyrosine, leucin, etc.), lipids (richer if it grows lacking nitrogen), carbohydrates (sucrose, maltose, etc.), minerals, vitamins (B_1, B_2, B_6, B_{12}, C, E, K, β-carotene = a provitamin A), phytosterols, carotenoids (β-carotene, loroxanthin, etc.), etc.
Properties and Uses: Processed chlorella is used as a mild tonic (supplement of proteins, minerals, incl. trace elements, and vitamins and carbohydrates). Chlorella has shown immunomodulant and antibacterial effects.
Caution: There are no reports of contraindications or side effects when used properly.

References: (5) Vol. 2, p. 4; (41) Vols. 1-7; (42) Vol. 1, p. 46; (49) Vol. 1, p. 357; (69) p. 50.

CINCHONA

Other Common Name(s): red cinchona
Botanical Name(s): *Cinchona pubescens* Vahl = *Cinchona succirubra* Pavon; *Cinchona officinalis* L. [Fam.: Rubiaceae]
Bark
Constituents: Quinoline alkaloids, including (−)-quinine, (+)-quinidine, etc., bitter principles (triterpenoid glycosides: collectively referred to as quinovin; quinine), tannins (condensed t.), phlobaphenes (cinchona red), phenolic acids (quinic acid, etc.), etc.
Properties: Bitter tonic, antimalarial, antipyretic, astringent. Except the astringent effect, which is due to tannins, quinine accounts in large part for the other mentioned effects. Quinine is plasmodicidal, active against all *Plasmodium* spp. causatives of different malarias. Quinine is also a mild muscle relaxant. Quinidine is an antiarrhythmic drug.
Uses: Internally it is used (as a tea, h. p.) for loss of appetite and nonulcer dyspepsia (with fullness, flatulence, bloating), feverish states, and minor fatigue and convalescence. Quinine is still used for malarias, systremma (= cramp in the calf of the leg), and (as a combination product) for feverish states and the common cold. Quinidine is used for cardiac arrhythmias.
Caution: Cinchona should not be taken during pregnancy and lactation and in peptic ulcers. It should not be taken for a prolonged period as it may lead to a chronic intoxication, cinchonism (with disturbed vision and hearing, headache, dizziness, vomiting, urticaria, etc.). At higher doses than recommended it causes gastrointestinal irritations (with nausea, vomiting, diarrhea). Unless directed by a health professional, a combination of cinchona with anticoagulants (warfarin, etc.) should be avoided as it may potentiate their effect. Quinine and quinidine are prescription drugs.
Note: Yellow cinchona bark derives from *Cinchona calisaya* Wedd. = *Cinchona ledgeriana* Moens. It is chiefly used for the industrial production of quinine as quinine makes its chief alkaloid constituent.

References: (1) Vol. 4, p. 874; (3) Vol. 4, p. 13; (8) p. 159; (11) p. 157; (12) p. 1044; (13) p. 250; (17) p. 150; (19) p. 64; (36) p. 397; (37) p. 332; (46) p. 289; (47) p. 946; (48) p. 1029; (72) nr. 63034.

CINNAMON

Other Common Name(s): Ceylon cinnamon, true cinnamon
Botanical Name(s): *Cinnamomum verum* J. Presl. = *Cinnamomum zeylanicum* Nees [Fam.: Lauraceae]
Bark
Constituents: Volatile oil (chiefly with cinnamic aldehyde, also eugenol, etc.), tannins (proanthocyanidins), mucilage, mannitol, phenolic acids, etc.

Properties: Aromatic, gastrointestinal tonic (increases gastric secretion and bowel motility), mild tonic, antibacterial, antifungal, astringent, demulcent, antioxidant. Cinnamic aldehyde has been shown to be indirect-acting sympathomimetic. This explains its tonic effect especially on the cardiovascular system, among others. Cinnamic acid, normally an oxidation product of cinnamic aldehyde, has shown cytostatic effect against certain tumors.

Uses: Cinnamon is extensively used as a flavor ingredient in culinary practice and food and pharmaceutical industries, and it is beneficial also due to its antioxidant effect. Internally it is used (as a tea, h. p.) for loss of appetite and nonulcer dyspepsia (with fullness, flatulence, minor cramps, sluggish bowels), inflammations of the gastrointestinal tract (minor diarrhea, etc.) and upper respiratory tract (esp. the common cold, also as a diaphoretic and tonic hot tea), minor fatigue, and it may be beneficial for low sexual drive and erectile dysfunction.

Caution: Unless consumed in small amounts as a flavor or advised by a health professional, it should not be taken during pregnancy. Due to cinnamic aldehyde it may cause allergic reactions when hypersensitive to it. Otherwise, there are no reports of contraindications or side effects when used properly.

Note: Chinese cinnamon or cassia derives from *Cinnamomum aromaticum* Nees = *Cinnamomum cassia* Nees ex Blume. Its volatile oil contains chiefly cinnamic aldehyde and very small amounts of eugenol.

References: (1) Vol. 4, p. 900; (3) Vol. 4, p. 50; (8) p. 167; (9) p. 167; (11) p. 96; (12) p. 666; (13) p. 130; (15) p. 68; (19) p. 251; (20) p. 76; (27) p. 70; (29) p. 31; (46) p. 218; (48) p. 548; (59) p. 95.

CINNAMON, WHITE

Other Common Name(s): canella, pepper cinnamon
Botanical Name(s): *Canella winterana* (L.) Gaertn. = *Canella alba* Murray [Fam.: Canellaceae]

Bark

Constituents: Volatile oil (with eugenol, 1,8-cineole, etc.), sesquiterpenes (canellal, etc.), resin (designated as canellin, probably of bitter taste), mannitol, phytosterols, etc.

Properties: Aromatic, stomachic, antimicrobial, tonic.

Uses: White cinnamon is chiefly used as a spice, also as a flavor ingredient in tobacco and liqueur / liquor industries. Internally it is used (as a tea, h. p.) for nonulcer dyspepsia (with flatulence, minor cramps) and as a diaphoretic hot tea for feverish states and the common cold. Externally it is used (as a gargle, mouthwash) for inflammations of the mouth and throat and (as a wet compress) for rheumatic pains.

Caution: White cinnamon should not be consumed in excessive amounts during pregnancy. Otherwise, there are no reports of contraindications or side effects when used properly.

References: (2) Vol. 2, p. 277; (3) Vol. 3, p. 650; (5) Vol. 1, p. 214; (35) p. 202; (36) p. 278; (45) p. 180; (52) p. 148.

CLARY SAGE

Other Common Name(s): clary, muscatel sage
Botanical Name(s): *Salvia sclarea* L. [Fam.: Lamiaceae (Labiatae)]
Aerial part
Constituents: Volatile oil (see Clary sage oil), Lamiaceae tannins (rosmarinic acid and other caffeic acid derivatives), a diterpenoid alcohol (sclareol), triterpenes (ursolic acid, etc.), wax, etc.
Properties: Aromatic, stomachic, antispasmodic, carminative, emmenagogue, sedative, antimicrobial.
Uses: Internally it is used (as a tea, h. p.) for nonulcer dyspepsia (with flatulence, cramps, etc.), primary dysmenorrhea (= painful menstruation without pathology), secondary amenorrhea and oligomenorrhea (= ceased / infrequent / scanty menstruation without pathology), and headache. Externally it is used (as a mouthwash, gargle) for inflammations of the mouth and throat and (as a wash, wet compress) for wounds. Clary sage is used as a flavor ingredient in liqueur / liquor industry.
Caution: Clary sage is best avoided during pregnancy. For gynecologic disorders the problem should be judged by a health professional. Otherwise, there are no reports of contraindications or side effects when used properly.
Clary sage oil, concrète, absolut
Clary sage oil is the volatile oil obtained by steam distillation from the fresh aerial parts. Concrète is a waxy residue obtained after removing the solvent from a hydrocarbon extract of clary sage. Absolute is a waxy residue obtained after removing the alcohol from an alcoholic extract of clary sage.
Constituents: Clary sage oil contains chiefly linalyl-acetate and linalool, but very small amounts of sclareol. Concrète and absolut contain sclareol in a very high percentage.
Properties and Uses: Clary sage oil is used as a fragrance ingredient, while concrète and absolut are used as fixatives in cosmetics and perfumery.
Caution: There are no reports of skin irritations when applying products of clary sage oil and concrète.

References: (1) Vol. 6, p. 565; (3) Vol. 6b, p. 249; (5) Vol. 1, p. 960; (9) p. 173; (10) p. 78; (35) p. 203; (45) p. 263; (52) p. 692.

CLOVE

Other Common Name(s): clove tree
Botanical Name(s): *Syzygium aromaticum* (L.) Merr. et L.M. Perry = *Eugenia caryophyllata* Thunb. [Fam.: Myrtaceae]
Clove (flower bud)

102

Constituents: Volatile oil (see Clove oil), triterpenes (oleanolic acid, etc.), flavonoids, tannins (hydrolyzable t.), phenolic acids, etc.

Properties: Aromatic, antioxidant, local anesthetic, antibacterial, antiviral, antifungal, antispasmodic, anti-inflammatory (by inhibiting biosynthesis of prostaglandins and leukotrienes), astringent, antiulcer (= prevents or helps in healing peptic ulcers), platelet aggregation inhibitory, and possibly liver protective.

Uses: Externally it is used (as a mouthwash, gargle) for inflammations of the mouth and throat, (as a mouthwash, chewing) for bad breath, (as a cotton swab or pasty mass applied to the tooth, or by chewing the herb) for toothache, and (as a liniment, paint) for fungal skin infections. Internally it is used (as a tea, h. p.) for inflammatory and spastic conditions of the gastro-intestinal tract (nausea, flatulence, cramps, diarrhea, minor peptic ulcers) and upper respiratory tract (bronchitis, laryngitis with hoarseness, the common cold, influenza). Clove may be helpful for primary dysmenorrhea (= painful menstruation without pathology) by taking it 24-48 hours before menstrual flow, then continuing through 1-2 days of the cycle. Clove is widely used as a flavor ingredients in food industry.

Caution: There are no reports of contraindications or side effects when used properly.

Clove oil

It is the volatile oil obtained by steam distillation from the cloves.

Constituents: Chiefly eugenol, also eugenyl acetate, β-caryophyllene, etc.

Properties: Aromatic, antioxidant, local anesthetic, counterirritant, antibacterial, antifungal, antiviral.

Uses: Externally it is used (clove oil, eugenol) in dentistry for topical anesthesia and as an antiseptic. Clove oil is used in flavoring food and drug products. Eugenol is used for the semisynthetic production of vanillin.

Caution: Clove oil and eugenol should be used in moderate amounts as they irritate the mucous membranes.

References: (1) Vol. 6, p. 855; (3) Vol. 6b, p. 714; (9) p. 174; (10) p. 79; (17) p. 136; (19) p. 90; (20) p. 79; (22) p. 176; (27) p. 124; (28) p. 193; (46) p. 633; (48) p. 553; (68) p. 55.

CLUBMOSS

Other Common Name(s): club moss
Botanical Name(s): *Lycopodium clavatum* L. [Fam.: Lycopodiaceae]
Aerial part
Constituents: Alkaloids (lycopodium a.: lycopodine, clavatine, etc.), flavonoids, phenolic acids, minerals (aluminum, etc.), sugars, triterpenes, fixed oil, phytosterols, etc.

Properties: Diuretic, antispasmodic. Lycopodium alkaloids have been shown to be toxic.

Uses: Clubmoss is used only in traditional medicine and as directed by ex perienced practitioners. Internally the aerial part is used (as an h. p.; usually combined with other herbs) for inflammatory and spastic conditions of the genitourinary tract (cystitis, gravel, nonobstructive stones) and primary dysmenorrhea (= painful menstruation without pathology). To enhance the effects in problems of the genitourinary tract, the fluid intake (incl. herbal teas) should be more than 2 liters per day.

Caution: Clubmoss should be used only as directed by an experienced practitioner and not for prolonged period. At higher doses than recommended it causes gastrointestinal irritations (with nausea, vomiting, diarrhea).

Lycopodium (vegetable sulfur)

With lycopodium or vegetable sulfur is to be understood the spores separated from the clubmoss or other related *Lycopodium* spp. Lycopodium is very rich in fixed oil and is used in pharmaceutical and cosmetic industries as an ingredient in nonstick dusting powders, among others.

References: (2) Vol. 3, p. 122; (3) Vol. 5, p. 601; (8) p. 347; (13) p. 417; (17) p. 360; (36) p. 364; (37) p. 846; (47) p. 1802; (49) Vol. 1, p. 372; (51) p. 230; (55) p. 115; (65) p. 110; (66) p. p. 333.

CNIDIUM

Botanical Name(s): *Cnidium monnieri* (L.) Cusson ex Juss. [Fam.: Apiaceae (Umbelliferae)]

Fruit

Constituents: Coumarins (osthol, etc.), furanocoumarins (bergaptene, oroselone, imperatorin, edultin), volatile oil (chiefly with monoterpenes, also polyacetylenes) and very possibly the interesting alkyl-phthalides.

Properties: Antifungal (against *Tinea* spp. and other dermatophytes), antibacterial, antiprotozoal (agaist *Trichomonas* spp., *Plasmodium* spp.), antitumoral, diuretic, emmenagogue, tonic, and it is claimed to be aphrodisiac.

Uses: Externally it is used (as an ointment, lotion) for fungal skin infections and (as a vaginal irrigation / sitz bath / wash) for leukorrhea and vulvovaginitis. Internally it is used (as an h. p.) for trichomoniasis and erectile dysfunction.

Caution: Cnidium should not be taken during pregnancy and lactation. When handling the herb avoid contact with skin and when taking its products avoid exposure to strong sunrays as it may cause phototoxic skin irritations. Otherwise, there are no reports of contraindications or side effects when used properly.

References: (3) Vol. 4, p. 172; (5) Vol. 1, p. 311; (42) Vol. 6, pp. 561, 563; (45) p. 190; (52) p. 201.

COCILLANA

Botanical Name(s): *Guarea rusbyi* (Britton) Rusby [Fam.: Meliaceae]

Bark

Constituents: Triterpenes, volatile oil, alkaloids, flavonoids, phytosterols, tannins, etc. Cocillana may contain bitter principles (nortriterpenes of limonoid type).

Properties: (At low doses): Expectorant, laxative. (At high doses): Emetic, drastic purgative, emmenagogue.

Uses: Internally it is used (as a tea, h. p.) for inflammations of the upper respiratory tract (bronchitis, etc.; coughs due to thickened bronchial secretion), similar to Ipecac.

Caution: Cocillana should not be taken during pregnancy and lactation and is best used as directed by an experienced practitioner. At higher doses than recommended it causes gastrointestinal irritations (with nausea, vomiting, diarrhea).

References: (2) Vol. 2, p. 821; (3) Vol. 4, p. 1209; (10) p. 82; (14) p. 63; (15) p. 108; (36) p. 379; (41) Vols. 1-7; (52) p. 352; (61) p. 301.

CODONOPSIS

Other Common Name(s): 1) bellflower; 2) bellflower, Sichuan dang shen
Botanical Name(s): 1) *Codonopsis pilosula* (Franch.) Nannf.; 2) *Codonopsis tangshen* Oliv. [Fam.: Campanulaceae]
Root (= dang shen)
Constituents: Triterpenoid saponins (tangshenosides), phytosterols (7-sterols: α-spinasterol, etc.), water-soluble polysaccharides (compounds CP-1, etc.), a β-carboline alkaloid (perlolyrine), a phenol glycoside (syringin), sesquiterpenes (atractylenolide, etc.), polyacetylenes, inulin, etc.

Properties: Adaptogenic (= increases adaptation and resistance to stress). Dang shen increases plasma levels of corticosterone, exerts immunomodulant, mild CNS stimulant and antiulcer (= prevents or helps in healing peptic ulcers) effects. Tangshenosides may account for the increase of corticosterone levels. Water-soluble polysaccharides account in large part for the immunomodulant and antiulcer effects. Possibly, through hydrolysis (in the intestinal tract) and oxidation (chiefly in the liver), syringin is converted to sinapic acid (as with the conversion of salicin of willow bark to salicylic acid). Sinapic acid has shown liver protective, antibacterial and antifungal effects. Many polyacetylenes have shown antimicrobial effects.

Uses: Internally it is used as an invigorator (tea, h. p.) for minor fatigue, feeling of weakness, decreased mental and physical performance, decreased concentration and mood, convalescence, and for chronic inflammations of the gastrointestinal tract (loss of appetite, gastritis, diarrhea), genitourinary tract (chronic nephritis) and upper respiratory tract (bronchitis, etc., bronchial asthma). Due also to 7-sterols (see PUMPKIN) it may be beneficial for early stages of benign prostatic hyperplasia (= BPH).

Caution: Normally, codonopsis should not be taken for more than 6-8 weeks. Before a possible resuming, a break for 2-3 weeks is required (see

ECHINACEA; LICORICE; GINSENG). Otherwise, there are no reports of contraindications or side effects when used properly.

References: (5) Vol. 3, p. 132; (9) p. 185; (13) p. 429; (31) pp. 46, 487; (36) p. 509; (41) Vols. 1-7; (45) p. 82; (53) p. 58.

COFFEE

Other Common Name(s): 1) Arabian coffee 2) robusta coffee
Botanical Name(s): 1) *Coffea arabica* L. 2) *Coffea canephora* Pierre ex A. Froehner = *Coffea robusta* Linden [Fam.: Rubiaceae]
Coffee charcoal
Constituents: Coffee charcoal contains less caffeine than roasted coffee.
Properties: Adsorbent, astringent.
Uses: Internally for diarrhea, gastroenteritis, flatulence and heartburn.
Caution: Coffee charcoal may impair the absorption of some drugs. In view of this, when under a vital oral medication, drugs should be taken about one hour apart from coffee charcoal.
Roasted coffee
Constituents: Purine alkaloids (chiefly caffeine, some theophylline), trigonelline, phenolic acid derivatives (chlorogenic acid, etc.), fixed oil (coffee oil), choline, aromatic substances (α-furfurylmercaptan, kahweofuran, etc.), etc.
Properties: The effects of coffee are due in large part to caffeine. Caffeine is a stimulant of the central nervous system, respiration and skeletal muscles. Its effects include cardiac stimulation, coronary dilation, smooth muscle relaxation and diuresis. Coffee, taken as a beverage, has been shown to increase gastrointestinal secretions.
Uses: Coffee is consumed as a popular stimulant beverage and its effects vary depending on the amount used and the individual, among others (see Properties).
Caution: Due to caffeine, the consumption of coffee to extensive amounts may cause nervous irritability, muscular tremor and a premature contraction of the heart. In persons with hypersensitive gastrointestinal tract, it may cause belching, cramps and diarrhea. During pregnancy coffee consumption should be in moderation.

References: (1) Vol. 4, p. 926; (3) Vol. 4, p. 186; (8) p. 176; (9) p. 187; (12) p. 1064; (13) p. 265; (16) p. 150; (19) p. 118; (22) p. 174; (36) p. 403; (46) p. 175; (48) p. 1079; (67) p. 464.

COLA

Other Common Name(s): kola
Botanical Name(s): *Cola acuminata* (Pall.) Schott et Endl.; *Cola nitida* (Vent.) A. Chev. [Fam.: Sterculiaceae]
Seed (cotyledon)

106

Constituents: Purine alkaloids (chiefly caffeine, some theobromine), tannins (proanthocyanidins), phlobaphenes (collectively referred to as kola red), flavonoids (catechins), etc. In the fresh seed, caffeine is combined with catechins and their derivatives, but during drying it is mostly freed of them.

Properties: CNS and respiratory stimulant (see COFFEE), gastrointestinal tonic (increases gastric acid secretion and bowel motility), promotes the breakdown of fats into free fatty acids and glycerol (= lipolytic effect), increases slightly the rate of the heartbeat (= positive chronotropic effect), mild diuretic (see CACAO). In cola, caffeine remains partly combined with catechins therefore it acts slower than coffee. Due to catechins and proanthocyanidins it may exert antioxidant effect.

Uses: Internally it is used as an invigorator (usually as a combination product) for minor fatigue and feeling of weakness, short-term decreased mental and physical performance and convalescence. Cola is an important ingredient in a number of soft drinks.

Caution: Cola should not be taken in cases of peptic ulcers. See COFFEE.

References: (1) Vol. 4, p. 941; (3) Vol. 4, p. 229; (8) p. 180; (9) p. 332; (13) p. 268; (14) p. 64; (19) p. 131; (23) p. 316; (36) p. 403; (46) p. 339; (48) p. 1081; (49) Vol. 2, p. 256.

COLOCYNTH

Other Common Name(s): bitter apple

Botanical Name(s): *Citrullus colocynthis* (L.) Schrad. [Fam.: Cucurbitaceae]

Fruit

Constituents: Bitter principles (triterpenes: chiefly glycosides of cucurbitacin E), phenolic acids (caffeic and chlorogenic acids, etc.), resin, volatile oil, salts of organic acids, etc.

Properties: Laxative / drastic purgative (depending on doses).

Uses: Internally it is used (only incorporated in small amounts in combination products) for constipation.

Caution: Cucurbitacin E is very toxic. Colocynth should not be taken during pregnancy and lactation and in cases of impaired renal function. Large doses cause severe gastroenteritis and kidney damage.

References: (3) Vol. 4, p. 79; (8) p. 168; (10) p. 33; (37) p. 336; (46) p. 373; (47) p. 1060; (65) p. 180; (66) p. 247.

COLTSFOOT

Botanical Name(s): *Tussilago farfara* L. [Fam.: Asteraceae (Compositae)]

Leaf

Constituents: Polysaccharides (mucilaginous polysaccharides, inulin), tannins, triterpenes, flavonoids, coumarins, phenolic acids, minerals (rich in potassium), unsaturated pyrrolizidine alkaloids (= UPAs, hepatotoxic and carcinogenic!), saturated pyrrolizidine alkaloids (non-toxic), etc.

Properties: Demulcent, antitussive (mucosal protective effect), emollient, anti-inflammatory, antibacterial. Its main effects, namely demulcent, antitussive and emollient are due to mucilaginous polysaccharides. Unsaturated pyrrolizidine alkaloids (= UPAs) have shown hepatotoxic and carcinogenic effects (see Caution).

Uses: Internally it is used (as a tea, h. p.) for inflammations of the upper respiratory tract (bronchitis, bronchial asthma, laryngitis with hoarseness; irritating dry coughs). Externally it is used (as a mouthwash, gargle) for inflammations of the mouth and throat and (as a poultice, wet compress) for skin inflammations (incl. milk crust = infantile eczema).

Caution: Coltsfoot should not be taken during pregnancy and lactation. In coltsfoot products the UPAs content should be within limits. For internal use, the daily dose of a leaf extract or expressed juice should not contain more than 1μg (= one microgram = one thousandth of milligram) UPAs. The daily dose of the leaf itself, when used as a tea, should not contain more than 10 μg UPAs. For external applications, the daily dose of the leaf should not contain more than 100 μg UPAs. Even following these limits, coltsfoot should not be used for more than 14 days in a row, and 4-6 weeks / year.

References: (1) Vol. 6, p. 1017; (3) Vol. 6c, p. 324; (6) pp. 99, 100; (8) p. 566; (15) p. 220; (17) p. 214; (20) p. 85; (23) p. 209; (27) p. 127; (28) p. 76; (35) p. 212; (47) p. 1338; (51) p. 214.

COLUMBO, AMERICAN

Botanical Name(s): *Frasera caroliniensis* Walter = *Swertia carolinensis* (Walt.) Ktze. [Fam.: Gentianaceae]

Root

Constituents: Bitter principles (iridoids: gentiopicrin, loganic acid, etc.), xanthones (methoxy derivatives: swerchirin and its glucoside, etc.), tannins (hydrolyzable t.), sugars, possibly mucilage but no starch.

Properties: Bitter tonic. Swerchirin has shown moderate MAO inhibiting and liver protective effects.

Uses: Internally it is used (as a tea, h. p.) for loss of appetite and nonulcer dyspepsia (with flatulence, minor cramps), minor fatigue and convalescence. American columbo has been used as a substitute for Calumba (q. v.).

Caution: Unless advised by a health professional, it should not be taken during pregnancy and lactation. It should not be combined with MAOI antidepressant drugs (e. g. phenelzine) or herbs (e. g. St. John's wort) as it may potentiate their effect. At higher doses than recommended it causes gastrointestinal irritations (with nausea, vomiting, diarrhea). Otherwise, there are no reports of contraindications or side effects when used properly.

References: (3) Vol. 4, p. 1049; (10) p. 86; (31) p. 538; (41) Vols. 1-7; (44) p. 237; (52) p. 318.

COMBRETUM MICRANTHUM

Other Common Name(s): kinkéliba
Botanical Name(s): *Combretum micranthum* G. Don. = *Combretum altum* Guill. et Perr. [Fam.: Combretaceae]

Leaf

Constituents: Tannins (proanthocyanidins; rich), flavonoids (vitexin, iso-vitexin), phenolic acids, a proline-betaine (hydroxy-stachydrine), choline, a sugar alcohol (sorbitol), a cyclitol (myo-inositol), minerals (potassium), etc. It possibly contains stilbenoids as they are found in other *Combretum* spp.

Properties: Astringent, choleretic, cholagogue, antioxidant, diuretic, antimicrobial. The hepatobiliary effects may be due to phenolic acids, choline and myo-inositol. Here contribute also proanthocyanidins with their antioxidant effect. To the diuretic effect possibly contribute flavonoids, sorbitol and potassium. The astringent effect is due in large part to tannins. Stilbenoids, if present, may account for its antimicrobial effect.

Uses: Internally it is used (as a tea, h. p.; combined with other herbs) for minor hepatobiliary disorders (with impaired bile secretion and flow) and complaints associated with them (impaired digestion, flatulence, minor gastrointestinal cramps, vomiting, minor diarrhea). Combretum is also used as an antidyscratic (= blood purifier; tea, h. p.) for atopic eczema (= chronic eczema of internal origin) and chronic rheumatic complaints.

Caution: There are no reports of contraindications or side effects when used properly.

References: (3) Vol. 4, p. 253; (5) Vol. 1, p. 326; (8) p. 183; (31) p. 509; (41) Vols. 1-7; (48) pp. 302, 340; (49) Vol. 2, p. 455; (52) p. 208.

COMFREY

Botanical Name(s): *Symphytum officinale* L. [Fam.: Boraginaceae]

Root

Constituents: Allantoin, mucilaginous polysaccharides (rich), tannins (condensed t.), unsaturated pyrrolizidine alkaloids (= UPAs, hepatotoxic and carcinogenic!), etc.

Properties: Anti-inflammatory, emollient, astringent, wound-healing. The wound-healing effect is due in large part to allantoin and partly due to tannins. The other effects are due in large part to mucilage and tannins.

Uses: Externally it is used (as an ointment, paste, poultice, wet compress) for minor skin inflammations, bruises, sprains, injuries, fractures, and boils.

Caution: Due to the risk of hepatotoxic and carcinogenic effects, the internal use is no longer recommended. In comphrey products, the UPAs content should be within limits. For dosage limits of UPAs see COLTSFOOT.
Comphrey should not be applied when the skin is damaged, during pregnancy and in infacts. Comphrey applications should be limited to 4-6 weeks.

References: (3) Vol. 6b, p. 706; (8) p. 541; (9) p. 190; (13) p. 270; (14) p. 66; (16) p. 40; (17) p. 568; (19) p. 41; (20) p. 87; (23) p. 337.

CONDURANGO

Other Common Name(s): condor vine
Botanical Name(s): *Marsdenia cundurango* Reichb. f. [Fam.: Asclepiadaceae]
Bark
Constituents: Bitter principles (saponin-like glycosides: collectively referred to as condurangin), phenolic acids (chlorogenic acid, etc.), coumarins, flavonoids, a cyclitol (conduritol), etc.
Properties: Bitter tonic, gastric sedative.
Uses: Internally it is used (as a tea, h. p.; usually combined with other herbs) for loss of appetite and nonulcer dyspepsia and it is beneficial also when these complaints are of nervous origin (due to stress, etc.). It is also recommended for patients with stomach tumors as it improves appetite and at the same time has been shown to decrease nausea.
Caution: There are no reports of contraindications or side effects when used properly. As condurangin is soluble in cold water, not in hot water, the prepared decoction should be strained at room temperature.

References: (1) Vol. 5, p. 782; (3) Vol. 5, p. 706; (6) pp. 132, 290; (8) p. 356; (12) p. 600; (13) p. 165; (15) p. 138; (16) p. 136; (17) p. 160; (23) p. 60; (37) p. 864; (46) p. 380; (47) p. 1070; (48) p. 754.

COPAIBA

Botanical Name(s): *Copaifera officinalis* (Jacq.) L. = *Copaifera jacquini* Desf.; *Copaifera langsdorfii* Desf.; *Copaifera multijuga* Hayne [Fam.: Fabaceae (Caesalpiniaceae)]
Balsam of copaiba (copaiba)
It is obtained by tapping the trunks. Copaiba is in fact an oleoresin as it doesn't contain benzoic and cinnamic acids.
Constituents: Volatile oil (copaiba oil), which consists chiefly of β-bisabolene, caryophyllene and copaene, and a resin, which consists of diterpenoid acids (copalic and copaiferic acids).
Properties: Diuretic, antimicrobial, carminative, stimulant.
Uses: Internally it is used (as an h. p.; usually combined with other herbs) for chronic inflammations of the genitourinary tract (cystitis, urethritis, prostatitis, leukorrhea), gastrointestinal tract (flatulence, sluggish bowels, minor constipation) and upper respiratory tract (bronchitis, etc.; coughs). To enhance the effects in problems of the genitourinary tract, the fluid intake (incl. herbal teas) should be more than 2 liters per day. It has also been used for chronic skin diseases (psoriasis, etc.). Externally it is used (as a liniment, ointment) for minor skin inflammations, wounds and ulcers. Both balsam and oil are used in cosmetics and perfumery.

110

Caution: Copaiba should not be taken in cases of impaired renal function. Dosed higher than recommended cause gastrointestinal irritations (with nausea, vomiting, diarrhea), genitourinary tract (nephritis) and nervous system (nervousness, insomnia). Topically, copaiba may cause allergic reactions and if applied in higher concentrations or left on site longer than advised it may cause blisters.

References: (2) Vol. 2, p. 422; (3) Vol. 4, p. 283; (8) p. 190; (9) p. 61; (10) p. 89; (36) p. 288; (37) p. 175; (47) p. 656; (49) Vol. 2, p. 25; (66) p. 251.

COPALCHI

Other Common Name(s): 1) copalchi 2) Coutarea latiflora, copalchi
Botanical Name(s): 1) *Hintonia latiflora* (Sessé et Moç. ex DC.) Bullock 2) *Coutarea latiflora* Moç. et Sessé [Fam.: Rubiaceae]
Bark
Constituents: Bitter principles (cucurbitacins), flavonoids, neoflavonoids (= 4-phenyl-coumarins), phenolic acids, tannins (condensed t.), etc., but no quinine.
Properties: Bitter tonic, antiprotozoal (against *Plasmodium falciparum* = causative for malignant tertian malaria), mild antihyperglycemic.
Uses: Internally it is used (as a tea, h. p.) for nonulcer dyspepsia, feverish states and malaria and as an adjuvant for diabetes.
Caution: There are no reports of contraindications or side effects when used properly. Nevertheless, it should be avoided during pregnancy and lactation. At higher doses than recommended it causes nausea, vomiting and profuse perspiration.

References: (1) Vol. 5, p. 443; (5) Vol. 3, p. 281; (23) p. 142; (41) Vols. 1-7; (52) p. 374; (72) nr. 11082.

COPTIS

Other Common Name(s): 1) Chinese goldthread, coptis 2) Japanese goldthread 3) Indian / Tibetian goldthread 4) Greenlandic goldthread
Botanical Name(s): 1) *Coptis chinensis* Franch.; *Coptis deltoidea* C.Y. Cheng et P.K. Hsiao; 2) *Coptis japonica* (Thunb.) Makino; 3) *Coptis teeta* Wall.; 4) *Coptis groenlandica* (Oed.) Fernald [Fam.: Ranunculaceae]
Root (rhizome)
Constituents: Alkaloids chiefly of protoberberine type (chiefly berberine, also coptisine, berberastine, etc.), also benzophenanthridine type (palmatine, etc.), etc.
Properties: See BARBERRY.
Uses: See BARBERRY. From the root is isolated berberine, which as berberine sulfate is used for most of the indications given for barberry. Ber-

berine sulfate is sometimes used for conjunctivitis and Oriental sore (= cutaneous leishmaniasis).
Caution: See BARBERRY.

References: (3) Vol. 4, p. 295; (5) Vol. 1, p. 338; (10) p. 132; (12) p. 990; (13) p. 234; (29) p. 36; (37) p. 197; (59) p. 105; (89) p. 162.

CORIANDER

Botanical Name(s): *Coriandrum sativum* L. [Fam.: Umbelliferae]
Fruit (commonly called seed)
Constituents: Volatile oil (see Coriander oil), coumarins (scopoletin, umbelliferone), phenolic acids (caffeic and chlorogenic acids, etc.), flavonoids, fixed oil, proteins, etc.
Properties: Aromatic, stomachic, antispasmodic, carminative. Most of the effects are attributed to its volatile oil. Coriander oil has also shown antimicrobial effect.
Uses: Coriander is chiefly used as a spice. Internally it is used (as a tea, h. p.) for loss of appetite and nonulcer dyspepsia (with flatulence, minor cramps) and gastrointestinal inflammations (gastritis, diarrhea, etc.). In pharmaceutical and food industries it is used as a flavor ingredient and it is added to anthranoid laxatives (Cascara sagrada, etc.) to prevent their griping effect. Externally it is used (as a mouthwash, chewing) for bad breath.
Caution: There are no reports of contraindications or side effects when used properly. In rare cases it may cause contact allergic reactions.
Coriander oil
It is the volatile oil obtained by steam distillation from the freshly crushed fruits.
Constituents: Chiefly linalool, also geraniol, pinenes and other monoterpenes.
Properties and Uses: Coriander oil is chiefly used as a flavor and fragrance ingredient in liqueur / liquor and cosmetic / perfume industries.
Caution: There are no reports of contraindications or side effects when used properly.

References: (1) Vol. 4, p. 996; (3) Vol. 4, p. 300; (8) p. 192; (9) p. 193; (12) p. 661; (13) p. 124; (16) p. 125; (17) p. 165; (19) p. 132; (23) p. 84; (37) p. 361; (46) p. 396; (48) p. 518; (51) p. 126.

CORN

Other Common Name(s): maize
Botanical Name(s): *Zea mays* L. [Fam.: Poaceae (Gramineae)]
Cornsilk
Constituents: Saponins, minerals (rich in potassium), tannins, flavonoids (6-C-glycosyl-flavones: maysin, etc.), volatile oil (with carvacrol, thymol),

mucilaginous polysaccharides, sugars, allantoin, phytosterols (β-sitosterol, etc.), fixed oil, hydrocarbons, etc.

Properties: Mild diuretic, urinary demulcent, anti-inflammatory.

Uses: Internally it is used (usually combined with other herbs) as a flushing-out treatment (= herbal tea or product + liquids: more than 2 liters per day; sometimes combined with a medication) for inflammations of the genitourinary tract (cystitis, ureteritis, pyelitis, etc.), urinary gravel and nonobstructive stones, to prevent relapsing urinary infections / gravel / stones, and (as a tea, h. p.) for any condition where diuresis is advisable.

Caution: There are no reports of contraindications or side effects when used properly. Nevertheless, a flushing-out treatment is contraindicated in cases of obstructive urinary stones, edema due to impaired heart or kidney function and kidney inflammations (here can be used on health professional's advice to enhance the effects of an antimicrobial therapy).

References: (3) Vol. 6c, p. 550; (10) p. 91; (14) p. 69; (15) p. 238; (17) p. 362; (20) p. 90; (27) p. 163; (28) p. 163; (35) p. 225; (37) p. 1490; (41) Vols. 1-7; (46) p. 908; (47) p. 2618.

CORNFLOWER

Other Common Name(s): bechelor's button, cyani
Botanical Name(s): *Centaurea cyanus* L. [Fam.: Asteraceae (Compositae)]
Flower
Constituents: Flavonoids (anthocyanins, flavones), a bitter principle (a sesquiterpene lactone: cnicin = centaurin), a coumarin (cichoriin), mucilaginous polysaccharides, triterpenes, steroids, polyacetylenes, etc.

Properties and Uses: Cornflower is chiefly used as a safe coloring ingredient in herbal teas. In traditional medicine it is used internally (as a tea) for loss of appetite, hepatobiliary disorders, constipation, and feverish states (as a diaphoretic hot tea), and externally (as an eyewash) for eye inflammations (conjunctivitis, keratitis).

Caution: There are no reports of contraindications or side effects when used properly. For hygienic reasons, its application as eyewash should be avoided.

References: (1) Vol. 4, p. 752; (3) Vol. 3, p. 784; (5) Vol. 1, p. 253; (8) p. 131; (24) p. 201; (27) p. 138; (35) p. 223.

CORYDALIS

Other Common Name(s): hollow-root birthwort
Botanical Name(s): *Corydalis cava* (L.) Schweigg. et Koerte. [Fam.: Papaveraceae]
Root (tuber)

Constituents: Aporphine alkaloids (corydaline, bulbocapnine, tetrahydro-palmatine), etc.

Properties: Sedative, hypnotic, antispasmodic. At low doses corydaline is sedative and at high doses it causes spinal cord paralysis. Bulbocapnine at small doses is sedative.

Uses: Internally it is used only as an additive in some combination products, which are used for nervous system disorders (Parkinson's disease, sleep problems, etc.) and Ménière's disease (= a sudden attack, with violent dizziness, nausea and vomiting, ringing in the ear, etc.).

Caution: Corydalis is toxic and not for self-treatment. Combinations with sedative and hypnotic drugs should be made with caution and only by a health professional. Alcoholic drinks may interact with corydalis.

Note: Root (tuber) of *Corydalis yanhusuo* W.T. Wang = *C. turtschaninovii* Bess. f. *yanhusuo* Y.H. Chou et C.C. Hsu, known also as Chinese fumewort, contains closely related alkaloids and is used for much the same problems.

References: (1) Vol. 4, p. 1018; (3) Vol. 4, p. 311; (6) pp. 214, 215; (8) p. 193; (13) p. 234; (31) p. 198; (37) p. 364; (46) p. 399; (47) p. 1103; (48) p. 921; (72) nr. 48057.

COSTUS

Other Common Name(s): aucklandia

Botanical Name(s): *Saussurea costus* (Falc.) Lipsch. = *Saussurea lappa* Decne. = *Aucklandia costus* Falc. [Fam.: Asteraceae (Compositae)]

Root

Constituents: Volatile oil (with sesquiterpenes, monoterpenes), bitter principles (sesquiterpene lactones, chiefly steam distilling: dehydrocostus lactone, costunolide, etc.), alkaloid-like compounds (saussureamines), resin, inulin, etc.

Properties: Aromatic, bitter tonic, anti-inflammatory, antispasmodic, diuretic, antimicrobial, and it is claimed to be aphrodisiac.

Uses: Costus is chiefly used as a fragrance ingredient in cosmetics and perfumery, also as a flavor ingredient in food industry. Internally it is used (as a tea, h. p.) for loss of appetite, inflammatory and spastic conditions of the gastrointestinal tract (gastritis, impaired digestion with flatulence, cramps, diarrhea, etc.) and upper respiratory tract (bronchitis, bronchial asthma; coughs). In traditional medicine it is valued as a general tonic and aphrodisiac. Externally it is used (as a wet compress, poultice) for minor skin inflammations and wounds.

Caution: Costus may cause allergic contact dermatitis to persons hypersensitive to other Asteraceae plants (e. g. arnica, chamomile, feverfew, ragweed, tansy, yarrow) that contain sesquiterpene lactones. Otherwise, there are no reports of contraindications or side effects when used properly.

References: (1) Vol. 6, p. 620; (3) Vol. 6b, p. 300; (9) p. 196; (36) p. 494; (41) Vols. 1-7; (45) p. 265; (52) p. 702.

COUCH GRASS

Other Common Name(s): dog grass, quack grass, twitch grass, graminis
Botanical Name(s): *Elymus repens* (L.) Gould = *Agropyron repens* (L.) P.
Beauv. [Fam.: Poaceae (Gramineae)]
__Root__ (rhizome)
Constituents: Polysaccharides (rich in triticin = a fructose polymer, some
mucilaginous polysaccharides), steroidal saponins, a sugar alcohol (mannitol), minerals (silicic acid: free and water-soluble), volatile oil (with carvacrol, thymol, etc.), vanillin-glucoside, etc.
Properties: Diuretic, demulcent, nutrient, mild laxative, antibacterial, antifungal (against *Trichophyton* spp. and other dermatophytes). Saponins and
silicic acid may account at least in part for the diuretic effect. Volatile oil
and its phenolic constituents may account in large part for the antibacterial
and antifungal effects.
Uses: __Internally__ it is used as a flushing-out treatment (= herbal tea or product + liquids: more than 2 liters per day; sometimes combined with a medication) for inflammations of the genitourinary tract (cystitis, urethritis, prostatitis, etc.), urinary gravel and nonobstructive stones, to prevent relapsing
urinary infections / gravel / stones, (as a tea, h. p.) for inflammations of the
gastrointestinal tract (with minor constipation), and as an antidyscratic (=
blood purifier) for atopic eczema (= chronic eczema of internal origin) and
chronic rheumatic complaints. Due to triticin, it is recommended as a dietetic aid to diabetics. __Externally__ it is used (as a wash, wet compress) for hair
loss due to fungal infections and for other skin fungal infections.
Caution: There are no reports of contraindications or side effects when used
properly. Nevertheless, a flushing-out treatment is contraindicated in cases
of obstructive urinary stones, edema due to impaired heart or kidney function and kidney inflammations (here can be used on health professional's
advice to enhance the effects of an antimicrobial therapy).

References: (1) Vol. 4, p. 138; (3) Vol. 2, p. 1153; (6) p. 185; (9) p. 213; (16) p. 164; (17) p. 265; (19) p. 184; (20) p. 91; (27) p. 160; (28) p. 163; (35) p. 370; (37) p. 32; (47) p. 2733; (48) p. 86; (49) Vol. 2, p. 14; (51) p. 46.

COW PARSNIP, AMERICAN

Botanical Name(s): *Heracleum maximum* Bartr. = *Heracleum lanatum*
Michx. [Fam.: Apiaceae (Umbelliferae)]
__Root__
Constituents: Furanocoumarins, coumarins, phenolic acids, phytosterols,
etc. Furanocoumarins found here are of linear type (strong phototoxic) and
angular type (weak phototoxic), with quality and ratio depending on origin /
varieties.
Properties: Antimicrobial, antispasmodic, stomachic, carminative, rubefacient.

115

Uses: Internally it is used (as a tea, h. p.) for minor inflammatory and spastic conditions of the upper respiratory tract (pharyngitis, laryngitis, bronchial asthma; coughs) and gastrointestinal tract (impaired digestion, flatulence, minor cramps, diarrhea). Externally it is used (as a poultice, h. p.) for bruises, sprains, boils, wounds and rheumatic pains, and (as a hair rinse) for dandruff.

Caution: American cow parsnip should not be taken during pregnancy and lactation. When handling the herb avoid contact with skin and when taking its products avoid exposure to strong sunrays as it may cause phototoxic skin irritations.

References: (1) Vol. 5, p. 433; (3) Vol. 5, p. 52; (25) p. 60; (41) Vols. 1-7; (44) p. 260.

COWSLIP

Other Common Name(s): true cowslip
Botanical Name(s): *Primula veris* L. = *Primula officinalis* (L.) Hill.; *Primula elatior* (L.) Hill. [Fam.: Primulaceae]
Root, flower
Constituents: Triterpenoid saponins (root, flower: primulic acid A, etc.), phenol glycosides (root: primulaverin, etc.), free salicylates (root: methyl salicylate, etc.; liberated from phenol glycosides), flavonoids (flower), carotenoids (flower), volatile oil, etc.

Properties: (Root, flower): Expectorant (bronchial secretagogue effect); (root): anti-inflammatory (NSAID-like effect), antifungal (against *Candida albicans*). The bronchial secretagogic and the antifungal effects are attributed to saponins. The liberated salicylates (from root: during drying or after a product is ingested) account for the mild aspirin-like anti-inflammatory effect.

Uses: Internally it is used (as a tea, h. p.) for inflammations of the upper respiratory tract (bronchitis, laryngitis, pharyngitis, bronchial asthma; coughs: due to thickened bronchial secretion, whooping cough). Root is also used for rheumatic complaints (incl. rheumatoid arthritis). Externally it is used (root: as a mouthwash, paint, gel) for fungal infections (with *Candida albicans*) of the oral cavity.

Caution: Flowers may cause contact allergic reactions if hypersensitive to cowslip. At higher doses than recommended it causes gastrointestinal irritations (with nausea, vomiting, diarrhea). Otherwise, there are no reports of contraindications or side effects when used properly.

References: (1) Vol. 6, p. 277; (3) Vol. 6a, p. 872; (6) p. 101; (8) p. 461; (12) p. 537; (13) p. 206; (16) p. 62; (17) pp. 254, 257; (19) pp. 183, 202; (20) p. 92; (23) p. 214; (24) p. 291; (35) p. 229; (48) p. 702; (87) Vol. 2, p. 10.

116

CRAMP BARK

Other Common Name(s): guelder rose, high-bush cranberry, wild snowball
Botanical Name(s): *Viburnum opulus* L. [Fam.: Caprifoliaceae]
Bark
Constituents: Not well known. It is reported to contain a bitter principle (viburnin = glucoside of valerianic acid?), flavonoids (flavan-3-ols = catechins), coumarins, an alkaloid (?), resin (with valerianic acid, etc.), triterpenes (ursolic and oleanolic acids, etc.), etc.
Properties and Uses: Cramp bark has been used for the same indications as black haw, including threatened abortion, false labor pains and primary dysmenorrhea (= painful menstruation without pathology). Due to insufficient data on its constituents, black haw should be used instead (see BLACK HAW).
Caution: There are no reports of contraindications or side effects when used properly. Nevertheless, before using cramp bark the gynecologic problem should be judged by a health professional. At high doses and when taken for long periods, cramp bark extracts have been shown to cause dizziness and stomach irritations (nausea, vomiting).

References: (2) Vol. 3, p. 771; (3) Vol. 6c, p. 430; (15) p. 230; (37) p. 1449; (47) p. 2807; (66) p. 498.

CRANBERRY

Other Common Name(s): American cranberry, large cranberry
Botanical Name(s): *Vaccinium macrocarpon* Aiton [Fam.: Ericaceae]
Berries
Constituents: Tannins (proanthocyanidins), flavonoids (catechin, leptosin, oxycoccin), organic acids (citric acid, quinic acid, some benzoic acid), sugars (fructose, etc.), a bitter principle (vacciniin = 6-benzoyl-glucose), triterpenes, vitamin C, etc.
Properties: Antibacterial, acidulous, refrigerant, antioxidant. The antibacterial effect in the urinary tract is widely accepted to be due in large part to the ability of cranberry to prevent the adhering of certain bacteria (*Escherichia coli*, etc.) to the epithelium of urinary passages. Its antioxidant effect is due in large part to polyphenolic compounds (tannins and flavonoids).
Uses: Internally it is used (as a tea, h. p.) chiefly to enhance the effects of an antimicrobial therapy or for the prevention of inflammations of the genitourinary tract (cystitis, urethritis). To enhance the effects, the fluid intake (incl. herbal / craneberry teas) should be more than 2 liters per day. Cranberry is widely consumed as a refreshing drink with beneficial effects on the genitourinary and gastrointestinal tracts.
Caution: There are no reports of contraindications or side effects when used properly.

References: (5) Vol. 1, p. 1109; (9) p. 198; (22) p. 96; (48) p. 363; (52) p. 835; (68) p. 61.

CRANESBILL

Other Common Name(s): alumroot, American cranesbill, spotted cranesbill, spotted geranium, storksbill, wild geranium
Botanical Name(s): *Geranium maculatum* L. [Fam.: Geraniaceae]
Root, aerial part
Constituents: Tannins (root: rich in condensed t., also hydrolyzable t.; aerial part: rich in hydrolyzable t., also condensed t.), volatile oil (with sesquiterpenes: chiefly germacrol, also germazone, etc.). Root contains also phlobaphenes and starch.
Properties: Astringent, anti-inflammatory, hemostatic, wound-healing. The effects are due in large part to tannins. It is also claimed to exert aphrodisiac effects.
Uses: Internally it is used (as a tea, h. p.) for inflammations of the gastrointestinal tract (diarrhea, ulcerative colitis, incl. hemorrhoids; also when minor hemorrhages are present, but on professional's advice) and as an adjuvant for menorrhagia / hypermenorrhea (= prolonged / heavy menstruation). Externally it is used (as a vaginal irrigation / sitz bath / wash) for leukorrhea, (as a wash, wet compress, poultice) for minor skin inflammations, burns, wounds and ulcers, (as a wet compress, an enema) for hemorrhoids, (as a mouthwash, gargle) for inflammations of the mouth and throat, and (as a paint) for inflamed and bleeding gums, denture sores and canker sores.
Caution: There are no reports of contraindications or side effects when used properly. Nevertheless, before using it for gynecologic disorders, the problem should be judged by a health professional. At higher doses than recommended it may cause gastrointestinal irritations (with nausea, vomiting, constipation).

References: (1) Vol. 5, p. 252; (3) Vol. 4, p. 1125; (5) Vol. 1, p. 531; (15) p. 101; (18) p. 217; (35) p. 233; (37) p. 586; (41) Vols. 1-7; (44) p. 246; (46) p. 656; (49) Vol. 2, p. 279; (66) p. 290; (85) p. 799; (87) Vol. 1, p. 274.

CRESS, GARDEN

Other Common Name(s): pepperweed
Botanical Name(s): *Lepidium sativum* L. [Fam.: Brassicaceae (Cruciferae)]
Aerial part (fresh)
Constituents: Glucosinolates (glucotropaeolin = benzyl-glucosinolate, etc.; mainly in the intact fresh material; cf. CRESS, INDIAN and HORSERADISH TREE, INDIAN), volatile oil (with benzyl-isothiocyanate, etc.; mainly in processed / dried material), vitamins (A, C), minerals (iodine, nickel, cobalt; rich in potassium), enzymes, etc.
Properties: Stomachic, diuretic, antimicrobial, antioxidant, rubefacient, counterirritant. Under the action of enzymes (when the fresh material is crushed; partly with drying) glucotropaeolin liberates the volatile benzyl-

isothiocyanate, responsible for the pungent flavor and most of the mentioned effects.

Uses: <u>Internally</u> it is chiefly used as a spicy salad and as a natural supplement of vitamin C and minerals (incl. Potassium). Garden cress is beneficial for nonulcer dyspepsia, sluggish bowels, constipation and minor inflammations of the respiratory and genitourinary tracts. To enhance the effects in problems of the genitourinary tract, the fluid intake (incl. herbal teas) should be more than 2 liters per day. <u>Externally</u> it is used (as a wash, wet compress) for infected wounds, ulcers, (as a poultice) for minor muscular and arthritic pains, and (as a mouthwash) for inflammations of the mouth.

Caution: Garden cress should be collected during the early flowering stage (not with seeds). It should not be taken during pregnancy, in cases of impaired renal function, in peptic ulcers, biliary obstruction, and in children under 4 years of age. In cases of nonobstructive gallstones it can be used but only on health professional's advice. It should not be used or consumed for more than 4-6 weeks without breaks of a few days because it may cause goiter and irritations of the mucous membrane of the stomach. The distilled oil should not be taken internally. When used externally (as a poultice, etc.), it should not be applied in excessive amounts and left too long on the painful site as it may cause blisters.

References: (1) Vol. 5, p. 656; (3) Vol. 5, p. 487; (5) Vol. 1, p. 644; (19) p. 187; (29) p. 78; (37) p. 820; (49) Vol. 2, p. 221; (51) p. 86.

CRESS, INDIAN

Other Common Name(s): garden nasturtium
Botanical Name(s): *Tropaeolum majus* L. [Fam.: Tropaeolaceae]
<u>Aerial part</u> (fresh)
Constituents: Glucosinolates (chiefly glucotropaeolin = benzyl-glucosinolate; cf. CRESS, GARDEN; HORSERADISH TREE), vitamin C (rich), phenolic acids (chlorogenic acid, etc.), flavonoids (quercetin, etc.), enzymes, etc. Under the action of myrosinase (see MUSTARD) glucotropaeolin liberates the volatile benzyl-isothiocyanate, responsible for the pungent flavor and which is the main constituent of the volatile oil (chiefly in processed / dried material).

Properties: Antimicrobial, antifungal, antiviral, antioxidant, rubefacient, counterirritant. Isothiocyanates are responsible for most of the effects.

Uses: <u>Internally</u> it is used (juice, fresh herb, h. p.) for inflammations of the genitourinary and upper respiratory tracts. To enhance the effects in problems of the genitourinary tract, the fluid intake (incl. herbal teas) should be more than 2 liters per day. <u>Externally</u> it is used (as a wash, wet compress) for infected wounds, bacterial / fungal skin infections (incl. cases of hair loss), and (as a poultice) for minor muscular and arthritic pains. It is also used as a spicy salad and natural supplement of vitamin C.

Caution: See CRESS, GARDEN.

References: (1) Vol. 6, p. 1006; (3) Vol. 6c, p. 305; (6) pp. 116, 117, 188; (8) p. 564; (19) p. 123; (23) p. 474; (27) p. 230; (37) pp. 195, 1408; (47) p. 2739; (51) p. 110.

CRESS, SCURVY

Other Common Name(s): scurvy grass, spoonwort
Botanical Name(s): *Cochlearia officinalis* L. [Fam.: Brassicaceae (Cruciferae)]
Aerial part (dried)
Constituents: Volatile oil (with isobutyl-isothiocyanate, etc.; mainly in the processed / dried material), glucosinolates (glucocochlearin = isobutyl-glucosinolate, etc.; mainly in the intact fresh material), flavonoids (flavones, etc.), phenolic acids, vitamin C, a tropane alkaloid (cochlearine), etc.
Properties: Stomachic, mild cholagogue, diuretic, antibacterial, antioxidant, rubefacient, counterirritant. Isothiocyanates, which are liberated from glucosinolates, are responsible for the pungent flavor and most of the mentioned effects. See CRESS, GARDEN; MUSTARD.
Uses: Internally it is used (as a tea, h. p.) for loss of appetite and nonulcer dyspepsia (with flatulence, sluggish bowels, minor constipation, etc.), which are often associated with impaired bile flow. It is also consumed fresh as a spicy salad, with beneficial effects on the digestive system in general and as a natural vitamin C supplement. Externally it is used (as a poultice) for minor muscular and arthritic pains, (as a wash, compress) for infected wounds and ulcers, and (as a mouthwash, gargle) for inflammations of the mouth and throat.
Caution: See CRESS, GARDEN.

References: (1) Vol. 4, p. 923; (3) Vol. 4, p. 179; (24) p. 223; (27) p. 97; (37) p. 349; (46) p. 331; (47) p. 1023; (51) p. 88.

CRESS, WATER

Other Common Name(s): watercress
Botanical Name(s): *Rorippa nasturtium-aquaticum* (L.) Hayek = *Nasturtium officinale* W.T. Aiton [Fam.: Brassicaceae (Cruciferae)]
Aerial part (fresh, dried)
Constituents: Glucosinolates (gluconasturtiin = phenylethyl-glucosinolate, etc.; mainly in the intact fresh material), volatile oil (with phenylethyl-isothiocyanate, etc.; mainly in the processed / dried material), vitamins (C, B_1, B_2, E), minerals (K, Mn, Zn, Cu, As, I), enzymes, etc.
Properties: Stomachic, mild diuretic, mild cholagogue, antibacterial, antioxidant. Isothiocyanates, which are liberated from glucosinolates, are responsible for the pungent flavor and most of the mentioned effects. See CRESS, GARDEN; MUSTARD. **Uses:** Internally it is used (as a tea, h. p.)

for loss of appetite and nonulcer dyspepsia (with sluggish bowels, minor constipation), which are often associated with impaired bile flow, and for minor inflammations of the respiratory and genitourinary tracts. To enhance the effects in problems of the genitourinary tract, the fluid intake (incl. herbal teas) should be more than 2 liters per day. It is also used as an anti-dyscratic (= blood purifier; salad, juice, tea, h. p.) for atopic eczema (= chronic eczema of internal origin). Watercress is consumed as a spicy salad and natural supplement of vitamins and minerals. Externally it is used (as a poultice) for minor muscular and arthritic pains and (as a mouthwash) for inflammations of the mouth.
Caution: See CRESS, GARDEN.

References: (1) Vol. 5, p. 916; (3) Vol. 6a, p. 39; (8) p. 381; (17) p. 408; (19) p. 58; (24) p. 104; (27) p. 102; (35) p. 845; (37) p. 945; (46) p. 974; (47) p. 1965; (51) p. .

CROTON

Other Common Name(s): purging croton
Botanical Name(s): *Croton tiglium* L. [Fam.: Euphorbiaceae]
Croton oil
It is the fixed oil obtained by expression from the seed.
Constituents: Chiefly glycerides (fatty acids component: palmitic, oleic acids, etc.) and esters of phorbol (a diterpenoid alcohol) with fatty acids (tiglic and crotonic acids, etc.).
Properties: Local irritant (vesicant!), drastic purgative.
Uses: Today croton oil is used (incorporated in some test products applied to the skin) to cause a local irritation and inflammation and then to test the new anti-inflammatory drugs. Internally has been used (1 drop croton oil mixed with 30 grams castor oil) for obstinate constipation. Externally has been used (as a liniment combination product) for rheumatic and neuralgic pains, among others.
Caution: It should not be taken internally, even as a combination product, in cases of bowel obstruction and inflammations of the gastrointestinal tract. Croton oil should be handled with extreme caution, because phorbol esters are strong vesicants and carcinogenic. 20 drops of croton oil can be fatal to an adult.

References: (2) Vol. 2, p. 469; (3) Vol. 4, p. 346; (6) pp. 237, 271; (8) p. 200; (12) p. 1254; (13) p. 393; (36) p. 187; (37) p. 370; (55) p. 214; (65) pp. 138, 179; (66) p. 492.

CROW KILLER

Botanical Name(s): *Anamirta cocculus* (L.) Wight et Arn. [Fam.: Menispermaceae]
Fruit (Indian cockles, Indian berries, fish berries)

Constituents: Seed contains picrotoxin, which is a mixture of two bitter principles (sesquiterpene dilactones: picrotoxinin, highly toxic, and picrotin, non-toxic).

Properties: Picrotoxin is a central nervous system stimulant, due to its GABA (= gamma-aminobutyrric acid) antagonistic effect.

Uses: Picrotoxin has been used as an antidote to poisonings by sedative-hypnotic drugs. Due to its toxicity and as there are available other drug alternatives, picrotoxin is no longer used.

Caution: Seeds are extremely toxic. Ingestion of even 2-3 grams of seeds can be fatal to an adult.

References: (1) Vol. 4, p. 268; (3) Vol. 3, p. 72; (8) p. 52; (12) p. 472; (36) p. 327; (37) p. 1077; (55) p. 291; (65) p. 203; (66) p. 390; (67) p. 463.

CUBEB

Other Common Name(s): tailed pepper
Botanical Name(s): *Piper cubeba* L. f. [Fam.: Piperaceae]
Fruit
Constituents: Volatile oil (with sesquiterpenes: β-cubebene, copaene, cubebol, etc.; monoterpenes: 1,8-cineole, α-pinene, etc.), lignans (cubebin, etc.), resin (with resin acids: cubebic acid, etc.), fixed oil, minerals, etc.

Properties: Aromatic, bitter tonic, diuretic, antimicrobial, antiprotozoal (against *Entameba*), carminative, expectorant, and it is claimed to be aphrodisiac. Its antimicrobial effect is also exhibited in the genitourinary tract.

Uses: Cubeb is chiefly used as a spice. Internally it is used (as a tea, h. p.) for inflammations of the genitourinary tract (cystitis, urethritis, prostatitis, epididymitis, leukorrhea), nonulcer dyspepsia (with flatulence, sluggish bowels), diarrhea and amebic dysentery, and for inflammations of the upper respiratory tract (bronchitis, pharyngitis, etc.; coughs due to thickened bronchial secretion; also as a lozenge). To enhance the effects in problems of the genitourinary tract, the fluid intake (incl. herbal teas) should be more than 2 liters per day.

Caution: There are no reports of contraindications or side effects when used properly. Nevertheless, cubeb is best avoided during pregnancy. Dosed higher than recommended cause irritations of the genitourinary and gastrointestinal tracts, skin rash, tachycardia and headache, among others.

References: (1) Vol. 6, p. 194; (3) Vol. 6a, p. 705; (5) Vol. 1, p. 840; (8) p. 437; (9) p. 199; (10) p. 97; (12) p. 810; (29) p. 86; (41) Vols. 1-7; (46) p. 417; (47) p. 1135; (66) p. 256.

CUCUMBER

Botanical Name(s): *Cucumis sativus* L. [Fam.: Cucurbitaceae]
Fruit, **seed oil**

Constituents: The fruit pulp consists chiefly of water and contains minerals (rich in variety), vitamins (A, C, B complex), phytosterols, proteins, fat, carbohydrates and fragrant compounds, among others. Seed oil is a fixed oil with fatty acids component chiefly oleic acid, also linoleic acid, etc.

Properties and Uses: The juice of the ripe cucumber and the cucumber seed oil are ingredients in many cosmetic products (milks, ointments, cold creams). In traditional medicine the juice of the ripe cucumber (mixed with nutmeg) is used internally for inflammations of the genitourinary tract, while the seed is used as an anthelmintic.

Caution: There are no reports of contraindications or side effects when used properly.

References: (1) Vol. 4, p. 1066; (3) Vol. 4, p. 357; (5) Vol. 1, p. 366.

CUDWEED, FRAGRANT

Other Common Name(s): fragrant everlasting, gordolobo, rabbit tobacco, sweet balsam
Botanical Name(s): *Pseudognaphalium obtusifolium* (L.) Hillard et Burtt = *Gnaphalium obtusifolium* L. = *Gnaphalium polycephalum* Milchx. [Fam.: Asteraceae (Compositae)]
Aerial part (leaves and flowers)
Constituents: Volatile oil (with polyacetylenes and possibly phenols), flavonoids (methoxy-flavones, flavonols, biflavones). Among other possible constituents are sesquiterpene lactones, carotenoids and tannins.
Properties: Anti-inflammatory, antimicrobial, antispasmodic, diuretic, astringent. Among methoxy-flavones, which are found in fragrant everlasting, there are compounds with anti-inflammatory, antimicrobial, antispasmodic and strong antioxidant effects. Many polyacetylenes have shown antimicrobial effect.
Uses: Internally it is used (as a tea, h. p.) for minor inflammatory and spastic conditions of the upper respiratory tract (bronchitis, etc.; coughs; also as a diaphoretic hot tea), gastrointestinal tract (cramps, vomiting, diarrhea) and genitourinary tract (cystitis, urethritis, prostatitis), and for primary dysmenorrhea (= painful menstruation without pathology). To enhance the effects in problems of the genitourinary tract, the fluid intake (incl. herbal teas) should be more than 2 liters per day. Externally it is used (as a mouthwash, gargle) for inflammations of the mouth and throat, (as a vaginal irrigation / sitz bath / wash) for leukorrhea and vulvovaginitis, (as a wash, wet compress) for minor skin inflammations and wounds.
Caution: There are no reports of contraindications or side effects when used properly. Nevertheless, before using it for dysmenorrhea, the gynecologic problem should be judged by a health professional. If sesquiterpene lactones are present, it may cause allergic contact dermatitis to persons hyper-

123

sensitive to other Asteraceae plants (e. g. arnica, chamomile, feverfew, rag-weed, tansy, yarrow) that contain them.

References: (3) Vol. 4, p. 1177; (18) p. 284; (25) p. 82; (31) pp. 46, 388; (35) p. 80; (37) p. 1137; (41) Vols. 1-7; (42) Vol. 3, p. 495; (44) p. 250; (47) p. 1474; (52) p. 341.

CUDWEED, MARSH

Botanical Name(s): *Gnaphalium uliginosum* L. [Fam.: Asteraceae (Compositae)]
Aerial part
Constituents: Volatile oil, tannins, carotenoids, phytosterols, alkaloids (traces), vitamins (B$_1$, C, K) and a resin. Among other possible constituents are flavonoids (methoxy-flavones, flavonols, chalcones), polyacetylenes (normally in volatile oil), sesquiterpene lactones, and carotenoids. See CUDWEED, FRAGRANT.
Properties: Anti-inflammatory, antimicrobial, astringent, antispasmodic, diuretic.
Uses: <u>Internally</u> it is used (as a tea, h. p.) for inflammations of the gastrointestinal tract (incl. gastritis, peptic ulcers) and upper respiratory and genitourinary tracts. To enhance the effects in problems of the genitourinary tract, the fluid intake (incl. herbal teas) should be more than 2 liters per day. It is also used for minor cases of hypertension. <u>Externally</u> it is used (as a mouthwash, gargle) for inflammations of the mouth and throat. Between marsh cudweed and fragrant cudweed there are slight differences in constituents, particularly if marsh cudweed contains the reported alkaloids. Possibly, some of the indications mentioned under fragrant cudweed may apply also to marsh cudweed. See CUDWEED, FRAGRANT.
Caution: See CUDWEED, FRAGRANT.

References: (3) Vol. 4, p. 1176; (5) Vol. 1, p. 544; (10) p. 98; (15) p. 221; (18) p. 284; (36) p. 478; (41) Vols. 1-7; (42) Vol. 3, p. 495; (44) p. 250; (52) p. 341; (86) Vol. 1, p. 309; (87) Vol. 2, p. 228.

CULVER'S ROOT

Other Common Name(s): blackroot
Botanical Name(s): *Veronicastrum virginicum* (L.) Farw. = *Leptandra virginica* (L.) Nutt. [Fam.: Scrophulariaceae]
Root (rhizome)
Constituents: Volatile oil, phenolic acids, bitter principles (collectively referred to as leptandrin), phytosterols, tannins, resin, saponins, etc. The reported bitter principles are possibly iridoids, while saponins may be of triterpenoid type. It is also possible to contain flavonoids.
Properties: Bitter tonic, cholagogue, laxative. Fresh root is a strong purgative and emetic, but when dried becomes milder in action. Iridoids, which very possibly are present, have shown bitter tonic, choleretic, liver protec-

tive, laxative, diuretic, anti-inflammatory, antibacterial, antiviral, antifungal and immunomodulant effects, among others. To the hepatobiliary effects may contribute phenolic acids.

Uses: Internally it is used (as a tea, h. p.) for loss of appetite, nonulcer dyspepsia and chronic constipation associated with impaired bile secretion and flow.

Caution: Unless advised by an experienced practitioner, it should not be taken during pregnancy and lactation. At higher doses than recommended it causes gastrointestinal irritations (with nausea, vomiting, diarrhea), particularly when used fresh. Otherwise, there are no reports of contraindications or side effects when used properly.

References: (1) Vol. 6, p. 1121; (3) Vol. 6c, p. 431; (10) p. 37; (12) p. 438; (15) p. 229; (18) p. 255; (31) p. 569; (35) p. 111; (36) p. 437; (44) p. 593; (52) p. 846; (65) p. 180; (66) p. 328.

CUMIN

Botanical Name(s): *carrotum cyminum* L. [Fam.: Apiaceae (Umbelliferae)]
Fruit (commonly called seed)
Constituents: Volatile oil (with cuminaldehyde, etc.), flavonoids (flavones: luteolin and apigenin glycosides), tannins, fixed oil, sugars, proteins, but no starch.
Properties: Aromatic, stomachic, antispasmodic, carminative, antimicrobial, emmenagogue.
Uses: It is chiefly used as a spice, similar to caraway and is an ingredient of curry powder. Cumin fruit and cumin oil are used as flavor ingredients in liqueur / liquor industry. Internally it is used (as a tea, h. p.) for nonulcer dyspepsia (with flatulence, minor cramps) and minor diarrhea, and for secondary amenorrhea and oligomenorrhea (= ceased / infrequent / scanty menstruation without pathology).
Caution: Unless advised by an experienced practitioner, cumin should not be taken during pregnancy and lactation. Before using it for gynecologic disorders, the problem should be judged by a health professional. It should be avoided in cases of estrogen receptor-positive (ER+) tumors. Otherwise, there are no reports of contraindications or side effects when used properly.

References: (1) Vol. 4, p. 1079; (3) Vol. 4, p. 363; (9) p. 201; (10) p. 98; (24) p. 455; (35) p. 242.

CURRANT, BLACK

Other Common Name(s): cassis
Botanical Name(s): *Ribes nigrum* L. [Fam.: Grossulariaceae]
Leaf
Constituents: Flavonoids (flavonols: astragalin, rutin, etc.), tannins (proanthocyanidins), minerals (potassium), organic acids, volatile oil (traces), etc.

Properties: Diuretic, astringent. The diuretic effect is due to potassium, organic acids, and flavonols. It is astringent due to tannins.

Uses: Internally it is used (as a tea, h. p.; usually combined with other herbs) as a flushing-out treatment (= herbal tea or product + liquids: more than 2 liters per day; sometimes combined with a medication) for inflammations of the genitourinary tract (cystitis, etc.), urinary gravel and nonobstructive stones, to prevent relapsing urinary infections / gravel / stones, and (as a tea, h. p.) for inflammations of the gastrointestinal tracts. It is also used as an antidyscratic (= blood purifier; tea, h. p.) for chronic rheumatic complaints.

Caution: There are no reports of contraindications or side effects when used properly. Nevertheless, a flushing-out treatment is contraindicated in cases of obstructive urinary stones, edema due to impaired heart or kidney function and kidney inflammations (here can be used on health professional's advice to enhance the effects of an antimicrobial therapy).

Fruit

Constituents: Organic acids (citric acid, etc.), vitamin C (rich), invert sugar, pectin, flavonoids (anthocyanins, flavonols), phenolic acids, etc.

Properties: Acidulous, refrigerant, diuretic, antidiarrheal.

Uses: Internally it is used (as a tea, h. p.) for feverish and thirsty states, minor diarrhea and as a vitamin C supplement (also in jams or preserves). Cassis is extensively used in food industry in the production of jellies, wines, etc.

Caution: There are no reports of contraindications or side effects when used properly.

References: (1) Vol. 6, p. 467; (3) Vol. 6b, p. 133; (6) p. 186; (10) p. 35; (19) p. 114; (24) p. 180; (27) p. 287; (35) p. 243; (48) p. 364.

CURRY, INDIAN

Botanical Name(s): *Murraya koenigii* (L.) Spreng. [Fam.: Rutaceae]
Leaf

Constituents: Volatile oil (with isosafrole, caryophyllene, etc.), indole alkaloids (mukonicine, murrayanine, etc.), coumarins (scopolin = murrayin, etc.), tannins, etc.

Properties: Aromatic, stomachic, carminative, tonic, astringent.

Uses: Indian curry leaf is chiefly used as a spice, with beneficial effect on the digestive system, and as a general tonic. Internally it is used (as a tea, h. p.) for nonulcer dyspepsia (with flatulence, nausea, etc.) and diarrhea. Externally it is used (as a poultice, wet compress) for minor wounds and burns.

Caution: There are no reports of contraindications or side effects when used properly. Nevertheless, Indian curry is best avoided during pregnancy and lactation since it contains alkaloids and isosafrole.

References: (5) Vol. 2, p. 731; (31) p. 482; (41) Vols. 1-7; (45) p. 235; (52) p. 513.

DAISY, GARDEN

Other Common Name(s): daisy, English daisy
Botanical Name(s): *Bellis perennis* L. [Fam.: Asteraceae (Compositae)]
Flower
Constituents: Flavonoids, saponins, mucilage, volatile oil, tannins (condensed t.), bitter principles (possibly diterpenoid lactones), organic acids, inulin, resin, etc. It possibly contains coumarins and polyacetylenes.
Properties: Anti-inflammatory, emollient, mild astringent, wound-healing, expectorant, demulcent, diuretic, mild bitter tonic.
Uses: Externally it is used (as a wet compress, poultice) for minor skin inflammations, boils, wounds, and ulcers (incl. varicose ulcers = ulcus cruris), (as a paint: tincture) for common acne (= acne vulgaris), and (as a mouthwash, gargle) for inflammations of the mouth and throat. Internally it is used (as a tea, h. p.) for inflammations of the upper respiratory tract (bronchitis, etc.; minor irritating dry coughs), gastrointestinal tract (gastritis, loss of appetite, minor constipation) and genitourinary tract (cystitis, etc.). To enhance the effects in problems of the genitourinary tract, the fluid intake (incl. herbal teas) should be more than 2 liters per day. It is also used as an anti-inflammatory and antidyscratic (= blood purifier; tea, h. p.; combined with other herbs) for atopic eczema (= chronic eczema of internal origin) and chronic rheumatic complaints.
Caution: There are no reports of contraindications or side effects when used properly.

References: (3) Vol. 3, p. 376; (5) Vol. 1, p. 159; (6) p. 360; (18) p. 282; (24) p. 143; (27) p. 210; (37) p. 186; (47) p. 691; (51) p. 202; (87) Vol. 2, p. 228.

DAMIANA

Botanical Name(s): *Turnera diffusa* Willd. ex Schult. var. *aphrodisiaca* (Ward) Urb. = *Turnera aphrodisiaca* Ward [Fam.: Turneraceae]
Leaf
Constituents: Volatile oil (with 1,8-cineole, pinenes, thymol, δ-cadinene, etc.), a phenol glycoside (arbutin), a cyanogenic glycoside (tetraphyllin B), a bitter principle (damianin), hydrocarbons (triacontane, etc.), phytosterols, flavonoids, tannins, resin, etc.
Properties: Aromatic, bitter tonic, mild laxative, urinary antiseptic, diuretic, mild CNS stimulant.
Uses: Internally it is used (as a tea, h. p.) for loss of appetite and nonulcer dyspepsia (with impaired digestion, sluggish bowels, minor constipation), minor fatigue and depressive mood, inflammations of the genitourinary tract (cystitis, etc., with urinary incontinence). Damiana is claimed to exhibit aphrodisiac effect (in males and females), so it can be tried for low sexual drive in both sexes. To enhance the effects in problems of the genitourinary

tract, the fluid intake (incl. herbal teas) should be more than 2 liters per day. **Caution:** Damiana should not be taken during pregnancy. Doses higher than recommended should be avoided as tetraphyllin B is toxic. Otherwise, there are no reports of contraindications or side effects when used properly.

References: (3) Vol. 6c, p. 323; (6) p. 293; (8) p. 565; (9) p. 204; (10) p. 100; (12a) p. 630; (14) p. 71; (15) p. 219; (20) p. 94; (31) p. 91; (36) p. 290; (37) p. 1415; (46) p. 428; (47) p. 1171; (66) p. 261; (71) p. 234; (75) p. 173.

DANDELION

Other Common Name(s): lion's tooth, blow ball, puff ball
Botanical Name(s): *Taraxacum officinale* Web. ex F.H. Wigg. = *Taraxacum dens-leonis* Desf. = *Leontodon taraxacum* L. [Fam.: Asteraceae (Compositae)]
<u>Root, leaf</u>
Constituents: (Root and leaf): Bitter principles (sesquiterpene lactones), triterpenes, phytosterols, phenolic acids, minerals (rich in potassium); (root): inulin (richer in autumn), fructose (richer in spring); (leaf): flavonoids, etc.
Properties: Bitter tonic, cholagogue, choleretic, mild laxative, diuretic, antioxidant. Its bitter tonic and hepatobiliary effects are due in large part to bitter principles and phenolic acids. To the diuretic effect possibly contribute potassium salts (leaf is richer) and flavonoids (in leaf).
Uses: <u>Internally</u> it is used (as a tea, h. p.) for loss of appetite and nonulcer dyspepsia (with fullness, heartburn, burping, flatulence, bloating, sluggish bowels, minor constipation, incl. hemorrhoids) associated with impaired bile secretion and flow, and as an antidyscratic (= blood purifier) and mild diuretic for chronic rheumatic complaints, atopic eczema (= chronic eczema of internal origin) and minor inflammatory conditions of the genitourinary tract. To enhance the effects in problems of the genitourinary tract, the fluid intake (incl. herbal teas) should be more than 2 liters per day.
Caution: Dandelion should not be taken in cases of biliary obstruction and biliary abscess. In cases of nonobstructive gallstones it can be used but only on health professional's advice. The milky juice may cause allergic contact dermatitis to persons hypersensitive to other Asteraceae plants (e. g. arnica, chamomile, feverfew, ragweed, tansy, yarrow). Otherwise, there are no reports of contraindications or side effects when used properly.

References: (1) Vol. 6, p. 897; (3) Vol. 6c, p. 16; (6) pp. 148, 186; (8) p. 548; (9) p. 205; (12) p. 481; (14) pp. 73, 76; (15) p. 206; (16) p. 138; (17) p. 571; (19) p. 144; (20) p. 96; (23) pp. 135, 260; (46) p. 1593; (47) p. 2675; (48) p. 86.

DEER'S TONGUE
Other Common Name(s): Carolina vanilla
Botanical Name(s): *Carphephorus odoratissimus* (J.F. Gmel.) Herbert = *Trilisa odoratissima* (Walter ex J. F. Gmel.) Cass. [Fam.: Asteraceae (Compositae)]

Leaf

Constituents: Coumarins (chiefly coumarin), lignans (eudesmin, epieudesmin), mucilaginous polysaccharides, triterpenes (lupeol, etc.), 2,3-benzofuran, volatile oil (with geranylacetone, etc.), resin, wax, etc.

Properties: Aromatic, demulcent, antipyretic, sedative, diuretic. Coumarin has been shown to cause liver injuries, but only in animal tests. There are new data on immunomodulant effects of coumarin, with hopes for treating certain tumors. There are lignans that have shown immunomodulant, cytotoxic and antimicrobial effects, among others.

Uses: Deer's tongue is chiefly used as a flavor ingredient (substitute of tonka bean) in tobacco industry and as a fragrance ingredient in perfumery and cosmetics. Externally it is used (as a wet compress, poultice) for bruises. Internally it is used (only as a combination product) for feverish states, inflammatory conditions of the upper respiratory tract (the common cold, etc.) and minor nervousness.

Caution: Internally, deer's tongue should be used only as directed by an experienced practitioner. At higher doses than recommended it may cause headache.

References: (3) Vol. 6c, p. 277; (5) Vol. 1, p. 649; (9) p. 207; (10) p. 101; (12) p. 800; (25) p. 196; (31) p. 435; (35) p. 255; (41) Vols. 1-7; (52) p. 816.

DEVIL'S BIT

Other Common Name(s): corn scabious, field scabious, bachelor buttons, blue buttons

Botanical Name(s): *Knautia arvensis* (L.) Coult. = *Scabiosa arvensis* L. [Fam.: Dipsacaceae]

Aerial part

Constituents: Bitter principles (iridoids: rich in different types), β-methylglucoside, saponins, flavonoids (flavones), phenolic acids, tannins, etc.

Properties: Mild bitter tonic, expectorant, antimicrobial, astringent, wound-healing.

Uses: Internally it is used (as a tea, h. p.) for inflammations of the upper respiratory tract (bronchitis, the common cold, etc.; coughs), gastrointestinal tract (diarrhea, etc.) and genitourinary tract (cystitis, etc.), and as an antidyscratic (= blood purifier; tea, h. p.) for atopic eczema (= chronic eczema of internal origin). To enhance the effects in problems of the genitourinary tract, the fluid intake (incl. herbal teas) should be more than 2 liters per day. Externally it is used (as a wet compress, poultice) for minor skin inflammations, itching, wounds and ulcers.

Caution: There are no reports of contraindications or side effects when used properly.

References: (1) Vol. 5, p. 612; (3) Vol. 5, p. 408; (18) p. 268; (37) p. 768; (47) p. 2471; (51) p. 196.

DEVIL'S CLAW

Other Common Name(s): grapple plant, wool spider
Botanical Name(s): *Harpagophytum procumbens* (Burch.) DC. ex Meisn. [Fam.: Pedaliaceae]
Root (dried transverse slices of peripheral tubers)
Constituents: Iridoids (chiefly harpagoside = cinnamoyl-harpagide, very bitter; some harpagide, slightly sweet; etc.), phenylethanoid glycosides (acteoside = verbascoside, etc.), water-soluble oligosaccharides (stachyose, etc.), harpagoquinone, etc.
Properties: Anti-inflammatory, antiedematous, analgesic, bitter tonic, choleretic. Harpagoside has shown NSAID-like effect by inhibiting the biosynthesis of prostaglandins. It also accounts in large part for the bitter tonic and choleretic effects. Acteoside has been shown to be anti-inflammatory (by inhibiting the biosynthesis of leukotrienes) and liver protective.
Uses: Internally it is used (as an h. p.) for rheumatic complaints (incl. rheumatoid arthritis), neuralgic pains, headaches and feverish states. It is also used (as a tea, h. p.) for loss of appetite and nonulcer dyspepsia (with fullness, flatulence, minor cramps, etc.) associated with minor hepatobiliary disorders. As a bitter tonic, devil's claw is also recommended for the elderly.
Caution: Devil's claw should not be used in cases of peptic ulcers, during pregnancy and lactation, biliary obstruction, and in children under 12 years of age. In cases of nonobstructive gallstones it can be used but only on health professional's advice. Devil's claw products should be standardized to iridoids (expressed as harpagoside). Unless advised by an experienced practitioner, it should not be taken for more than three months.

References: (1) Vol. 5, p. 384; (3) Vol. 5, p. 18; (6) p. 241; (7) p. 292; (8) p. 297; (12) p. 444; (13) p. 411; (14) p. 78; (16) p. 53; (17) p. 277; (19) p. 226; (20) p. 98; (23) p. 279; (31) pp. 488, 574; (48) p. 600.

DEVIL'S COTTON

Other Common Name(s): abroma
Botanical Name(s): *Abroma augusta* (L.) L.f. [Fam.: Sterculiaceae]
Root bark, root
Constituents: Mucilaginous polysaccharides, triterpenes (friedelin, etc.), phytosterols (5-sterols: abromasterols A and B), minerals (rich in magnesium), biogenic amines (choline, betaine), tannins (condensed t.), phlobaphenes, phenolic acids, etc.
Properties: Emmenagogue, mild uterotonic, diuretic, antimicrobial.
Uses: Internally it is used (as a tea, h. p.) for secondary amenorrhea and oligomenorrhea (= ceased / infrequent / scanty menstruation without pathol-

ogy). Combined with other herbs it is also used (as a tea, h. p.) for primary dysmenorrhea (= painful menstruation without pathology).

Caution: Before using devil's cotton, the gynecologic problem should be judged by a health professional. Normally, it should not be taken during pregnancy and lactation.

References: (1) Vol. 4, p. 24; (3) Vol. 2, p. 871; (5) Vol. 1, p. 1; (41) Vols. 1-7; (52) p. 3.

DIGITALIS

Other Common Name(s): 1) purple foxglove, foxglove 2) woolly foxglove, Grecian foxglove
Botanical Name(s): 1) *Digitalis purpurea* L. 2) *Digitalis lanata* Ehrh. [Fam.: Plantaginaceae; formerly, Scrophulariaceae]
Leaf
Constituents: Its most important constituents are cardiac glycosides. Purple foxglove contains chiefly purpurea glycosides A and B, which through enzymatic hydrolysis yield digitoxin and gitoxin respectively. Woolly foxglove contains chiefly lanatosides C and A, which through enzymatic + alkaline hydrolysis yield digoxin and digitoxin respectively. It also contains steroidal saponins, flavonoids and mucilaginous polysaccharides.
Properties: Increases the contractility of the heart muscle (= positive inotropic effect), slows the rate of the heartbeat (= negative chronotropic effect), decreases the conductivity of the heart muscle (= negative dromotropic effect) and increases the excitability of the heart muscle (= positive bathmotropic effect). A rational therapy with digitalis or its cardiac glycosides results in an increase of cardiac output, renal blood flow and diuresis, and a decrease of cardiac filling pressure, heart size, venous and capillary pressures and edema.
Uses: Internally it is used for heart failure, to control an atrial fibrillation and flutter and for paroxysmal atrial tachycardia. Today the secondary glycosides, namely digoxin and digitoxin, are used mostly.
Caution: Digitalis and its glycosides are toxic and not for self-treatment. They should be standardized to the cardiac glycosides content and used only as directed by a health professional. Digitalis products or its glycosides, at higher doses than recommended, cause irregular pulse, nausea, vomiting and diarrhea, which are symptoms characteristic for intoxications with cardiac glycosides. A concomitant use of digitalis or its glycosides, with quinidine, calcium, potassium depleting diuretics (e. g. hydrochlorthiazide) or laxatives (e. g. Senna), or glucocorticoids, causes an increased effectiveness and / or side effects.

References: (1) Vol. 4, pp. 1171, 1179; (3) Vol. 4, p. 553; (7) p. 108; (8) p. 222; (11) p. 117; (12) pp. 586, 589; (13) p. 181; (19) p. 323; (46) p. 430; (48) p. 735; (50) p. 95.

DILL

Botanical Name(s): *Anethum graveolens* L. [Fam.: Apiaceae (Umbelliferae)]
Fruit (commonly called seed)
Constituents: Volatile oil (with carvone, also limonene, α-phellandrene, etc.), coumarins (scopoletin, etc.), furanocoumarins (bergaptene, etc.), phenolic acids, fixed oil, proteins, etc.
Properties: Aromatic, stomachic, carminative, antispasmodic, diuretic, antimicrobial, galactagogue.
Uses: Internally it is used (as a tea, h. p.) for loss of appetite and nonulcer dyspepsia (with flatulence, minor cramps, nausea, vomiting) and for minor diarrhea, also recommended for infants. It is also used for minor inflammations of the upper respiratory tract (bronchitis, etc.; coughs) and to promote the secretion of milk in nursing mothers. Externally it is used (as a mouthwash, gargle) for inflammations of the mouth and throat and (as a mouthwash, chewing) for bad breath. Dill seed and herb as well as their volatile oils are used as flavor ingredients in food industry.
Caution: Unless advised by a health professional, dill should not be taken during pregnancy. When handling the herb avoid contact with skin and when taking its products avoid exposure to strong sunrays as it may cause phototoxic skin irritations. Otherwise, there are no reports of contraindications or side effects when used properly.

References: (3) Vol. 3, p. 85; (5) Vol. 1, p. 82; (8) p. 58; (9) p. 210; (10) p. 102; (15) p. 24; (19) p. 67; (27) p. 31; (35) p. 255; (47) p. 520; (51) p. 136.

DITTANY, WHITE

Other Common Name(s): European dittany, dittany
Botanical Name(s): *Dictamnus albus* L. [Fam.: Rutaceae]
Leaf, **root**
Constituents: Furoquinoline alkaloids (dictamnine, etc.), bitter principles (nortriterpenes), volatile oil, furanocoumarins (bergaptene, etc.), coumarins, etc.
Properties: Diuretic, antispasmodic, carminative, emmenagogue, sedative.
Uses: Dittany is chiefly used in traditional medicine. Internally it is used (as a tea; at low doses or combined with other herbs) for spastic conditions of the urinary tract (incl. nonobstructive urinary stones) and gastrointestinal tract (flatulence, intestinal worms), primary dysmenorrhea (= painful menstruation without pathology), and for nervous disorders (epilepsy, nervousness, hysteria), among others. Externally it is used (as a wash, wet compress) for minor skin inflammations and itching.
Caution: Furoquinoline alkaloids and furanocoumarins have shown mutagenic and phototoxic effects. In view of this, an absolute contraindica-

132

tion should be pregnancy and lactation. Before using it for dysmenorrhea, the gynecologic problem should be judged by a health professional. When handling the herb avoid contact with skin and when taking its products avoid exposure to strong sunrays as it may cause phototoxic skin irritations.

References: (1) Vol. 4, p. 1159; (3) Vol. 4, p. 541; (8) p. 221; (24) p. 106; (35) p. 147; (47) p. 1178; (51) p. 114.

DOCK, YELLOW

Other Common Name(s): curled dock, curly dock, dock
Botanical Name(s): *Rumex crispus* L. [Fam.: Polygonaceae]
Root
Constituents: Anthranoids (chrysophanol, emodin, etc.; free, their glycosides), tannins (condensed t.), a 1,8-naphthalenediol (nepodin and its glycoside), sugars, mucilaginous polysaccharides, starch, minerals (calcium oxalate, oxalic acid, iron), fatty acids, etc.
Properties: Mild laxative (large intestine stimulant laxative; See SENNA.), cholagogue, astringent. Anthranoids account for the laxative and cholagogic effects, while tannins are astringent (cf. RHUBARB, CHINESE). Nepodin has shown antibacterial effect.
Uses: Internally it is used (as a tea, h. p.) for minor constipation (atonic, non-spastic) associated with impaired bile flow, and as an intestinal "detoxifier" for chronic skin diseases. Externally it is used (as a mouthwash, paint, gel) for inflammations of the oral cavity (gingivitis, stomatitis, etc.; cf. RHUBARB), (as a gargle) for sore throat, (as a poultice) for small cuts, minor wounds and ulcers, and (as a wash, wet compress) for hemorrhoids.
Caution: See SENNA. Yellow dock should not be taken in cases of bowel and gallbladder obstructions and in cases of a known history of oxalate kidney stones. In cases of nonobstructive gallstones it can be used but only on health professional's advice. Before using it internally, yellow dock root is best stored for at least 1 year.
Note: Leaves of yellow dock have constituents and are used very much like those of sorrel (see SORREL).

References: (3) Vol. 6b, p. 192; (16) p. 183; (20) p. 274; (27) p. 291; (29) p. 100; (31) p. 546; (35) p. 259; (36) p. 478; (44) p. 496; (47) p. 2365; (66) p. 419.

DODDER

Other Common Name(s): 1) European dodder 2) Indian dodder
Botanical Name(s): 1) *Cuscuta epithymum* L.; *Cuscuta europaea* L. 2) *Cuscuta reflexa* Roxb. [Fam.: Cuscutaceae (Convolvulaceae)]
Whole plant
Constituents: An isocoumarin (bergenin = cuscutin), phenolic acids (caffeic acid derivatives), tannins, flavonoids (flavonols), saponins, resin. In

133

Cuscuta spp. have been found ergot alkaloids. It may contain also constituents of the host plant whereon it grows.

Properties: Cholagogue, mild laxative, mild diuretic. The cholagogic effect is due to phenolic acids and the diuretic effect is due in large part to saponins and flavonoids. Bergenin has shown anti-inflammatory effect.

Uses: Internally it is used (as a tea, h. p.; combined with other herbs) for sluggish bowels, minor constipation and flatulence associated with impaired bile secretion and flow. It is also used (as a tea, h. p.) to induce diuresis when this is advisable and as an antidyscratic (= blood purifier) for chronic rheumatic complaints. Externally it is used (as a poultice) for boils.

Caution: There are no reports of contraindications or side effects when used properly. In the manufacture of dodder products it should be considered the origin of the raw material, i. e. its host plant as it may contain a part of its constituents.

References: (3) Vol. 4, p. 390; (5) Vol. 1, p. 373; (10) p. 103; (18) p. 242; (27) p. 105; (31) p. 541; (35) p. 260; (37) p. 374; (46) p. 426; (51) p. 152.

DOGWOOD, ASIATIC

Other Common Name(s): Asiatic cornel, Japanese cornel
Botanical Name(s): *Cornus officinalis* Siebold et Zucc. [Fam.: Cornaceae]
Fruit (dried fruit pulp)
Constituents: Bitter principles (seco-iridoids: cornuside, sweroside, etc.), tannins (ellagitannins, gallotannins), flavonoids (anthocyanins), organic acids, triterpenes (oleanolic and ursolic acids), etc.

Properties: Bitter tonic, diuretic, astringent, anti-inflammatory, antimicrobial, mild immunomodulant. Iridoids have shown bitter tonic, choleretic, liver protective, laxative, diuretic, anti-inflammatory, antimicrobial and immunomodulant effects, among others. Gallic acid has shown antimicrobial, anti-inflammatory and choleretic effects. Ellagic and gallic acids are phenols with antioxidant effect.

Uses: Internally it is used (as a tea, h. p.) for loss of appetite and nonulcer dyspepsia associated with chronic hepatobiliary disorders, for minor fatigue, decreased resistance to diseases, convalescence, erectile dysfunction and spermatorrhea, inflammatory conditions of the genitourinary tract (leukorrhea, irritable bladder with urinary incontinence), menorrhagia / hypermenorrhea (= prolonged / heavy menstruation), and as an adjuvant for diabetes.

Caution: There are no reports of contraindications or side effects when used properly. Nevertheless, before using it for gynecologic disorders, the problem should be judged by a health professional. At higher doses than recommended it may cause irritations of the genitourinary tract.

References: (1) Vol. 4, p. 1008; (12) pp. 438, 876; (31) pp. 457, 569; (41) Vols. 1-7; (45) p. 193; (48) p. 385; (52) p. 218; (82) p. 150.

134

DOGWOOD, FLOWERING

Other Common Name(s): American dogwood
Botanical Name(s): *Cornus florida* L. [Fam.: Cornaceae]
Bark
Constituents: Bitter principles (iridoids: cornin = verbenalin, etc.), steroidal saponins, triterpenes (betulinic acid, etc.), tannins (possibly hydrolyzable t.), etc.

Properties: Biter tonic, stomachic, antipyretic, astringent. Dogwood extracts have shown quinine-like plasmodicidal effect.

Uses: Internally it is used (as a tea, h. p.; only combined with other herbs) for loss of appetite and nonulcer dyspepsia (with fullness, flatulence), chronic diarrhea, feverish states and minor fatigue. It has been used as a substitute of cinchona bark for malaria, under the name of dogwoodchinin. Externally it is used (as a wet compress, poultice) for wounds and ulcers.

Caution: Flowering dogwood should not be taken during pregnancy and lactation. Verbenalin has shown parasympathomimetic activity therefore it may affect many organs (heart, bronchi, uterus, etc.; see VERVAIN, EUROPEAN). In view of this, flowering dogwood should be used only as a combination product and as directed by an experienced practitioner.

References: (1) Vol. 4, p. 1004; (3) Vol. 4, p. 306; (5) Vol. 1, p. 343; (9) p. 214; (10) p. 42; (12) p. 522; (31) p. 578, (35) p. 122; (44) p. 177; (66) p. 252.

DOGWOOD, JAMAICA

Other Common Name(s): fishpoison tree
Botanical Name(s): *Piscidia piscipula* (L.) Sarg. = *Piscidia erythrina* L. [Fam.: Fabaceae (Leguminosae)]
Root bark
Constituents: Flavonoids (flavanones: glabranin, etc.; isoflavones: jamaicin, piscidone, etc.), rotenoids (rotenone, milletone, etc.), organic acids (piscidic acid, etc.), tannins, phytosterols, etc.

Properties: Sedative, hypnotic, anti-inflammatory, analgesic, antispasmodic. It has been shown to be cardiovascular stimulant (at low doses) or depressant (at high doses).

Uses: Internally it is used (as a tea, h. p.; usually combined with other herbs) for anxiety, insomnia, neuralgic pains, migraine, spastic conditions of the upper respiratory tract (spastic bronchitis, bronchial asthma; whooping cough) and primary dysmenorrhea (= painful menstruation without pathology). It has also been used to ease the symptoms of opium withdrawal.

Caution: Jamaica dogwood should not be taken during pregnancy and lactation and in cases of heart problems. Before using it for dysmenorrhea, the gynecologic problem should be judged by a health professional. Alcoholic drinks may interact with Jamaica dogwood. A possible combination of Jamaica dogwood with sedative, hypnotic and antidepressant drugs should be made only by a health professional. At higher doses than recommended it causes cause nausea, dizziness and excessive salivation. Toxic doses lead to convulsions and respiratory paralysis.

References: (3) Vol. 6a, p. 726; (6) pp. 214, 215; (8) p. 442; (9) p. 214; (12a) p. 663; (14) p. 139; (15) p. 163; (20) p. 174; (31) p. 430; (46) p. 1113; (47) p. 2155; (65) p. 262; (66) p. 395.

DONG QUAI

Other Common Name(s): Chinese angelica, dang gui
Botanical Name(s): *Angelica sinensis* (Oliv.) Diels = *Angelica polymorpha* Maxim. var. *sinensis* Oliv. [Fam.: Apiaceae (Umbelliferae)]
Root
Constituents: Volatile oil, alkyl-phthalides (ligustilide, etc.), coumarins, furanocoumarins (bergaptene, imperatorin), phenolic acids (coniferyl-ferulate, etc.), polyacetylenes (falcarinol, etc.), water-soluble polysaccharides, etc.
Properties: Antispasmodic, anti-inflammatory, analgesic, mild sedative, bitter tonic, carminative, cholagogue, liver protective, platelet aggregation inhibitory, peripheral vasodilatory, diuretic, antihypertensive, antibacterial, immunomodulant. The relatively strong antispasmodic effect, also anti-inflammatory, analgesic, mild sedative effects are attributed to ligustilide and related compounds. Pharmacological findings (more recent report: β-sympathomimetic activity; earlier report: parasympatholytic activity) justify the traditional use of dong quai for spasms of the uterine and upper respiratory tracts and explain its peripheral vasodilatory properties.
Uses: Internally it is used (as a tea, h. p.) for primary dysmenorrhea (= painful menstruation without pathology), PMS (= premenstrual syndrome), menopausal syndrome, loss of appetite and nonulcer dyspepsia (with flatulence, burping, heartburn, bloating, cramps, spastic constipation), inflammatory and spastic conditions of the upper respiratory tract (the common cold, sinusitis, bronchitis, bronchial asthma), inflammations of the liver (chronic hepatitis, adjuvant for cirrhosis) and kidneys (chronic nephritis), and for neuralgic and arthritic pains. Based on the reported properties, dong quai seems to be valuable for minor cases of coronary heart disease (= a condition associated with decreased blood supply to the heart) and hypertension, to prevent or alleviate angina pectoris (= chest pain due to insufficient blood supply to the heart), and it may be helpful for intermittent claudication (= pain / cramp / weakness in the legs on walking) and Raynaud's disease (= pale or red-blue patchy fingers). Externally it is used (as a poultice) for rheumatic pains, and boils.
Caution: For gynecologic disorders as well as during pregnancy and lactation it should be used on health professional's advice. A possible combination of dong quai products with anticoagulants (warfarin, etc.) and / or platelet aggregation inhibitors (aspirin, etc.) should be made only by a

136

health professional. When handling the herb avoid contact with skin and when taking its products avoid exposure to strong sunrays as it may cause phototoxic skin irritations. Otherwise, there are no reports of contraindications or side effects when used properly.

References: (2) Vol. 2, p. 117; (3) Vol. 3, p. 98, Vol. 4. p. 170; (9) p. 33; (13) p. 426; (20) p. 28; (29) p. 11; (50) p. 54; (53) p. 65; (68) p. 68; (70) p. 181; (71) p. 158.

DUCKWEED

Other Common Name(s): lesser duckweed
Botanical Name(s): *Lemna minor* L. [Fam.: Lemnaceae]
Whole plant
Constituents: Flavonoids (luteolin and apigenin glycosides, etc.), acyclic diterpenes (1-phytene-3, 4-diol, etc.), mucilaginous polysaccharides, tannins, vitamins (B_1, B_2, C), unsaturated fatty acids (incl. some closely related to prostaglandins), etc.
Properties: Anti-inflammatory, diuretic. Flavonoids may account at least in part for the anti-inflammatory and diuretic effects. Possibly, the unsaturated fatty acids are involved in the biosynthesis of prostaglandins by modifying their ratio in favor of PGE_1. PGE_1 has shown anti-inflammatory, bronchodilatory, and immunomodulant effects, among others. This may justify the reported anti-inflammatory effect.
Uses: Internally it is used (as an h. p.; usually combined with other herbs) for inflammations of the upper respiratory tract (pharyngitis, chronic rhinitis, etc.) and as an anti-inflammatory and antidyscratic (= blood purifier) for chronic rheumatic complaints. Externally it is used (as a poultice) for rheumatic pains and carbuncles.
Caution: There are no reports of contraindications or side effects when used properly. It may accumulate toxic chemicals of the water on which it grows therefore manufacturers should run tests accordingly.

References: (1) Vol. 5, p. 644; (3) Vol. 5, p. 481; (12a) p. 87; (18) p. 300; (37) p. 820; (41) Vols. 1-7; (47) p. 1734; (51) p. 52.

DULSE

Other Common Name(s): dillisk, Irish dulse, purple dulse, varette, sea kale
Botanical Name(s): *Palmaria palmata* (L.) Kuntze = *Rhodymenia palmata* (L.) Grev. [Fam.: Palmariaceae (Rhodymeniaceae)]; Class: Rhodophyceae (red algae)
Alga
Constituents: Polysaccharides (xylans), proteins (with essential and non-essential amino acids), non-protein amino acids (histidine, citrulline), vitamins (C, provitamin A = carotene, B-complex, α-tocopherol), minerals (including trace elements: iodine, etc.), phytosterols (5-sterols: desmosterol, etc.), etc.

137

Properties: Bulk laxative. It is considered rich in non-digestible polysaccharides, in vitamins and minerals (including trace elements), at the same time to be very poor in lipids.

Uses: Raw dulse is beneficial for constipation and as an aid to a weight-loss diet.

Caution: There are no reports of contraindications or side effects when used properly.

References: (5) Vol. 2, p. 95; (41) Vols. 1-7; (48) p. 46; (52) p. 667.

DYER'S BROOM

Other Common Name(s): dyer's greenwood
Botanical Name(s): *Genista tinctoria* L. [Fam.: Fabaceae (Leguminosae)]
Aerial part
Constituents: Flavonoids (flavones: luteolin, etc.; isoflavones: genistein, etc.), quinolizidine alkaloids (N-methylcytisine, cytisine, etc.), mucilaginous polysaccharides, tannins, etc.

Properties: Diuretic, mild laxative, antimicrobial. Flavonoids may account for the diuretic effect. Its alkaloids have shown effects very similar to nicotine, and may account at least in part for the increase of bowel motility.

Uses: Internally it is used as a flushing-out treatment (= herbal tea or product + liquids: more than 2 liters per day; sometimes combined with a medication) for inflammations of the genitourinary tract (cystitis, etc.), urinary gravel and nonobstructive stones, to prevent relapsing urinary infections / gravel / stones, as an antidyscratic (= blood purifier; tea, h. p.) for chronic rheumatic complaints and atopic eczema (= chronic eczema of internal origin), and (as a tea, h. p.) for minor constipation. Dyer's broom is chiefly used in traditional medicine.

Caution: Dyer's broom should not be taken during pregnancy and lactation and in cases of hypertension. A flushing-out treatment is contraindicated in cases of obstructive urinary stones, edema due to impaired heart or kidney function and kidney inflammations (here can be used on health professional's advice to enhance the effects of an antimicrobial therapy).

References: (2) Vol. 2, p. 794; (3) Vol. 4, p. 1110; (10) p. 104; (17) p. 251; (37) p. 584; (47) p. 1431.

EASTERN HEMLOCK

Other Common Name(s): Canada hemlock
Botanical Name(s): *Tsuga canadensis* (L.) Carr. = *Picea canadensis* (L.) Link. = *Pinus canadensis* L. [Fam.: Pinaceae]
Eastern hemlock oil
It is the volatile oil obtained by steam distillation from the fresh twig tips with leaves.

138

Constituents: Chiefly bornyl acetate, also α-pinene and other monoterpenes.

Properties: Aromatic, antimicrobial, expectorant (bronchial secretagogue effect).

Uses: Needle oil of Eastern hemlock is chiefly used in cosmetics and perfumery. Internally it is used (as an inhalation combination product) for inflammations of the upper respiratory tract (the common cold, bronchitis, etc.; coughs due to thickened bronchial secretion).

Caution: Needle oil of Eastern hemlock should not be taken in cases of spastic conditions of the upper respiratory tract (bronchial asthma, whooping cough). There are no reports available, but it may contain 3-carene. Oxidation products of 3-carene are skin and mucosal irritants. In view of this 3-carene should be contained within limits.

Bark (inner bark)

Constituents: Tannins (condensed t.: rich in hemlock-tannin = a flavan-4-ol dimer), stilbenoids (piceatannol, etc.), polysaccharides, etc.

Properties: Astringent, antimicrobial. Among stilbenoids there are compounds that have shown antifungal and antibacterial effects. Piceatannol is very closely related to resveratrol, which is known for its antioxidant effect.

Uses: Internally it is used (as a tea, h. p.) for inflammations of the gastrointestinal tract (diarrhea, gastroenteritis, ulcerative colitis, incl. hemorrhoids; also when minor hemorrhages are present). Externally it is used (as a mouthwash, gargle) for inflammations of the mouth and throat, (as a wash, wet compress, poultice) for minor skin inflammations and wounds and (as a vaginal irrigation / sitz bath / wash) for leukorrhea and vulvovaginitis.

Caution: There are no reports of contraindications or side effects when used properly. For minor hemorrhages it should be used on professional's advice.

References: (3) Vol. 6c, p. 317; (5) Vol. 2, p. 240; (10) p. 217; (15) p. 218; (25) p. 290; (31) p. 516; (36) p. 478; (37) p. 1411; (44) p. 570; (66) p. 396.

ECHINACEA

Other Common Name(s): 1) narrow-leaf echinacea, narrow-leaf purple coneflower, Kansas snakeroot 2) pale-flower echinacea, pale purple coneflower 3) purple coneflower

Botanical Name(s): 1) *Echinacea angustifolia* DC. 2) *Echinacea pallida* (Nutt.) Nutt. 3) *Echinacea purpurea* (L.) Moench [Fam.: Asteraceae (Compositae)]

Root (three species), **aerial part** (*E. purpurea*)

Constituents: Phenolic acids (cichoric acid = 2,3-dicaffeoyl-tartaric acid, etc.) and a closely related phenylethanoid glycoside (echinacoside), alkylamides = alkamides (no echinacein, but closely related butylamides), polysaccharides, polyacetylenes, volatile oil, pyrrolizidine alkaloids (tussilagine: non-toxic), etc. Roots of *E. angustifolia* and *E. pallida* contain echinacoside, while *E. angustifolia* contains additionally cynarin (= 1,3-dicaffeoyl-quinic acid; see ARTICHOKE). In root and aerial part of *E. purpurea* no echinacoside is found present, but cichoric acid) instead. Aerial parts of all three species contain flavonoids.

Properties: (Internally): Immunomodulant. (Topically): Anti-inflammatory, antimicrobial, antiviral, vulnerary, anesthetic. Echinacea, when taken for a short period and with proper dosage, has been shown to increase the phagocytic activity of macrophages and granulocytes, and the leukocyte count. To the effects contribute almost all the mentioned constituents (polysaccharides, alkyl-amides, phenolic acids and related compounds, polyacetylenes).

Uses: Internally it is used (as an h. p.; often combined with a medication) to ease and shorten the duration of the common cold and flu and other viral or bacterial infections (often of relapsing nature) of the upper respiratory and genitourinary tracts. Externally it is used (as a wash, wet compress, ointment) for inflammatory and painful skin problems such as wounds, minor burns and ulcers (incl. varicose ulcers), eczema, (as a poultice, ointment) for rheumatic pains, (as a mouthwash, gargle) for inflammations of the mouth and throat, (as a mouthwash, chewing) for dry mouth, (as a cotton swab or pasty mass applied to the tooth, or by chewing the herb) for toothache, (as a paint) for denture sores and canker sores, and (as an ointment, lipstick) for cold sores (= herpes simplex).

Caution: Echinacea should not be taken in cases of chronic debilitating illnesses such as multiple sclerosis, tuberculosis, diffuse connective tissue diseases (rheumatoid arthritis, scleroderma, systemic lupus erythematosus, Behçet's syndrome, etc.), AIDS, etc. Echinacea should not be taken for more than 2 weeks and before a possible resuming, a break for 2 weeks is required. As a member of the Heliantheae tribe, echinacea may contain sesquiterpene lactones. If so, it may cause allergic contact dermatitis to persons hypersensitive to other Asteraceae plants (e. g. arnica, chamomile, feverfew, ragweed, tansy, yarrow) that contain them.

References: (1) Vol. 5, p. 1; (3) Vol. 4, p. 751; (6) p. 261; (7) p. 307; (8) p. 233; (9) p. 216; (12) p. 1305; (13) p. 551; (14) p. 81; (16) p. 195; (17) pp. 191, 195; (18) p. 284; (19) pp. 68, 212; (20) p. 101; (22) p. 253; (26) p. 81; (37) p. 446; (44) p. 205; (46) p. 492; (48) p. 173; (59) pp. 125, 136.

ECLIPTA

Other Common Name(s): false daisy, trailing eclipta
Botanical Name(s): *Eclipta prostrata* (L.) L. = *Eclipta alba* (L.) Hassk. [Fam.: Asteraceae (Compositae)]
Aerial part
Constituents: Coumestans (= coumarono-coumarins: wedelolactone, etc.), flavonoids (flavones), thiophenes (tigloyl and angeloyl esters of bithienyl- and terthienyl methanol), nicotine, phytosterols, triterpenes, etc.

Properties: Choleretic, liver protective, anti-inflammatory, antibacterial, antifungal, analgesic, anthelmintic (against *Ascaris* spp., *Oxyuris* spp., *Ancylostoma* spp.) Wedelolactone has shown liver protective effect.

Uses: Internally it is chiefly used (as a tea, h. p.) for hepatobiliary disorders (chronic hepatitis, intoxications), nonulcer dyspepsia (with change of bowel habits), intestinal worms (see Properties), and for respiratory disorders (spastic bronchitis, etc.). It is also used as an anti-inflammatory and anti-dyscratic (= blood purifier; tea, h. p.) for chronic rheumatic complaints and atopic eczema (= chronic eczema of internal origin). Externally it is used (as a poultice, wet compress, wash; h.p.) for minor wounds and burns and fungal skin infections (incl. Tinea capitis = fungal infection of the scalp, Tinea pedis = athlete's foot) and (as a vaginal irrigation / sitz bath / wash) for vulvovaginitis.

Caution: Eclipta should not be taken during pregnancy and lactation. As a member of the Heliantheae tribe, eclipta may contain sesquiterpene lactones. If so, it may cause allergic contact dermatitis to persons hypersensitive to other Asteraceae plants (e. g. arnica, chamomile, feverfew, ragweed, tansy, yarrow) that contain them. The toxic unsaturated pyrrolizidine alkaloids are seldom found in the Heliantheae tribe. Nevertheless, manufacturers should run tests for them. For their limits see COLTSFOOT. Otherwise, there are no reports of contraindications or side effects when used properly.

References: (1) Vol. 5, p. 34; (5) Vol. 3, p. 193; (6) p. 146; (31) p. 434; (36) p. 437; (41) Vols. 1-7; (45) p. 202; (52) p. 271.

ELDER, DWARF

Other Common Name(s): danewort
Botanical Name(s): *Sambucus ebulus* L. [Fam.: Caprifoliaceae]
Root
Constituents: Bitter principles (iridoids: ebuloside, etc.), a lignan, saponins, phytosterols, tannins (condensed t.), a phenol glycoside (an arbutin derivative), a cyanogenic glycoside, etc.

Properties: Diuretic, laxative, expectorant. The effects are mild.

Uses: Internally it is used as an adjuvant (tea, h. p.; combined with other herbs) for genitourinary disorders (cystitis, gravel, nonobstructive urinary stones, etc.), minor constipation and inflammations of the upper respiratory tract (laryngitis, etc.; coughs). To enhance the effects in problems of the genitourinary tract, the fluid intake (incl. herbal teas) should be more than 2 liters per day.

Caution: There are no reports of contraindications or side effects when used properly. Doses higher than recommended should be avoided as they cause gastrointestinal irritations (with nausea, vomiting, diarrhea) and as it may contain cyanogenic glycoside (toxic!).

References: (1) Vol. 6, p. 575; (3) Vol. 6b, p. 260; (8) p. 506; (24) p. 368; (35) p. 276; (47) p. 2410.

141

ELDER, EUROPEAN

Other Common Name(s): black elder, elder
Botanical Name(s): *Sambucus nigra* L. [Fam.: Caprifoliaceae]
Flower
Constituents: Flavonoids (chiefly flavonols: rutin, isoquercitrin, etc.), mucilaginous polysaccharides, tannins, phenolic acids (caffeic acid derivatives), volatile oil, triterpenes, minerals (rich in potassium), etc.
Properties: Expectorant (bronchial secretagogue effect), diuretic, laxative (milder than fruit), demulcent, emollient.
Uses: Internally it is used (as a tea, h. p.) for inflammations of the upper respiratory tract (esp. as a diaphoretic hot tea for the common cold and feverish states; bronchitis, etc.; minor coughs) and gastrointestinal tract (with minor constipation), and as an antidyscratic (= blood purifier) for atopic eczema (= chronic eczema of internal origin). Externally it is used (as a mouthwash, gargle) for inflammations of the mouth and throat, and (as a wet compress, poultice) for minor skin inflammations.
Caution: It should be used dried and without peduncle. Otherwise, there are no reports of contraindications or side effects when used properly.
Note: Flowers of the American / Canadian / sweet elder: *Sambucus nigra* L. ssp. *canadensis* (L.) R. Bolli = *Sambucus canadensis* L. are used the same.
Fruit (berry; ripe)
Constituents: Flavonoids (anthocyanins, rutin, etc.), organic acids (citric and malic acids), sugars, vitamins (C, B-complex), cyanogenic glycosides (in seed), lectins (in seed), etc.
Properties: Acidulous, refrigerant, laxative, diuretic.
Uses: Internally it is used (as a tea, h. p.) for inflammatory conditions of the upper respiratory tract (the common cold, feverish states), minor constipation, and inflammations of the genitourinary tract. Well-processed fresh berry products, with a known content of lectins and cyanogenetic glycosides, are reported to exert immunomodulant and antiviral effects and are used for the common cold and flu. Elderberry is also used in food industry as a coloring ingredient.
Caution: Raw berries and fresh berry products if not well processed cause gastrointestinal irritations (with nausea, vomiting). Otherwise, there are no reports of contraindications or side effects when used properly.

References: (1) Vol. 6, p. 579; (3) Vol. 6b, p. 254; (7) p. 154; (8) p. 507; (9) p. 220; (12) p. 856; (13) p. 314; (14) p. 84; (16) p. 76; (17) pp. 528, 531; (19) p. 107; (20) p. 104; (27) p. 304; (35) p. 265; (46) p. 1421; (47) p. 2415; (48) p. 366; (68) p. 71.

ELECAMPANE

Other Common Name(s): scabwort
Botanical Name(s): *Inula helenium* L. [Fam.: Asteraceae (Compositae)]
Root

Constituents: Volatile oil (with sesquiterpene lactones), bitter principles (sesquiterpene lactones, collectively designated "helenin": alantolactone, etc.), triterpenes, phytosterols, polyacetylenes, a polysaccharide (inulin), etc.

Properties: Expectorant, bitter tonic, choleretic, cholagogue, antimicrobial, anthelmintic, diuretic. The mentioned effects are due in large part to helenin (= a mixture of alantolactone and its derivatives; steam distilling).

Uses: Internally it is used (as a tea, h. p.; only combined with other herbs) for inflammations of the upper respiratory tract (the common cold, bronchitis, minor bronchial asthma; coughs) and for loss of appetite and nonulcer dyspepsia (with change of bowel habits; incl. hemorrhoids) associated with hepatobiliary disorders (chronic cholecystitis, nonobstructive gallstones, impaired bile secretion and flow). Elecampane is also used (as a tea, h. p.) for intestinal worms, inflammations of genitourinary tract and as an anti-dyscratic (= blood purifier) for chronic rheumatic complaints, among others. To enhance the effects in problems of the genitourinary tract, the fluid intake (incl. herbal teas) should be more than 2 liters per day.

Caution: Elecampane should not be taken during pregnancy and lactation. It may cause allergic contact dermatitis to persons hypersensitive to other Asteraceae plants (e. g. arnica, chamomile, feverfew, ragweed, tansy, yarrow) that contain sesquiterpene lactones. At higher doses than recommended it may cause gastrointestinal irritations (with nausea, vomiting, diarrhea). Otherwise, there are no reports of contraindications or side effects when used properly.

References: (1) Vol. 5, p. 526; (3) Vol. 5, p. 246; (8) p. 323; (13) p. 414; (14) p. 87; (17) p. 283; (20) p. 106; (23) p. 218; (27) p. 114; (29) p. 64; (31) p. 601; (46) p. 549; (47) p. 1619; (48) p. 629; (51) p. 204.

ELECAMPANE, BRITISH / JAPANESE

Other Common Name(s): 1) British elecampane 2) Japanese elecampane
Botanical Name(s): 1) *Inula britannica* L. 2) *Inula japonica* Thunb. = *Inula britannica* L. var. *japonica* (Thunb.) Franch. et Sav. [Fam.: Asteraceae (Compositae)]

Flowering top

Constituents: Bitter principles (sesquiterpene lactones: gaillardin, etc.), flavonoids (flavonols, flavones), phenolic acids (caffeic and chlorogenic acids), triterpenes, volatile oil (with sesquiterpenes), etc.

Properties: Bitter tonic, anti-inflammatory, expectorant.

Uses: Internally it is used (as a tea, h. p.) for loss of appetite and nonulcer dyspepsia (with minor cramps, vomiting) and inflammations of the upper respiratory tract (bronchitis, pharyngitis, etc.; coughs) and genitourinary tract (cystitis, etc.). To enhance the effects in problems of the genitourinary tract, the fluid intake (incl. herbal teas) should be more than 2 liters per day.

Caution: There are no reports of contraindications or side effects when used properly. Nevertheless, it is best to avoid it during pregnancy and lactation.

It may cause allergic contact dermatitis to persons hypersensitive to other Asteraceae plants (e. g. arnica, chamomile, feverfew, ragweed, tansy, yarrow) that contain sesquiterpene lactones.

References: (1) Vol. 5, p. 523; (3) Vol. 5, p. 249; (41) Vols. 1-7; (45) p. 221; (52) p. 396.

EPAZOTE

Other Common Name(s): American wormseed, Mexican tea
Botanical Name(s): *Chenopodium ambrosioides* L., especially varieties rich in ascaridol such as var. *anthelminticum* A. Gray (American wormseed) [Fam.: Chenopodiaceae]
Chenopodium oil (= oil of American wormseed)
It is the volatile oil obtained by steam distillation from the aerial part collected when the seeds are ripe.
Constituents: Chiefly ascaridol (an unsaturated monoterpene peroxide), also p-cymene, limonene, camphor, etc.
Properties: Ascaridol exerts anthelmintic effect against roundworms (= *Ascaris* spp.) and hookworms (= *Ancylostoma* spp. and *Necator* spp.).
Uses: Internally it has been used as an anthelmintic for infestations with the mentioned parasites and (in veterinary practice) it is sometimes used for lungworm infestations. Externally it is sometimes used for athlete's foot.
Caution: Chenopodium oil is toxic (esp. for children). Miscalculated administrations have led to lethal intoxications. When taking chenopodium oil products, follow the manufacturer's instructions, which say that after 2 hours from the last dose to take a saline purgative (not oily purgatives!).

References: (2) Vol. 2, p. 344; (3) Vol. 3, p. 842; (8) p. 146; (9) p. 152; (13) p. 119; (37) p. 305; (46) p. 283; (55) p. 411.

EPHEDRA

Other Common Name(s): 1) Chinese ephedra 2) Indian / Pakistani ephedra
Botanical Name(s): 1) *Ephedra equisetina* Bunge = *Ephedra shennungiana* Tang; *Ephedra sinica* Stapf 2) *Ephedra intermedia* Schrenk et C.A. Meyer; *Ephedra gerardiana* Wall ex Stapf. [Fam.: Ephedraceae]
Aerial part (ma huang)
Constituents: Non-heterocyclic alkaloids: chiefly (−)-ephedrine, along with (−)-norephedrine, (−)-N-methylephedrine, (+)-pseudoephedrine, (+)-norpseudoephedrine, (+)-N-methylpseudoephedrine, etc. It also contains tannins (proanthocyanidins), flavonoids, and phenolic acids, among others.
Properties: (−)-Ephedrine is sympathomimetic (primarily indirect by releasing norepinephrine from sympathetic nerve endings, partly direct), due to which it exerts bronchodilatory, nasal decongestant and cardiac stimulant effects, stimulates central nervous system, increases arterial pressure, skele-

144

tal muscle strength and tone of vesicle sphincter, and relaxes smooth muscle of the gastrointestinal tract, among others. Ephedrine promotes the breakdown of glycogen into glucose (= glycogenolytic effect). Pseudoephedrine is weaker in action and less toxic than ephedrine.

Uses: <u>Internally</u> it is used (as an h. p. standardized to ephedrine content; ephedrine; pseudoephedrine) for spastic and inflammatory conditions of the upper respiratory tract (minor bronchial asthma, hay fever, bronchitis, the common cold, etc.), and for brief hypotensive (= low blood pressure) and sleepy states.

Caution: Ephedra products should be standardized to ephedrine content. Ephedrine and ephedra are contraindicated in hypertension, glaucoma, diabetes, micturition problems, among others. They should not be combined with MAOI antidepressant drugs (e. g. phenelzine) or herbs (e. g. St. John's wort). Unless directed by a health professional, they should not be combined with caffeine or caffeine rich herbs / drinks (coffee, cola, guaraná, maté, tea) as it may result in a risky overstimulation of the nervous system. Depending on doses and extension of time used, they may cause nervousness, insomnia, tachycardia (= rapid heartbeat; at excessive doses, cardiac arrest), headache, hypertension (at excessive doses, cerebral hemorrhage), and dry mouth, nausea, vomiting, among others.

References: (1) Vol. 5, p. 48; (3) Vol. 4, p. 782; (6) p. 110; (7) p. 164; (8) p. 241; (11) p. 180; (12) p. 1091; (13) p. 271; (15) p. 82; (22) p. 112; (46) p. 507; (48) p. 880; (50) p. 25; (59) p. 145; (67) p. 493.

EPIMEDIUM

Other Common Name(s): Horny goat weed
Botanical Name(s): *Epimedium brevicornu* Maxim.; *E. grandiflorum* C. Morren; other *Epimedium* species [Fam.: Berberidaceae]
<u>Aerial part</u> (mostly leaves)
Constituents: Flavonoids (rich in 8-prenyl flavonol glycosides: icariin and related compounds), water-soluble polysaccharides, tannins, volatile oil, etc. It possibly contains benzyl-isoquinoline alkaloids.
Properties: Peripheral vasodilatory, mild antihypertensive, estrogenic, platelet aggregation inhibitory, antioxidant, anti-inflammatory, immuno-modulant, antitussive (possibly cough suppressant effect). Icariin has been shown to promote bone formation and together with other flavonoids accounts for most of the effects. If present, benzyl-isoquinoline alkaloids certainly contribute to the overall effect. They have shown vasodilatory, anti-hypertensive and antitussive effects.
Uses: <u>Internally</u> it is used (as a tea, h. p.) for postmenopausal hypertension, low sexual drive, postmenopausal osteoporosis, erectile dysfunction, coronary heart disease, inflammations of the liver (chronic hepatitis) and upper respiratory tract (bronchitis, etc.; with irritating dry coughs). It may be helpful for alcoholism, intermittent claudication and Raynaud's disease.

Caution: There are no reports of contraindications or side effects when used properly. Manufacturers should evaluate the alkaloids content in raw materials (natural or cured) and / or their products.

References: (3) Vol. 4, p. 788; (5) Vol. 1, p. 458; (9) p. 230; (18) p. 128; (31) p. 188; (36) p. 38; (41) Vols. 1-7.

ERGOT

Other Common Name(s): ergot of rye, rye ergot
Ergot (Lat. Secale cornutum) is the dried sclerotium of the fungus *Claviceps purpurea* (Fries) Tulasne [Fam.: Clavicipitaceae] that grows parasitically on rye (*Secale cereale* L.; Fam.: Poaceae) by replacing many of its grains.
Constituents: Ergoline alkaloids of which those most important can be classified: a) ergotamine group (ergotamine, ergosine), b) ergotoxine group (ergocristine, ergokryptine, ergocornine), and c) ergometrine group (ergometrine = ergobasine). It also contains amino acids (histidine, etc.), biogenic amines (tyramine, choline, betaine), carbohydrates, fixed oil, phytosterols, etc.
Properties: The genuine alkaloids of peptide type (ergotamine and ergotoxine groups) are α-adrenergic blockers but possess also an agonistic active component, particularly proven for ergotamine, which leads to vasoconstriction. The six mentioned alkaloids exert oxytocic effect.
Uses: Ergot extracts are no longer used. Ergotamine and dihydroergotamine are used for migraine headache. A mixture of hydrogenated alkaloids of ergotoxine group is used for cerebral insufficiency in geriatric patients. Methylergometrine (a semisynthetic derivative of ergometrine) exerts only oxytocic effect and is chiefly used to decrease postpartum hemorrhage (= h. following childbirth).
Caution: Ergot is toxic. Ergot products as well as isolated alkaloids and their changed derivatives are used only by prescription. In the past, the consumption of ergot-infected rye has caused poisoning (= egotism), which has led to gangrene of extremities.

References: (1) Vol. 4, p. 911; (3) Vol. 4, p. 102; (8) p. 171; (11) p. 172; (12) p. 1015; (13) p. 243; (36) p. 385; (37) p. 1248; (46) p. 1454; (47) p. 2501; (48) p. 983; (72) nrs. 18050, 36016; (74) p. 398.

ERYNGO

Other Common Name(s): 1) plains eryngo 2) field e. 3) eryngo, sea holly
Botanical Name(s): 1) *Eryngium planum* L. 2) *Eryngium campestre* L. 3) *Eryngium maritimum* L. [Fam.: Apiaceae (Umbelliferae)]
Root, aerial part
Constituents: Triterpenoid saponins, tannins, phenolic acids (caffeic acid

146

derivatives), volatile oil, flavonoids (aerial part). Among the mentioned species as well as between root and aerial part there are slight differences.

Properties: Diuretic, antispasmodic, expectorant, anti-inflammatory.

Uses: Internally it is used (as a tea, h. p.; usually combined with other herbs) for minor inflammatory and spastic conditions of the genitourinary tract (cystitis, urethritis, prostatitis, gravel, nonobstructive urinary stones) and upper respiratory tract (bronchitis, etc.; coughs: irritating cough, whooping cough). To enhance the effects in problems of the genitourinary tract, the fluid intake (incl. herbal teas) should be more than 2 liters per day.

Caution: There are no reports of contraindications or side effects when used properly.

References: (1) Vol. 5, p. 76; (3) Vol. 4, p. 804; (8) p. 248; (10) p. 109; (15) p. 84; (23) p. 403; (24) p. 233; (27) p. 65; (35) p. 407; (36) p. 476; (47) p. 1294.

ERYSIMUM

Botanical Name(s): *Erysimum diffusum* Ehrh. = *Erysimum canescens* Roth.; *Erysimum crepidifolium* Rchb. [Fam.: Brassicaceae (Cruciferae)]
Aerial part
Constituents: Cardiac glycosides (erysimoside, helveticoside, etc., with aglycone k-strophanthidin), glucosinolates, etc.

Properties: Erysimum exerts strophanthus-like cardiotonic effect. Helveticoside (= k-strophanthidin-digitoxoside) acts similar to k-strophanthin (see STROPHANTHUS). See DIGITALIS.

Uses: Internally it is used (as an injection: isolated and purified helveticoside) for heart failure. *E. diffusum* and *E. crepidifolium* are considered among the richest herbs in cardiac glycosides.

Caution: Erysimum and its cardiac glycosides are toxic and not for self-treatment. Helveticoside is used as directed by a health professional. See DIGITALIS. Erysimum is not to be confused with hedge mustard or bank cress: *Sisymbrium officinale* (L.) Scop. = *Erysimum officinale* L. (See MUSTARD, HEDGE).

References: (1) Vol. 5, p. 85; (3) Vol. 4, p. 808; (8) p. 249; (13) p. 192; (36) p. 319; (37) p. 482.

EUCALYPTUS

Botanical Name(s): *Eucalyptus globulus* Labill. [Fam.: Myrtaceae]
Leaf
Constituents: Volatile oil (see Eucalyptus oil), tannins, flavonoids (flavonols: quercetin, rutin, etc.), triterpenes, phenolic acids, etc.

Properties: Expectorant (bronchial secretagogue effect), antimicrobial, astringent, anti-inflammatory, mild antispasmodic. Most of the effects are due to the volatile oil and its eucalyptol content.

Uses: <u>Internally</u> it is used (as a tea, h. p.) chiefly for inflammations of the upper respiratory tract (the common cold, bronchitis, tracheitis, pharyngitis, laryngitis, sinusitis, rhinitis; coughs due to thickened bronchial secretion) and to a lesser extent those of the genitourinary tract (cystitis, urethritis, prostatitis, etc.) and gastrointestinal tract (diarrhea, etc., incl. hemorrhoids). To enhance the effects in problems of the genitourinary tract, the fluid intake (incl. herbal teas) should be more than 2 liters per day. <u>Externally</u> it is used (as a wash, wet compress) for minor wounds, ulcers and burns and (as a mouthwash, gargle) for inflammations of the mouth and throat.

Caution: See Eucalyptus oil.

Eucalyptus oil

It is the volatile oil obtained by steam distillation from the crushed leaves.

Constituents: 1,8-cineole (= eucalyptol = cajeputol) as its major constituent, also myrtenol, pinenes, α-phellandrene, etc.

Properties: Expectorant (bronchial secretagogue effect), antimicrobial, rubefacient.

Uses: Rectified eucalyptus oil (with α-phellandrene content in minimum) and eucalyptol are used <u>internally</u> (as a cough drop, inhalation) and <u>externally</u> (as a liniment, ointment) for inflammations of the upper respiratory tract and rheumatic pains. Both are important ingredients in oral hygiene products (toothpastes, mouthwashes) and fragrances.

Caution: Botanicals very rich in cineole should not be taken in cases of inflammatory conditions of the gastrointestinal and biliary tracts, severe liver disorders, in infants, and are best avoided during pregnancy, lactation and when on a vital medication (cineole causes enzyme induction in the liver and an increased metabolism of some drugs). For infants and young children eucalyptus oil products should be rubbed on chest and throat, avoiding face and nostrils. Avoid inhalations in bronchial asthma and whooping cough.

References: (1) Vol. 5, p. 116; (3) Vol. 4, p. 854; (6) pp. 95, 97; (8) p. 254; (9) p. 232; (11) p. 93; (12) p. 723; (13) p. 106; (16) pp. 48, 72; (17) p. 208; (19) pp. 74, 75; (20) p. 108; (46) p. 560; (47) p. 1302; (48) p. 555; (49) Vol. 2, p. 438.

EUCOMMIA

Other Common Name(s): Chinese rubber tree, hardy rubber tree
Botanical Name(s): *Eucommia ulmoides* Oliv. [Fam.: Eucommiaceae]

Bark

Constituents: Bitter principles (iridoids: aucubin, ulmoside, etc.), lignans (pinoresinol and medioresinol glycosides), phenolic acids (caffeic acid, etc.), flavonoids (leucoanthocyanidins), minerals (potassium, etc.), etc.

Properties: Bitter tonic, anti-inflammatory, analgesic, antimicrobial, mild immunomodulant, antioxidant, liver protective, diuretic, peripheral vasodilatory, antihypertensive, sedative, and it is reported to be aphrodisiac. Iridoids have shown bitter tonic, choleretic, liver protective, laxative, diuretic, anti-inflammatory, antibacterial, antiviral, antifungal and immunomodulant effects, among others. The diuretic effect is due at least in part to flavonoids and potassium salts. The peripheral vasodilatory and antihypertensive effect is due in large part to pinoresinol glycosides. Lignans have shown anti-inflammatory, antioxidant, liver protective, immunomodulant, antibacterial, antiviral, and estrogen-like effects, among others.

Uses: Internally it is used (as a tea, h. p.) for loss of appetite and nonulcer dyspepsia, inflammations of the liver (chronic hepatitis) and kidneys (chronic nephritis), chronic rheumatic complaints, minor cases of hypertension and fatigue, and it may be beneficial for low sexual drive and erectile dysfunction.

Caution: There are no reports of contraindications or side effects when used properly. Nevertheless, before using eucommia for gynecologic disorders, the problem should be judged by a health professional.

References: (3) Vol. 4, p. 861; (5) Vol. 1, p. 479; (12) p. 438; (13) p. 430; (31) pp. 435, 569; (41) Vols. 1-7; (42) Vol. 4, p. 100; (45) p. 205; (52) p. 294; (53) p. 249.

EVENING PRIMROSE

Botanical Name(s): *Oenothera biennis* L. [Fam.: Onagraceae (Oenotheraceae)]
Evening primrose oil (= EPO)
It is the fixed oil obtained by cold expression from the seeds.
Constituents: Chiefly glycerides, with fatty acids component high proportions of linoleic acid and gamma-linolenic acid (= GLA = gamolenic acid), which are omega-6 fatty acids, and oleic acid.
Properties: Linoleic acid and gamma-linolenic acid, the so-called essential fatty acids (= EFAs), are involved in the biosynthesis of prostaglandins by modifying their ratio in favor of PGE_1. PGE_1 has shown anti-inflammatory, immunomodulant, vasodilatory, antihypertensive, cholesterol reducing, platelet aggregation inhibitory and bronchodilatory effects, and it stimulates the smooth-muscle contraction in the gastrointestinal tract.
Uses: Internally it is used as a rich natural supplement of the essential fatty acids, which are recommended for conditions associated with an imbalance of prostaglandin biosynthesis, including atopic eczema (= eczema of internal origin) and premenstrual syndrome = PMS (with breast pain = mastodynia, etc., see Therapeutic Checklist). EFAs are beneficial also for high cholesterol and cardiovascular diseases in general, bronchial asthma, rheumatic complaints (incl. rheumatoid arthritis) and endometriosis (= abnormal growth of endometrial tissue outside the uterus), among others. Externally it is used (as a paint, liniment: undiluted oil) for atopic eczema and other skin inflammatory disorders.
Caution: Evening primrose oil should not be used internally in infants under one year of age. It should be standardized to the GLA content. In rare

cases it may cause gastrointestinal discomfort (nausea, impaired digestion), headache, or skin rash. It should not be combined with phenothiazine antipsychotic / antihistamine drugs. Before using evening primrose oil for PMS with breast pain (= mastodynia), the problems should be judged by a health professional.

References: (1) Vol. 5, p. 929; (3) Vol. 6a, p. 303; (6) p. 355; (7) p. 287; (8) p. 386; (12) p. 266; (13) p. 394; (19) p. 162; (22) p. 192; (23) p. 335; (26) p. 97; (48) p. 157; (67) p. 807; (68) p. 76; (71) p. 84; (72) nr. 31354; (75) p. 210.

EYEBRIGHT

Botanical Name(s): *Euphrasia rostkoviana* F. Hayne; *Euphrasia stricta* J.P. Wolf ex J. F. Lehm. = *Euphrasia officinalis* L.; etc. [Fam.: Scrophulariaceae]
Aerial part
Constituents: Bitter principles (iridoids: aucubin, catalpol, euphroside, eurostoside, etc.), flavonoids (flavonols, flavones), phenolic acids, phenylethanoid glycosides (eukovoside, etc.), lignans, phytosterols, etc.
Properties: Bitter tonic, anti-inflammatory, astringent, mild antimicrobial.
Uses: Internally it is used (as a tea, h. p.) for inflammations of the gastrointestinal tract (gastritis, loss of appetite, impaired digestion) and upper respiratory tract (bronchitis, laryngitis with hoarseness, tracheitis, etc.). Externally it is chiefly used in traditional medicine (as an eye-wash, eye-bath) for eye inflammations, (as a poultice) for sty, and (as a wash, wet compress) for minor skin inflammations.
Caution: There are no reports of contraindications or side effects when used properly. Topical applications of eyebright preparations for eye problems for hygienic reasons are best avoided, or at least should be supervised by an experienced practitioner.

References: (2) Vol. 2, p. 667; (3) Vol. 4, p. 886; (6) p. 376; (8) p. 258; (9) p. 237; (12) p. 443; (13) p. 408; (15) p. 89; (17) p. 211; (20) p. 114; (47) p. 1328; (51) p. 188.

FALSE UNICORN

Other Common Name(s): blazing star, fairy wand, helonias
Botanical Name(s): *Chamaelirium luteum* (L.) A. Gray = *Helonias dioica* Pursh. = *Veratrum luteum* L. [Fam.: Liliaceae]
Root (rhizome)
Constituents: It is not well studied. It is reported to contain steroidal saponins (diosgenin glycosides: chamaelirin, etc.), also free diosgenin. As a member of Melanthioideae subfamily, it possibly contains alkaloids.
Properties: Uterotonic, emmenagogue, diuretic.
Uses: Internally it is used (as a tea, h. p.) for secondary amenorrhea and oligomenorrhea (= ceased / infrequent / scanty menstruation without pathol

150

ogy), hypotonic uterus, menopausal syndrome, and to induce diuresis when this is advisable.

Caution: Before using false unicorn for gynecologic disorders, the problem should be judged by a health professional. Unless advised by a health professional, it should not be taken during pregnancy and lactation. At higher doses than recommended it causes gastrointestinal irritations (with nausea, vomiting). Manufacturers should evaluate the presence of alkaloids (see Constituents).

References: (2) Vol. 2, p. 341; (3) Vol. 3, p. 831; (14) p. 125; (15) p. 59; (20) p. 116; (36) pp. 51, 475; (37) p. 300; (42) Vol. 2, pp. 280, 286, 484; (46) p. 548; (47) p. 1533; (49) Vol. 2, p. 30; (71) p. 234.

FENNEL

Other Common Name(s): 1) bitter fennel 2) sweet fennel
Botanical Name(s): 1) *Foeniculum vulgare* Mill. ssp. *vulgare* var. *vulgare* 2) *Foeniculum vulgare* Mill. ssp. *vulgare* var. *dulce* (Mill.) Batt. et Trab. [Fam.: Apiaceae (Umbelliferae)]
<u>Fruit</u> (commonly called seed)
Constituents: Volatile oil (see below), phenolic acids (caffeic acid, etc.), flavonoids, furanocoumarins, fixed oil, etc. Compared to the sweet variety, bitter variety contains more fenchone (bitter!) and less anethole (sweet!).
Properties: Aromatic, stomachic, gastrointestinal tonic (at lower doses: increases bowel motility) and antispasmodic (at higher doses), carminative, expectorant (chiefly bronchial secretagogue effect), emmenagogue, galactagogue, antimicrobial.
Uses: Sweet variety is extensively used as a spice (in culinary practice and spice industry). Fennel (esp. fennel oil) is also used in liqueur / liquor industry. For medicinal purposes the bitter variety is preferred. <u>Internally</u> it is used (as a tea, h. p.) for nonulcer dyspepsia (with fullness, flatulence), irritable bowel syndrome and inflammations of the upper respiratory tract (bronchitis, etc.; coughs due to thickened bronchial secretion), and to promote milk secretion in nursing mothers.
Caution: In rare cases it may cause allergic reactions of the skin and respiratory tract. Otherwise, there are no reports of contraindications or side effects when used properly.
<u>Fennel oil</u>
It is the volatile oil obtained by steam distillation from the freshly crushed fruits.
Constituents: Chiefly trans-anethole, also fenchone and some estragole (= methylchavicol), etc.
Uses: <u>Internally</u> it is used (as a combination product) much like fennel fruit.
Caution: Same as fennel fruit.

References: (1) Vol. 5, p. 157; (6) pp. 95, 128; (7) p. 199; (8) p. 265; (12) p. 695; (13) p. 127; (16) p. 73; (17) p. 200; (19) p. 78; (23) p. 82; (27) p. 135; (28) p. 102, 119; (37) p. 549; (46) p. 605; (48) p. 515.

FENUGREEK

Botanical Name(s): *Trigonella foenum-graecum* L. [Fam.: Fabaceae (Leguminosae)]

Seed

Constituents: Mucilages (very rich), steroidal saponins (with aglycone: diosgenin; cf. YAM, WILD), bitter principles (chiefly saponins), trigonelline (= nicotinic acid N-methyl-betaine), free amino acids (4-hydroxy-isoleucine, etc.), proteins, lipids (fixed oil, phospholipids), flavonoids, etc.

Properties: Demulcent, expectorant, emollient, stomachic, tonic, cholesterol and triglyceride reducing, mild antihyperglycemic. The expectorant, demulcent, emollient effects are due in large part to mucilages and saponins. The cholesterol reducing effect is due to mucilages (see PSYLLIUM) and saponins, by acting upon the gastrointestinal tract. Steroidal saponins have been shown to lower elevated cholesterol levels (cf. SARSAPARILLA). They may inhibit the absorption of dietary cholesterol and at the same time may bind available bile salts and increase their fecal excretion. Then the liver to synthesize biliary acids will utilize the excessive LDL-cholesterol. The mild antihyperglycemic effect may be due to 4-hydroxy-isoleucine.

Uses: Internally it is used (as an h. p., powdered seed) for inflammations of the gastrointestinal tract (loss of appetite, gastritis, irritable bowel syndrome) and upper respiratory tract (bronchitis, etc.; coughs) and as a tonic. Fenugreek has shown beneficial effects for high cholesterol and triglycerides, and diabetes. Externally it is used (as a poultice) for minor skin inflammations and indurations, eczema, ulcers, and boils.

Caution: Fenugreek may impair the absorption of some drugs. In view of this, when taking a vital oral medication, drugs should be taken about one hour apart from fenugreek products. Otherwise, there are no reports of contraindications or side effects when used properly.

References: (1) Vol. 6, p. 994; (3) Vol. 6c, p. 268; (6) p. 99; (8) p. 562; (9) p. 243; (12) p. 367; (13) p. 372; (16) p. 28; (17) p. 221; (19) p. 50; (20) p. 117; (37) p. 1401; (46) p. 599; (47) p. 1362; (48) p. 105.

FEVER BARK TREE, AUSTRALIAN

Other Common Name(s): fever tree, Australian fever tree

Botanical Name(s): *Alstonia constricta* F. v. Muell. [Fam.: Apocynaceae]

Bark (bitter bark, fever bark)

Constituents: Indole alkaloids, including alstonine, serpentine (steroisomer of alstonine), reserpine, alstonidine and alstoniline, among others.

Properties: Bitter tonic, antipyretic, antispasmodic, diuretic, antihypertensive.

Uses: Internally it is used (as a tea, h. p.) for feverish states, the common cold, diarrhea, and minor hypertension.

Caution: Fever bark should be used only as directed by an experienced practitioner as it contains potential alkaloids. Normally, it should not be taken during pregnancy and lactation.

References: (3) Vol. 2, p. 1235; (5) Vol. 1, p. 61; (10) p. 9; (35) p. 30; (36) p. 396; (37) p. 52; (45) p. 163; (50) p. 118; (66) p. 268.

FEVERFEW

Botanical Name(s): *Tanacetum parthenium* (L.) Sch. Bip. = *Chrysanthemum parthenium* (L.) Bernh. [Fam.: Asteraceae (Compositae)]
Leaf
Constituents: Sesquiterpene lactones (chiefly parthenolide, etc.), flavonoids (flavones), volatile oil (with camphor, chrysanthenyl acetate, etc.), etc. Parthenolide concentration varies widely depending on geographical origin, crop, drying process and storage. Its concentration in the extracts depends on the extraction process.
Properties: Migraine preventive, anti-inflammatory. It has been shown to inhibit the release of serotonin from blood platelets, which explains at least in part the anti-migraine properties.
Uses: Internally it is used as a preventive (standardized product) for migraine and rheumatic complaints (incl. rheumatoid arthritis). Feverfew should be taken for at least 3 months. A treatment for more than 4 months should be monitored by a health professional.
Caution: Feverfew should not be taken during pregnancy and lactation. It should be used on health professional's advice and only as a standardized product to parthenolide content. Feverfew may cause allergic contact dermatitis to persons hypersensitive to other Asteraceae plants (e. g. arnica, chamomile, ragweed, tansy, yarrow) that contain sesquiterpene lactones. Otherwise, there are no reports of contraindications or side effects when used properly.

References: (2) Vol. 3, p. 618; (3) Vol. 3, p. 906; (9) p. 246; (12) p. 491; (13) p. 404; (22) p. 173; (48) p. 631.

FIG

Botanical Name(s): *Ficus carica* L. [Fam.: Moraceae]
Fruit (ripe, dried)
Constituents: Carbohydrates (chiefly invert sugar and sucrose, also pectin and mucilaginous polysaccharides), organic acids, fat, proteins, minerals, vitamins, furanocoumarins, etc.
Properties: Nutrient, mild laxative, demulcent.
Uses: Internally it is used for minor constipation, for which is often combined with other laxatives such as Senna (q. v.), Manna (q. v.) and Tamarind (q. v.). It is also used as a natural sweetener of herbal teas, and (roasted) as a coffee substitute.

Caution: Fig should not be taken in cases of bowel obstruction. In rare cases it may cause allergic reactions. When handling fresh figs avoid contact with skin and after eating fresh figs avoid exposure to strong sunrays as it may cause phototoxic skin irritations.

Note: Milky juice of the unripe fruit contains proteolytic enzymes and is used <u>externally</u> (as a paint) for corns.

References: (2) Vol. 2, p. 714; (3) Vol. 4, p. 990; (8) p. 262; (10) p. 116; (13) p. 346; (27) p. 132; (37) p. 530.

FIGWORT

Other Common Name(s): brownwort
Botanical Name(s): *Scrophularia nodosa* L. [Fam.: Scrophulariaceae]
Aerial part
Constituents: Iridoids (aucubin, catalpol, harpagide and its esters, etc.), saponins, phenolic acids (caffeic acid, etc.), flavonoids (diosmin, hesperidin, etc.), tannins, etc.
Properties: Mild diuretic, bitter tonic, laxative, anti-inflammatory, wound-healing. Iridoids have shown bitter tonic, choleretic, cholagogic, liver protective, laxative, diuretic, anti-inflammatory, analgesic, antibacterial, antiviral, antifungal and immunomodulant effects, among others. Diosmin and hesperidin have shown anti-inflammatory effect. Saponins and flavonoids may account at least in part for the diuretic effect.
Uses: <u>Internally</u> it is chiefly used as an antidyscratic (= blood purifier) and anti-inflammatory for atopic eczema (= chronic eczema of internal origin), and for loss of appetite and nonulcer dyspepsia (with sluggish bowels, minor constipation, hemorrhoids). <u>Externally</u> it is used (as a wet compress, poultice) for minor skin inflammations, eczemas (incl. milk crust), wounds, ulcers and hemorrhoids, and (as a vaginal irrigation / sitz bath / wash) for vulvovaginitis. In traditional medicine it is also used for minor cases of scrofula (= tuberculosis of lymph nodes, esp. those in the neck). Based on constituents and their effects, this seems justifiable.
Caution: There are no reports of contraindications or side effects when used properly.

References: (3) Vol. 6b, p. 336; (8) p. 515; (10) p. 116; (12) p. 438; (15) p. 193; (20) p. 122; (24) p. 98; (31) pp. 396, 474, 569; (35) p. 313; (37) p. 1247; (47) p. 2493; (51) p. 182.

FIR

Other Common Name(s): 1) silver fir, European silver fir 2) North Japanese fir 3) Siberian fir 4) spruce fir, white fir, European (Norway) spruce
Botanical Name(s): 1) *Abies alba* Mill. = *Abies pectinata* (Lam.) DC. 2) *Abies sachalinensis* (Schmidt) Masters 3) *Abies sibirica* Ledebour 4) *Picea abies* (L.) Karsten = *Picea excelsa* (Lam.) Link. [Fam. Pinaceae]

154

Fir needle oil

It is the volatile oil obtained by steam distillation from the fresh twig tips with leaves of any species mentioned above.

Constituents: Chiefly bornyl acetate, also other monoterpenes such as α- and β-pinene, etc. It may contain small amount of another monoterpene, 3-carene.

Properties: Aromatic, antimicrobial, expectorant (bronchial secretagogue effect), rubefacient.

Uses: Internally it is used (as an inhalation, drops on sugar, lozenge) for inflammations of the upper respiratory tract (the common cold, bronchitis, tracheitis, etc.; coughs due to thickened bronchial secretion). Externally it is used (as an ointment, liniment) for inflammations of the upper respiratory tract and for neuralgic and rheumatic pains. It is widely used in cosmetics and perfumery.

Caution: Fir needle oil should not be used in cases of spastic conditions of the upper respiratory tract (bronchial asthma, whooping cough). Oxidation products of 3-carene are skin and mucosal irritants. In view of this 3-carene should be contained within limits.

Buds (fresh)

They are obtained from European silver fir and spruce fir (= white fir = European / Norway spruce).

Constituents: Volatile oil, chiefly with bornyl acetate, also free borneol and other monoterpenes.

Properties: Expectorant (bronchial secretagogue effect), antimicrobial, rubefacient.

Uses: Internally it is used for inflammations of the upper respiratory tract (the common cold, bronchitis, tracheitis, etc.; coughs due to thickened bronchial secretion). Externally it is used (as a poultice, partial / full bath) for neuralgic and rheumatic pains.

Caution: There are no reports of contraindications or side effects when used properly.

References: (1) Vol. 4, pp. 7, 20; (3) Vol. 2, p. 869; (5) Vol. 2, pp. 185, 187; (8) p. 15; (9) p. 60; (16) p. 74; (19) pp. 80, 81; (36) p. 269; (37) p. 2; (48) p. 584.

FLAX

Botanical Name(s): *Linum usitatissimum* L. [Fam.: Linaceae]

Seed (flaxseed, linseed)

Constituents: Fixed oil, mucilaginous polysaccharides, proteins, crude fiber, lignans, phenyl-ethanoid glycosides, phosphatides, phytosterols, enzymes, cyanogenic glycosides, etc.

Properties: Demulcent, emollient, bulk laxative. Flaxseed lignans have shown anticarcinogenic property. Flaxseed enzymes are destroyed by the gastric juice hence no hydrocyanic acid is liberated from the cyanogenic glycosides.

Uses: Internally it is used (whole seed, crushed seed, prepared mucilage) for chronic constipation, irritable bowel syndrome, (prepared mucilage) for chronic inflammations of the gastrointestinal tract (gastritis, peptic ulcers, irritable bowel syndrome), and as a dietary aid to the prevention of cancer. Externally it is used (as a poultice) for boils and carbuncles.

Caution: Flaxseed should not be taken in cases of bowel obstruction and acute inflammations of the gastrointestinal tract. It should be taken with plenty of fluids (about 10 times its amount). To avoid calories take the seeds uncrushed. As with other mucilage rich herbs, it may slow the absorption of drugs, which should be taken about one hour apart from flax seed products.

Flaxseed oil (= linseed oil)

Constituents: Chiefly glycerides (= esters of glycerin with fatty acids), with fatty acids component high proportions of essential fatty acids (= EFAs) including alpha-linolenic acid (an omega-3 fatty acid) and linoleic acid (an omega-6 fatty acid), etc.

Properties: Cholesterol and triglyceride reducing, laxative, demulcent, emollient, and other effects attributed to EFAs (see EVENING PRIMROSE).

Uses: Internally it is used as a mild laxative for minor constipation and inflammations of the lower intestinal tract, as a dietary supplement of EFAs, recommended for high cholesterol and the prevention of cardiovascular disease, among others (see EVENING PRIMROSE). Externally it is used (as a liniment) for eczemas (incl. milk crust). In traditional medicine it is still used (mixed with lime-wash) for minor burns.

Caution: There are no reports of contraindications or side effects when used properly.

References: (1) Vol. 5, p. 671; (3) Vol. 5, p. 517; (6) p. 168; (7) pp. 186, 222; (8) p. 344; (11) p. 73; (12) pp. 267, 370; (13) p. 390; (17) p. 346; (36) p. 188; (37) pp. 528, 831; (48) p. 117.

FLEABANE, CANADA

Other Common Name(s): Canadian butterweed, Canadian coltstail, Canadian horseweed

Botanical Name(s): *Conyza canadensis* (L.) Cronquist = *Erigeron canadensis* L. [Fam.: Asteraceae (Compositae)]

Aerial part

Constituents: Volatile oil (with limonene, etc.), polyacetylenes (matricaria-methylester, etc.), flavonoids, tannins, phenolic acids (caffeic acid, gallic acid, etc.), phytosterols, etc.

Properties: Anti-inflammatory, antimicrobial, astringent, diuretic, hemostatic.

Uses: Internally it is used (as a tea, h. p.) for chronic inflammations (also when minor hemorrhages are present) of the gastrointestinal tract (diarrhea,

156

etc., incl. hemorrhoids), upper respiratory tract (bronchitis, etc.) and genitourinary tract (cystitis, urethritis, etc.). To enhance the effects in problems of the genitourinary tract, the fluid intake (incl. herbal teas) should be more than 2 liters per day. Externally it is used (as a wash, wet compress, poultice) for skin inflammations, wounds, ulcers and hemorrhoids and (as a mouthwash, gargle) for inflammations of the mouth and throat.

Caution: There are no reports of contraindications or side effects when used properly. For minor hemorrhages it should be used on professional's advice.

References: (1) Vol. 4, p. 990; (3) Vol. 4, p. 797; (10) p. 117; (35) p. 320; (37) p. 360; (44) p. 173; (45) p. 203; (47) p. 1284; (51) p. 203.

FLY TRAP

Other Common Name(s): Venus' fly trap
Botanical Name(s): *Dionaea muscipula* Ellis [Fam.: Droseraceae]
Aerial part
Constituents: Naphthoquinones (plumbagin derivatives: free and glycosidic), flavonoids (flavonols, leucoanthocyandins, anthocyanidins), tannins (gallotannins, ellagitannins), minerals, etc.
Properties, Uses, and Caution: See SUNDEW.

References: (2) Vol. 2, p. 525; (5) Vol. 3, p. 176; (6) p. 284; (8) p. 228; (52) p. 256.

FORSKOHLII

Other Common Name(s): coleus
Botanical Name(s): *Plectranthus barbatus* Andrews = *Coleus barbatus* (Andrews) Benth. = *Coleus forskohlii* auct. [Fam.: Lamiaceae (Labiatae)]
Root
Constituents: The most interesting constituents are diterpenes, particularly forskolin (= colforsin), also plectrin, plectrinone A, etc.
Properties: Forskolin is an adenylate cyclase stimulant, which explains its positive inotropic (= cardiotonic) effect. It has also shown peripheral vasodilatory and antihypertensive, to lower intraocular pressure, antispasmodic (bronchial active) and strong platelet aggregation inhibitory effects.
Uses: Forskolin is very promising for the treatment of heart failure, hypertension, glaucoma and bronchial asthma. A therapy with forskolin is not yet established, while forskohlii root is used in traditional medicine for most of the mentioned problems.
Caution: Forskohlii is best used on health professional's advice and if possible as a standardized product.

References: (10) p. 85; (11) p. 88; (12) p. 499; (36) p. 328; (37) p. 354; (41) Vols. 1-7; (48) p. 652; (67) p. 783.

FO-TI

Other Common Name(s): fleeceflower
Botanical Name(s): *Polygonum multiflorum* Thunb. [Fam.: Polygonaceae]
Root (unprocessed-dried-aged = he shou wu)
Constituents: Anthranoids (chrysophanol, chrysophanol anthrone, etc.: free and glycosidic), stilbenoids (rhaponticin, polygonimitin C), a xanthone (polygonimitin B), acetophenones (polygoacetophenoside, etc.), tannins (galloyl-catechins, galloyl-procyanidins), etc.
Properties: Laxative, antioxidant, liver protective, cholesterol and triglyceride reducing, antimicrobial. Anthranoids exert laxative effect (see SENNA) and in moderate amounts contribute to the overall "detoxifying" effect. Stilbenoids have shown antifungal, antibacterial and antioxidant effects, among others. Acetophenones have shown inhibitory effect on platelet aggregation and biosynthesis of prostaglandins and leukotrienes. Galloyl-catechins and -procyanidins are antioxidants. Among xanthones there are compounds that have shown anti-inflammatory and MAO inhibitory effects.
Uses: Internally it is used (as a tea, h. p.) for constipation (atonic, not spastic), high cholesterol and triglycerides and minor hepatobiliary disorders. It is also used as an antidyscratic (= blood purifier; tea, h. p.; mainly combined with other herbs) for atopic eczema (= chronic eczema of internal origin) and other chronic inflammatory skin diseases (with itching, etc.).
Caution: See SENNA. Unprocessed fo-ti at higher doses than recommended may cause gastrointestinal irritations (with abdominal pain, nausea, vomiting, diarrhea).
Note: There are available different cured fo-ti products (zhi he shou wu). With curing the effects are modified. For example, anthranoids are oxidized and the laxative effect becomes much milder, tannins are mostly oxidized to insoluble phlobaphenes and their constipating effect becomes much weaker. Generally, cured fo-ti products exert milder and safer tonic and antidyscratic effects, with much less irritations (in the gastrointestinal and genitourinary tracts, etc.).

References: (3) Vol. 6a, p. 823; (9) p. 250; (31) pp. 467, 509, 533; (41) Vols. 1-7; (48) p. 302; (53) p. 79; (54) p. 121; (68) p. 91.

FRANGULA

Other Common Name(s): alder buckthorn
Botanical Name(s): *Frangula alnus* Mill. = *Rhamnus frangula* L. [Fam.: Rhamnaceae]
Bark
Constituents: Anthranoids (glycosides: glucofrangulins A, B, frangulins A, B; some dianthrones; some free anthraquinones), etc.
Properties: Laxative (large intestine stimulant laxative). See SENNA.

158

Uses: <u>Internally</u> it is used (as a tea, h. p.; often combined with other herbs) for constipation (atonic, non-spastic). See SENNA. It is one of the anthranoid herbs most incorporated in herbal teas.

Caution: See SENNA.

References: (1) Vol. 6, p. 397; (3) Vol. 6b, p. 71; (6) p. 165; (7) p. 230; (8) p. 477; (12) p. 907; (13) p. 295; (17) p. 227; (22) p. 59; (46) p. 611; (47) p. 1369; (48) p. 430.

FRANKINCENSE TREE

Other Common Name(s): 1) frankincense tree 2) boswelia, Indian frankincense tree

Botanical Name(s): 1) *Boswellia sacra* Flueck. = *Boswellia carteri* Birdw.; *Boswellia frereana* Birdw. 2) *Boswellia serrata* Roxb. [Fam.: Burseraceae]

Frankincense (incense, olibanum); **Indian olibanum** (Salai guggul)
They are the hardened gum-oleoresins obtained by incision from the bark. Frankincense is obtained from the first species, while Indian olibanum is obtained from the second species.

Constituents: Resin (with boswellic acids: α- and β-boswellic acid, 11-keto-β-boswellic acid, 3-acetyl-11-keto-β-boswellic acid, etc.; their ratio depends on species), volatile oil (1: with n-octyl acetate, etc.; 2: with thujone, etc.) and gum. They partly dissolve in ethanol, but in water mostly swell (only a small part of the gum is water-soluble).

Properties: Anti-inflammatory and analgesic, immunosupressive, antibacterial, demulcent, antidiarrheal, emollient. Most of the effects are due to boswellic acids, which have been shown to inhibit the biosynthesis of the inflammatory prostaglandins and leukotrienes. Indian olibanum is richer in 11-keto derivatives, which have shown stronger anti-inflammatory and immunosuppressive effects. It is demulcent and emollient due to the gum.

Uses: <u>Internally</u> they are used (as an h. p. standardized to boswellic acids) for rheumatic complaints (incl. rheumatoid arthritis), inflammatory and spastic conditions of the upper respiratory tract (pharyngitis, laryngitis, tracheitis, spastic bronchitis, bronchial asthma; also as an inhalation), gastrointestinal tract (diarrhea, stomachache, ulcerative colitis, Crohn's disease) and genitourinary tract (cystitis, urethritis, etc.). To enhance the effects in problems of the genitourinary tract, the fluid intake (incl. herbal teas) should be more than 2 liters per day. They are also used as an aid to a weight-loss diet and may be beneficial to high cholesterol. <u>Externally</u> are used (as an ointment) for wounds, bacterial and fungal infections, ulcers, hemorrhoids, etc. Both are still used in incense and fumigating products, and in perfumery.

Caution: In rare cases they may cause gastrointestinal complaints or allergic reactions. Otherwise, there are no reports of contraindications or side effects when used properly.

References: (2) Vol. 2, p. 245; (3) Vol. 3, p. 491; (6) p. 240; (8) p. 104; (12) p. 521; (13) p. 138; (19) p. 242; (29) p. 21; (36) p. 289; (37) p. 230; (47) p. 2016; (48) p. 580; (50) p. 164.

FRINGE TREE

Other Common Name(s): white fringetree
Botanical Name(s): *Chionanthus virginicus* L. [Fam.: Oleaceae]
Root bark
Constituents: Saponins (possibly of triterpenoid type), a lignan glucoside (phillyrin = chionanthin). It possibly contains a phenol glycoside (syringin = glucoside of sinapyl alcohol) and iridoids, found in many other plants of Oleaceae family.
Properties: Cholagogue, liver protective, laxative, antioxidant, diuretic. Many lignans have shown liver protective, anti-inflammatory, antioxidant, immunomodulant, antibacterial and antiviral effects. If syringin is present, it is possible that in our body it is converted to sinapic acid (as with the conversion of salicin of willow bark to salicylic acid). Sinapic acid has shown liver protective, antibacterial and antifungal effects.
Uses: Internally it is used (as a tea, h. p.) for inflammatory conditions of the hepatobiliary tract (chronic cholecystitis, nonobstructive gallstones, chronic hepatitis, incl. first stages of cirrhosis) and genitourinary tract. Externally it is used (as a wash, wet compress) for wounds and (as a poultice) for cuts and bruises.
Caution: There are no reports of contraindications or side effects when used properly.

References: (2) Vol. 2, p. 352; (3) Vol. 3, p. 859; (15) p. 63; (25) p. 270; (29) p. 29; (31) pp. 435, 487; (35) p. 328; (36) p. 475; (37) p. 309; (42) Vol. 5, p. 236; (44) p. 158; (46) p. 301; (47) p. 966.

FROSTWEED

Other Common Name(s): frostwort, Canadian rock-rose
Botanical Name(s): *Helianthemum canadense* (L.) Michx. [Fam.: Cistaceae]
Aerial part
Constituents: It is not well studied. It is reported to contain tannins (hydrolyzable t.: ellagitannins, ellagic acid), volatile oil, flavonoids (flavonols, leucoanthocyanidins), etc.
Properties: Astringent, anti-inflammatory, antioxidant, diuretic.
Uses: Internally it is used (as a tea, h. p.) for inflammations of the gastrointestinal tract (diarrhea, gastroenteritis, ulcerative colitis, etc.; also when minor hemorrhages are present, but on professional's advice), upper respiratory tract (chiefly as a diaphoretic hot tea for the common cold) and genitourinary tract. Externally it is used (as a wash, wet compress) for minor skin inflammations, (as a poultice) for wounds and ulcers, and (as a mouthwash, gargle) for inflammations of the mouth and throat.
Caution: There are no reports of contraindications or side effects when used properly.

160

References: (3) Vol. 5, p. 27; (18) p. 200; (25) p. 98; (35) p. 328; (42) Vol. 3, p. 429; (44) p. 257; (47) p. 1003.

FUMITORY

Other Common Name(s): earth smoke, fume weed
Botanical Name(s): *Fumaria officinalis* L. [Fam.: Papaveraceae]
Aerial part
Constituents: Isoquinoline alkaloids (protopine = fumarine, etc.), phenolic acids (caffeic, chlorogenic, and ferulic acids), fumaric acid, flavonoids, mucilaginous polysaccharides, etc.
Properties: Antispasmodic (biliary and gastrointestinal active), cholagogue, choleretic, mild laxative, antibacterial, liver protective, mild diuretic. The antispasmodic and cholagogic effects are due in large part to alkaloids. Depending on doses and especially hepatobiliary conditions, it has shown balancing effect on bile secretion. Due in large part to phenolic acids it exerts antibacterial, antioxidant and liver protective effects.
Uses: Internally it is used (as a tea, h. p.) for spastic and inflammatory conditions of the hepatobiliary tract (irregular bile secretion and flow, nonobstructive gallstones, cholecystitis) and gastrointestinal tract (incl. minor constipation). It is also used as an antidyscratic (= blood purifier; tea, h. p.) mainly for atopic eczema (= chronic eczema of internal origin).
Caution: There are no reports of contraindications or side effects when used properly. Nevertheless, during pregnancy and lactation it can be used but only on health professional's advice. Doses higher than recommended should be avoided (alkaloid containing herb!).

References: (1) Vol. 5, p. 207; (3) Vol. 4, p. 1066; (6) pp. 148, 360; (8) p. 271; (13) p. 234; (14) p. 102; (16) p. 121; (17) p. 234; (19) p. 74; (20) p. 127; (23) p. 133; (27) p. 143; (31) pp. 216, 472; (35) p. 329; (46) p. 621; (47) p. 1391; (48) p. 915.

GALANGAL, GREATER

Other Common Name(s): galanga, Java galanga, Siamese galanga
Botanical Name(s): *Alpinia galanga* (L.) Sw. = *Maranta galanga* L. [Fam.: Zingiberaceae]
Root (rhizome)
Constituents: Volatile oil (with eugenol, 1,8-cineole, etc.), pungent principles, flavonoids, starch, a water-insoluble gum (bassorin), tannins (condensed t.), phlobaphenes, resin, fat, etc.
Properties: Aromatic, stomachic, carminative, antimicrobial, expectorant, tonic, and it is claimed to be aphrodisiac. Compared to lesser galangal it contains about 3 times more volatile oil, but of different aroma.
Uses: Greater galangal is chiefly used as a spice, but its flavor is considered inferior to lesser galangal. Internally it is used (as a tea, h. p.; better red root: less astringent) for nonulcer dyspepsia (with flatulence) and inflammations

161

of the gastrointestinal tract (diarrhea) and upper respiratory tract (the common cold, bronchitis, etc.; coughs). In traditional medicine it is also used as a tonic for low sexual drive and as an adjuvant for diabetes and hypertension.

Caution: There are no reports of contraindications or side effects when used properly. Nevertheless, greater galangal should be avoided during pregnancy and lactation.

References: (3) Vol. 2, p. 1234; (5) Vol. 1, p. 60; (36) p. 504; (37) p. 51; (52) p. 36.

GALANGAL, LESSER

Other Common Name(s): Chinese galangal, Chinese ginger
Botanical Name(s): *Alpinia officinarum* Hance [Fam.: Zingiberaceae]
Root (rhizome)
Constituents: Volatile oil (with 1,8-cineole, etc.; eugenol, etc.; acetoxy-chavicol, etc.; sesquiterpenes), pungent principles (chiefly diaryl-heptanoids, also aryl-alkanones: gingerol, etc.), tannins (condensed t.), phlobaphenes ("galangal red"), flavonoids, starch (rich), etc.
Properties: Aromatic, stomachic, antispasmodic, carminative, anti-inflammatory and analgesic (NSAID-like effect, by inhibiting biosynthesis of prostaglandins), antimicrobial, antitumoral, tonic (also aphrodisiac?). Pungent principles have been shown to inhibit the biosynthesis of prostaglandins. Cineole is antimicrobial, while acetoxychavicol acetate has shown antitumoral effects. It acts much like ginger, including the antiemetic effects.
Uses: It is widely used as a spice, much like ginger, and is an important flavor ingredient in a number of beverages and bitters. Internally it is used (as a tea, h. p.) for loss of appetite and nonulcer dyspepsia (with flatulence, cramps, nausea, vomiting), minor spastic conditions of the biliary tract, inflammations of the gastrointestinal tract (diarrhea) and upper respiratory tract (chronic bronchitis, etc.; coughs), and for minor fatigue. Lesser galangal may be helpful for primary dysmenorrhea (= painful menstruation without pathology) by taking it 24-48 hours before menstrual flow, then continuing through 1-2 days of the cycle. Externally it is used (as a mouthwash, gargle) for inflammations of the mouth and throat, and (as a liniment) for rheumatic pains .
Caution: Unless consumed in small amounts as a flavor, lesser galangal should not be taken in cases of obstructive gallstones. In cases of nonobstructive gallstones it can be used but only on health professional's advice. Before using it for dysmenorrhea, the gynecologic problem should be judged by a health professional. Otherwise, there are no reports of contraindications or side effects when used properly.

References: (3) Vol. 2, p. 1232; (5) Vol. 1, p. 60; (6) p. 47; (8) p. 44; (12) p. 655; (13) p. 143; (15) p. 21; (17) p. 237; (19) p. 87; (23) p. 66; (31) p. 473; (35) p. 339; (37) p. 51; (45) p. 58; (46) p. 624; (47) p. 1397.

162

GALBANUM

Other Common Name(s): galbanum giant fennel
Botanical Name(s): *Ferula gummosa* Boiss. = *Ferula galbaniflua* Boiss. et Buhse [Fam.: Apiaceae (Umbelliferae)]

Galbanum

It is the gum-oleoresin obtained by incisions made to the stems near the ground or the upper part of the roots and then drying.

Constituents: Volatile oil (= galbanum oil: with β- and α-pinene, also 3-carene, some guaiazulene, alkylated pyrazines, the strong aromatic galbanols, etc.), gum, resin (with so-called resinic acids, and a coumarin derivative, umbelliferone), etc.

Properties: Aromatic, antispasmodic, carminative, expectorant, antibacterial (against *Staphylococcus aureus*), rubefacient.

Uses: Galbanum and galbanum oil are chiefly used as fragrance and fixative ingredients in cosmetics and perfumery, and as flavor ingredients in food industry. Internally it has been used (combined with other herbs) for inflammatory and spastic conditions of the gastrointestinal tract (with flatulence, intestinal colics), upper respiratory tract (spastic bronchitis, etc.; coughs due to thickened bronchial secretion) and genitourinary tract, and for primary dysmenorrhea (= painful menstruation without pathology). Externally it is used (as a plaster, ointment) for rheumatic pains, bruises and sprains, and (as an ointment) for wounds.

Caution: Oxidation products of 3-carene are skin and mucosal irritants. In view of this 3-carene should be contained within limits. Otherwise, there are no reports of contraindications or side effects when used properly.

References: (2) Vol. 2, p. 705; (3) Vol. 4, p. 984; (9) p. 254; (12) p. 1109; (24) p. 442; (37) p. 523; (48) p. 581; (49) Vol. 2 p. 479; (66) p. 288.

GALE, SWEET

Other Common Name(s): bog myrtle, Dutch myrtle
Botanical Name(s): *Myrica gale* L. [Fam.: Myricaceae]

Leaf

Constituents: Volatile oil (with 1,8-cineole, α-pinene, cadinenes, etc.), flavonoids (flavones, dihydrochalcones), phenolic acids, tannins (hydrolyzable t.), triterpenes, etc.

Properties: Aromatic, astringent, diuretic, antimicrobial, emmenagogue, insect-repellent.

Uses: Internally it is used (as a tea, h. p.) for inflammations of the gastrointestinal tract (diarrhea, etc.) and genitourinary tract (cystitis, urethritis, etc.) and as an antidyscratic (= blood purifier) for chronic skin diseases. To enhance the effects in problems of the genitourinary tract, the fluid intake (incl. herbal teas) should be more than 2 liters per day.

Externally it is used (as a wash, wet compress) for minor wounds and skin inflammations and (as a wash) for parasitic skin infections (scabies = the itch, etc.). It is also used as an insect-repellent (against moths, etc.). Sweet gale has been used as a flavor ingredient in the production of beer and is still included in some herbal alcoholic drinks.

Caution: Sweet gale should not be taken during pregnancy, and in severe liver and kidney disorders. At higher doses than recommended it may cause gastrointestinal irritations (with nausea, vomiting). Sweet gale volatile oil should not be used internally.

References: (3) Vol. 5, p. 918; (5) Vol. 1, p. 734; (10) p. 123; (18) p. 158; (25) p. 254; (31) p. 367; (35) p. 341; (37) p. 933; (42) Vol. 5, p. 141; (44) p. 352; (52) p. 518.

GAMBOGE

Other Common Name(s): Hanbury's garcinia, Siam gamboge
Botanical Name(s): *Garcinia hanburyi* Hook. f. [Fam.: Clusiaceae (Guttiferae)]
Gamboge (gutta gamba)
It is a gum-resin, the dried exudate obtained by incisions made to the bark.
Constituents: Resin (rich in xanthones: gambogic acid, etc., of yellow to red color) and a gum (water-soluble).
Properties: Purgative, anthelmintic, antibacterial.
Uses: Internally it is used almost only in veterinary medicine, as a drastic purgative and for intestinal worms.
Caution: In human medicine gamboge is almost no longer used. In any event, it should not be taken during pregnancy and lactation. Even 4 grams can be fatal to an adult.

References: (2) Vol. 2, p. 762; (3) Vol. 4, p. 1100; (10) p. 124; (36) p. 290; (37) p. 574; (49) Vol. 2, p. 237; (65) p. 181; (66) p. 197.

GARDENIA

Other Common Name(s): Cape jasmine
Botanical Name(s): *Gardenia augusta* Merr. = *Gardenia jasminoides* J. Ellis [Fam.: Rubiaceae]
Fruit
Constituents: Bitter principles (iridoids: gardenoside, geniposide = genipinglucoside, genipin, etc.), volatile oil, pectin, tannins, phytosterols, carotenoids (crocin, etc.), hydrocarbons, etc.
Properties: Bitter tonic, antipyretic, choleretic, cholagogue, liver protective, laxative, diuretic, anti-inflammatory, antimicrobial. Gardenoside and geniposide have shown laxative effect. Genipin has shown cholagogic effect. Iridoids have shown bitter tonic, choleretic, cholagogic, liver protec-

164

tive, laxative, diuretic, anti-inflammatory, analgesic, antibacterial, antiviral, antifungal and immunomodulant effects, among others.

Uses: <u>Internally</u> it is used (as a tea, h. p.; at low doses) for feverish states, inflammations of the liver (chronic hepatitis), gastrointestinal tract (with impaired digestion, minor constipation), genitourinary tract (cystitis, etc.), and as an antidyscratic (= blood purifier) and anti-inflammatory for atopic eczema (= chronic eczema of internal origin) and chronic rheumatic complaints. As a yellow coloring ingredient (due to crocin) it is also used in food industry. To enhance the effects in problems of the genitourinary tract, the fluid intake (incl. herbal teas) should be more than 2 liters per day. <u>Externally</u> it is used (as a wet compress) for minor skin inflammations and wounds.

Caution: At higher doses than recommended it causes gastrointestinal irritations (with nausea, vomiting, diarrhea). Otherwise, there are no reports of contraindications or side effects when used properly.

References: (3) Vol. 4, p. 1103; (5) Vol. 1, p. 523; (12) p. 438; (31) pp. 569, 574; (36) p. 507; (45) p. 213; (52) p. 327; (53) p. 185; (57) p. 364.

GARLIC

Botanical Name(s): *Allium sativum* L. [Fam.: Liliaceae (Alliaceae)]
<u>Bulb</u> (cloves)

Constituents: The most important constituent is still considered a sulfur compound, namely alliin, which is non-odoriferous and its content varies very much. When garlic cloves are crushed, under the action of an enzyme (alliinase), alliin is converted to allicin, which is highly odoriferous but unstable. Allicin on its part yields other strong-smelling compounds (ajoenes, etc.). So, the most important active compounds are still considered allicin and ajoenes. Other important constituents are sulfur-containing peptides (γ-glutamyl-cysteine peptides), amino acids, biogenic amines (choline, etc.), glycolipids, phospholipids, etc.

Properties: Cholesterol (total and LDL) and triglyceride reducing, antioxidant, platelet aggregation inhibitory, anticoagulant, vasodilatory, antihypertensive (the effects are seen after about 6 months) , antibacterial (against *Staphylococcus aureus*, *Mycobacterium tuberculosis*, *Escherichia coli*, *Bacillus* spp., *Proteus* spp., etc.), antifungal (against *Candida* spp., *Aspergillus* spp., *Trichophyton* spp.), anthelmintic (against pinworms = *Oxyuris* spp.).

Uses: <u>Internally</u> it is used (as an h. p., raw) for high cholesterol and triglycerides and the prevention of arteriosclerosis, minor cases of hypertension and coronary heart disease (= a condition associated with decreased blood supply to the heart), bacterial and fungal infections of the respiratory tract (the common cold and flu, bronchitis, etc.), gastrointestinal tract (with flatulence, cramps, diarrhea) and genitourinary tract (cystitis, etc.), chronic rheumatic complaints, and for infestations with pinworms (= *Oxyuris* spp.).

To enhance the effects in problems of the genitourinary tract, the fluid intake (incl. herbal teas) should be more than 2 liters per day. Garlic may be helpful for intermittent claudication (= pain / cramp / weakness in the legs on walking) and Raynaud's disease (= pale or red-blue patchy fingers). Externally it is used for bacterial and fungal infections of the mouth (as a mouthwash, gargle), ear (as oily eardrops), skin (as a wet compress for Tinea capitis = fungal infection of the scalp, Tinea pedis = athlete's foot), vagina and external female genitalia (as a vaginal irrigation / sitz bath / wash; combined with other herbs), common and plantar warts and corns (as a poultice, ointment), wounds (as a wet compress, poultice), and rheumatic and neuralgic pains (as a poultice, liniment, ointment).

Caution: In rare cases it may cause contact skin or mucosal irritations. It also may cause gastrointestinal discomfort (heartburn, nausea), especially when taken at higher doses than recommended or on an empty stomach. Other than this and its unpleasant smell, there are no reports of contraindications or side effects when used properly. A possible combination of garlic products with antihypertensives, anticoagulants (warfarin, etc.) and / or platelet aggregation inhibitors (aspirin, etc.) should be made only by a health professional.

References: (1) Vol. 4, p. 190; (3) Vol. 2, p. 1210; (6) pp. 59, 62; (7) p. 116; (8) p. 35; (13) p. 151; (14) p. 105; (16) p. 108; (19) p. 130; (20) p. 129; (22) p. 132; (24) p. 195; (26) p. 107; (27) p. 22; (46) p. 21; (47) p. 465; (48) p. 208; (49) Vol. 2, p. 62; (59) p. 16.

GAYFEATHER

Other Common Name(s): dense gayfeather
Botanical Name(s): *Liatris spicata* (L.) Willd. [Fam.: Asteraceae (Compositae)]
Root (rhizome)
Constituents: Sesquiterpene lactones (spicatin, prespicatin) and a diterpenoid lactone (hydroxybacchotricuneatin A) that are mainly steam distilling. It also contains benzofurans (euparin, etc.), coumarin, and volatile oil.
Properties: Aromatic, bitter tonic, diuretic, expectorant, carminative, antimicrobial. Spicatin has shown cytotoxic and antitumoral effects. Benzofurans have shown antifungal and antibacterial effects.
Uses: Internally it is used (as a tea, h. p.) for inflammations of the genitourinary tract (cystitis, urethritis, etc.), upper respiratory tract (bronchitis, etc.; coughs) and gastrointestinal tract (flatulence, cramps, diarrhea). To enhance the effects in problems of the genitourinary tract, the fluid intake (incl. herbal teas) should be more than 2 liters per day. Externally it is used (as a gargle) for throat inflammations and (as a wet compress, poultice) for wounds and ulcers.
Caution: It may cause allergic contact dermatitis to persons hypersensitive to other Asteraceae plants (e. g. arnica, chamomile, feverfew, ragweed,

tansy, yarrow) that contain sesquiterpene lactones. Otherwise, there are no reports of contraindications or side effects when used properly.

References: (3) Vol. 5, p. 506; (10) p. 53; (31) pp. 340, 637; (35) pp. 255, 746; (44) p. 305; (47) p. 1753.

GELSEMIUM

Other Common Name(s): yellow jasmine, yellow jessamine, poison jasmine
Botanical Name(s): *Gelsemium sempervirens* (L.) J.St.-Hil. [Fam.: Loganiaceae]
Root (rhizome)
Constituents: Indole alkaloids (gelsemine, gelsemicine, etc.), iridoids (gelsemide, etc.), coumarins (scopoletin, etc.), tannins, anthranoids, volatile oil, resin, etc.
Properties: Analgesic, antispasmodic, sedative.
Uses: Internally it is used (as a tea, h. p.; only combined with other herbs) for neuralgic pains (nervous headaches, migraine, trigeminal neuralgias) and rheumatic pains (incl. arthritic pains). It has also been used for spastic conditions of the genitourinary tract (dysmenorrhea = painful menstruation without pathology, irritable bladder (with urinary incontinence) and upper respiratory tract (bronchial asthma), and for nervousness, restlessness, anxiety.
Caution: Gelsemium is a highly toxic herb. It should be handled by experienced practitioners and used as directed by them. It should not be taken during pregnancy and lactation, fatigue and low blood pressure. High doses have shown depressive effect on the cardiovascular system. Toxic doses depress the respiratory system and lead to death due to its arrest.

References: (3) Vol. 4, p. 1107; (6) p. 73; (8) p. 279; (9) p. 264; (10) p. 125; (13) p. 409; (15) p. 98; (23) p. 185; (31) p. 364; (37) p. 582; (41) Vols. 1-7; (46) p. 637; (48) p. 1014; (65) p. 353; (66) p. 288.

GENTIAN

Other Common Name(s): yellow gentian
Botanical Name(s): *Gentiana lutea* L. [Fam.: Gentianaceae]
Root
Constituents: Bitter principles (seco-iridoids: chiefly gentiopicrin, also amarogentin, sweroside, etc.), sugars (invert sugar; two bitter sugars: gentiobiose, gentianose), yellow pigments (xanthones: gentisin, etc.), etc.
Properties: Bitter tonic, digestive secretagogue (increases secretions of the mouth, stomach, liver and pancreas), mild immunomodulant. Due to gentiopicrin, gentian exerts also mild antipyretic and antimalarial effects, for which it has been used since ancient times. Iridoids have shown bitter tonic,

choleretic, liver protective, laxative, diuretic, anti-inflammatory, antibacterial, antiviral, antifungal and immunomodulant effects, among others.

Uses: <u>Internally</u> it is used (as a tea, h. p.) for loss of appetite and nonulcer dyspepsia (with fullness, belching, heartburn, flatulence, minor cramps, sluggish bowels). Gentian is also helpful for convalescence, minor fatigue and decreased resistance to infections. It is extensively used in food industry as a flavor ingredient in some alcoholic and non-alcoholic bitters. Gentian brandies are produced from the fermented root (fresh root, cut / ground, mixed with water, fermented, distilled) and retain only the aroma but do not taste bitter.

Caution: Gentian should not be taken in cases of peptic ulcers as well as during pregnancy and lactation. In very seldom cases, in hypersensitive persons, it may cause headache. At higher doses than recommended it causes gastrointestinal irritations (with nausea, vomiting, diarrhea). Otherwise, there are no reports of contraindications or side effects when used properly.

References: (1) Vol. 5, p. 230; (3) Vol. 4, p. 1112; (8) p. 280; (12) p. 452; (13) p. 161; (14) p. 109; (16) p. 137; (17) p. 254; (20) p. 134; (23) p. 59; (27) p. 150; (46) p. 646; (47) p. 1436; (48) p. 604.

GERMANDER

Other Common Name(s): 1) germander, common germander 2) wood germander, wood sage 3) marum-germander, cat thyme 4) poley-germader, poley 5) water germander

Botanical Name(s): 1) *Teucrium chamaedrys* L. 2) *Teucrium scorodonia* L. 3) *Teucrium marum* L. 4) *Teucrium polium* L. 5) *Teucrium scordium* L. [Fam.: Lamiaceae (Labiatae)]

<u>Aerial part</u>

Constituents: Bitter principles (diterpenoid lactones; iridoids), volatile oil, Lamiaceae tannins (rosmarinic acid and other caffeic acid derivatives), flavonoids, triterpenes (ursolic acid, etc.), etc.

Properties: Bitter tonic, aromatic, choleretic, astringent, wound-healing. Diterpenoid lactones found in the above mentioned species are chiefly of furano-neoclerodane type, which have shown hepatotoxic effect.

Uses: <u>Internally</u> they have been used (as teas, h. p.) for loss of appetite and nonulcer dyspepsia associated with biliary disorders and for minor diarrhea and hemorrhoids, among others. <u>Externally</u> they have been used (as a wash, wet compress, poultice) for minor skin inflammations, wounds and hemorrhoids and (as a mouthwash) for inflammations of the mouth.

Caution: Due to the hepatotoxic effect, germanders (*Teucrium spp.* in general) are no longer advisable.

References: (1) Vol. 6, p. 929-940; (3) Vol. 6c, pp. 70-77; (8) p. 552; (10) p. 126; (15) pp. 208, 209; (20) p. 239; (24) pp. 442, 460; (27) p. 67; (35) pp. 351, 352; (48) p. 649; (51) p. 161.

GINGER

Botanical Name(s): *Zingiber officinale* Roscoe [Fam.: Zingiberaceae]
<u>Root</u> (rhizome)
Constituents: Volatile oil (with zingiberene, also bisabolene, etc.), pungent principles (chiefly aryl-alkanones: gingerols, shogaols; also diaryl-heptanoids), lipids, glycolipids, starch, etc. Shogaols are more pungent than gingerols. They are formed from gingerols during drying and storage of the root in good conditions, and during the production of the oleoresin. Poorly dried and stored ginger contains chiefly the non-pungent zingerone.
Properties: Aromatic, stomachic (salivary and gastric secretagogue effect), gastrointestinal tonic and antiemetic (gastrointestinal active, i. e. acts through autonomic nervous system, not CNS), anti-inflammatory and analgesic (by inhibiting biosynthesis of prostaglandins and leukotrienes), platelet aggregation inhibitory, carminative, cholagogue, cholesterol reducing, mild cardiotonic (increases the contractility of the heart muscle = positive inotropic effect), antispasmodic, antibacterial, antifungal, rubefacient. The effects (incl. the NSAID-like effect: anti-inflammatory, analgesic, platelet aggregation inhibitory) are due to the volatile oil and pungent principles.
Uses: Ginger is extensively used as a flavor ingredient in culinary practice and food industry. <u>Internally</u> it is used (as a tea, h. p.) for nausea and vomiting (due to motion sickness, morning sickness, medications, nonulcer dyspepsia, etc.; also as a preventive), nonulcer dyspepsia (with fullness, flatulence, minor cramps and heartburn, nausea), inflammations of the gastrointestinal tract (chronic diarrhea, sluggish bowels, irritable bowel syndrome) and upper respiratory tract (the common cold, bronchitis, etc.; dry coughs), minor fatigue, high cholesterol, and rheumatic complaints (incl. rheumatoid arthritis). Ginger may be helpful for primary dysmenorrhea (= painful menstruation without pathology) by taking it 24-48 hours before menstrual flow, then continuing through 1-2 days of the cycle. <u>Externally</u> it is used (as a gargle, lozenge) for sore throat and (as a liniment) for rheumatic pains.
Caution: In cases of obstructive gallstones, ginger should be consumed in small amounts as a flavor. In cases of nonobstructive gallstones, morning sickness and dysmenorrhea, it should be used on health professional's advice, and a possible combination with anticoagulants (warfarin, etc.) and / or platelet aggregation inhibitors (aspirin, etc.) should be made only by them. Ginger products are best used standardized to the pungent principles content. Otherwise, there are no reports of side effects when used properly.

References: (2) Vol. 3, p. 838; (3) Vol. 6c, p. 568; (6) pp. 128, 225; (8) p. 598; (9) p. 271; (11) p. 103; (12) p. 657; (13) p. 142; (14) p. 112; (17) p. 631; (19) pp. 113, 717; (20) p. 135; (22) p. 47; (23) p. 65; (26) p. 242; (37) p. 1496; (46) p. 1807; (47) p. 2837; (48) p. 299; (59) p. 277; (71) p. 187; (88) p. 245.

GINGER, AMERICAN WILD

Other Common Name(s): Canadian wild ginger, Canada snakeroot

169

Botanical Name(s): *Asarum canadense* L. [Fam.: Aristolochiaceae]
Root
Constituents: It is reported to contain volatile oil (with methyleugenol, etc., or α-terpineol, etc.; depending on chemotype). It possibly contains tannins, mucilaginous polysaccharides, starch, sugars and phenolic acids.
Properties: Aromatic, stomachic, carminative, tonic, antiseptic, antispasmodic.
Uses: It is chiefly used as a flavor ingredient in wine industry and as a fragrance ingredient in perfumery. Internally it is used (as a tea, h. p.) for nonulcer dyspepsia (with flatulence, minor cramps) and minor inflammations of the upper respiratory tract (bronchitis, the common cold, etc.; irritating dry coughs).
Caution: Canadian wild ginger should not be taken during pregnancy and lactation. At higher doses than recommended it may cause gastrointestinal irritations (with nausea, vomiting). Manufacturers should run tests for aristolochic acids and evaluate them (see BIRTHWORT).

References: (1) Vol. 4, p. 378; (3) Vol. 3, p. 283; (10) p. 128; (18) p. 109; (25) p. 138; (29) p. 16; (31) pp. 480, 567; (35) p. 354; (37) p. 147; (44) p. 105; (52) p. 78.

GINGER, CREPE

Other Common Name(s): cane reed
Botanical Name(s): *Costus speciosus* (J. König) Sm. [Fam.: Costaceae (Zingiberaceae)]
Root (rhizome)
Constituents: Steroidal saponins (chiefly diosgenin-glycosides), curcuminoids (rich in curcumin), phytosterols (5-sterols: β-sitosterol, etc.), triterpenes, long chain alkanes, etc.
Properties: Anti-inflammatory, antimicrobial, demulcent, choleretic, diuretic, uterotonic, emollient. The anti-inflammatory, antimicrobial and choleretic effects are due in large part to curcuminoids.
Uses: Internally it is used (as a tea, h. p.) for nonulcer dyspepsia, inflammations of the upper respiratory tract (the common cold, bronchitis, etc.; coughs), as an anti-inflammatory and antidyscratic (= blood purifier; tea, h. p.) for atopic eczema (= chronic eczema of internal origin), menorrhagia / hypermenorrhea (= prolonged / heavy menstruation), postpartum hemorrhage (= h. following childbirth), and a hypotonic uterus. Due to steroidal saponins it may be beneficial for high cholesterol (see FENUGREEK). Externally it is used (as a poultice) for minor skin inflammations.
Caution: There are no reports of contraindications or side effects when used properly. Nevertheless, before using it for gynecologic disorders, the problem should be judged by a health professional.

References: (1) Vol. 4, p. 1032; (18) p. 322; (31) p. 489; (41) Vols. 1-7; (49) Vol. 1, p. 78; (52) p. 221; (57) p. 234.

GINKGO

Other Common Name(s): maidenhair tree
Botanical Name(s): *Ginkgo biloba* L. [Fam.: Ginkgoaceae]
Leaf
Constituents: Terpenoid lactones (diterpenoid lactones: ginkgolides A, B, C, etc.; a sesquiterpene lactone: bilobalide), flavonoids (flavonols, flavones, flavanonols, biflavones, flavan-3-ols = catechins), tannins (proanthocyanidins, etc.), organic acids (ginkgolic acid, etc.), lignans, etc.

Properties: Standardized special extracts of ginkgo have been shown to improve peripheral and central blood flow, to prevent and resolve edemas (esp. in the brain tissue), to protect the brain tissue from damaging effects of free radicals and toxins and to increase its hypoxic tolerance, with nootropic effect (= increases cognitive function), among others. Terpenoid lactones have shown anti-PAF (= anti-platelet-activating factor) effect, due to which blood viscosity is decreased and smooth muscles (esp. vascular, also tracheo-bronchial, intestinal) are relaxed. Ginkgo flavonoids exert strong antioxidant and "vitamin P"-like (= help in normalizing an increased microvascular permeability and fragility; P = permeability) effect. By crossing the so-called blood-brain barrier they are available for the protection of the brain tissue from damaging effects of free radicals, therefore are considered neuro-protective. By normalizing an increased microvascular permeability and fragility they prevent and resolve edemas (esp. in the brain tissue). Ginkgolic acid is toxic and allergenic (see Caution).

Uses: <u>Internally</u> it is used (only as a standardized special extract) for cerebrovascular disease (= a complex condition associated with changes in the brain blood flow), impaired cognitive function, depressive mood, headache, tinnitus (= subjective perception of noise in the ears), impaired hearing, vertigo (= a type of dizziness), Ménière's disease (= a sudden attack, with violent dizziness, nausea and vomiting, ringing in the ear, etc.), intermittent claudication (= pain / cramp / weakness in the legs on walking), Raynaud's disease (= pale or red-blue patchy fingers / toes), age-related macular degeneration (= AMD), and for any condition where an improvement of peripheral blood flow is sought. Ginkgo is also used as an adjuvant for bronchial asthma.

Caution: Before using a ginkgo product the problem should be judged by a health professional. Only special extracts standardized to flavonoids and terpenoid lactones (ginkgolides and bilobalide) should be used. Ginkgolic acid is toxic and allergenic and in ginkgo extracts should not exceed 5 ppm. In rare cases ginkgo products may cause skin allergic reactions, mild gastrointestinal irritations or headache. Most of the indications require at least 6-8 weeks to develop the beneficial effects. A possible combination of ginkgo products with anticoagulants (warfarin, etc.) and / or platelet aggregation inhibitors (aspirin, etc.) should be made only by a health professional. Otherwise, there are no reports of contraindications or side effects when used

properly.

References: (1) Vol. 5, p. 270; (3) Vol. 4, p. 1134; (6) p. 51; (7) p. 42; (8) p. 284; (9) p. 274; (12) p. 849; (13) pp. 310, 410; (16) p. 106; (19) p. 92; (20) p. 238; (22) p. 141; (23) p. 178; (26) p. 129; (48) p. 329; (59) p. 154.

GINSENG

Other Common Name(s): 1) Asian ginseng, Korean ginseng, Chinese ginseng 2) American Ginseng
Botanical Name(s): 1) *Panax ginseng* C. A. Meyer = *Panax schinseng* T. Nees 2) *Panax quinquefolius* L. [Fam.: Araliaceae]
<u>Root</u> (white ginseng)
Constituents: Triterpenoid saponins (ginsenosides R_X = panaxosides R_X; X: $_0$, a_1, a_2, a_3, b_1, b_2, b_3, c, d, e, f, g_1, g_2, etc.), glycopeptides (panaxanes), polysaccharides, polyacetylenes, volatile oil, starch, etc. Lateral roots are richer in active constituents. Between Asian and American ginsengs there are differences, particularly in regard to some sapogenins and the proportions of saponins.
Properties: Adaptogenic (= increases adaptation and resistance to stress). Ginseng increases plasma levels of corticosterone, exerts nootropic effect (= increases cognitive function), immunomodulant (chiefly by stimulating the activity of T-lymphocytes and the interferon production), antihyperglycemic and cholesterol reducing, liver protective, platelet aggregation inhibitory, antioxidant, anti-inflammatory and peripheral vasodilatory effects. All the mentioned constituents contribute to the overall effect, particularly ginsenosides and panaxanes. Asian ginseng exerts mild CNS stimulating effect, while American ginseng has shown mild sedative effect.
Uses: <u>Internally</u> it is used as an invigorator (h. p., tea) for fatigue and feeling of weakness, decreased mental performance (incl. cognitive function) and physical performance, decreased concentration and mood, convalescence, as an adjuvant for diabetes and high cholesterol, and for decreased immune response in general. Ginseng seems to decrease elevated prolactin levels, so it is beneficial for erectile dysfunction and secondary amenorrhea and oligomenorrhea (= ceased / infrequent / scanty menstruation without pathology). Ginseng exerts also beneficial effects on the cardiovascular system, respiratory tract, and may increase chances of survival in cases of breast cancer. The best ginseng products should be those standardized to their ginsenosides content.
Caution: There are no reports of contraindications or side effects when used properly. Doses higher than recommended should be avoided. Normally, it should be used for 1-3 months and limited to adults. Before a possible resuming a break is necessary. Consider differences in effects between two ginsengs (see Properties), and choose accordingly. When taking it as a tea, ginseng root is best freshly ground.

172

Note: Red ginseng or Hongshen is Asian ginseng, which before drying has undergone a curing process.

References: (1) Vol. 6, p. 13; (3) Vol. 6a, p. 390; (6) p. 295; (7) p. 302; (8) p. 399; (9) p. 277; (12) pp. 533, 554; (13) p. 214; (14) p. 115; (16) p. 201; (19) p. 94; (20) p. 145; (22) p. 236; (23) p. 314; (36) p. 300; (37) p. 1022; (47) p. 1457; (48) p. 706; (59) p. 168.

GINSENG, SIBERIAN

Other Common Name(s): eleuthero
Botanical Name(s): *Eleutherococcus senticosus* (Rupr. & Maxim.) Maxim. = *Acanthopanax senticosus* (Rupr. et Maxim.) Harms [Fam.: Araliaceae]
Root (rhizome and root)
Constituents: Eleutherosides A - G (= glycosides with aglycones: lignans, phenolic acid derivatives, coumarins, phytosterols), triterpenoid saponins, polysaccharides (incl. water-soluble p.), etc. It doesn't contain ginsenosides, the triterpenoid saponins of ginseng (q. v.).
Properties: Adaptogenic (= increases adaptation and resistance to stress). Siberian ginseng exerts immunomodulant effect (chiefly by increasing T-lymphocyte count), increases levels of glucocorticoids and sex hormones and then exerts anabolic effect (= promotes biosynthesis of macromolecular body substances such as proteins), decreases elevated levels of cholesterol and glucose, and exerts mild CNS stimulating, platelet aggregation in-hibitory and antioxidant effects. Responsible for its main effects are consid-ered eleutherosides (incl. eleutheroside B). Eleutheroside B (= syringin) is one of its main active constituents. Possibly, through hydrolysis (in the in-testinal tract) and oxidation (chiefly in the liver), syringin is converted to sinapic acid (as with the conversion of salicin of willow bark to salicylic ac-id). Sinapic acid has shown liver protective, antibacterial and antifungal ef-fects. Water-soluble polysaccharides account at least in part for the immu-nomodulating effect.
Uses: Internally it is used as an invigorator (h. p., tea) for fatigue and feel-ing of weakness, decreased mental and physical performance, decreased concentration, depressive mood, convalescence (incl. cases of underweight), as an adjuvant for diabetes and high cholesterol, and for decreased immune response in general.
Caution: Siberian ginseng should not be taken in cases of hypertension. Normally, it should be used for 1-3 months and limited to adults. Before a possible resuming a break is necessary. At higher doses than recommended it may cause headache, irritability, insomnia, cardiac arrhythmias and ele-vated blood pressure. Otherwise, there are no reports of contraindications or side effects when used properly.

References: (2) Vol. 2, p. 557; (6) pp. 269, 297, 308; (7) p. 305; (8) p. 238; (9) p. 225; (12) p. 811; (13) p. 407; (14) p. 89; (16) p. 203; (19) p. 222; (20) p. 141; (22) p. 239; (23) p. 315; (31) p. 487; (48) p. 709; (68) p. 72.

GOA TREE

Other Common Name(s): Angeleen tree, Bahia powder tree, goa angelin tree
Botanical Name(s): *Vataireopsis araroba* (Aguiar) Ducke = *Andira araroba* Aguiar [Fam.: Fabaceae (Leguminosae)]

Chrysarobin

Chrysarobin is obtained from Goa powder by extraction with hot benzene and then crystallization. Goa powder, which is formed and deposited in the center of the wood, is scraped out with a tool.

Constituents: Anthranoids, particularly chrysophanol and physcion. Both are found in their reduced and oxidized forms.

Properties: Irritant antiseptic, keratolytic.

Uses: Externally has been used (as an ointment) for psoriasis and fungal skin infections. Today it is almost totally replaced by a synthetic related compound, dithranol (= anthralin = cignolin), which acts stronger and dyes the skin and clothes much less.

Caution: Chrysarobin should be used only externally and on health professional's advice. If taken internally, even in small amounts (a few centigrams), may cause severe gastroenteritis, and kidney inflammation with proteinuria. This may happen even when it is applied to a body surface area larger than recommended.

References: (3) Vol. 3, p. 77; (8) p. 56; (11a) p. 66; (12a) p. 722; (35) p. 51; (36) p. 247; (37) p. 83; (55) p. 149; (65) p. 139.

GOAT'S RUE

Botanical Name(s): *Galega officinalis* L. [Fam.: Fabaceae]

Aerial part

Constituents: Guanidine derivatives (galegine, hydroxy-galegine), quinazoline alkaloids (peganine = vasicine, etc.), flavonoids (flavones), minerals (chromium, etc.), etc.

Properties: Antihyperglycemic, diuretic, galactagogue. Metformin (= glucophage), an antihyperglycemic drug still in use, has the basic structure of guanidine. Chromium is an essential trace element required for normal glucose metabolism.

Uses: Internally it is used as an adjuvant for diabetes, inflammations of the genitourinary tract, and to promote the secretion of milk in nursing mothers.

Caution: There are no reports of contraindications or side effects when used properly. Nevertheless, goat's rue is best avoided during pregnancy.

References: (2) Vol. 2, p. 741; (3) Vol. 4, p. 1082; (8) p. 273; (15) p. 96; (17) p. 240; (23) p. 141; (36) pp. 440, 476; (37) p. 569; (46) p. 626; (47) p. 1402; (71) p. 234.

GOLDENROD

Other Common Name(s): 1) European goldenrod / virgaurea 2) giant / early goldenrod 3) Canadian goldenrod
Botanical Name(s): 1) *Solidago virgaurea* L. 2) *Solidago gigantea* Aiton 3) *Solidago canadensis* L. [Fam.: Asteraceae (Compositae)]
Aerial part
Constituents: Flavonoids (chiefly flavonols: quercetin glycosides; giant g. is richer), triterpenoid saponins (giant g. is richer; different aglycones), phenol glycosides (leicarposide, virgaureoside A; only in European g.), diterpenes (not present in European g.), phenolic acids (caffeic acid derivatives), tannins (condensed t.), polysaccharides, volatile oil, etc.
Properties: Diuretic, anti-inflammatory, mild antispasmodic, antibacterial, antifungal, astringent, immunomodulant. Its main active constituents are considered flavonoids, saponins, and phenol glycosides, but also other constituents (volatile oil, tannins, polysaccharides, etc.) contribute to the effects. European goldenrod is better studied and mostly preferred.
Uses: Internally it is used as a flushing-out treatment (= herbal tea or product + liquids: more than 2 liters per day; sometimes combined with a medication) for inflammations of the genitourinary tract (cystitis, urethritis, prostatitis, etc.), urinary gravel and nonobstructive stones, to prevent relapsing urinary infections / gravel / stones, (as a tea, h. p.) for inflammations of the gastrointestinal tract (diarrhea, etc., incl. hemorrhoids) and upper respiratory tract (bronchitis, etc., as a diaphoretic hot tea for the common cold). It is also used as an antidyscratic (= blood purifier) and anti-inflammatory (tea, h. p.) for chronic rheumatic complaints. Externally it is used (as a mouthwash, gargle) for inflammations of the mouth and throat and (as a wash, wet compress) for minor wounds and skin inflammations.
Caution: There are no reports of contraindications or side effects when used properly. Nevertheless, a flushing-out treatment is contraindicated in cases of obstructive urinary stones, edema due to impaired heart or kidney function and kidney inflammations (here can be used on health professional's advice to enhance the effects of an antimicrobial therapy).

References: (1) Vol. 6, p. 752; (3) Vol. 6b, p. 452; (6) p. 184; (8) p. 527; (12) p. 860; (13) p. 219; (15) p. 234; (16) p. 160; (17) p. 561; (19) p. 97; (22) p. 90; (37) p. 1277; (47) p. 1571; (48) p. 253; (51) p. 200.

GOLDENSEAL

Other Common Name(s): yellow puccoon, yellow root
Botanical Name(s): *Hydrastis canadensis* L. [Fam.: Ranunculaceae]
Root (rhizome)
Constituents: Isoquinoline alkaloids (chiefly of phthalide-isoquinoline type: hydrastine, etc.; also protoberberine type: berberine, berberastine, canadine, etc.), phenolic acids (chlorogenic acid, etc.), resin, etc.

Properties: Bitter tonic; cholagogue, antibacterial, antifungal and antiprotozoal, which are due in large part to berberine; peripheral vasoconstrictor, oxytocic and hemostatic, which are due in large part to hydrastine.

Uses: Internally it is used (as a tea, h. p.) for loss of appetite and nonulcer dyspepsia, especially when they are associated with hepatobiliary disorders (impaired bile secretion and flow, minor inflammations of the biliary tract, possibly hepatic amebiasis) and inflammations of the gastrointestinal tract (diarrhea, amebic dysentery, etc., incl. hemorrhoids; also when minor hemorrhages are present, but on professional's advice). It has also been used for menorrhagia / hypermenorrhea (= prolonged / heavy menstruation) and postpartum hemorrhage (= h. following childbirth). Externally it is used (as a mouthwash, paint) for inflammations of the mouth, inflamed and bleeding gums and canker sores, (as a wash) for minor skin inflammations, and (as a vaginal irrigation / sitz bath / wash, suppository) for vulvovaginitis.

Caution: Goldenseal should not be used internally during pregnancy and lactation and is best avoided in infants. Before using it for gynecologic disorders, the problem should be judged by a health professional. At higher doses than recommended it causes gastrointestinal irritations (with nausea, vomiting, diarrhea). Otherwise, there are no reports of contraindications or side effects when used properly.

References: (3) Vol. 5, p. 160; (8) p. 312; (9) p. 282; (11) p. 161; (12a) p. 525; (13) p. 234; (14) p. 119; (20) p. 151; (22) p. 225; (29) p. 62; (41) Vols. 1-7; (46) p. 731; (47) p. 1559; (48) p. 914; (66) p. 308; (71) p. 282.

GOTU KOLA

Other Common Name(s): Asiatic pennywort, Indian pennywort
Botanical Name(s): *Centella asiatica* (L.) Urb. = *Hydrocotyle asiatica* L. [Fam.: Apiaceae (Umbelliferae)]

Aerial part
Constituents: Triterpenes (free triterpenoid acids: asiatic acid, madecassic acid; their ester glycosides: asiaticoside, madecassoside), flavonoids (flavonols), polyacetylenes, phytosterols, volatile oil, tannins, etc.

Properties: Wound-healing, cicatrizant and venotonic (chiefly by increasing collagen production), antibacterial, antifungal, anti-inflammatory, mild CNS depressant (by elevating levels of GABA = GABA-mimetic effect), antiulcer (= prevents or helps in healing peptic ulcers, esp. when they are associated with stress). Its most important active constituents are triterpenes, especially in regard to the increase of collagen production and the CNS depressant and antiulcer effects.

Uses: Externally it is used (as an ointment, liniment, poultice) for wounds, burns, scars, ulcers (incl. varicose ulcers) and other skin lesions (after surgery, leprotic / syphilitic lesions, eczema, psoriasis, acne, etc.). Internally it is used (as a tea, h. p.) for peripheral venous disorders (varicose veins in the

176

legs, hemorrhoids, etc.). The beneficial results are due in large part to the increase of collagen production. Gotu kola is also used for minor cases of impaired mental performance (incl. cognitive function), anxiety, epilepsy, hypertension, peptic ulcers, and for low sexual drive and orgasm problems. Here the beneficial results are due in large part to the GABA-mimetic effect. **Caution:** Gotu kola is best avoided during pregnancy and lactation. A combination of gotu kola products with sedative-hypnotic or antihypertensive drugs should be made only by a health professional. It possibly contains sesquiterpene lactones. If so, it may cause contact dermatitis to persons hypersensitive to other Asteraceae plants (e. g. arnica, chamomile, feverfew, ragweed, tansy, yarrow) that contain them. Otherwise, there are no reports of contraindications or side effects when used properly.

References: (1) Vol. 4, p. 764; (3) Vol. 3, p. 792; (8) p. 133; (9) p. 284; (13) p. 219; (20) p. 170; (36) p. 503; (37) p. 296; (41) Vols. 1-7; (45) p. 74; (48) p. 703; (59) p. 77; (63) Vol. 3, p. 145; (68) p. 111; (69) p. 38; (71) p. 234; (74) p. 832; (75) p. 219.

GRAINS-OF-PARADISE

Botanical Name(s): *Aframomum melegueta* K. Schum. = *Amomum melegueta* Roscoe [Fam.: Zingiberaceae]
Seed (Guinea grain, melegueta pepper)
Constituents: Volatile oil (with paradol = a phenol of pungent flavor, very closely related to gingerol of ginger), resin, tannins, starch, fixed oil, etc.
Properties: Aromatic, stomachic, tonic, antioxidant.
Uses: Guinea grain is chiefly used as a spice, and it is beneficial for nonulcer dyspepsia and as a general tonic. Its distilled volatile oil is used as an ingredient in some pungent flavored liqueurs.
Caution: There are no reports of contraindications or side effects when used properly. Nevertheless, Guinea grain is best avoided during pregnancy and lactation.

References: (3) Vol. 2, p. 1139; (5) Vol. 1, p. 36; (10) p. 133; (31) p. 485; (45) p. 159; (48) p. 302; (52) p. 20.

GRAPE

Botanical Name(s): *Vitis vinifera* L. [Fam.: Vitaceae]
Seed
It is obtained from the red variety: *Vitis vinifera* L. ssp. vinifera var. *tinctoria* DC.
Constituents: Oligomeric proanthocyanidins (= OPCs: oligomers of catechin and epicatechin, which on their part are flavan-3-ol derivatives; rich), flavonoids (flavonols), fixed oil (with glycerides of linoleic acid, etc.), etc.
Properties: Antioxidant, anti-inflammatory, "vitamin P"-like (= helps in

normalizing an increased microvascular permeability and fragility; P = permeability). The effects are attributed chiefly to OPCs and flavonoids.

Uses: Internally are used (proanthocyanidins isolated from the seed) for increased microvascular permeability and fragility (with hemorrhagic patches in the skin, vascular retinopathy), with beneficial effects on the cardiovascular system in general. It is reported that proanthocyanidins cross the so-called blood-brain barrier therefore their benefits as antioxidants are also brought to the brain tissue.

Caution: Grape seed extract should't be used during pregnancy and lactation. No other reports of contraindications or side effect when used properly.

Leaf

It is obtained from the red variety (see Seed).

Constituents: Flavonoids (rich in anthocyanins, also flavonols: quercetin, rutin, etc.), tannins (gallocatechins, proanthocyanidins), minerals (rich in potassium), phenolic acids (caffeic acid derivatives), triterpenes (oleanolic acid), etc.

Properties: Venotonic, anti-inflammatory, antioxidant, "vitamin P"-like.

Uses: Internally it is used (as a tea, h. p.) for increased microvascular permeability and fragility (with hemorrhagic patches in the skin, vascular retinopathy), varicose veins in the legs, and hemorrhoids. It is also recommended for minor inflammations of the gastrointestinal tract and the liver and menopausal complaints, with beneficial effects on the cardiovascular system in general.

Caution: There are no reports of contraindications or side effect when used properly.

Fruit (raisin)

Constituents: Invert sugar, pectin, organic acids (free: tartaric acid, etc.; salts: potassium tartrate, etc.), flavonoids (anthocyanins, catechins, etc.), tannins (condensed t.), phenolic acids (caffeic acid, etc.), etc.

Properties: Mild laxative, demulcent, diuretic, antioxidant.

Uses: Internally it is chiefly used (as a tea) for minor constipation.

Caution: There are no reports of contraindications or side effect when used properly.

References: (3) Vol. 6c, p. 499; (5) Vol. 1, p. 1138; (8) p. 595; (9) p. 288; (12) p. 837; (13) p. 305; (22) p. 250; (28) p. 152; (36) p. 504; (37) p. 1466; (48) p. 399; (49) Vol. 2, p. 334; (56) p. 92.

GRINDELIA

Other Common Name(s): gumweed, field gumweed, Great Valley gumweed, gum plant

Botanical Name(s): *Grindelia camporum* Greene = *Grindelia robusta* Nutt.; *Grindelia hirsuta* Hook. et Arn. = *Grindelia humilis* Hook. et Arn.; *Grindelia squarrosa* Pursh (Dun.); etc. [Fam.: Asteraceae (Compositae)]

Aerial part

178

Constituents: Resin (with diterpenoid acids: grindelic acid, etc.), volatile oil, triterpenoid saponins, flavonoids, polyacetylenes, tannins (hydrolyzable t.), phenolic acids, etc.

Properties: Expectorant, mild antispasmodic (esp. bronchial active), anti-inflammatory, antibacterial.

Uses: Internally it is chiefly used (as a tea, h. p.; often combined with other herbs) for inflammations and minor spastic conditions of the upper respiratory tract (bronchitis, etc., bronchial asthma; coughs: irritating cough, whooping cough). It is also used (combined with other herbs) for minor inflammations of the gastrointestinal, hepatobiliary and genitourinary tracts. Externally it is used (as a wet compress, poultice) for poison ivy dermatitis.

Caution: There are no reports of contraindications or side effects when used properly. At higher doses than recommended it causes irritations of the gastrointestinal and genitourinary tracts.

References: (2) Vol. 2, p. 813; (3) Vol. 4, p. 1189; (7) p. 168; (8) p. 292; (15) p. 106; (19) p. 98; (29) p. 59; (35) p. 376; (36) p. 291; (37) p. 623; (46) p. 706; (47) p. 1493; (48) p. 647.

GROUND IVY

Other Common Name(s): alehoof, field balm, cat's foot
Botanical Name(s): *Glechoma hederacea* L. [Fam.: Lamiaceae (Labiatae)]
Aerial part
Constituents: Volatile oil, bitter principles (sesquiterpene lactones), Lamiaceae tannins (rosmarinic acid and other caffeic acid derivatives), triterpenoid saponins, flavonoids, etc.

Properties: Astringent, anti-inflammatory, stomachic, expectorant, diuretic. Rosmarinic acid and related caffeic acid derivatives have been shown to inhibit the biosynthesis of leukotrienes and prostaglandins, and to exert choleretic, antibacterial and antiviral effects.

Uses: Internally it is used (as a tea, h. p.) for minor inflammations of the gastrointestinal tract (gastritis, diarrhea, etc., incl. hemorrhoids), upper respiratory tract (bronchitis, etc.) and genitourinary tract (cystitis, etc.). To enhance the effects in problems of the genitourinary tract, the fluid intake (incl. herbal teas) should be more than 2 liters per day. Externally it is used (as a wash, wet compress, poultice) for minor skin inflammations, ulcers.

Caution: There are no reports of contraindications or side effects when used properly. It doesn't seem to contain allergenic sesquiterpene lactones.

References: (1) Vol. 5, p. 293; (3) Vol. 4, p. 1138; (6) p. 102; (12) p. 782; (14) p. 121; (14) p. 121; (20) p. 154; (27) p. 112; (35) p. 442; (36) p. 477; (37) p. 597; (48) p. 651; (51) p. 162.

GUAIACUM

Other Common Name(s): Brazilian wood, pockwood
Botanical Name(s): *Guaiacum officinale* L.; *Guaiacum sanctum* L. [Fam.:

Zygophyllaceae]
Guaiac wood (lignum vitae)
Guaiac wood consists of the dried heartwood chips.
Constituents: Volatile oil (with guaiol, etc.), resin (= guaiacum resin = guaiac), triterpenoid saponins, gum, etc. Guaiacum resin (= guaiac), obtained by rendering or extraction, contains lignans (guaiaretic acid, nordihydroguaiaretic acid = NDGA, etc.) and guaiacol. Cf. CHAPARRAL.
Properties: Anti-inflammatory and analgesic (NSAID-like effect, by inhibiting the biosynthesis of prostaglandins), mild diuretic and laxative, antimicrobial, rubefacient. The NSAID-like effect is due to lignans and the volatile oil. It is antimicrobial due to phenols (guaiacol, guaiaretic acid, etc.; cf. CHAPARRAL).
Uses: Internally it is used (as a tea, h. p.) for rheumatic complaints (incl. rheumatoid arthritis), as an anti-inflammatory and antidyscratic (= blood purifier; tea, h. p.) for chronic skin diseases (atopic eczema = chronic eczema of internal origin, psoriasis, incl. disorders of syphilitic origin), and for inflammations of the urinary tract (urethritis, cystitis, etc.) and upper respiratory tract (the common cold, bronchitis, etc.; coughs; also as a diaphoretic hot tea). Guaiacum may be helpful for primary dysmenorrhea (= painful menstruation without pathology) by taking it 24-48 hours before menstrual flow, then continuing through 1-2 days of the cycle. Externally it is used (as an ointment) for rheumatic pains, and (as a gargle) for sore throat. Guaiac (= guaiacum resin) is also used in food industry as an antioxidant.
Caution: There are no reports of contraindications or side effects when used properly. Nevertheless, guaiacum is best avoided during pregnancy and lactation. Before using it for dysmenorrhea, the gynecologic problem should be judged by a health professional.

References: (1) Vol. 5, p. 349; (3) Vol. 4, p. 1197; (8) p. 293; (9) p. 292; (12) p. 816; (13) p. 123; (14) p. 123; (16) p. 49; (19) p. 99; (20) p. 156; (24) p. 389; (27) p. 163; (36) p. 291; (37) p. 624; (46) p. 709; (47) p. 1497; (66) p. 650.

GUAR

Other Common Name(s): cluster bean
Botanical Name(s): *Cyamopsis tetragonoloba* (L.) Taub. = *Cyamopsis psoralioides* DC., nom. illeg. [Fam.: Fabaceae (Papilionaceae)]
Guar gum (guar, guar powder, guar flour)
It is the powdered endosperm, which makes about 40 % of the seed. Guaran, which makes about 80 % of guar gum, is the refined product obtained by water extraction, precipitation with alcohol and then drying.
Constituents: Chiefly guaran, also proteins, lipids, minerals, etc. **Guaran** is a galactomannan (a mucilaginous polysaccharide).
Properties: Bulk laxative, demulcent, gelling. Guar gum possesses a high swelling capacity.

Uses: <u>Internally</u> it is used to control appetite as an aid to a weight-loss diet, and for constipation. As it has been shown to delay the absorption of sugars from the bowels, it is also recommended as a dietetic aid to diabetics (esp. overweight diabetics). It has also shown mild cholesterol reducing effect due to mucilaginous polysaccharides (see PSYLLIUM). In pharmaceutical and food industries guar gum is used as a thickening and gelling ingredient.

Caution: The recommended amount should be reached step-by-step and taken with sufficient liquid. It may impair the absorption of some drugs. In view of this, when taking a vital oral medication, drugs should be taken about one hour apart from guar products.

References: (1) Vol. 4, p. 1103; (3) Vol. 4, p. 393; (8) p. 210; (9) p. 289; (11) p. 46; (12) p. 368; (13) p. 373; (23) p. 142; (36) p. 215; (37) p. 375; (72) nr. 11079.

GUARANÁ

Other Common Name(s): guaraná shrub, Brazilian cocoa
Botanical Name(s): *Paullinia cupana* Kunth [Fam.: Sapindaceae]
<u>Guaraná</u>
It is the dried paste made from the crushed kernels.

Constituents: Purine alkaloids (chiefly caffeine, richer than coffee, tea, cola and maté; some theobromine and theophylline), tannins (rich in oligomeric proanthocyanidins = OPCs), flavonoids (catechins), starch (very rich), saponins, fat, etc.

Properties: Stimulant of the central nervous system (due to caffeine), astringent and antioxidant (due to OPCs and catechins). It acts slower than coffee because caffeine is combined with tannins.

Uses: <u>Internally</u> it is used (as an h. p.) for short-term decreased mental and physical performance and for diarrhea. Guaraná extract is used as a flavor ingredient in some soft drinks and alcoholic beverages.

Caution: See COFFEE.

References: (1) Vol. 6, p. 53; (3) Vol. 6a, p. 481; (8) p. 409; (9) p. 293; (11) p. 184; (12) p. 1063; (13) p. 270; (36) p. 403; (37) p. 1034; (48) p. 1084.

GUGGUL

Other Common Name(s): bdellium tree, Indian bdellium tree, false myrrh, mukul myrrh tree
Botanical Name(s): *Commiphora mukul* (Hook. ex Stocks) Engl. [Fam.: Burseraceae]
<u>Guggul</u>
Guggul is the hardened gum-oleoresin that exudes after incisions made to the bark.

Constituents: Chiefly a resin (with phytosteroids: guggulsterones) and gum (mucilaginous polysaccharides) and some volatile oil (with myrcene, etc.).

Properties and Uses: Guggul is chiefly used for the extraction of guggulipid. In traditional medicine guggul is used for rheumatic complaints (incl. rheumatoid arthritis; justifiable due to the anti-inflammatory and antiexudative effects of guggulsterones) and overweight (justifiable due to the swelling capacity of gum).

Caution: Raw guggul may cause allergic reactions and gastrointestinal irritations. See Guggulipid. Guggul may impair the absorption of some drugs. In view of this, when taking a vital oral medication, drugs should be taken about one hour apart from guggul products.

Guggulipid

Guggulipid is the dried ethyl acetate extract of guggul.

Constituents: Chiefly guggulsterones (*E*- and *Z*- guggulsterone, etc.), also long-chain tetrahydric alcohols, etc.

Properties: LDL-cholesterol and triglyceride reducing, HDL-cholesterol increasing, platelet aggregation inhibitory, anti-inflammatory and antiedematous, thyroid stimulant. The effects are due in large part to guggulsterones.

Uses: Internally guggulipid is used for high cholesterol and triglycerides and rheumatic complaints (incl. rheumatoid arthritis).

Caution: Guggulipid should not be taken during pregnancy and lactation and hyperthyroidism (= Basedow's disease). The lipid lowering effect is due to a liver-active mechanism. In view of this, as with cholesterol reducing drugs (clofibrate, lovastatin, etc.), it should not be taken in severe liver disorders. In cases of minor liver problems it can be used but monitored by a health professional. Guggulipid products should be standardized to guggulsterones. Guggulipid needs about 4 weeks to develop the effects.

References: (1) Vol. 4, p. 966; (6) p. 71; (13) p. 411; (22) p. 227; (29) p. 35; (48) p. 752; (68) p. 122; (75) p. 221; (79) p. 279.

GUM ARABIC TREE

Other Common Name(s): thorny acacia
Botanical Name(s): *Acacia senegal* (L.) Willd. [Fam.: Fabaceae (Mimosaceae)]

Gum Arabic (acacia, acacia gum, Senegal gum)

It is the dried natural exudate of the stem and branches.

Constituents: Chiefly a polysaccharide (arabin = mineral salts of arabic acid), enzymes, but no starch. Arabin is water-soluble.

Properties: Suspending and emulsifying, thickening, demulcent, emollient.

Uses: It is chiefly used in the production of emulsions and suspensions, tablets and lozenges. To the products that it is incorporated it adds demulcent effect therefore it is beneficial for inflammations of the gastrointestinal tract. Gum Arabic is an important ingredient in Cola Flavor Emulsion.

Caution: There are no reports of contraindications or side effects when used properly.

References: (1) Vol. 4, p. 36; (3) Vol. 4, p. 1211; (8) p. 17; (9) p. 4; (11) p. 42; (12) p. 351; (13) p. 363; (37) p. 627; (48) p. 93.

GYMNEMA

Other Common Name(s): gurmar
Botanical Name(s): *Gymnema silvestre* (Retz.) R. Br. ex Schult. [Fam.: Asclepiadaceae]
Leaf
Constituents: Triterpenoid saponins (gymnemic acids), an alkaloid (gymnamine, closely related to lycopodium alkaloids), biogenic amines, amino acids (including GABA = gamma aminobutyrric acid), etc.
Properties: Taste suppressant. By topical application (chewing, etc.), gymnema has been shown to block the sweet taste and some of the bitter taste, but not salt and acid tastes. By keeping off the sweet taste it helps to control a craving for sugar. Responsible for this are considered saponins. Gymnema has also shown mild antihyperglycemic effect.
Uses: Topically (applied to the tongue, mainly to the tip; or by chewing) it is used to control a craving for sugar, recommended as an aid to a weight-loss diet and diabetes. Internally it is used as an adjuvant (tea, h. p.) for diabetes.
Caution: There are no reports of contraindications or side effects when used properly.

References: (3) Vol. 4, p. 1221; (5) Vol. 1, p. 555; (13) p. 159; (36) p. 439; (37) p. 629; (48) p. 683; (65) p. 23.

HARONGA

Botanical Name(s): *Harungana madacascariensis* Lam. ex Poir. = *Haronga madacascariensis* (Lam. ex Poir.) Choisy. [Fam.: Hypericaceae (Guttiferae)]
Bark and leaf
Constituents: Anthranoids (bark: harunganin, chrysophanol, etc.; leaf: madacascarin = an anthrone dimer), naphthodiantrones (leaf: hypericin, etc.), flavonoids (leaf: flavonols; bark: catechins), tannins (proanthocyanidins), triterpenes, etc.
Properties: Digestive secretagogue (increases secretions of the stomach, liver and pancreas), liver protective, cholagogue, carminative, antibacterial.
Uses: Internally it is used (as a tea, h. p.; often combined with other herbs or enzymes) for nonulcer dyspepsia (with fullness, flatulence, including intolerance of sweets) due to insufficiency of digestive secretions (incl. pancreatic juice = external secretion of pancreas that passes into duodenum).
Caution: Haronga should not be taken for more than 2 months. When taking haronga products, avoid exposure to strong sunrays as it may cause pho-

183

totoxic skin irritations, due to hypericinoids (see ST. JOHN'S WORT). It should not be taken in cases of severe liver disorders, biliary and bowel obstructions, biliary abscess and acute pancreatitis. In cases of nonobstructive gallstones it can be used but only on health professional' s advice. Haronga products should be standardized to the anthranoids content.

References: (1) Vol. 5, p. 391; (3) Vol. 5, p. 16; (8) p. 299; (13) p. 412; (23) p. 88; (24) p. 391; (37) p. 643; (41) Vols. 1-7; (42) Vol. 4, pp. 223, 471; (72) nr. 59338.

HART'S TONGUE FERN

Botanical Name(s): *Asplenium scolopendrium* L. = *Phyllitis scolopendrium* (L.) Newman = *Scolopendrium vulgare* Sm. [Fam.: Polypodiaceae]
Fronds (full-developed)
Constituents: Tannins (possibly of condensed type), mucilage, flavonoids (leucoanthocyanidins), amino acids (aspartic acid, glutamic acid), etc.
Properties: Astringent, wound-healing, demulcent, diuretic.
Uses: Internally it is used (as a tea, h. p.; usually combined with other herbs) for minor inflammations (also when minor hemorrhages are present) of the gastrointestinal tract (diarrhea, etc., incl. hemorrhoids), respiratory tract (bronchitis, etc.; minor irritating dry coughs) and genitourinary tract (gravel, nonobstructive urinary stones; as an adjuvant for chronic nephritis). To enhance the effects in problems of the genitourinary tract, the fluid intake (incl. herbal teas) should be more than 2 liters per day. Externally it is used (as a wash, wet compress, poultice, ointment) for wounds and hemorrhoids, and (as a mouthwash, gargle) for inflammations of the mouth and throat (incl. bleeding gums).
Caution: There are no reports of contraindications or side effects when used properly. For minor hemorrhages it should be used on professional's advice.

References: (3) Vol. 6a, p. 635; (15) p. 191; (27) p. 310; (35) p. 304; (36) p. 478; (42) Vol. 1, p. 282; (47) p. 2489; (49) Vol. 2, p. 370.

HAWTHORN

Other Common Name(s): 1) hawthorn, May thorn, white thorn 2) one-seed hawthorn, white thorn
Botanical Name(s): 1) *Crataegus laevigata* (Poir.) DC. = *C. oxyacantha* L. = *C. oxyacanthoides* Thuill. 2) *Crataegus monogyna* Jacq. [Fam.: Rosaceae]
Leaf and flowers
Constituents: Flavonoids (chiefly flavones: vitexin = apigenin-8-C-glucoside, vitexin-rhamnoside, etc.; also: flavonols: rutin and other quercetin glycosides), oligomeric proanthocyanidins (= OPCs: oligomers of catechin and epicatechin, which on their part are flavan-3-ol derivatives), triterpenoid sapogenins (ursolic and crataegolic acids), biogenic amines (choline, β-phenylethylamine, etc.), etc.

184

Properties: The effects of hawthorn on the heart muscle include increased contractility (= positive inotropic effect), increased conductivity (= positive dromotropic effect), decreased excitability (= negative bathmotropic effect), a normalized rate of the heartbeat, and antioxidant (= cardioprorecticve effect). Hawthorn dilates peripheral blood vessels, especially coronary vessels. This results in improved coronary blood flow and mild antihypertensive effect. Responsible for most of the effects are flavonoids and oligomeric proanthocyanidins, which act synergistically. Hawthorn exerts also mild sedative-antianxiety effect, due in large part to flavones (vitexin derivatives).

Uses: Internally it is used (as an h. p.) for heart failure (= a clinical condition associated with insufficient cardiac output) in early stages (stages I and II, according to NYHA), minor coronary heart disease (= a condition associated with decreased blood supply to the heart) and to prevent or alleviate angina pectoris (= chest pain due to insufficient blood supply to the heart) associated with it, as an adjuvant for cardiac arrhythmias and hypertension, and (as a tea, h. p.; often combined with other herbs) for minor cases of insomnia. Hawthorn is also recommended for minor cardiac insufficiencies associated with infective conditions or age-related cases (presbycardia = senile heart).

Caution: There are no reports of contraindications or side effects when used properly. Hawthorn is a safe herb. Nevertheless, due to the seriousness of heart problems, it is best used on health professional's advice. Hawthorn should not be taken for an acute attack as it needs at least 6 weeks to develop the effects. Hawthorn products should be standardized to flavonoids or / and oligomeric proanthocyanidins. A possible combination with cardioactive glycosides or herbs (digoxin, lily-of-the-valley, etc.) should be made only by a health professional.

Note: Hawthorn leaf with flower is seldom obtained from other *Crataegus* spp. such as *C. pentagyna* Waldst. et Kit. ex Willd.; *C. nigra* Waldst. et Kit.; and *C. azarolus* L. (azarole).

Fruit (berry)

Constituents: Oligomeric proanthocyanidins (= OPCs), flavonoids (chiefly quercetin glycosides; less than leaf with flower), triterpenoid sapogenins, etc.

Properties: Mild peripheral vasodilatory and antihypertensive, and antioxidant.

Uses: Internally it is used as an adjuvant (h. p.) for minor cases of hypertension. It is also incorporated in different products that contain the extract of hawthorn leaf with flower.

Caution: See Leaf with flower.

References: (1) Vol. 4, p. 1040; (3) Vol. 4, p. 324; (6) p. 38; (7) p. 99; (8) p. 195; (12) p. 844; (13) p. 311; (16) p. 100; (17) p. 168; (19) p. 243; (23) p. 156; (26) p. 145; (27) p. 55; (28) pp. 138, 144, 217; (46) p. 143; (47) p. 1113; (48) p. 396.

HAZEL, EUROPEAN

Other Common Name(s): European filbert
Botanical Name(s): *Corylus avellana* L. [Fam.: Betulaceae]
Leaf
Constituents: Flavonoids (myricitrin, etc.), tannins (proanthocyanidins), triterpenes (taraxerol, etc.), phenolic acids (chlorogenic acid, etc.), volatile oil, etc.
Properties: Astringent, anti-inflammatory, hemostatic (topical action). It has been claimed to exert witch hazel-like effects.
Uses: Externally it is used (as a wash, wet compress) for minor cuts, wounds, ulcers, hemorrhoids, and (as a mouthwash, gargle) for inflammations of the mouth and throat (incl. bleeding gums). Internally it is used (as a tea, h. p.) for minor inflammations of the gastrointestinal tract (diarrhea, ulcerative colitis, incl. hemorrhoids; also when minor hemorrhages are present, but on professional's advice).
Caution: There are no reports of contraindications or side effects when used properly.

References: (1) Vol. 4, p. 1027; (3) Vol. 4, p. 315; (5) Vol. 1, p. 348; (8) p. 194; (27) p. 233; (35) p. 233; (37) p. 364; (48) p. 395; (87) Vol. 1, p. 73.

HEAL ALL

Other Common Name(s): self heal, all heal
Botanical Name(s): *Prunella vulgaris* L. [Fam.: Lamiaceae (Labiatae)]
Aerial part
Constituents: Bitter principles (possibly iridoids), Lamiaceae tannins (rosmarinic acid and other caffeic acid derivatives), triterpenes (arjunolic, ursolic and oleanolic acids), flavonoids (flavonols, anthocyanins), etc.
Properties: Bitter tonic, astringent, wound-healing, and possibly mild choleretic, antioxidant, antibacterial and antiviral (against *Herpes*). The bitter tonic effect is due to bitter principles (possibly iridoids) and bitter triterpenes. The rest of the effects are due in large part to Lamiaceae tannins, enhanced by flavonoids.
Uses: Internally it is used (as a tea, h. p.) for nonulcer dyspepsia and inflammations of the gastrointestinal tract (diarrhea, ulcerative colitis, etc., incl. hemorrhoids; also when minor hemorrhages are present, but on professional's advice). Externally it is used (as a mouthwash, gargle) for inflammations of the mouth and throat and (as a wash, wet compress) for wounds and hemorrhoids (also as an enema).
Caution: There are no reports of contraindications or side effects when used properly.

References: (3) Vol. 6a, p. 937; (18) p. 259; (27) p. 61; (31) p. 472; (35) p. 731; (36) p. 48; (41) Vols. 1-7; (42) Vol. 4, pp. 322, 331; (51) p. 160; (87) Vol. 2, p. 128.

186

HEARTSEASE

Other Common Name(s): European wild pansy, Johny-jump-up, wild violet

Botanical Name(s): *Viola tricolor* L. [Fam.: Violaceae]

Aerial part

Constituents: Flavonoids (flavonols: quercetin, rutin; flavones: luteolin, vitexin; anthocyanins), phenolic acids (salicylic, gentisic and caffeic acids; methyl-salicylate), phenol glycosides (violutoside, etc.), mucilaginous polysaccharides (rich), tannins, coumarins, peptides, etc.

Properties: Anti-inflammatory, antioxidant, diuretic, expectorant, demulcent, mild laxative, emollient. Heartsease is reported to exert cortisone-like and NSAID-like effects.

Uses: Internally it is used (usually combined with other herbs) chiefly as an anti-inflammatory and antidyscratic (= blood purifier; tea, h. p.) for atopic eczema (= chronic eczema of internal origin, incl. milk crust = infantile eczema), common acne (= acne vulgaris) and chronic rheumatic complaints, and for inflammations of the upper respiratory tract (the common cold, bronchitis, etc.; coughs; also as a diaphoretic hot tea) and minor constipation. Externally it is used (as a wash, wet compress) for chronic skin disorders (eczema, milk crust, dandruff, common acne) and bacterial skin infections, and (as a vaginal irrigation / sitz bath / wash) for vulvovaginitis.

Caution: There are no reports of contraindications or side effects when used properly.

References: (1) Vol. 6, p. 1148; (3) Vol. 6c, p. 482; (6) pp. 101, 184, 233, 330; (8) p. 589; (15) p. 233; (16) p. 30; (17) p. 619; (19) p. 219; (28) p. 191; (37) p. 1453; (51) p. 120; (73) pp. 204, 1238.

HEATHER

Botanical Name(s): *Calluna vulgaris* (L.) Hull. [Fam.: Ericaceae]

Flowering top

Constituents: Flavonoids (flavonols, catechins), a phenol glycoside (arbutin = hydroquinone-glucoside), tannins (oligomeric proanthocyanidins), phenolic acids (chlorogenic acid, etc.), triterpenes (ursolic acid, etc.), etc.

Properties: Anti-inflammatory, diuretic, urinary antiseptic, astringent. Heather is anti-inflammatory and diuretic due in large part to flavonoids and urinary antiseptic due to hydroquinone liberated from arbutin (see UVA-URSI).

Uses: Internally it is used (as a tea, h. p.; combined with other herbs) chiefly for inflammations of the genitourinary tract (cystitis, urethritis, prostatitis, pyelonephritis). To enhance the effects, urine should be slightly alkaline (this can be done by consuming a diet rich in vegetables and / or taking about a teaspoonful / day of baking soda) and the fluid intake (incl. herbal teas) should be more than 2 liters per day. It is also used for minor inflammations of the gastrointestinal tract (diarrhea, etc.) and as a diaphoretic hot tea for the common cold.

Caution: There are no reports of contraindications or side effects when used properly.

References: (1) Vol. 4, p. 617; (3) Vol. 3, p. 610; (13a) p. 243; (15) p. 45; (24) p. 156; (36) p. 475; (37) p. 260; (47) p. 1279; (51) p. 272.

HELLEBORE, AMERICAN

Other Common Name(s): American white hellebore, false hellebore, Indian poke
Botanical Name(s): *Veratrum viride* Aiton [Fam.: Liliaceae (Melanthiaceae)]
<u>Root</u> (rhizome)
Constituents: Steroidal alkaloids (free alkamines: jervine, etc.; esters: germidine, protoveratrines A and B, etc.; glycoalkaloids: pseudojervine, veratrosine, etc.), etc.
Properties: Antihypertensive.
Uses: <u>Internally</u> it has been used for hypertension (at low doses only!).
Caution: American hellebore is very toxic and not for self-treatment. It is no longer used for medicinal purposes.

References: (2) Vol. 3, p. 754; (3) Vol. 6c, p. 406; (11) p. 178; (37) p. 1445; (46) p. 1680; (47) p. 2786; (48) p. 1062.

HELLEBORE, BLACK

Other Common Name(s): Christmas rose
Botanical Name(s): *Helleborus niger* L. [Fam.: Ranunculaceae]
<u>Root</u> (rhizome)
Constituents: (Dried or fresh): steroidal saponins (collectively referred to as helleborin), phytosterols (phytoectysterones), etc.; (dried): anemonin (= protoanemonin dimer); (fresh): protoanemonin (an unstable compound). The reports on cardiac glycosides (hellebrin, etc.) remain controversial.
Properties: (Dried root): Diuretic, antimicrobial, laxative. Saponins are responsible for the diuretic and laxative effects. They irritate the nasal mucosa and cause sneezing. Anemonin is non-toxic and has shown antimicrobial activity. Protoanemonin is toxic and a strong local irritant (cf. PULSATILLA).
Uses: <u>Internally</u> it is used (only dried!) mainly as a flushing-out treatment (= herbal tea or product + liquids: more than 2 liters per day; sometimes combined with a medication) for inflammations of the genitourinary tract (cystitis, etc.), urinary gravel and nonobstructive stones, to prevent relapsing urinary infections / gravel / stones, and (as a tea, h. p.) for inflammations of the gastrointestinal tract (with sluggish bowels, constipation). It is also incorporated in some sniffing powders.

Caution: Internally should be used only dried herb and as directed by an experienced practitioner. Even dried, black hellebore should not be taken during pregnancy as it may still contain protoanemonin (teratogenic, abortifacient!; cf. PULSATILLA). Fresh herb should be handled with care (see Properties). If taken internally, fresh herb (also dried herb at higher doses than recommended) causes strong gastrointestinal irritations (with vomiting, diarrhea), etc. A flushing-out treatment is contraindicated in cases of obstructive urinary stones, edema due to impaired heart or kidney function and kidney inflammations (here can be used on health professional's advice to enhance the effects of an antimicrobial therapy).

References: (1) Vol. 5, p. 421; (3) Vol. 5, p. 43; (6) p. 38; (8) p. 304; (11) p. 120; (13) p. 194; (18) p. 125; (23) p. 396; (36) p. 320; (37) p. 648; (47) p. 1526; (48) p. 747.

HELLEBORE, WHITE

Other Common Name(s): European hellebore
Botanical Name(s): *Veratrum album* L. [Fam.: Liliaceae (Melanthiaceae)]
<u>Root</u> (rhizome)
Constituents: Steroidal alkaloids (free alkamines: jervine, etc. and their glycosides; esters: protoveratrines, etc.), etc.
Properties: Antihypertensive.
Uses: <u>Internally</u> it has been used for hypertension (at low doses only!).
Caution: White hellebore is very toxic and not for self-treatment.

References: (2) Vol. 3, p. 742; (3) Vol. 6c, p. 401; (11a) p. 238; (37) p. 1444; (46) p. 1679; (47) p. 2778; (48) p. 1061.

HEMIDESMUS

Other Common Name(s): East Indian sarsaparilla
Botanical Name(s): *Hemidesmus indicus* (L.) W.T. Aiton = *Periploca indica* L. [Fam.: Asclepiadaceae]
<u>Root</u>
Constituents: Triterpenes (esterified triterpenes), phytosterols (free, glycosidic), volatile oil (with p-methoxy-salicylaldehyde), tannins, coumarin derivatives (hemidesminine, etc.), etc.
Properties: Diuretic, anti-inflammatory, tonic.
Uses: <u>Internally</u> it has been used much like sarsaparilla as an antidyscratic (= blood purifier), anti-inflammatory and tonic (tea, h. p.) for venereal diseases, atopic eczema and chronic rheumatic complaints, and as a diaphoretic hot tea for the common cold and feverish states.
Caution: There are no reports of contraindications or side effects when used properly. In plants of Asclepiadaceae family are found alkaloids and cardiac glycosides therefore manufacturers should evaluate them.

References: (3) Vol. 5, p. 48; (18) p. 253; (35) p. 714; (36) pp. 47, 492; (42) Vol. 3, p. 222; (41) Vols. 1-7.

HEMLOCK, POISON

Other Common Name(s): spotted hemlock
Botanical Name(s): *Conium maculatum* L. [Fam.: Apiaceae (Umbelliferae)]
Aerial part
Constituents: Piperidine alkaloids (chiefly coniine, which decreases on drying and storage), polyacetylenes, flavonoids, furanocoumarins.
Properties: Coniine is very toxic, with nicotine-like and curare-like effects.
Uses: Internally it is no longer used. Externally it is used (only incorporated in a few products) for neuralgic pains and lymphedema, among others.
Caution: With toxic amounts, firstly occurs the paralysis of motor endings of skeletal muscles, later comes a respiratory paralysis and death (death of Socrates, 399 B.C.). Poison hemlock resembles some other plants of the same family, due to which its leaves are mistaken for parsley, root for western osha or parsnip, and seed for anise, among others. Poison hemlock has a very unpleasant odor.

References: (1) Vol. 4, p. 970; (3) Vol. 4, p. 262; (6) p. 342; (8) p. 186; (11a) p. 440; (13) p. 276; (23) p. 345; (37) p. 358; (46) p. 307; (47) p. 1075; (48) p. 863.

HEMP AGRIMONY

Other Common Name(s): hemp thoroughwort, water hemp
Botanical Name(s): *Eupatorium cannabinum* L. [Fam.: Asteraceae (Compositae)]
Aerial part
Constituents: Bitter principles (sesquiterpene lactones: eupatoriopicrin, etc.), phenolic acids, water-soluble polysaccharides, a benzofuran (euparin), volatile oil, flavonoids, tannins, unsaturated pyrrolizidine alkaloids (= UPAs), etc.
Properties: Bitter tonic, choleretic, cholagogue, mild laxative, antipyretic, mild immunomodulant, diuretic, wound-healing. The bitter tonic and hepatobiliary effects may be attributed to bitter principles and phenolic acids. The immunomodulant effect is due to water-soluble polysaccharides, potentiated by bitter principles.
Uses: Internally it is used (as a tea, h. p.) for loss of appetite and nonulcer dyspepsia (with sluggish bowels, minor constipation), hepatobiliary disorders (impaired bile secretion and flow, nonobstructive gallstones, chronic cholecystitis) and feverish states. It is also used for decreased resistance to infections, especially in the upper respiratory tract. Externally it is used (as a wash, wet compress) for minor skin inflammations and wounds.

190

Caution: Hemp agrimony should not be taken in cases of biliary and bowel obstructions, and it is best to avoid it during pregnancy and lactation. In cases of nonobstructive gallstones it can be used but on health professional's advice. At higher doses than recommended it may cause gastrointestinal irritations (with nausea, vomiting, diarrhea). In hemp agrimony products, the UPAs content should be within limits. For dosage limits of UPAs see COLTSFOOT. Otherwise, there are no reports of contraindications or side effects when used properly.

References: (3) Vol. 4, p. 869; (6) p. 262; (10) p. 142; (27) p. 70; (35) p. 15; (37) p. 499; (46) p. 204; (47) p. 1310; (51) p. 200.

HEMP NETTLE

Botanical Name(s): *Galeopsis segetum* Neck. = *Galeopsis ochroleuca* Lam. [Fam.: Lamiaceae (Labiatae)]
Aerial part
Constituents: Triterpenoid saponins, iridoids (harpagide, 8-O-acetylharpagide), Lamiaceae tannins (rosmarinic acid and other caffeic acid derivatives; rich), flavonoids, minerals (silicic acid: free and water-soluble), volatile oil, etc.
Properties: Expectorant, astringent, diuretic. The expectorant and diuretic effects are due in large part to saponins, and it is astringent due to Lamiaceae tannins.
Uses: Internally it is used (as a tea, h. p.; usually combined with other herbs) for chronic inflammations of the respiratory tract. Due to Lamiaceae tannins (= caffeic acid derivatives) it may exert beneficial effects on the digestive system.
Caution: There are no reports of contraindications or side effects when used properly.

References: (3) Vol. 4, p. 1084; (8) p. 274; (12a) p. 567; (17) p. 243; (19) p. 106; (23) p. 235; (24) p. 168; (37) p. 570; (47) p. 1408.

HENBANE

Botanical Name(s): *Hyoscyamus niger* L. [Fam.: Solanaceae]
Leaf
Constituents: Tropane alkaloids: chiefly (–)-hyosciamine and atropine = (±)-hyosciamine, also (–)-scopolamine = hyoscine, etc.; biogenic amines (choline, etc.), tannins, flavonoids, etc. Cf. BELLADONNA
Properties: Due to the parasympatholytic activity of hyosciamine / atropine and scopolamine, henbane exerts antispasmodic and antisecretory effects, among others. Scopolamine is a CNS depressant and as it is contained in higher ratio than in belladonna, henbane exerts also sedative effect.

Uses: Internally it is used (usually as a standardized combination product) for spastic conditions of the gastrointestinal tract (irritable bowel syndrome, spastic constipation, peptic ulcers, vomiting, griping due to anthranoid laxatives) and motion sickness. Externally it is used (as a liniment) for neuralgic pains. In these formulations is incorporated henbane oil, which itself is prepared by extracting leaves with ethanol, ammonia and peanut oil.

Caution: Henbane is toxic. Today are used extracts (standardized to hyosciamine / atropine content) and especially the isolated alkaloids, which are given by prescription only. It should not be taken in cases of tachycardia, glaucoma, retention of urine due to prostatic hyperplasia, bowel obstruction and during pregnancy, among others.

References: (1) Vol. 5, p. 464; (3) Vol. 5, p. 203; (8) p. 313; (11) p. 151; (12) p. 970; (13) p. 240; (14) p. 131; (19) p. 45; (37) pp. 690, 997; (46) p. 693; (47) p. 1578; (48) p. 811; (74) p. 320.

HENNA

Botanical Name(s): *Lawsonia inermis* L. = *Lawsonia alba* Lam. [Fam.: Lythraceae]

Leaf

Constituents: Pigments (1,4- naphthoquinones: lawsone = isojuglone, etc.), tannins (chiefly gallotannins, also free gallic acid), flavonoids, xanthones, coumarins, sugars, etc.

Properties: Astringent, antimicrobial, diuretic. Lawsone has shown antibacterial, antifungal and antitumoral effects.

Uses: Externally it is chiefly used as an ingredient in the production of many hair dyes. Henna is also used for eczema, fungal skin infections and ulcers. Internally it is chiefly used in traditional medicine (as a tea) for inflammations of the gastrointestinal tract (diarrhea, etc.) and gastrointestinal ulcers.

Caution: Henna should not be taken during pregnancy and lactation. Otherwise, there are no reports of contraindications or side effects when used properly.

References: (3) Vol. 5, p. 468; (9) p. 297; (17) p. 291; (29) p. 68; (36) pp. 248, 498; (37) p. 812; (46) p. 721; (48) p. 419; (49) Vol. 2, p. 453.

HERB-ROBERT

Botanical Name(s): *Geranium robertianum* L. [Fam.: Geraniaceae]

Aerial part

Constituents: Tannins (ellagitannins, gallotannins), flavonoids (flavonols: quercetin, rutin, kaempferol, etc.), organic acids (malic and citric acids), etc.

Properties: Astringent, anti-inflammatory, hemostatic, wound-healing.

Uses: Internally it is used (as a tea, h. p.) for inflammatory conditions of the gastrointestinal tract (diarrhea, gastroenteritis, ulcerative colitis, incl. hemorrhoids; also when minor hemorrhages are present, but on professional's advice). Externally it is used (as a wash, wet compress, poultice) for wounds, ulcers, hemorrhoids and (as a mouthwash, gargle) for inflammations of the mouth and throat.

Caution: There are no reports of contraindications or side effects when used properly.

References: (1) Vol. 5, p. 254; (3) Vol. 4, p. 1126; (8) p. 282; (6) p. 315; (23) p. 374; (27) p. 91; (37) p. 586; (47) p. 1444; (51) p. 88.

HIBISCUS

Other Common Name(s): karkadé, red sorrel, roselle
Botanical Name(s): *Hibiscus sabdariffa* L. [Fam.: Malvaceae]
Flower (here: calyx, i.e. all sepals of the flower, colectivelly)
Constituents: Organic acids (very rich; chiefly hibiscus acid = a lactone of hydroxycitric acid, also citric and malic acids, etc.), flavonoids (an anthocyanin: hibiscin of red color; flavonols of yellow color; etc.), phenolic acids, mucilaginous polysaccharides, etc.
Properties: Acidulous, refrigerant, diuretic, antihypertensive (ACE-inhibitory effect), antioxidant, cholesterol reducing..
Uses: Internally it is used (as a tea, h. p.) as a refreshing drink, for feverish and thirsty states, and for minor cases of hypertension and high cholesterol.
Caution: There are no reports of contraindications or side effects when used properly. At higher doses, it exerts laxative effect.

References: (3) Vol. 5, p. 77; (6) p. 186; (8) p. 307; (9) p. 444; (13) p. 412; (17) p. 297; (21) p. 209; (37) p. 663; (48) p. 24.

HOLLY

Other Common Name(s): English holly
Botanical Name(s): *Ilex aquifolium* L. [Fam.: Aquifoliaceae]
Leaf
Constituents: Triterpenes (27-cumaroxyursolic acid, etc.), flavonoids (flavonols: quercetin, rutin, etc.), a bitter principle (a sesquiterpene lactone, designated as ilicin), phytosterols (5-sterols: β-sitosterol, etc.), phenolic acids (chlorogenic acid, etc.), etc., but no theobromine.
Properties: Mild diuretic and bitter tonic.
Uses: Internally it is used as a diaphoretic hot tea for feverish states and the common cold and as an antidyscratic (= blood purifier; tea, h. p.) for chronic rheumatic complaints. It has been claimed to be a tea substitute (see MATÉ = *Ilex paraguariensis* A. St. Hil.) but it cannot replace it because holly leaf doesn't contain any purine alkaloids (caffeine, theophylline, theobromine).
Caution: There are no reports of contraindications or side effects when used properly.

References: (1) Vol. 5, p. 506; (3) Vol. 5, p. 226; (5) Vol. 1, p. 603; (24) p. 462; (27) p. 24; (35) p. 405; (37) p. 697; (41) Vols. 1-7; (47) p. 1609; (48) p. 190.

HOLLYHOCK

Botanical Name(s): *Alcea rosea* L. = *Althaea rosea* (L.) Cav [Fam.: Malvaceae]

Flower

Constituents: It is not well studied. It is reported to contain mucilaginous polysaccharides, flavonoids (anthocyanins), etc.

Properties: Demulcent, emollient.

Uses: Internally it is used (as a tea, h. p.; usually combined with other herbs) for inflammations of the upper respiratory, gastrointestinal and genitourinary tracts. Externally it is used (as a mouthwash, gargle) for inflammations of the mouth and throat and (as a wash, poultice) for minor skin inflammations and ulcers. It can be used much like flowers of high mallow (*Malva sylvestris* L.; see MALLOW). It is widely used to improve the appearance of herbal teas and to give color to wines and fruit juices, for which *Alcea rosea* var. *nigra* L. is preferred.

Caution: There are no reports of contraindications or side effects when used properly.

References: (1) Vol. 4, p. 159; (3) Vol. 2, p. 1246; (12a) p. 125; (24) p. 321; (27) p. 206; (37) p. 36.

HOLY BASIL

Other Common Name(s): sacred basil, tulsi

Botanical Name(s): *Ocimum tenuiflorum* L. = *Ocimum sanctum* L. [Fam.: Lamiaceae (Labiatae)]

Aerial part

Constituents: Volatile oil (with eugenol, methylchavicol = estragole, etc.; depending on the origin, etc.), flavonoids (flavones: luteolin, apigenin, molludistin, etc.), Lamiaceae tannins (rosmarinic acid and other caffeic acid derivatives), triterpenes (oleanolic and ursolic acids), etc.

Properties: Adaptogenic, antihyperglycemic, anti-inflammatory, antioxidant, antimicrobial, expectorant, antispasmodic.

Uses: Internally it is used (as a tea, h. p.) for minor cases of fatigue and feeling of weakness, diabetes, inflammatory and spastic conditions of the upper respiratory tract (the common cold, bronchitis, asthma, etc.; coughs; also as a diaphoretic hot tea) and gastrointestinal tract (peptic ulcers, diarrhea, etc.), with beneficial effects also in improving cerebral blood flow and memory.

Caution: Holy basil should not be taken during pregnancy and lactation. Otherwise, there are no reports of contraindications or side effects when used properly.

References: (3) Vol. 6a, p. 291; (5) Vol. 1, p. 756; (41) Vols. 1-7; (45) p. 114; (52) p. 536; (96) p. 167.

HOLY THORN

Other Common Name(s): mayten
Botanical Name(s): *Maytenus ilicifolia* Reissek [Fam.: Celastraceae]
Leaf
Constituents: Macrolide alkaloids (maytansinoids: maytansine, etc.), triterpenoid quinones (monomers: ilicifoline, congoronine; dimers: congorosins A, B, etc.), tannins, etc.
Properties: Antiulcer (= prevents or helps in healing peptic ulcers), analgesic, gastrointestinal antiseptic, astringent, wound-healing, contraceptive. Maytansine has shown antitumoral effect, but it is toxic and not used.
Uses: Internally it is used (as a tea, h. p.) for peptic ulcers and dyspeptic disorders (heartburn, stomach pain, flatulence). In traditional medicine it is used for its claimed contraceptive effect. Externally it is used (as a wash) for ulcers and chronic skin diseases (eczema, etc.).
Caution: Holy thorn should not be taken during pregnancy. Unless advised by a health professional, it should not be taken during lactation. Otherwise, there are no reports of contraindications or side effects when used properly.

References: (1) Vol. 5, p. 795; (3) Vol. 5, p. 723; (31) p. 317; (36) p. 417; (41) Vols. 1-7; (48) p. 1069; (52) p. 483; (57) p. 517.

HONEYSUCKLE

Other Common Name(s): 1) Japanese honeysuckle 2) wild honeysuckle 3) honeysuckle
Botanical Name(s): 1) *Lonicera japonica* Thunb. 2) *Lonicera confusa* (Sweet) DC. 3) *Lonicera dasystyla* Rehder; *Lonicera hypoglauca* Miq. [Fam.: Caprifoliaceae]
Flower bud
Constituents: Flavonoids (flavones: luteolin glycosides), bitter principles (iridoids), phenolic acids (caffeic acid derivatives), volatile oil (with linalool, geraniol, aromadendrenes), saponins (possibly triterpenoid s.), etc.
Properties: Anti-inflammatory, antioxidant, diuretic, bitter tonic, astringent, antibacterial, antiviral, antitumoral, mild immunomodulant. The effects are due in large part to flavonoids (esp. luteolin), iridoids, and phenolic acids. The diuretic effect is due to saponins, flavonoids and volatile oil.
Uses: Internally it is used (as a tea, h. p.) for feverish states, inflammatory conditions (esp. due to relapsing infections) of the upper respiratory tract, also genitourinary and gastrointestinal tracts, and as a minor general tonic. Externally it is used (as a wash, wet compress) for minor skin inflammations and wounds and (as a poultice) for boils. In traditional medicine it is also used for certain tumors.
Caution: There are no reports of contraindications or side effects when used properly.

References: (3) Vol. 5, p. 574; (9) p. 536; (31) pp. 404, 475; (36) p. 507; (41) Vols. 1-7; (52) p. 455; (53) p. 292.

HOP TREE

Other Common Name(s): wafer ash
Botanical Name(s): *Ptelea trifoliata* L. [Fam.: Rutaceae]
Root bark
Constituents: Furoquinoline alkaloids (pteleatine, kokusaginine, skimmianine, dictamnine, etc.), furanocoumarins (isopimpinellin, phellopterin, etc.), lignans (arctigenin-methylether, maculatin), a quinolone derivative, etc.
Properties: Bitter tonic, antipyretic, antispasmodic, antibacterial, antifungal, anthelmintic. Pteleatine and isopimpinellin account for its strong antibacterial and antifungal effects. Isopimpinellin, a linear furanocoumarin, exerts strong phototoxic effect.
Uses: Internally it is used (as a tea, h. p.) for loss of appetite and nonulcer dyspepsia, feverish states, and inflammatory and spastic conditions of the upper respiratory tract (bronchitis, bronchial asthma), biliary tract (nonobstructive gallstones, chronic cholecystitis) and gastrointestinal tract (spastic constipation). Externally it is used (as a mouthwash, gargle) for inflammations of the mouth and throat and (as a wash) for wounds.
Caution: Hop tree should not be taken during pregnancy and lactation. When handling the herb avoid contact with skin and when taking its products avoid exposure to strong sunrays as it may cause phototoxic skin irritations.

References: (3) Vol. 6a, p. 962; (10) p. 277; (25) p. 272; (31) pp. 279, 359; (35) p. 71; (37) p. 1139; (44) p. 452; (48) p. 1043; (51) p. 258; (52) p. 639.

HOPS

Botanical Name(s): *Humulus lupulus* L. [Fam.: Cannabaceae]
Hops (strobiles)
Constituents: Bitter principles (acyl-phloroglucinols: humulone derivatives), resin (with bitter humulones and pro-bitter lupulones), volatile oil (with myrcene, humulene, methylbutenol, etc.), flavonoids (flavonols; flavanones: 8-prenyl-naringenin, which is one of the most potent phytoestrogens; chalcones: xanthohumol, etc.), tannins (proanthocyanidins), etc.
Properties: Sedative, hypnotic, antispasmodic, bitter tonic, aromatic, antibacterial, antifungal, estrogen-like (possibly due to some flavonoids; cf. RED CLOVER; SOY). The sedative effects are due in large part to volatile oil with its constituents (humulene, methylbutenol, etc.), and partly due to bitter priciples. Bitter principles have also shown antibacterial effect.

Uses: Internally it is used (as an h. p., tea; usually combined with other herbs) for nervousness, anxiety, insomnia, minor spastic conditions of the genitourinary tract (irritable urinary bladder with urinary incontinence), primary dysmenorrhea (= painful menstruation without pathology), hyperactive sexual desires, and for loss of appetite and nonulcer dyspepsia, especially when they are associated with nervous tension.

Caution: Alcoholic drinks may interact with hops. A possible combination of hops with sedative, hypnotic and antidepressant drugs should be made only by a health professional. Before using it for dysmenorrhea, the gynecologic problem should be judged by a health professional. Otherwise, there are no reports of contraindications or side effects when used properly.

References: (1) Vol. 5, p. 447; (3) Vol. 5, p. 101; (12) p. 669; (13) p. 413; (14) p. 128; (16) p. 179; (17) p. 356; (19) p. 107; (20) p. 162; (22) p. 160; (23) p. 292; (27) p. 201; (46) p. 893; (47) p. 1794; (48) p. 455; (71) p. 188.

HOREHOUND

Other Common Name(s): white horehound
Botanical Name(s): *Marrubium vulgare* L. [Fam.: Lamiaceae (Labiatae)]
Aerial part
Constituents: Bitter principles (diterpenoid lactones: marrubiin = an artifact of premarrubiin, and premarubiin, etc.), phenolic acids (chlorogenic acid, etc.), flavonoids, a proline-betaine (betonicine), a biogenic amine (choline), volatile oil (traces), etc.

Properties: Aromatic, bitter tonic, choleretic, expectorant (bronchial secretagogue effect), antispasmodic. The mentioned effects are mild and attributed chiefly to marrubiin and related compounds.

Uses: Internally it is used (as a tea, h. p.; usually combined with other herbs) for loss of appetite and nonulcer dyspepsia (with fullness, flatulence) associated with impaired bile secretion and flow and for minor inflammatory and spastic conditions of the upper respiratory tract (spastic bronchitis, tracheitis, laryngitis with hoarseness, bronchial asthma; minor coughs due to thickened bronchial secretion).

Caution: There are no reports of contraindications or side effects when used properly.

References: (1) Vol. 5, p. 778; (3) Vol. 5, p. 703; (8) p. 355; (12) p. 502; (14) p. 218; (17) p. 370; (19) p. 27; (22) p. 122; (28) p. 78; (37) p. 864; (46) p. 921; (47) p. 1841; (48) p. 650.

HOREHOUND, BLACK

Other Common Name(s): fetid horehound
Botanical Name(s): *Ballota nigra* L. [Fam.: Lamiaceae (Labiatae)]
Aerial part
Constituents: Bitter principles (diterpenoid lactones: marrubiin, balloni-

grin, etc.), phenolic acids (chlorogenic acid, etc.), flavonoids, volatile oil (traces; of unpleasant smell), a proline-betaine (stachydrine), a biogenic amine (choline), saponins, etc.

Properties: Sedative, antispasmodic, stomachic, choleretic. The mild sedative effect may be due at least in part to volatile oil (unpleasant smelling!; cf. VALERIAN).

Uses: Internally it is used (as a tea, h. p.; usually combined with other herbs) for minor nervousness and anxiety, loss of appetite and nonulcer dyspepsia (with nausea, cramps, etc.), minor insomnia associated with nervous tension, and minor cases of whooping cough.

Caution: There are no reports of contraindications or side effects when used properly.

References: (1) Vol. 4, p. 454; (3) Vol. 349; (20) p. 164; (36) p. 475; (37) p. 175; (48) p. 650.

HORSE CHESTNUT

Botanical Name(s): *Aesculus hippocastanum* L. [Fam.: Hippocastanaceae]
Seed
Constituents: Cotyledons contain triterpenoid saponins (collectively referred to as aescin = escin: β-aescin, etc., with aglycones protoaescigenin and barringtogenol C), flavonoids (flavonols: quercetin, rutin, etc.), starch, fixed oil, phytosterols, etc. Skin contains coumarins (aesculin, etc.), tannins (oligomeric proanthocyanidins = OPCs), etc.

Properties: Vasotonic (esp. venotonic), diuretic, antiexudative, antiedematous, antioxidant, "vitamin P"-like (= helps in normalizing an increased microvascular permeability and fragility; P = permeability). Most of the effects are attributed to aescin. Flavonols, in synergism with OPCs and aesculin, contribute with their "vitamin P"-like and antioxidant effects.

Uses: Internally it is used (as a standardized product to aescin content) for peripheral venous disorders associated with chronic venous insufficiency (varicose veins in the legs, hemorrhoids), varicose ulcers, and postthrombotic syndrome (= symptoms associated with the presence of a blood clot / thrombus in a blood vessel or heart chamber). Externally it is used (as an ointment prepared with standardized extract or isolated aescin) for hemorrhoids and sprains.

Caution: There are no reports of contraindications or side effects when used properly. In rare cases it may cause stomach upset. It should be used only standardized products to aescin content. A possible combination of horse chestnut products with anticoagulants (warfarin, etc.) and / or platelet aggregation inhibitors (aspirin, etc.) should be made only by a health professional.

References: (1) Vol. 4, p. 110; (3) Vol. 2, p. 1110; (6) pp. 75, 101; (7) p. 140; (12) p. 551; (13) p. 210; (16) pp. 41, 114; (17) p. 305; (19) p. 193; (22) p. 147; (23) p. 199; (26) p. 157; (36) p. 304; (37) p. 28; (46) p. 763; (47) p. 418; (48) p. 694.

HORSE NETTLE

Other Common Name(s): Apple-of-Solomon, Carolina horse nettle, sand brier
Botanical Name(s): *Solanum carolinense* L. [Fam.: Solanaceae]
Fruit (berry)
Constituents: Very limited information is available. It is reported to contain glycosidic steroidal alkaloids (solasonine, solamargine). For berries of a closely related species, bittersweet (*Solanum dulcamara* L.) it is reported that the glycosidic steroidal alkaloids with ripening are dismantled or transformed into saponins.
Properties and Uses: Horse nettle has been chiefly used in traditional medicine. Internally it has been used as a sedative and antispasmodic (tea) for epilepsy. Externally it has been used (as an ointment) for the itch (in cats, dogs).
Caution: As with berries of other wild Solanaceae (Nightshade Family) plants, horse nettle berries are toxic.

References: (1) Vol. 6, p. 736; (3) Vol. 6b, p. 447; (25) p. 182; (35) p. 417; (44) p. 534; (52) p. 734.

HORSERADISH

Botanical Name(s): *Armoracia rusticana* P. Gaertn. et al. = *Armoracia lapathifolia* Gilib. = *Cochlearia armoracia* L. = *Cochlearia rusticana* Lam. [Fam.: Brassicaceae (Cruciferae)]
Root (fresh, dried)
Constituents: Glucosinolates (chiefly sinigrin = allyl-glucosinolate, etc.; mainly in the intact fresh material; cf. MUSTARD), volatile oil (with allyl-isothiocyanate, etc.; mainly in the processed / dried material), vitamin C (rich), amino acids (asparagine, etc.), enzymes, etc.
Properties: Stomachic, diuretic, antispasmodic, antibacterial (B. subtilis, E, coli, S. aureus), antioxidant, rubefacient, counterirritant. Isothiocyanates, which are liberated from glucosinolates, are responsible for the pungent flavor and most of the mentioned effects. See CRESS, GARDEN; MUSTARD.
Uses: Internally it is used (as a tea, h. p.) for loss of appetite and nonulcer dyspepsia (with flatulence, sluggish bowels, minor constipation), minor hepatobiliary disorders (with impaired bile flow), inflammations of the upper respiratory tract (bronchitis, laryngitis, the common cold, etc.; coughs) and genitourinary tract (cystitis, urethritis, prostatitis, leukorrhea), and as an antidyscratic (= blood purifier) for chronic rheumatic complaints. To enhance the effects in problems of the genitourinary tract, the fluid intake (incl. herbal teas) should be more than 2 liters per day. Externally it is used (as a poultice) for inflammations of the upper respiratory tract, rheumatic and neuralgic pains (incl. sciatica), and (as a wet compress, poultice) for headache.

Caution: See CRESS, GARDEN.

References: (1) Vol. 4, p. 339; (3) Vol. 3, p. 213; (6) pp. 116, 188, 189; (8) p. 72; (19) p. 154; (20) p. 168; (27) p. 282; (28) p. 225; (37) p. 128; (46) p. 1200; (51) p. 90.

HORSERADISH TREE

Other Common Name(s): Indian horseradish, moringa
Botanical Name(s): *Moringa oleifera* Lam. [Fam.: Moringaceae]
Root (fresh, dried)
Constituents: Glucosinolates (glucotropaeolin = benzyl-glucosinolate, etc.; mainly in the intact fresh material; cf. CRESS, GARDEN; CRESS, INDI-AN), volatile oil (with benzyl-isothiocyanate, etc.; mainly in the processed / dried material), a biogenic amine (moringine = benzylamine = phenyl-methylamine), phytosterols, enzymes, etc.
Properties: Antibacterial, cardiovascular tonic, rubefacient, counterirritant. Isothiocyanates, which are liberated from glucosinolates, are responsible for the pungent flavor and the mentioned effects, except the sympathomimetic activity. Moringine is sympathomimetic, acting much like tyramine (see CEREUS, NIGHT-BLOOMING) but possibly weaker, and may be responsible for most of the cardiovascular tonic effects.
Uses: <u>Internally</u> it is used (as a tea, h. p.) for inflammations of the gastrointestinal and upper respiratory tracts, feverish states, and (usually combined with other herbs) for minor cardiac and coronary insufficiencies (see CEREUS, NIGHT-BLOOMING). It may be beneficial for minor cases of hypotension (= low blood pressure), and fatigue and feeling of weekness. <u>Externally</u> it is used (as a wash, wet compress) for wounds and skin infections, (as a wet compress, poultice) for rheumatic pains, and (as a mouthwash) for inflammations of the mouth.
Caution: See CRESS, GARDEN; CEREUS, NIGHT-BLOOMING
Seed
Constituents: Glucosinolates (richer than root), moringine, fixed oil, enzymes, etc.
Properties: Antibacterial, rubefacient, counterirritant (stronger than root), and it is claimed to be aphrodisiac.
Uses: <u>Externally</u> it is used for rheumatic and neuralgic pains. <u>Internally</u> it is used (as a tea, h. p.) for inflammations of the gastrointestinal and upper respiratory tracts.
Caution: See CRESS, GARDEN; CEREUS, NIGHT-BLOOMING.
Ben oil (= behen oil, moringa oil)
It is the fixed oil obtained by expression from the seeds.
Constituents: Chiefly glycerides (fatty acids component: chiefly oleic acid, also palmitic and behenic acids, etc.), etc.
Uses: Behen oil is edible oil and is also used in the production of ointments and creams.

References: (1) Vol. 5, p. 852; (3) Vol. 5, p. 893; (5) Vol. 1, p. 728; (32) Vol. 1, p. 142; (37) p. 921; (41) Vols. 1-7; (52) p. 508; (67) p. 192.

HORSETAIL

Other Common Name(s): field horsetail, shave grass, shavetail grass
Botanical Name(s): *Equisetum arvense* L. [Fam.: Equisetaceae]
Aerial part
Constituents: Minerals (free silicic acid, water-soluble silicates, potassium), flavonoids (flavonols, flavones), phenolic acids (caffeic acid derivatives), polyacetylenes (equisetolic acid, etc.), phytosterols, alkaloids (nicotine, etc.; very small amounts), etc., but no saponins.
Properties: Diuretic, wound-healing. The diuretic effect is due in large part to flavonoids. Horsetail has been shown to strengthen connective tissue for which, silicic acid is considered responsible.
Uses: Internally it is used as a flushing-out treatment (= herbal tea or product + liquids: more than 2 liters per day; sometimes combined with a medication) for inflammations of the genitourinary tract (cystitis, etc.), urinary gravel and nonobstructive stones and to prevent relapsing urinary infections / gravel / stones. Due to its silicic acid content, it has been used as an adjuvant for pulmonary tuberculosis. Silicic acid is recommended for inflammatory changes in the connective tissue of joints, muscles, blood vessels, skin and other organs. Horsetail is used as a natural supplement of silicic acid (as water-soluble silicate). Externally it is used (as a wash, wet compress, poultice) for wounds and ulcers and (as a mouthwash, gargle) for inflammations of the mouth and throat.
Caution: There are no reports of contraindications or side effects when used properly. Nevertheless, a flushing-out treatment is contraindicated in cases of obstructive urinary stones, edema due to impaired heart or kidney function and kidney inflammations (here can be used on health professional's advice to enhance the effects of an antimicrobial therapy).

References: (1) Vol. 5, p. 65; (3) Vol. 4, p. 790; (12) p. 81; (13) p. 317; (14) p. 92; (16) p. 165; (17) p. 203; (19) p. 199; (23) p. 257; (27) p. 98; (46) p. 333; (47) p. 1267; (48) p. 340; (51) p. 229; (69) p. 28.

HYDRANGEA

Other Common Name(s): seven barks, wild hydrangea
Botanical Name(s): *Hydrangea arborescens* L. [Fam.: Hydrangeaceae (Saxifragaceae)]
Root (rhizome)
Constituents: Coumarins (hydrangin = umbelliferone, etc.), saponins (possibly triterpenoid s.), stilbenoids (hydrangenol, etc.), carbohydrates (gum, starch, sugars), a quinazoline alkaloid (febrifugine), etc.
Properties: Diuretic. Umbelliferone and hydrangenol have shown antim

icrobial effect. Febrifugine is a known natural antipyretic.

Uses: <u>Internally</u> it is used (usually combined with other herbs) as a flushing-out treatment (= herbal tea or product + liquids: more than 2 liters per day; sometimes combined with a medication) for inflammations of the genitourinary tract (cystitis, urethritis, prostatitis, etc.), urinary gravel and nonobstructive stones and to prevent relapsing urinary infections / gravel / stones.

Caution: Hydrangea should be used only as directed by an experienced practitioner. It should not be taken during pregnancy and lactation. At higher doses than recommended it may cause dizziness and gastrointestinal irritations, among others. A flushing-out treatment is contraindicated in cases of obstructive urinary stones, edema due to impaired heart or kidney function and kidney inflammations (here can be used on health professional's advice to enhance the effects of an antimicrobial therapy).

References: (3) Vol. 5, p. 112; (9) p. 309; (12) p. 949; (15) p. 113; (18) p. 235; (20) p. 169; (31) pp. 274, 365, 513; (36) p. 476; (37) pp. 405, 515; (42) Vol. 6, p. 321); (44) p. 270; (47) p. 1556; (66) p. 300.

HYPOXIS ROOPERI

Other Common Name(s): African potato
Botanical Name(s): *Hypoxis rooperi* T. Moore [Fam.: Hypoxidaceae]
<u>Root</u> (tuberous rhizome)
Constituents: Phytosterols (5-sterols: β-sitosterol, β-sitosterolin = β-sitosterol-glucoside, campesterol, etc.), lignans (hypoxoside = rooperol-glucoside, etc.), carbohydrates (sugars, starch), etc.

Properties: Anti-inflammatory, antiexudativ, cholesterol reducing. Phytosterols obtained from hypoxis rooperi have been shown to inhibit the biosynthesis of prostaglandins and leukotrienes. To this may contribute also lignans. Additionally, hypoxis phytosterols are competitive inhibitors of the absorption of dietary cholesterol, which like them is a 5-sterol. This results in an increased fecal excretion of cholesterol, and then the liver to synthesize biliary acids utilizes the excessive LDL-cholesterol. Lignans have shown liver protective, anti-inflammatory and immunomodulant effects.

Uses: <u>Internally</u> it is used (as an h. p. with extract standardized to sterols) for micturition problems associated with early stages of benign prostatic hyperplasia (= BPH: stages I and II). Rational treatments with Hypoxis extract (standardized to sterols) have resulted in an increase of urine flow, decrease of frequency of urination and decrease of residual urine. It is also used for rheumatic complaints (incl. rheumatoid arthritis) and high cholesterol.

Caution: Hypoxis rooperi products should be standardized to sterols. Before using them for BPH, the prostate problem should be judged by a health professional. Otherwise, there are no reports of contraindications or side effects when used properly.

References: (1) Vol. 5, p. 496; (6) p. 198; (7) p. 256; (8) p. 318; (12) p. 513; (13) p. 414; (19) p. 110; (23) p. 266; (36) p. 52; (48) p. 291; (67) p. 618; (77) p. 160.

HYSSOP

Other Common Name(s): garden hyssop
Botanical Name(s): *Hyssopus officinalis* L. [Fam.: Lamiaceae (Labiatae)]
Aerial part
Constituents: Volatile oil (with isopinocamphone, β-pinene, pinocamphone), Lamiaceae tannins (rosmarinic acid and other caffeic acid derivatives), flavonoids (diosmin, hesperidin), bitter principles (marrubiin, diosmin, ursolic acid), triterpenes (ursolic acid, etc.), etc.
Properties: Expectorant, mild antispasmodic, antibacterial, antifungal, antiviral, anti-inflammatory, "vitamin P"-like, bitter tonic, mild neurocirculatory stimulant. Rosmarinic acid and related caffeic acid derivatives have been shown to inhibit the biosynthesis of prostaglandins and leukotrienes, and to exert choleretic, antibacterial and antiviral effects.
Uses: Internally it is used (as a tea, h. p.) for inflammatory and spastic conditions of the upper respiratory tract (the common cold, bronchitis, laryngitis, tracheitis, bronchial asthma; coughs; also as a diaphoretic hot tea) and gastrointestinal tract (loss of appetite, impaired digestion, flatulence and minor cramps, minor diarrhea, etc.). Hyssop is also used for minor cases of hypotension (= low blood pressure), fatigue and convalescence. Externally it is used (as a gargle) for sore throat with hoarseness, (as a poultice) for bruises, and (as a wash) for minor skin inflammations and wounds. Hyssop is also used in spice and liqueur / liquor industries, and hyssop oil in cosmetics and perfumery.
Caution: There are no reports of contraindications or side effects when used properly. Nevertheless, hyssop is best avoided during pregnancy and lactation. Hyssop oil should not be taken internally.

References: (2) Vol. 2, p. 868; (3) Vol. 5, p. 219; (6) p. 102; (8) p. 319; (9) p. 312; (12) p. 782; (24) p. 363; (27) p. 170; (28) pp. 77, 78; (29) p. 63; (37) pp. 420, 694; (47) p. 1595; (51) p. 168.

INDIAN PIPE

Other Common Name(s): bird's nest, corps plant, fit root
Botanical Name(s): *Monotropa uniflora* L. [Fam.: Monotropaceae (Ericaceae)]
Aerial part, root
Constituents: Not well known and may vary (saprophytic plant!). It is reported to contain phenol glycosides (arbutin, monotropitoside = methyl salicylate glycoside), an iridoid (monotropein), phytosterols, phenolic acids (p-coumaric acid, etc.), triterpenes (ursolic acid, etc.), and andromedotoxin related compounds (reported in 1899).
Properties: Sedative, anticonvulsant, antispasmodic, antibacterial.
Uses: Indian pipe is chiefly used in traditional medicine. Internally it is used (as a tea) for epilepsy and other convulsive states in children, for nervous-

ness, rheumatic complaints (incl. arthritic pains), colds and feverish states, etc.

Caution: Indian pipe may contain the toxic andromedotoxin therefore is not for self-treatment. If andromedotoxin derivatives are absent, there shouldn't be contraindications or side effects when used properly.

References: (3) Vol. 5, p. 887; (18) p. 230; (25) p. 28; (42) Vol. 4, pp. 80, 451, 454; (44) p. 349; (57) p. 541.

INDIGO, WILD

Other Common Name(s): false indigo
Botanical Name(s): *Baptisia tinctoria* (L.) R. Br. [Fam.: Fabaceae (Leguminosae)]
Root
Constituents: Water-soluble polysaccharides, glycoproteins, quinolizidine alkaloids (sparteine, cytisine, etc.), flavonoids (isoflavones: baptisin, etc.), coumarins (scopoletin, etc.), etc.
Properties: Immunomodulant, antipyretic, cholagogue, mild cardioactive (due to alkaloids; see SCOTCH BROOM), and possibly estrogen-like (due to isoflavones; see SOY). The immunomodulating effect is attributed to the water-soluble polysaccharides and glycoproteins. Scopoletin has shown anti-inflammatory, antispasmodic, antibacterial and antifungal effects.
Uses: Internally it is used (as an h. p.; usually combined with other herbs, to enhance the effects of a therapy) to ease and shorten the duration of the common cold and flu and other viral or bacterial infections (often of relapsing nature) of the upper respiratory and genitourinary tracts. Externally it is used (as a mouthwash, gargle) for inflammations of the mouth and throat, (as an ointment) for wounds and ulcers, and (as a vaginal irrigation / sitz bath / wash) for leukorrhea.
Caution: Wild indigo should not be taken during pregnancy and lactation. Due to its cardioactive effect, wild indigo is best used on health professional's advice. As with other immunomodulant herbs, it should be used for a short term (see ECHINACEA). For surer results there are available standardized products to polysaccharides / glycoproteins content. At higher doses than recommended it causes gastrointestinal irritations (with nausea, vomiting, diarrhea), with effects also on the cardiovascular and nervous systems. Otherwise, there are no reports of side effects when used properly.

References: (1) Vol. 4, p. 463; (3) Vol. 3, p. 355; (6) p. 262; (8) p. 95; (12a) p. 648; (13) p. 554; (15) p. 38; (16) p. 193; (29) p. 18; (31) p. 286; (35) p. 432; (37) p. 177; (44) p. 120; (46) p. 127; (47) p. 666.

IPECAC

Other Common Name(s): ipecacuanha; 1) Brazilian / Matto-Grosso / Rio ipecac 2) Cartegena / Costa Rica / Panama ipecac
Botanical Name(s): 1) *Cephaelis ipecacuanha* (Brot.) Tussac 2) *Cephaelis acuminata* H. Karst. [Fam.: Rubiaceae]
Root (rhizome and root)
Constituents: Isoquinoline alkaloids (chiefly emetine and cephaeline, localized chiefly in root-bark), starch, etc. The ratio emetine: cephaeline is higher in the first species than in the second one.
Properties: (At low doses, about $1/5^{th}$ of the emetic doses): Expectorant. (At high doses): Emetic, amebicidal. Emetine exerts more expectorant and less emetic effects compared to cephaeline.
Uses: Internally it is used (as a tea, h. p.; at low doses; combined with other herbs) for coughs associated with chronic inflammations of the upper respiratory tract, and (at higher doses, as Ipecac Syrup) to induce vomiting in cases of intoxications. Emetine, for its amebicidal effect, has been used for the treatment of amebic dysentery.
Caution: To induce vomiting, Ipecac Syrup should not be given to an unconscious intoxicated person, during pregnancy, in cases of peptic ulcers, severe heart problems, etc. In view of this, as an emetic drug Ipecac Syrup should be used only as directed by a health professional. If not vomited it can lead to toxic effects (e. g. cardiac arrhythmias, etc.). In these cases it is recommended to take enough fluids and activated charcoal.

References: (1) Vol. 4, p. 774; (3) Vol. 3, p. 795; (8) p. 135; (11) p. 160; (12) p. 1005; (13) p. 248; (14) p. 133; (17) p. 313; (37) p. 296; (46) p. 739; (48) p. 961.

IVY, ENGLISH

Other Common Name(s): common ivy, ivy
Botanical Name(s): *Hedera helix* L. [Fam.: Araliaceae]
Leaf
Constituents: Triterpenoid saponins (hederasaponin C = hederacoside C, etc.), flavonoids (flavonols: rutin; etc.), polyacetylenes (falcarinol, etc.), phenolic acids (caffeic acid, etc.), coumarins (scopolin, etc.), etc.
Properties: Expectorant (bronchial secretagogue effect), antispasmodic (esp. bronchial active), antibacterial, antifungal, antiexudative, anti-inflammatory. The expectorant effect is due in large part to saponins. Polyacetylenes are considered plant antibiotics. The antispasmodic effect is due to scopolin and flavonoids.
Uses: Internally it is used (as an h. p.) for inflammatory and spastic conditions of the upper respiratory tract (spastic bronchitis, etc.; coughs: spastic dry cough, whooping cough). Externally it is used (as a poultice, wet compress) for boils, wounds, ulcers, and burns.

Caution: Internally, for best results should be used extracts standardized to the antispasmodic effect, and not teas. When applying externally, English ivy products may cause skin allergic reactions, which disappear easily after stopping the application. Otherwise, there are no reports of contraindications or side effects when used properly.

References: (1) Vol. 5, p. 398; (3) Vol. 5, p. 21; (6) p. 101; (8) p. 300; (16) p. 61; (17) p. 280; (19) p. 68; (22) p. 124; (24) p. 111; (27) p. 110; (37) p. 645; (46) p. 503; (47) p. 1512; (48) p. 701.

JABORANDI

Botanical Name(s): *Pilocarpus jaborandi* Holmes; *Pilocarpus microphyllus* Stapf; *Pilocarpus pennatifolius* Lem. [Fam.: Rutaceae]
Leaf
Constituents: Imidazole alkaloids (chiefly pilocarpine), volatile oil, etc. Pilocarpine decomposes very easily and after two years of storage is almost not found in leaves.
Properties: Due to pilocarpine, a parasympathomimetic, it acts as secretagogue (increases secretions of sweat, saliva, bronchi, stomach, tears), increases peristalsis (with vomiting, diarrhea), and caused contractions of the smooth musculature (bronchial, biliary, gastrointestinal, and urinary tracts). When applied locally to the eye, pilocarpine causes miosis (= contraction of the pupil) and a fall in intraocular pressure.
Uses: Jaborandi leaf is used only for the extraction of pilocarpine. Pilocarpine hydrochloride is used (in eyedrops) for the treatment of glaucoma.
Caution: Jaborandi leaf products (tea, tincture) have been used to induce diaphoresis (= profuse sweating) in cases of common cold. Due to its toxicity Jaborandi leaf is no longer used as such.

References: (1) Vol. 6, p. 128; (3) Vol. 6a, p. 658; (8) p. 424; (11) p. 177; (12) p. 1075; (13) p. 274; (37) p. 1078; (47) p. 1641; (48) p. 1046; (49) Vol. 2, p. 302.

JALAP

Other Common Name(s): true jalap
Botanical Name(s): *Ipomoea purga* (Wender.) Hayne = *Exogonium purga* (Wender.) Benth. = *Convolvulus jalapa* Schiede non L. [Fam.: Convolvulaceae]
Jalap (jalap tuber, jalap root), **jalap resin**
Jalap resin is the dried purified extract of the tuber.
Constituents: Jalap root contains resin, glycoretins, free fatty acids, coumarins (scopoletin, etc.), starch, sugars, etc. Jalap resin consists of glycoretins (chiefly convolvulin, some jalapin), which are ester glycosides composed of hydroxy-fatty acids, volatile short chain fatty acids and sugars.
Properties: Drastic purgative (resin is much stronger).

Uses: Internally it is used (as an h. p.; only combined with other herbs) for habitual constipation (cf. SCAMMONY, MEXICAN).

Caution: Jalap should not be taken during pregnancy and lactation and inflammations of the gastrointestinal tract. At higher doses than recommended it causes gastrointestinal irritations (with nausea, cramps, pains).

References: (1) Vol. 5, p. 543; (3) Vol. 4, p. 895; (11a) p. 143; (13) p. 302; (29) p. 64; (36) p. 292; (37) pp. 612, 729; (46) p. 658; (47) p. 1650; (48) p. 180; (66) p. 324.

JALAP, INDIAN

Other Common Name(s): turpeth, St. Thomas lidpod
Botanical Name(s): *Operculina turpethum* (L.) Silva Manso = *Ipomoea turpethum* (L.) R. Br. [Fam.: Convolvulaceae]
Root
Constituents: Its main active constituent is a resin, which consists of glycoretins (chiefly turpethin, some α-turpethin), similar to those contained in jalap.
Properties: Drastic purgative, milder than jalap. See JALAP.
Uses: Internally it is used (as an h. p.; usually combined with other herbs) for constipation. In traditional medicine it is also used for other cases when purgation is sought (intoxications, intestinal worms, etc.).
Caution: Indian jalap should not be taken during pregnancy and lactation and inflammations of the gastrointestinal tract. At higher doses than recommended it causes gastrointestinal irritations (with nausea, vomiting, diarrhea).

References: (1) Vol. 5, p. 948; (3) Vol. 5, p. 268; (13) p. 302; (36) p. 494; (37) pp. 612, 1001; (48) p. 180.

JAMBOLAN

Other Common Name(s): Java plum, jumbul
Botanical Name(s): *Syzygium cumini* (L.) Skeels = *Syzygium jambolana* DC. = *Eugenia jambolana* Lam. [Fam.: Myrtaceae]
Bark
Constituents: Tannins (rich in gallotannins and ellagitannins), an isocoumarin (bergenin), triterpenes, phytosterols (5-sterols: β-sitosterol, etc.), flavonoids, etc.
Properties: Mild antihyperglycemic, astringent, anti-inflammatory. The antihyperglycemic effect may be due to the hydrolysable tannins. The anti-inflammatory effect is due in large part to bergenin, phytosterols and flavonoids.
Uses: Internally it is used as an adjuvant (tea, h. p.) for diabetes and inflammations of the gastrointestinal tract (diarrhea, enteritis, ulcerative coli-

tis). <u>Externally</u> it is used (as a mouthwash, gargle) for inflammations of the mouth and throat and (as a wash, wet compress) for minor skin inflammations, wounds and ulcers.

Caution: There are no reports of contraindications or side effects when used properly.

<u>Seed</u>

Constituents: Tannins (same type as bark), volatile oil, phenolic acids, fixed oil, etc.

Properties: Mild antihyperglycemic, astringent, anti-inflammatory, mild diuretic, mild sedative.

Uses: <u>Internally</u> it is used as an adjuvant (tea, h. p.) for diabetes.

Caution: There are no reports of contraindications or side effects when used properly.

References: (1) Vol. 6. p. 870; (3) Vol. 6b, p. 717; (8) p. 546; (15) p. 204; (19) p. 221; (27) p. 173; (31) p. 541; (36) p. 440; (37) p. 1339; (42) Vol. 5, p. 186; (46) p. 788; (47) p. 2655; (65) p. 66.

JASMINE

Other Common Name(s): poet's jasmine, common jasmine, white jasmine
Botanical Name(s): *Jasminum officinale* L. = *Jasminum grandiflorum* L.; etc. [Fam.: Oleaceae]

<u>Flower</u>

Constituents: It is reported to contain volatile oil (q. v.). As a member of Oleaceae family it possibly contains a phenylethanoid glycoside (acteoside = verbascoside) and bitter principles (iridoids; a triterpene: ursolic acid), among others.

Properties: Antispasmodic, sedative, and it is claimed to be aphrodisiac. Volatile oil may play an important role in the effects. Acteoside has been shown to be anti-inflammatory (by inhibiting the biosynthesis of leukotrienes) and liver protective. Iridoids have shown bitter tonic, choleretic, liver protective, laxative, diuretic, anti-inflammatory, antimicrobial, immunomodulant and antitumoral effects, among others.

Uses: Jasmine flower is chiefly used in traditional medicine. <u>Internally</u> it is used (as a tea, h. p.) for inflammatory and spastic conditions of the hepatobiliary tract (incl. chronic hepatitis), gastrointestinal tract (minor spastic states) and upper respiratory tract (spastic bronchitis, etc.), and for low sexual drive. <u>Externally</u> it is used (as a liniment) for rheumatic pains.

Caution: There are no reports of contraindications or side effects when used properly.

<u>Jasmine oil</u>, <u>jasmine absolute</u>

Jasmine oil is the volatile oil obtained by steam distillation from fresh flowers. Jasmine absolute is the waxy residue obtained after removing the alcohol from an alcoholic extract of jasmine flowers.

Constituents: Depending on the origin, jasmine oil and jasmine absolute

208

contain chiefly benzyl acetate and linalyl acetate, also benzyl alcohol, linalool, jasmolone, etc. Absolute contains also benzoic acid and fatty acids.

Properties and Uses: Oil and absolute are chiefly used as fragrance ingredients in cosmetics and perfumery and as flavor ingredients in food industry. Jasmine oil is used in aromatherapy for its relaxing effects.

Caution: There are no reports of skin-irritating effect.

References: (3) Vol. 5, p. 309; (9) p. 319; (18) p. 257; (41) Vols. 1-7; (42) Vol. 5, pp. 240, 241; (52) p. 406; (87) Vol. 2, p. 151.

JAVA TEA

Other Common Name(s): orthosiphon

Botanical Name(s): *Orthosiphon aristatus* (Blume) Miq. = *Orthosiphon stamineus* Benth. = *Orthosiphon spicatus* Backer [Fam.: Lamiaceae (Labiatae)]

Leaf (Java tea)

Constituents: Volatile oil (with β-caryophyllene, α-humulene, etc.), minerals (rich in potassium), flavonoids (methoxy-flavones: sinensetin, etc.), triterpenoid saponins, Lamiaceae tannins (rosmarinic acid and other caffeic acid derivatives), diterpenes (orthosiphols A-E), etc.

Properties: Diuretic, anti-inflammatory, mild antispasmodic, cholagogue, antimicrobial. The diuretic effect is due in large part to the high potassium content, enhanced by flavonoids, saponins and volatile oil. The antispasmodic effect is due to flavonoids and volatile oil. Rosmarinic acid and related caffeic acid derivatives have been shown to inhibit the biosynthesis of prostaglandins and leukotrienes, and to exert choleretic, antibacterial and antiviral effects. To the antimicrobial effect may contribute volatile oil.

Uses: Internally it is used as a flushing-out treatment (= herbal tea or product + liquids: more than 2 liters per day; sometimes combined with a medication) for inflammations of the genitourinary tract (cystitis, urethritis, etc.), urinary gravel and nonobstructive stones, to prevent relapsing urinary infections / gravel / stones, and as an antidyscratic (= blood purifier; tea, h. p.) and anti-inflammatory for chronic rheumatic complaints. Orthosiphon extract may be combined with a potassium depleting diuretic (e. g. hydrochlorthiazide) as it may enhance the effect, enable a decrease of doses of the diuretic drug, and supplement a part of the depleted potassium.

Caution: There are no reports of contraindications or side effects when used properly. Nevertheless, a flushing-out treatment is contraindicated in cases of obstructive urinary stones, edema due to impaired heart or kidney function and kidney inflammations (here can be used on health professional's advice to enhance the effects of an antimicrobial therapy). A combination with diuretic drugs should be made only by a health professional.

References: (1) Vol. 5, p. 966; (3) Vol. 6a, p. 338; (6) p. 184; (8) p. 395; (12) p. 782; (13) p. 104; (16) p. 163; (17) p. 413; (19) p. 167; (23) p. 249; (37) p. 1009; (46) p. 1050; (47) p. 2043; (48) p. 250.

JIMSON WEED

Other Common Name(s): stramonium, thorn apple
Botanical Name(s): *Datura stramonium* L. [Fam.: Solanaceae]
Leaf
Constituents: Tropane alkaloids: chiefly (−)-hyosciamine and (−)-scopolamine = hyoscine, also some atropine = (±)-hyosciamine; flavonoids (flavonols); coumarins (scopoletin, etc.); tannins, etc.. Compared to belladonna, it contains higher proportions of scopolamine (cf. BELLADONNA).
Properties: Due to the parasympatholytic activity of hyosciamine / atropine and scopolamine, jimson weed exerts antispasmodic and antisecretory effects, among others. Scopolamine is a CNS depressant and as it is contained in higher ratio than in belladonna, jimsonweed exerts also sedative effect. See HENBANE; BELLADONNA.
Uses: Internally it is sometimes used (usually in a standardized combination product) for spastic conditions of the upper respiratory tract (spastic bronchitis, bronchial asthma, laryngitis) and more seldom for those of the gastrointestinal tract.
Caution: Jimson weed is toxic. Smoking of asthma cigarettes that contain jimson weed today is discouraged. This is due also to the difficulty of calculating the alkaloids per smoke. The abusive smoking of jimson weed seeds has resulted in severe intoxications, even death.

References: (1) Vol. 4, p. 1142; (3) Vol. 4, p. 449; (8) p. 217; (11) p. 152; (12a) p. 513; (13a) p. 186; (14) p. 209; (22) p. 112; (31) p. 721; (36) p. 349; (44) p. 194; (46) p. 1526; (48) p. 811; (51) p. 182.

JOE PYE

Other Common Name(s): queen-of-the-meadow, sweet-scented Joe Pye weed
Botanical Name(s): *Eupatorium purpureum* L. [Fam.: Asteraceae (Compositae)]
Root (gravel root)
Constituents: Triterpenoid saponins, bitter principles (sesquiterpene lactones), a benzofuran (euparin), volatile oil, possibly polyacetylenes, etc.
Properties: Diuretic, bitter tonic. The diuretic effect may be due at least in part to saponins and flavonoids. Its bitter tonic effect is due in large part to sesquiterpene lactones. Benzofurans and polyacetylenes (if present) have shown antifungal and antibacterial effects.
Uses: Internally it is chiefly used as a flushing-out treatment (= herbal tea or product + liquids: more than 2 liters per day; sometimes combined with a medication) for inflammations of the genitourinary tract (cystitis, urethritis, prostatitis, etc.), urinary gravel and nonobstructive stones, to prevent relapsing urinary infections / gravel / stones, and as an antidyscratic (= blood purifier; tea, h. p.) for chronic rheumatic complaints.

Caution: There are no reports of contraindications or side effects when used properly. Nevertheless, gravel root is best avoided during pregnancy and lactation. A flushing-out treatment is contraindicated in cases of obstructive urinary stones, edema due to impaired heart or kidney function and kidney inflammations (here can be used on health professional's advice to enhance the effects of an antimicrobial therapy). There are no reports that it contains unsaturated pyrrolizidine alkaloids (= UPAs). Nevertheless, manufacturers should evaluate them. For dosage limits of UPAs see COLTSFOOT. It may cause allergic contact dermatitis to persons hypersensitive to other Asteraceae plants (e. g. arnica, chamomile, feverfew, ragweed, tansy, yarrow) that contain sesquiterpene lactones.

References: (3) Vol. 4, p. 872; (15) p. 87; (18) p. 284; (20) p. 153; (31) p. 338; (35) p. 374; (41) Vols. 1-7; (42) Vol. 3, pp. 453, 487; (44) p. 230; (45) p. 206; (82) p. 87.

JOJOBA

Other Common Name(s): jojoba bush, jojove
Botanical Name(s): *Simmondsia chinensis* (Link) C. K. Schneid. = *Simmondsia californica* Nutt. [Fam.: Simmondsiaceae (Buxaceae)]
Jojoba oil (= jojoba liquid wax)
It is the fixed oil obtained by cold expression from the ripe seeds.
Constituents: A mixture of esters of fatty acids (straight chain fatty acids; monounsaturated fatty acids: eicosenoic, docosenoic acids, etc.) with alcohols (chiefly eicosenol and docosenol).
Properties: Emollient.
Uses: Jojoba oil is an important ingredient in a number of creams and other skincare products. In traditional medicine jojoba oil is used as an emollient for skin problems (common acne = acne vulgaris, psoriasis, etc.). Through hydrogenation jojoba oil yields a waxy material of similar qualities to spermaceti, for which is widely used as a substitute in the manufacture of creams, lipsticks and other cosmetic products.
Caution: Jojoba oil should not be taken internally as it is non-digestible.

References: (1) Vol. 6, p. 699; (7) p. 296; (8) p. 522; (9) p. 322; (11) p. 76; (12) p. 292; (37) p. 1271; (48) p. 168.

JUBA'S BUSH

Botanical Name(s): *Iresine diffusa* Humb. et Bonpl. ex Willd. = *Iresine celosia* L. = *Iresine celosioides* L. = *Achyranthes calea* Ibañez [Fam.: Amaranthaceae]
Aerial part
Constituents: Bitter principles (sesquiterpene lactones: iresin, etc., non-allergenic), *n*-hexacosanol (= ceryl alcohol), phytosterols (5-sterols: β-sitosterol, etc.), flavonoids (an isoflavone: tlatlancuayin, etc.), etc.

Properties: Bitter tonic, antipyretic, diuretic.

Uses: Internally it is used (as a tea, h. p.) for feverish states and the common cold, also as a diaphoretic hot tea.

Caution: There are no reports of contraindications or side effects when used properly. Amaranthaceae plants are considered rich in soluble oxalates (large amounts are toxic!). In view of this, manufacturers should evaluate their presence in juba's bush.

References: (1) Vol. 5, p. 550; (3) Vol. 5, p. 273; (5) Vol. 3, p. 302; (18) p. 140; (41) Vols. 1-7; (42) Vol. 3, p. 86; (44) p. 277; (52) p. 399; (57) p. 432.

JUJUBE

Other Common Name(s): Chinese date, Chinese jujube, jujube date

Botanical Name(s): *Ziziphus jujuba* Mill. = *Ziziphus vulgaris* Lam. [Fam.: Rhamnaceae]

Fruit (ripe)

Constituents: Vitamin C, organic acids (malic and tartaric acids), invert sugar, mucilage, tannins, flavonoids (flavonols), coumarins, triterpenoids (saponins; betulinic, oleanolic and ursolic acids, etc.), cyclic AMP (reported to be rich), carotenoids, minerals (potassium, magnesium), phytosterols, etc.

Properties: Nutrient, demulcent, emollient, expectorant, liver protective, tonic, anti-inflammatory, antispasmodic, antibacterial. Cyclic AMP, a second messenger, participates in the activity of vital hormones (epinephrine, vasopressine, ACTH) and has been shown to inhibit platelet aggregation.

Uses: Internally it is used (as a tea, h. p.) for minor fatigue, loss of appetite, and as an adjuvant for minor inflammatory and spastic conditions of the upper respiratory and gastrointestinal tracts. Externally it is used as an ingredient in skin-care products and (as a gargle) for sore throat.

Caution: There are no reports of contraindications or side effects when used properly.

References: (3) Vol. 6c, p. 576; (9) p. 324; (37) p. 1501; (45) p. 281; (48) p. 1068; (49) Vol. 2, p. 333; (67) p. 623; (87) Vol. 1, p. 287.

JUNIPER

Other Common Name(s): common juniper

Botanical Name(s): *Juniperus communis* L. [Fam.: Cupressaceae]

Fruit (berry)

Constituents: Volatile oil (with α- and β-pinene, also terpinen-4-ol, etc.), invert sugar (rich), tannins (proanthocyanidins), flavonoids, organic acids, pectin, resin, etc.

Properties: Aromatic, diuretic, antibacterial, digestive stimulant, carminative, antispasmodic (gastrointestinal and bronchial active), expectorant. For the strong diuretic effect responsible is considered terpinen-4-ol. Responsi-

212

ble for the irritating effect to the kidneys are considered terpenoid hydrocarbons (pinenes, etc.), and not terpinen-4-ol.

Uses: Internally it is used (usually combined with other herbs) as a flushing-out treatment (= herbal tea or product + liquids: more than 2 liters per day; sometimes combined with a medication) for inflammations of the genitourinary tract (cystitis, etc.), urinary gravel and nonobstructive stones, to prevent relapsing urinary infections / gravel / stones, (as a tea, h. p.) for loss of appetite and nonulcer dyspepsia (with flatulence, etc.) and light inflammatory and spastic conditions of the upper respiratory tract (bronchitis, the common cold, etc.; coughs). Juniper is extensively used in spice and liquor industries. Externally it is used (as a mouthwash, chewing) for bad breath.

Caution: Juniper should not be taken during pregnancy. Overdosing may cause kidney damage (with proteinuria, hematuria), particularly if pinenes in the essential oil are contained in very high ratio to terpinen-4-ol. A flushing-out treatment is contraindicated in cases of obstructive urinary stones, edema due to impaired heart or kidney function and kidney inflammations (here can be used on health professional's advice to enhance the effects of an antimicrobial therapy).

References: (1) Vol. 5, p. 565; (3) Vol. 5, p. 333; (8) p. 328; (9) p. 325; (12) p. 711; (16) p. 166; (17) p. 322; (19) p. 236; (20) p. 176; (22) p. 93; (23) p. 253; (27) p. 153; (36) p. 270; (37) p. 741; (46) p. 662; (47) p. 1671; (48) p. 587.

KAVA

Other Common Name(s): awa, kava kava, kava pepper, yangona
Botanical Name(s): *Piper methysticum* G. Forst. [Fam.: Piperaceae]
Root (rhizome)
Constituents: Kavapyrones (= kavalactones: kawain, dihydrokawain, methysticin, dihydromethysticin, etc.), flavonoids (chalcones: flavokavins A, B, etc.), minerals, starch, etc. Kavapyrones are α-pyrone derivatives.
Properties: Standardized special extract of kava has shown anxiolytic (= relieves anxiety), mild sedative, muscle relaxant, antispasmodic, analgesic, local anesthetic and diuretic effects. Its main active constituents are considered the mentioned kavapyrones. Their mechanism of action is complex, but similar to benzodiazepines (e. g. Valium), possibly by exerting GABA-mimetic activity (increasing binding affinity of GABA to its receptors). Compared to benzodiazepines kava doesn't interfere with the concentration and cognitive function unless taken at high doses (sedative-hypnotic effect!), and there haven't been seen dependence or withdrawal problems.
Uses: Internally it is used (as an h. p. with standardized special extract) for anxiety, nervousness, impaired concentration, insomnia, nervous cardiac disorders (esp. tachycardia = rapid heartbeat) and depressive mood, mostly associated with stress, for nervous menopausal complaints (anxiety, emotional instability, depressive mood, insomnia), primary dysmenorrhea

213

(= painful menstruation without pathology), and for irritable urinary passages (associated with pyelitis, ureteritis, cystitis, urethritis), urinary incontinence and childhood enuresis.

Caution: It should not be taken during pregnancy, lactation and in endogenous depression. In rare cases it may cause stomach upset, skin allergic reactions and headache. Kava products should be standardized to kavapyrones. Unless advised by a health professional, kava should not be taken for more than 2 months, after which should be done a liver test. Alcoholic drinks may interact with kava. A combination of kava with sedative, hypnotic and antidepressant drugs should be made only by a health professional.

References: (1) Vol. 6, p. 201; (3) Vol. 6a, p. 708; (6) p. 312; (7) p. 71; (8) p. 438; (9) p. 330; (12) pp. 867, 1205; (13) p. 414; (16) p. 185; (19) p. 125; (22) p. 157; (23) p. 309; (26) p. 171; (37) p. 1085; (47) p. 2142; (48) p. 304.

KELP

Under kelp shall be included those brown algae (Class Phaeophyceae), which are used in the production of alginic acid and alginates. Among seaweeds there are used giant kelp, kelp: *Macrocystis pyrifera* (L.) C. Agardh [Fam.: Lessoniaceae]; and horsetail kelp, kelp, seawand, tangle: *Laminaria digitata* (Huds.) J.V. Lamour. [Fam.: Laminariaceae]. Among rockweeds there are used knotted wrack, kelp: *Ascophyllum nodosum* Le Jol.; and other species [Fam.: Fucaceae].

Alginic acid and alginates
Alginic acid is a polysaccharide, a polymer of D-mannuronic and L-guluronic acids, extracted from seaweeds and some rockweeds, then converted to water-soluble salts (esp. sodium alginate, also potassium alginate, ammonium alginate) or water insoluble calcium alginate.

Properties and Uses: Alginates are used in pharmaceutical and food industries as thickening and gelling ingredients in washable creams, ice creams and jellies, as suspending and emulsifying ingredients in emulsions and suspensions, and as binding and disintegrating ingredients in tablets and lozenges, exerting at the same time demulcent effect.

Caution: There are no reports of contraindications or side effects when used properly.

References: (1) Vol. 4, p. 393, Vol. 5, p. 740; (5) Vol. 2, pp. 13, 26, 40; (9) p. 16; (11) p. 43; (12) p. 380; (13) p. 362; (48) p. 47; (49) Vol. 1, p. 355.

KHAT

Other Common Name(s): kat, Abyssinian tea, Arabian tea
Botanical Name(s): *Catha edulis* (Vahl) Forssk. ex Endl. = *Celastrus edulis* Vahl [Fam.: Celastraceae]
Leaf

214

Constituents: Alkaloids, which are collectively referred to as khatamines. In fresh leaf is chiefly found cathinone (= α-aminopropiophenone), while in the dried and fully developed leaf is chiefly found (+)-nor-pseudoephedrine (= cathine), also some norephedrine, etc. It also contains tannins (condensed t.), flavonoids, and volatile oil.

Properties: Amphetamine-like, i. e. indirect-acting sympathomimetic, stimulant of the central nervous system, appetite suppressant, etc. Among khatamines, cathinone exerts stronger effects.

Uses: Khat is not used in medicine. In countries of cultivation, fresh leaves are chewed as a CNS stimulant to "frighten" fatigue, hunger and sleep, and for rhinitis and asthma, among others.

Caution: As with amphetamine, among side effects are dry mouth, tachycardia, elevated blood pressure, etc., and is developed tolerance and dependence. As with ephedra or ma huang (see EPHEDRA), khat should not be combined with caffeine or caffeine rich herbs / drinks (coffee, guaraná, tea, mate, cola, etc.) because it may result in a risky overstimulation of the nervous system.

References: (1) Vol. 4, p. 730; (3) Vol. 3, p. 770; (8) p. 125; (11a) p. 243; (12) p. 1095; (13) p. 272; (36) p. 366; (37) p. 286; (48) p. 883; (49) Vol. 2, p. 320; (81) p. 324.

KHELLA

Other Common Name(s): lesser bishop's weed, large bullwort, toothpick ammi, visnaga

Botanical Name(s): *Ammi visnaga* (L.) Lam. [Fam.: Apiaceae (Umbelliferae)]

Fruit (commonly called seed)

Constituents: Furanochromones (= γ-pyrones: khellin, khellol, khellol-glucoside, visnagin), pyranocoumarin esters (= visnagans: visnadin, samidin, etc.), flavonoids, volatile oil (with terpinen-4-ol, etc.), fixed oil, etc.

Properties: Smooth muscle relaxant (coronary, bronchial, urinary, gastrointestinal and biliary active), diuretic.

Uses: Internally it is used (usually the isolated active constituents or standardized extracts, usually as a combination product) for minor cases of angina pectoris (= chest pain due to insufficient blood supply to the heart), and for spastic conditions of the upper respiratory, urinary, gastrointestinal and biliary tracts.

Caution: It may cause skin allergic reactions. Khella products should be standardized to γ-pyrones, expressed as khellin. At higher doses than recommended it may cause nausea, loss of appetite, headache and dizziness, among others. Otherwise, there are no reports of contraindications or side effects when used properly.

References: (3) Vol. 3, p. 27; (6) pp. 44, 110, 190, 193; (8) p. 47; (12) p. 805; (13) p. 326; (17) p. 58; (19) p. 26; (23) p. 164; (37) p. 67; (46) p. 60; (47) p. 498; (48) p. 271; (49) Vol. 2, p. 465.

KINO, EUCALYPTUS

Botanical Name(s): *Eucalyptus rostrata* Schlecht; *Eucalyptus camaldulensis* Dehn.; etc. [Fam.: Myrtaceae]

Kino (eucalyptus kino, red gum)

It is the dried juice obtained by incisions made to the inner bark.

Constituents: Tannins (very rich in proanthocyanidins, collectively referred to as kino-tannic acid), small amounts of catechol (= pyrocatechol), gum, volatile oil (with citronellal, etc.), etc.

Properties: Astringent. Its astringent effect is very strong but weaker than Malabar kino as it contains almost half the amount of kino-tannic acid.

Uses: Externally it is used (as a mouthwash, gargle) for inflammations of the mouth and throat, and (as a mouthwash, paint) for gingivitis (= inflammation of the gums), denture sores and canker sores. Internally it is used (as a tea, powder, h. p.) for diarrhea. The same indications mentioned under Malabar kino (see KINO TREE, INDIAN) may apply to eucalyptus kino.

Caution: As with Malabar kino, both very rich in tannins, internally should be used in moderate amounts only. At higher doses than recommended it causes gastrointestinal irritations (with nausea, vomiting) and constipation.

References: (5) Vol. 1, p. 477; (10) p. 111; (35) p. 289; (49) Vol. 2, p. 442; (52) p. 293.

KINO TREE, INDIAN

Other Common Name(s): Indian padauk, Malabar kino, Vengai padauk

Botanical Name(s): *Pterocarpus marsupium* Roxb. [Fam.: Fabaceae (Papilionaceae)]

Wood

Constituents: Flavonoids (flavones, isoflavones, and chalcones such as isoliquiritigenin), stilbenoids (a resveratrol derivative), benzofurans (marsupin, carpusin), triterpenes (oleanolic acid, etc.), 2-propanol derivatives (propterol, etc.), etc.

Properties: Mild antihyperglycemic, antimicrobial, antioxidant, anti-inflammatory.**Uses:** Internally it is used as an adjuvant (tea, h. p.) for diabetes, and for minor inflammations of the gastrointestinal tract (diarrhea, etc.).

Caution: There are no reports of contraindications or side effects when used properly.

Kino (Malabar kino, East Indian kino, Cochin kino, black kino gum)

It is the dried juice obtained by incisions made to the inner bark.

Constituents: Tannins (very rich in proanthocyanidins, collectively referred to as kino-tannin or kino-tannic acid) and small amounts of free catechol (= pyrocatechol = pyrocatechin) and gallic acid.

Properties: Astringent (very strong).

Uses: Externally it is used (mouthwash, gargle) for inflammations of the mouth and throat, and (as a mouthwash, paint) for gingivitis (= inflammation of the gums), denture sores and canker sores. <u>Internally</u> it is used for diarrhea. Malabar kino is chiefly used in tanning industry.

Caution: It is a very strong astringent therefore when used internally it should be taken in moderate amounts (as recommended) and diluted, otherwise it may cause gastrointestinal irritations (with nausea, vomiting, constipation).

References: (2) Vol. 3, p. 414; (12) p. 835; (36) pp. 230, 439; (37) p. 1140; (41) Vols. 1-7; (55) p. 129; (66) p. 327.

KNOTWEED

Other Common Name(s): common knotgrass, erect knotgrass, prostrate knotweed
Botanical Name(s): *Polygonum aviculare* L. [Fam.: Polygonaceae]
Aerial part
Constituents: Flavonoids (chiefly flavonols: avicularin and other quercetin glycosides, etc.; also flavones), minerals (silicic acid: chiefly free, partly water-soluble), tannins (hydrolyzable and condensed t.), phenolic acids (caffeic and chlorogenic acids), coumarins (umbelliferone, scopoletin), mucilaginous polysaccharides, etc.
Properties: Anti-inflammatory, astringent, demulcent, diuretic. The effects are mild. Knotweed has also shown ACE-inhibitory (cf. LESPEDEZA) and platelet aggregation inhibitory effects, due in large part to flavonoids and tannins.
Uses: <u>Internally</u> it is used (as a tea, h. p.; usually combined with other herbs) for minor inflammations (also when minor hemorrhages are present, but on health professional's advice) of the upper respiratory tract (bronchitis, etc.), gastrointestinal tract (diarrhea, ulcerative colitis, etc., incl. hemorrhoids) and genitourinary tract (cystitis, etc., gravel, nonobstructive urinary stones). To enhance the effects in problems of the genitourinary tract, the fluid intake (incl. herbal teas) should be more than 2 liters per day. Due to its silicic acid content, it has been used as an adjuvant for pulmonary tuberculosis. Silicic acid is recommended for inflammatory changes in the connective tissue of joints, muscles, blood vessels, skin and other organs. <u>Externally</u> it is used (as a poultice) for wounds, (as a mouthwash, gargle) for inflammations of the mouth and throat, and (as a paint, mouthwash) for gingivitis (= inflammations of the gums).
Caution: For cases of minor hemorrhages it should be used on health professional's advice. Otherwise, there are no reports of contraindications or side effects when used properly.

References: (1) Vol. 6, p. 246; (3) Vol. 6a, p. 813; (6) pp. 184, 314; (8) p. 452; (17) p. 452; (19) p. 236; (27) p. 85; (37) p. 1103; (47) p. 2192; (51) p. 66; (69) p. 28.

KOUSSO

Other Common Name(s): brayera
Botanical Name(s): *Hagenia abyssinica* (Bruce) Gmelin = *Brayera anthelmintica* Kunth ex Brayer [Fam.: Rosaceae]
Flower (female flower)
Constituents: Phloroglucinol derivatives (acyl-phloroglucinols: α-kosin, protokosin, kosidin, etc.), tannins (possibly of condensed type), gum, resin and volatile oil.
Properties: Taeniafuge. Fresh flower is more active, because the effects decrease on drying and storage.
Uses: Internally it is still used (esp. the isolated α-kosin, combined with a saline purgative) for tapeworm infestations.
Caution: Kousso is a toxic herb. It should be used only as directed by a health professional. An absolute contraindication of kousso is pregnancy, and is best avoided in cases of heart and kidney problems.

References: (2) Vol. 2, p. 830; (3) Vol. 5, p. 4; (8) p. 294; (37) p. 635; (41) Vols. 1-7; (47) p. 1693; (49) Vol. 2, p. 423; (66) p. 261.

KUDZU

Botanical Name(s): *Pueraria montana* (Lour.) Merr. var. *lobata* (Willd.) Maesen et S.M. Almeida = *Pueraria lobata* (Willd.) Ohwi [Fam.: Fabaceae (Leguminosae)]
Root
Constituents: Flavonoids (rich in isoflavones: puerarin = daidzein-8-*C*-glucoside, daidzin = daidzein-7-*O*-glucoside, etc.), coumestans (= coumarono-coumarins: coumestrol, puerarol, etc.), coumarins (scoparone, etc.), phytosterols (possibly of miroestrol type), starch (rich), etc.
Properties: Peripheral vasodilatory, antispasmodic, antihypertensive, antiarrhythmic, antioxidant, liver protective, estrogenic, disulfiram-like (= antabuse-like: causes hangover even with small amounts of alcohol, by inhibiting the two steps of enzymatic degradation of alcohol to acetate). Most of the effects are due to daidzein and its glycosides (puerarin, daidzin) and scoparone. Coumestans have shown liver protective effect. Coumestrol exerts estrogen-like effect (stronger than genistein, much stronger than daidzein and formononetin; cf. ALFALFA; RED CLOVER; SOY).
Uses: Internally it is used (as a tea, h. p.) to prevent or alleviate angina pectoris (= chest pain due to insufficient blood supply to the heart) and cardiac arrhythmias (= altered rhythm of the heartbeat), and minor cases of hypertension. Products standardized to isoflavones and coumestrol may be used to alleviate menopausal syndrome, and to prevent postmenopausal problems (osteoporosis, breast and uterine cancer, etc.) and prostate cancer. It may also be helpful for chronic hepatitis, alcoholism, intermittent claudication (=

pain / cramp / weakness in the legs on walking), and Raynaud's disease (= pale or red-blue patchy fingers).

Caution: There are no reports of contraindications or side effects when used properly. For cautions of estrogen-like / phytoestrogenic products see SOY.

References: (3) Vol. 6a, p. 970; (5) Vol. 2, p. 888; (9) p. 333; (31) pp. 363, 419, 430; (41) Vols. 1-7; (45) p. 256; (50) pp. 5, 305; (67) p. 80; (68) p. 135.

LABRADOR TEA, MARSH

Other Common Name(s): wild rosemary
Botanical Name(s): *Ledum palustre* L. ssp. *decumbens* (Aiton) Hultén [Fam.: Ericaceae]
Aerial part
Constituents: Volatile oil (with ledol = ledum camphor, alloaromadendrene, cumin alcohol, carvacrol, thymol, etc.), flavonoids (flavonols, flavones), coumarins (palustroside, etc.), a phenol glycoside (arbutin), tannins (condensed t.), etc.
Properties: Anti-inflammatory (by inhibiting the biosynthesis of prostaglandins and possibly leukotrienes), antibacterial (against *Mycobacterium tuberculosis*), antifungal (against *Candida* spp., etc.), expectorant, diuretic, counterirritant.
Uses: Internally it is used (as an h. p. with the extract, as a tea) for inflammations of the upper respiratory tract (bronchitis, etc., bronchial asthma; coughs: due to thickened bronchial secretion, whooping cough; as an adjuvant for pulmonary tuberculosis), genitourinary tract (cystitis, etc.), and gastrointestinal tract (diarrhea), and as an anti-inflammatory and antidyscratic (= blood purifier) for atopic eczema (= chronic eczema of internal origin) and chronic rheumatic complaints. To enhance the effects in problems of the genitourinary tract, the fluid intake (incl. herbal teas) should be more than 2 liters per day. Externally it is used (as a poultice) for rheumatic pains, insect bites and bruises.
Caution: It should not be taken during pregnancy and lactation. At higher doses than recommended it causes gastrointestinal irritations (with nausea, vomiting), violent headache and symptoms of narcotic effects, much like Marsh Tea Beer of Vikings. Otherwise, there are no reports of contraindications or side effects when used properly.

References: (3) Vol. 5, p. 479; (6) pp. 107, 235; (8) p. 339; (13) p. 416; (23) p. 403; (35) p. 460; (37) p. 818; (47) p. 1727; (51) p. 268; (52) p. 435.

LADY'S MANTLE

Other Common Name(s): common lady's mantle, lion's foot
Botanical Name(s): *Alchemilla xanthochlora* Rothm. = *Alchemilla vulgaris* auct. [Fam.: Rosaceae]

219

Aerial part
Constituents: Tannins (ellagitannins, gallotannins), flavonoids (flavonols, leucoanthocyanidins), bitter principles, etc. The reported bitter principles possibly are triterpenes (oleanolic and ursolic acids).
Properties: Astringent, hemostatic, antispasmodic, wound-healing, bitter tonic, diuretic.
Uses: Internally it is used (as a tea, h. p.) for menorrhagia / hypermenorrhea (= prolonged / heavy menstruation), primary dysmenorrhea, metrorrhagia (= nonmenstrual uterine bleeding), for inflammations of the gastrointestinal tract (diarrhea, ulcerative colitis, etc., incl. hemorrhoids; also when minor hemorrhages are present, but on professional's advice) and genitourinary tract (leukorrhea). Externally it is used (as a wet compress, poultice) for wounds and ulcers, (as a vaginal irrigation / sitz bath / wash) for leukorrhea, and (as a mouthwash, gargle) for inflammations of the mouth and throat.
Caution: There are no reports of contraindications or side effects when used properly. Nevertheless, before using it for gynecologic disorders, the problem should be judged by a health professional.

References: (1) Vol. 4, p. 162; (3) Vol. 2, p. 1163; (6) pp. 306, 315; (8) p. 32; (15) p. 27; (17) p. 42; (18) p. 168; (19) p. 85; (23) p. 377; (27) p. 25; (37) p. 36; (47) p. 455; (51) p. 102.

LADY'S SLIPPER

Other Common Name(s): large yellow lady's slipper
Botanical Name(s): *Cypripedium parviflorum* Salisb. var. *pubescens* (Willd.) Knight = *Cypripedium calceolus* L. var. *pubescens* (Willd.) Correll = *Cypripedium pubescens* Willd. [Fam.: Orchidaceae]
Root (rhizome)
Constituents: It is reported to contain volatile oil, resin, tannins (hydrolyzable t.), carbohydrates and a glycoside. It is also reported to contain cypripedin, a benzo-naphthoquinone, which is considered responsible for the contact dermatitis caused by the leaves of lady's slipper.
Properties: It is reported to exert sedative and antispasmodic effects due to which it has been designated as "American valerian".
Uses: Internally it has been used (as a tea, h. p.) for nervousness, anxiety, insomnia, epilepsy, neuralgic pains and nervous headaches.
Caution: Based on the fact that in traditional medicine lady's slipper is usedas an anthelmintic, analgesic, strong sedative, and that it has shown hallucinogenic effects, it possibly contains potentially active constituents. Some plants of Orchidaceae family are known for the presence of alkaloids (indolizidine, indole, pyrrolidine and pyrrolizidine types), which exert their effects through nervous system. In view of this, it should not be used during pregnancy and lactation, and it is best used as directed by an experienced practitioner. As with other strong sedative herbs, it may interact with alcoholic drinks as well as sedative, hypnotic and antidepressant drugs.

References: (1) Vol. 4, p. 1122; (3) Vol. 4, p. 424; (15) p. 75; (18) p. 312; (20) p. 178; (31) p. 496; (36) p. 53; (37) p. 381; (42) Vol. 2, p. 387; (44) p. 191; (47) p. 1163; (66) p. 261.

LARKSPUR, FORKING

Other Common Name(s): field larkspur
Botanical Name(s): *Consolida regalis* Gray = *Delphinium consolida* L. [Fam.: Ranunculaceae]
Flower
Constituents: Flavonoids, chiefly as anthocyanins (delphinin* = delphinidin-glucoside: blue color; etc.), also flavonols (quercetin and kaempferol glycosides). Diterpenoid alkaloids of aconitine type are not found in flower but only in other aerial parts (esp. seed) and root. *) Delphinin is an anthocyanin and is not to be confused with delphinine, which is a diterpenoid alkaloid.
Properties: Mild diuretic, due in large part to flavonols.
Uses: It is used almost exclusively to improve the appearance of herbal teas and some food products. In traditional medicine it is chiefly used (as a tea) for its mild diuretic effect.
Caution: There are no reports of contraindications or side effects when used properly. Other parts of forking larkspur (root, seed, aerial part) contain diterpenoid alkaloids, which are very toxic. In view of this, manufacturers should determine the presence of other parts and evaluate alkaloids.

References: (2) Vol. 2, p. 418; (3) Vol. 4, p. 483; (8) p. 220; (17) p. 163; (35) p. 464; (37) p. 391; (41) Vols. 1-7.

LAVENDER

Other Common Name(s): true lavender
Botanical Name(s): *Lavandula angustifolia* Mill. = *Lavandula officinalis* Chaix. = *Lavandula vera* DC. [Fam.: Lamiaceae (Labiatae)]
Flower
Constituents: Volatile oil (see Lavender oil), Lamiaceae tannins (rosmarinic acid and other caffeic acid derivatives), coumarins (umbelliferone, herniarin), flavonoids, triterpenes (ursolic acid, etc.), etc.
Properties: Aromatic, sedative, choleretic, cholagogue, carminative, rubefacient, antimicrobial. Volatile oil accounts for most of the effects. The hepatobiliary effects are due in large part to caffeic acid derivatives.
Uses: Internally it is used (as a tea, h. p.) for minor cases of nervousness, insomnia, headache, depressive mood, and gastrointestinal complaints (irritable stomach, upper abdominal pains, flatulence, intestinal cramps). Externally it is used (as a full / partial bath) for rheumatic and neuralgic pains and (as a wash, wet compress) for minor wounds.
Caution: There are no reports of contraindications or side effects when used

properly.

Lavender oil

It is the volatile oil obtained by steam distillation from fresh flowering tops.

Constituents: Linalyl acetate and free linalool, also small amounts of 1,8-cineole, terpinen-4-ol, cymene, limonene, etc.

Properties: Aromatic, rubefacient, counterirritant, antimicrobial, mild sedative, antispasmodic.

Uses: Lavender oil is an important ingredient in perfumery and cosmetics. Externally it is used (as a liniment, partial / full bath) for rheumatic and neuralgic pains and (as a liniment, ointment) for headaches. Internally it is used (a few drops on sugar) for impaired digestion, gastrointestinal cramps, minor insomnia, and for inflammations of the upper respiratory tract (bronchitis, colds, etc.).

Caution: In rare cases it may cause contact allergic reactions. Otherwise, there are no reports of contraindications or side effects when used properly.

Lavandin oil

It is obtained from lavandin or Dutch lavender: *Lavandula* × *intermedia* Emeric ex Loisel., which is a hybrid of true lavender (*L. angustifolia* Mill.) with spike lavender (*L. latifolia* Medic.).

Constituents, Properties, Uses: Compared to the true lavender, besides linalyl acetate and linalool, it contains higher amounts of cineole and camphor. Lavandin oil is extensively used in perfumery and cosmetics.

Caution: There are no reports of contraindications or side effects when used properly.

References: (1) Vol. 5, p. 630; (3) Vol. 5, p. 464; (6) pp. 214, 215, 361; (8) p. 338; (13) p. 107; (15) p. 128; (16) p. 181; (17) p. 335; (19) p. 138; (23) p. 298; (27) p. 183; (35) p. 467; (37) p. 812; (47) p. 2721; (48) p. 528; (51) p. 274.

LEMON

Botanical Name(s): *Citrus* × *limon* (L.) Osbeck [Fam.: Rutaceae]

Peel

Constituents: Volatile oil (see Lemon oil), bitter principles (flavanones), flavonoids (bitter tasting flavanone neohesperidosides: neohesperidin, naringin; a tasteless flavanone glycoside: hesperidin), pectin, carotenoids, furanocoumarins (bergamottin, etc.), etc.

Properties: Aromatic, mild bitter tonic, antioxidant, "vitamin P"-like (= helps in normalizing an increased microvascular permeability and fragility).

Uses: Lemon peel is chiefly used as a flavor ingredient. Internally it is used (as a tea, h.p.; in combination products) for loss of appetite and nonulcer dyspepsia. Flavonoids (= bioflavonoids) isolated from the lemon peel are used (in combination products) for different disorders associated with an increased microvascular permeability and fragility (cardiovascular / cerebrovascular / ophthalmologic disorders).

Caution: There are no reports of contraindications or side effects when used properly.

Lemon oil

It is the volatile oil obtained by expression from the fresh peels, without the aid of heat.

Constituents: Chiefly limonene, also citral, β-pinene, γ-terpinene, furano-coumarins (bergamottin, etc.), etc.

Properties: Aromatic, carminative, tonic.

Uses: Lemon oil is used as a flavor ingredient, and it is beneficial due to its carminative and mild tonic effects.

Caution: When handling the oil avoid contact with skin, as it may cause phototoxic skin irritations, especially if exposed to strong sunrays. Otherwise, there are no reports of contraindications or side effects when used properly.

References: (3) Vol. 4, p. 93; (11a) p. 122; (17) p. 156; (29) p. 33; (37) p. 337; (46) p. 828.

LEMONGRASS

Other Common Name(s): 1) West Indian lemongrass 2) Java citronella
Botanical Name(s): 1) *Cymbopogon citratus* (DC. ex Nees) Stapf 2) *Cymbopogon winterianus* Jowitt [Fam.: Poaceae (Gramineae)]

Leaf

Constituents: Volatile oil (see Lemongrass oil), triterpenes, phytosterols, flavonoids, etc.

Properties: Aromatic, analgesic, antipyretic, sedative, antimicrobial, antioxidant.

Uses: Internally it is used (as a tea, h. p.) for spastic conditions of the gastrointestinal tract, as a diaphoretic hot tea for the common cold and feverish states, and for mild anxiety. It is also used as a flavor ingredient in herbal teas. Externally it is used (as a partial bath) for rheumatic pains.

Caution: It should not be taken during pregnancy and lactation. Otherwise, there are no reports of contraindications or side effects when used properly.

Lemongrass oil, citronella oil

It is the volatile oil obtained by steam distillation from the leaves.

Constituents: Citral a (= geranial), citral b (= neral), geraniol, citronellal, citronellol, etc., in different ratio, depending on species and chemical type.

Properties: Rubefacient, mild counterirritant.

Uses: Externally it is used (as a partial / full bath) for rheumatic pains, and as an insect-repellent spray. It is an important fragrance ingredient in cosmetics and perfumery.

Caution: It should not be taken internally. External applications have resulted to be non-irritating to the skin. **References:** (1) Vol. 4, p. 1110; (3) Vol. 4, p. 409; (9) p. 344; (13) p. 104; (37) p. 380; (41) Vols. 1-7; (52) p. 237.

LESPEDEZA

Other Common Name(s): round-head lespedeza
Botanical Name(s): *Lespedeza capitata* Michx. [Fam.: Fabaceae (Leguminosae)]
Leaf, aerial part (leafy stem)
Constituents: Flavonoids (chiefly flavone-C-glycosides: esp. lespecapitoside = iso-orientin = homoorientin = luteolin-6-C-glucoside, etc.; flavonols: kaempferol and quercetin glycosides), tannins (oligomeric proanthocyanidins = OPCs), hydrocarbons (hentriacontane, etc.), etc.
Properties: Diuretic, anti-inflammatory, mild antihypertensive, anti-uremic, cholesterol reducing, antioxidant. The diuretic effect is due in large part to flavonoids. Lespedeza OPCs have been shown to be ACE (= angiotensin-converting enzyme) inhibitors and may account in large part for its mild antihypertensive effect and the potentiation of diuretic effect.
Uses: Internally it is used as an adjuvant (h. p.) for impaired kidney function and benign nephrosclerosis, with oliguria, anuria and chronic uremia. It is also used for minor cases of high cholesterol and as a preventive for arteriosclerosis. Due to its ACE-inhibitory effect it may be beneficial for minor cases of hypertension, considering the other possible active constituents are absent (see Caution).
Caution: There are no reports of contraindications or side effects when used properly. At higher doses than recommended it may cause gastrointestinal irritations (with nausea, diarrhea). As the indications are serious conditions, it should be used on health professional's advice. Lespedeza products should be standardized to flavonoids. Manufacturers should evaluate alkaloids, biogenic amines (tryptamine derivatives), cyanogenic glycosides and lectins, especially if leaves / leafy stems contain other parts of the plant.

References: (3) Vol. 5, p. 491; (6) pp. 184, 185; (8) p. 341; (12a) p. 400; (13) p. 416; (18) p. 177; (23) p. 252; (32) Vol. 1, p. 175, Vol. 3, p. 1637; (37) p. 821; (41) Vols. 1-7; (49) Vol. 2, p. 377; (72) nr. 81168.

LETTUCE, WILD

Botanical Name(s): *Lactuca virosa* L. [Fam.: Asteraceae (Compositae)]
Lactucarium (lettuce opium)
It is the dried milky juice collected after cutting off the stems during the flowering period.
Constituents: Bitter principles (sesquiterpene lactones: lactucin, lactucopicrin; cf. CHICORY), triterpenes (taraxasterol = α-lactucerol: esterified and free; etc.), phytosterols, plant organic acids, etc.
Properties and Uses: It is claimed to be sedative and analgesic.
Caution: The above claimed effects remain doubtful and for this reason wild lettuce is obsolete.

References: (2) Vol. 3, p. 21; (3) Vol. 5, p. 432; (21) p. 237; (36) p. 476; (37) p. 806; (46) p. 805; (47) p. 1699; (48) p. 633.

LICORICE

Other Common Name(s): Russian / Spanish / Turkish licorice
Botanical Name(s): *Glycyrrhiza glabra* L. = *Glycyrrhiza glandulifera* Walst. et Kit. [Fam.: Fabaceae (Leguminosae)]
Root
Constituents: Triterpenoid saponins (collectively referred to as glycyrrhizin: a mixture of potassium and calcium salts of glycyrrhizic acid; glycyrrhizic acid = a glycyrrhetic acid glycoside), flavonoids (flavanones: liquiritin, liquiritigenin, etc.; chalcones: isoliquiritigenin; isoflavones: formononetin, etc.; etc.), polysaccharides, sugars, phytosterols, coumarins, etc.
Properties: Anti-inflammatory (corticosteroid-like effect), antiulcer (= prevents or helps in healing peptic ulcers), antispasmodic, expectorant (bronchial secretagogue effect), demulcent, liver protective, antioxidant, antibacterial (against *Staphylococcus aureus*, *Mycobacterium tuberculosis*, *Helicobacter pylori*, etc.), antiviral, antifungal (against *Candida albicans*). The effects are due in large part to glycyrrhizin and flavonoids. Glycyrrhizin has been shown to inhibit the dismantling of steroids and the biosynthesis of inflammatory prostaglandins and leukotrienes. Glycyrrhizin is about 50 times sweeter than sucrose. Licorice flavonoids play an important role in the effects (anti-ulcer, antispasmodic, antioxidant, etc.).
Uses: Internally it is used (as a tea, h. p.; often combined with other herbs, etc.) for inflammations of the upper respiratory tract (bronchitis, tracheitis, pharyngitis, laryngitis with hoarseness, etc.; coughs due to thickened bronchial secretion; bronchial asthma) and gastrointestinal tract (gastritis, incl. peptic ulcers; with impaired digestion, heartburn, upper abdominal pain, flatulence, minor constipation), and for fatigue, atopic eczema (= chronic eczema of internal origin) and rheumatic complaints (incl. rheumatoid arthritis). Licorice is widely used as a flavor ingredient in food and pharmaceutical industries.
Caution: Licorice should not be taken during pregnancy, in severe liver and kidney disorders, excessive potassium depletion (often caused by certain diuretics such as hydrochlorthiazide) and in hypertension. Doses higher than recommended when taken for prolonged periods cause water retention, edema, potassium depletion and hypertension. In view of this, unless advised and monitored by a health professional, licorice should not be taken for more than 4-6 weeks. The mentioned contraindications and side effects are due to glycyrrhizin and do not pertain to the almost glycyrrhizin-free products, rich in licorice flavonoids.

References: (1) Vol. 5, p. 312; (3) Vol. 4, p. 1160; (6) p. 138; (7) pp. 174, 203; (8) p. 287; (9) p. 346; (11) p. 55; (12) p. 542; (13) p. 212; (14) p. 145; (16) p. 63; (17) p. 301; (36) p. 305; (46) p. 840; (47) p. 1776; (48) p. 688; (59) p. 183.

225

LILY-OF-THE-VALLEY

Other Common Name(s): Mayflower, May-lily
Botanical Name(s): *Convallaria majalis* L. [Fam.: Asparagaceae; formerly, Convallariaceae (Liliaceae)]

Aerial part

Constituents: Cardiac glycosides (convallatoxin = k-strophanthidin rhamnoside, convallatoxol = strophanthidol rhamnoside, etc.), steroidal saponins, flavonoids, etc.

Properties: Lily-of-the-valley exerts strophanthus-like and digitalis-like effect, and is diuretic. Convallatoxin, one of the strongest cardiac glycosides, is eliminated very fast therefore does not cumulate. See DIGITALIS; STROPHANTHUS.

Uses: Internally it is used for early stages of heart failure (stages I and II, according to NYHA), chronic cor pulmonale (= heart hypertrophy and minor failure due to chronic pulmonary disorders), age-related cardiac insufficiency (presbycardia = senile heart), also when minor edemas are present.

Caution: Lily-of-the-valley is toxic and not for self-treatment. It is used only as directed by health professionals. Its products should be standardized to the cardiac glycosides content. See DIGITALIS.

References: (1) Vol. 4, p. 977; (3) Vol. 4, p. 270; (8) p. 187; (12) p. 595; (13) p. 188; (16) p. 97; (19) p. 149; (23) p. 168; (37) p. 359; (46) p. 382; (48) p. 746.

LIME

Other Common Name(s): key lime
Botanical Name(s): *Citrus* × *aurantifolia* (Christm.) Swingle [Fam.: Rutaceae]

Lime oil

It is the volatile oil obtained by steam distillation from the fresh peels.

Constituents: Chiefly limonene, also citral, α- and β-pinene, α-terpineol, bergamotene, sabinene, bisabolene, etc. If the oil is produced by expression, it will contain phototoxic furanocoumarins (bergamottin, isoimperatorin, bergaptene, etc.).

Properties: Aromatic.

Uses: Lime oil is used as a fragrance ingredient in cosmetics and perfumery and as a flavor ingredient in liqueur / liquor industry. It is preferred the rectified oil, with an improved lemon lime aroma and which doesn't contain the phototoxic furanocoumarins.

Caution: Lime oil obtained by steam distillation and rectified is not a skin irritant. Lime oil obtained by expression may cause phototoxic skin irritations, particularly if the skin is then exposed to strong sunrays.

References: (3) Vol. 4, p. 96; (9) p. 352; (37) p. 337; (41) Vols. 1-7.

LINDEN

Other Common Name(s): 1) large-leaf linden, summer linden, tilia 2) small-leaf lime tree, winter linden 3) European linden, European lime tree, tilia, which is the hybrid of the mentioned two species.
Botanical Name(s): 1) *Tilia platyphyllos* Scop. 2) *Tilia cordata* Mill. 3) *Tilia × vulgaris* Hayne = *Tilia europaea* L. [Fam.: Tiliaceae]
Flower (flowers with bract)
Constituents: Flavonoids (chiefly flavonols: quercetin glycosides, such as tiliroside, quercitrin, etc.; etc.), mucilaginous polysaccharides, tannins (condensed t.), volatile oil (with linalool, 1,8-cineole, eugenol, etc.), phenolic acids (caffeic acid, etc.), phytosterols (5-sterols: β-sitosterol, etc.), etc.
Properties: Demulcent, anti-inflammatory, expectorant, sedative (GABA-mimetic effect), astringent, antispasmodic, diuretic, antimicrobial. All the mentioned effects are mild.
Uses: Internally it is used (as a tea, h. p.) for inflammations of the upper respiratory tract (bronchitis, etc.; coughs; esp. as a diaphoretic hot tea for the common cold and feverish states), gastrointestinal tract (gastritis, minor cramps, etc.) and genitourinary tract (cystitis, etc.). It is also used (usually combined with other herbs) for minor cases of nervousness and insomnia.
Caution: There are no reports of contraindications or side effects when used properly.

References: (2) Vol. 3, p. 657; (3) Vol. 6c, p. 180; (6) p. 324; (8) p. 561; (12) p. 857; (13) p. 313; (14) p. 142; (17) p. 581; (19) p. 143; (24) p. 221; (27) p. 328; (35) p. 485; (46) p. 1606; (47) p. 2710; (48) p. 113.

LINGONBERRY

Other Common Name(s): cowberry, foxberry, northern mountain cranberry
Botanical Name(s): *Vaccinium vitis-idaea* L. [Fam.: Ericaceae]
Leaf
Constituents: Phenol glycosides (chiefly arbutin, also salidroside), some free hydroquinone, tannins (chiefly hydrolyzable t.), flavonoids, triterpenes, minerals (rich in manganese).
Properties: Urinary antiseptic, due to hydroquinone liberated from arbutin (= hydroquinone-glucoside; see UVA-URSI). Compared to uva-ursi, it contains less arbutin but also the constipating tannins are in lower concentrations.
Uses: Internally it is used (as a tea, h. p.) for inflammations of the genitourinary tract (cystitis, urethritis, prostatitis, pyelonephritis). To enhance the effects, urine should be slightly alkaline (this can be done by consuming a diet rich in vegetables and / or taking about a teaspoonful / day of baking soda) and the fluid intake (incl. herbal teas) should be more than 2 liters per day.

Caution: See UVA-URSI.

References: (1) Vol. 6, p. 1062; (3) Vol. 6c, p. 372; (6) p. 188; (8) p. 575; (13) p. 304; (19) p. 182; (28) p. 165; (37) p. 1433; (46) p. 959.

LIPPIA, MEXICAN

Other Common Name(s): hierba dulce, rough fogfruit
Botanical Name(s): *Phyla scaberrima* (Juss.) Moldenke = *Lippia dulcis* Trevir [Fam.: Verbenaceae]
Leaf
Constituents: Volatile oil, with camphor as its chief constituent, also hernandulcin (a sweet tasting sesquiterpene). It possibly contains flavonoids and bitter principles (iridoids), but no alkaloids.
Properties: Antitussive (possibly indirect cough suppressant effect), antispasmodic, stomachic, emmenagogue, antibacterial. Mexican lippia has a pleasant aromatic bittersweet taste. Hernandulcin is about 1,000 times sweater than sucrose.
Uses: Internally it is used (as a tea, h. p.) for minor inflammatory and spastic conditions of the upper respiratory tract (bronchitis, bronchial asthma; spastic and irritating coughs, whooping cough), gastrointestinal tract (with cramps), and for secondary amenorrhea and oligomenorrhea (= ceased / infrequent / scanty menstruation without pathology).
Caution: Due to its high camphor content, which acts upon the CNS, it should not be used in infants, and strong teas should be avoided. Before using it for gynecologic disorders, the problem should be judged by a health professional. Otherwise, there are no reports of contraindications or side effects when used properly.

References: (1) Vol. 5, p. 687; (3) Vol. 5, p. 526; (10) p. 172; (18) p. 259; (31) p. 588; (52) p. 589; (57) p. 480.

LIVERWORT

Other Common Name(s): American liverleaf, American liverwort
Botanical Name(s): *Hepatica nobilis* Schreber = *Anemone hepatica* L. [Fam.: Ranunculaceae]
Aerial part
Constituents: (Dried herb): anemonin (= protoanemonin dimer); (fresh herb): protoanemonin (an unstable compound); and (fresh or dried): tannins, flavonoids, saponins, etc.
Properties: (Dried herb): Antimicrobial, antispasmodic, diuretic. (Fresh herb): Counterirritant / vesicant (depending on concentration), analgesic. Anemonin is non-toxic and has shown antimicrobial effect. Protoanemonin is toxic and a strong local irritant (cf. PULSATILLA).

Uses: <u>Internally</u> it is used (only dried!; as a tea, h. p.) for inflammatory and spastic conditions of the hepatobiliary, upper respiratory and genitourinary tracts. To enhance the effects in problems of the genitourinary tract, the fluid intake (incl. herbal teas) should be more than 2 liters per day. <u>Externally</u> it is used (as a poultice, liniment: fresh herb) for rheumatic pains, (as a wash: dried herb) for bacterial and fungal skin infections.

Caution: Internally should be used only dried herb and as directed by an experienced practitioner. Even dried, liverwort should not be taken during pregnancy as it may still contain protoanemonin (teratogenic, abortifacient!; cf. PULSATILLA). Fresh herb should be handled with care (see Properties), even when used externally. If taken internally, fresh herb (also dried herb at higher doses than recommended) causes strong gastrointestinal irritations (with vomiting, diarrhea), etc.

References: (1) Vol. 5, p. 428; (3) Vol. 5, p. 49; (24) p. 213; (35) p. 493; (37) p. 650, 1133; (47) p. 1537; (48) p. 747; (51) p. 76.

LOBELIA

Other Common Name(s): Indian tobacco, puke weed
Botanical Name(s): *Lobelia inflata* L. [Fam.: Campanulaceae (Lobeliaceae)]
<u>Aerial part</u> (leaves and tops)
Constituents: Piperidine alkaloids (chiefly lobeline, also lobelanine, lobelanidine, isolobinine, norlobelanine, norlobelanidine, etc.), chelidonic acid, resin, volatile oil, etc.
Properties: (At low doses): Respiratory stimulant, antispasmodic, expectorant. (At high doses): Emetic. Lobeline exerts milder but similar effects to nicotine.
Uses: <u>Internally</u> it is used (as an h. p.) for spastic conditions particularly of the upper respiratory tract (spastic bronchitis, bronchial asthma, etc.), but also gastrointestinal tract. As lobeline resembles nicotine in effects, it has been used as a supportive aid to quit smoking but due to the side effects (stomach discomfort, nausea, vomiting, cardiovascular disturbances) and as there are other alternatives, it is no longer recommended.
Caution: It should not be taken during pregnancy and lactation. Lobelia products should be standardized to lobeline and used on health professional's advice. At higher doses than recommended it causes nausea, vomiting and tachycardia (= rapid heart beat). Toxic doses cause respiratory depression and death.

References: (2) Vol. 3, p. 96; (3) Vol. 5, p. 551; (11) p. 148; (13) p. 275; (14) p. 149; (15) p. 134; (20) p. 187; (46) p. 867; (47) p. 1782; (48) p. 859; (65) p. 352; (66) p. 332.

LOCUST, BLACK

Other Common Name(s): false acacia
Botanical Name(s): *Robinia pseudoacacia* L. [Fam.: Fabaceae (Leguminosae)]

Flower

Constituents: Flavonoids (robinin = a kaempferol glycoside, also acaciin = an acacetin glycoside), volatile oil (with farnesol, nerol, linalool, etc.), phytosterols (5-sterols: β-sitosterol, etc.), etc.

Properties: Aromatic, antispasmodic, cholagogue, diuretic. Robinin has shown antibacterial and strong diuretic effects.

Uses: Internally it is used (as a tea, h. p.; usually combined with other herbs) for minor inflammatory and spastic conditions of the genitourinary tract (cystitis, urethritis, prostatitis, gravel, nonobstructive urinary stones), upper respiratory tract (the common cold, etc., also as a diaphoretic hot tea) and gastrointestinal tract (gastritis, heartburn, belching) associated with minor hepatobiliary disorders (impaired bile flow). To enhance the effects in the inflammatory problems of the genitourinary tract, the fluid intake (incl. herbal teas) should be more than 2 liters per day. It is also an ingredient in aromatic waters used in the production of sorbet, among others.

Caution: There are no reports of contraindications or side effects when used properly. At higher doses than recommended it causes gastrointestinal irritations (with nausea, vomiting, diarrhea). Manufacturers should evaluate cardiac glycosides as there have been reports of their presence.

References: (3) Vol. 6b, p. 153; (5) Vol. 1, p. 935; (6) p. 183; (13) p. 320; (31) p. 410; (37) p. 1194; (41) Vols. 1-7; (47) p. 2330; (51) p. 256.

LOGWOOD

Other Common Name(s): bloodwood, campeachy wood, campeche
Botanical Name(s): *Haematoxylum campechianum* L. [Fam.: Caesalpiniaceae (Leguminosae)]

Logwood

It is the dried heartwood chips, which have not undergone fermentation before drying.

Constituents: Tannins (rich in hydrolyzable t.), phenolic compounds (chiefly hematoxylin: chiefly free, partly glycosidic; also hematein), volatile oil, etc.

Properties: Astringent, antimicrobial. Hematoxylin has shown antibacterial and platelet aggregation inhibitory effects. Hematoxylin is colorless, but under the influence of light and especially enzymes is oxidized to hematein of red color.

Uses: Internally it is used (as a tea, h. p.) for inflammations of the gastrointestinal tract (diarrhea, ulcerative colitis, etc.; also when minor hemorrhages are present, but on professional's advice). <u>Externally</u> has been used (as a vaginal irrigation) for leukorrhea. Hematoxylin is used in the practice of microscopy for staining the cell nuclei. It is also used as a dye for silk products and in the manufacture of inks.

Caution: There are no reports of contraindications or side effects when the unfermented material is used properly. Due to the presence of small amounts of hematein, logwood colors the stools and urine red. As with other herbs rich in tannins, at higher doses than recommended it causes gastrointestinal irritations (with nausea, vomiting) and constipation.

References: (2) Vol. 2, p. 827; (3) Vol. 1, p. 558; (5) Vol. 1, p. 558; (35) p. 496; (37) pp. 631, 632; (66) p. 297.

LOOSESTRIFE, PURPLE

Other Common Name(s): spiked loosestrife, striped loosestrife, red sally
Botanical Name(s): *Lythrum salicaria* L. [Fam.: Lythraceae]
Aerial part
Constituents: Tannins (rich in gallotannins), mucilaginous polysaccharides, pectin, flavonoids (flavones: vitexin = apigenin-8-C-glucoside, etc.; anthocyanins), phenolic acids, a biogenic amine (choline), phytosterols, etc.
Properties: Astringent, anti-inflammatory, antioxidant, antibacterial, antidiarrheal, demulcent, emollient, hemostatic, wound-healing.
Uses: <u>Internally</u> it is used (as a tea, h. p.) for minor inflammatory conditions of the gastrointestinal tract (diarrhea, ulcerative colitis, hemorrhoids; also when minor hemorrhages are present). <u>Externally</u> it is used (as a vaginal irrigation / sitz bath / wash) for leukorrhea and vulvovaginitis, (as a mouthwash, gargle, paint) for inflammations of the mouth and throat, and (as a wash, wet compress, poultice) for eczema, wounds and varicose ulcers.
Caution: There are no reports of contraindications or side effects when used properly. For minor hemorrhages use it only on health professional's advice.

References: (3) Vol. 5, p. 618; (27) p. 298; (28) p. 175; (35) p. 496; (46) p. 1393; (47) p. 1815; (49) Vol. 2, p. 452; (51) p. 122; (87) Vol. 1, p. 244.

LOUSEWORT, CANADIAN

Other Common Name(s): betony
Botanical Name(s): *Pedicularis canadensis* L. [Fam.: Scrophulariaceae]
Root
Constituents: No reports are available. In *Pedicularis* spp. have been found iridoids (aucubin, etc.), saponins, tannins and monoterpenoid alkaloids (pedicularine, boschniakine, etc.), among others.
Properties: Bitter tonic, expectorant, diuretic, astringent. Iridoids have shown bitter tonic, choleretic, liver protective, laxative, diuretic, anti-inflammatory, antibacterial, antiviral, antifungal, immunomodulant and antitu-

moral effects, among others. Saponins are known for their expectorant and diuretic effects, while tannins are astringent.

Uses: Canadian lousewort is chiefly used in traditional medicine. <u>Internally</u> it is used (as a tea) for inflammations of the gastrointestinal tract (with impaired digestion, stomachache, diarrhea, etc.) and respiratory tract (pharyngitis, bronchitis, etc.; coughs). <u>Externally</u> it is used (as a poultice) for swellings and (as a wash, wet compress) for minor skin inflammations.

Caution: It should not be taken during pregnancy and lactation. At higher doses than recommended it may cause gastrointestinal irritations (with nausea, vomiting, diarrhea). The fact that it may contain alkaloids and that in traditional medicine it is also used as an emetic, abortifacient and for heart problems, suggests for caution and to be used as directed by an experienced practitioner.

References: (3) Vol. 6a, p. 488; (18) p. 255; (25) p. 106; (31) p. 572; (36) p. 49; (41) Vols. 1-7; (44) p. 380; (52) p. 572; (57) p. 593.

LOVAGE

Other Common Name(s): American lovage
Botanical Name(s): *Levisticum officinale* Koch [Fam.: Apiaceae (Umbelliferae)]
<u>Root</u>
Constituents: Alkyl-phthalides (ligustilide, etc.), volatile oil (with alkyl-phthalides, also pinenes, etc.), coumarins (coumarin, umbelliferone), furanocoumarins (psoralene, bergaptene), organic acids (ferulic and benzoic acids, etc.), polyacetylenes (falcarinol, etc.), phytosterols (5-sterols: β-sitosterol, etc.), sugars, etc.

Properties: Diuretic, antispasmodic, stomachic, carminative, antibacterial, emmenagogue. Volatile oil and its constituents (ligustilide, etc.) play an important role in the effects. Ligustilide has shown β-sympathomimetic activity (in earlier reports: parasympatholytic), which may account at least in part for the antispasmodic effect.

Uses: <u>Internally</u> it is used as a flushing-out treatment (= herbal tea or product + liquids: more than 2 liters per day; sometimes combined with a medication) for inflammations of the genitourinary tract (cystitis, etc.), urinary gravel and nonobstructive stones, to prevent relapsing urinary infections / gravel / stones, (as a tea, h. p.) for loss of appetite and nonulcer dyspepsia (with fullness, burping, heartburn, minor upper abdominal pains), inflammations of the upper respiratory tract (bronchitis, etc.; coughs), and primary dysmenorrhea (= painful menstruation without pathology). Lovage is an ingredient in some bitter liqueurs.

Caution: Lovage should not be taken during pregnancy and lactation. Before using it for dysmenorrhea, the gynecologic problem should be judged by a health professional. A flushing-out treatment is contraindicated in cases

of obstructive urinary stones, edema due to impaired heart or kidney function and kidney inflammations (here can be used on health professional's
advice to enhance the effects of an antimicrobial therapy). When handling
the herb avoid contact with skin, and when taking its products avoid exposure to strong sunrays as it may cause phototoxic skin irritations.

References: (1) Vol. 5, p. 664; (3) Vol. 5, p. 497; (6) p. 183; (8) p. 342; (9) p. 357; (13) p. 328; (15) p.
130; (16) p. 162; (17) p. 340; (19) p. 142; (22) p. 94; (23) p. 255; (29) p. 69; (37) p. 823; (41) Vols.1-7;
(42) Vol. 6, pp. 564, 584, 611.

LOVAGE, CHINESE

Botanical Name(s): *Ligusticum sinense* Oliv. [Fam.: Apiaceae (Umbelliferae)]
Root (rhizome)
Constituents: Alkyl-phthalides (cnidilide, neocnidilide, senkyunolides,
etc.), volatile oil (with alkyl-phthalides, also monoterpenes, etc.), phenolic
acids (ferulic acid, etc.), polyacetylenes, phytosterols, etc.
Properties: Anti-inflammatory, analgesic, antipyretic, sedative, antifungal
(against *Tinea* spp., and other dermatophytes).
Uses: Internally it is used (as a tea, h. p.) for arthritic, abdominal and menstrual pains, headaches, and the common cold. Externally it is used (as a
wash) for athlete's foot (= Tinea pedis) and other skin fungal infections.
Caution: There are no reports of contraindications or side effects when used
properly.

References: (9) p. 539; (29) p. 70; (36) p. 507; (41) Vols. 1-7; (42) Vol. 6; (52) p. 444.

LOVAGE, SICHUAN

Other Common Name(s): chuanxiong
Botanical Name(s): *Ligusticum chuanxiong* Hort. = *Ligusticum wallichii*
auct. sin. non Franch. [Fam.: Apiaceae (Umbelliferae)]
Root (rhizome)
In commerce it is found under the name of chuan xiong.
Constituents: Alkyl-phthalides (monomers: senkyunolides, etc.; dimers;
etc.), alkaloids (tetramethylpyrazine, etc.), purine bases (adenine, etc.), volatile oil (with alkyl-phthalides, etc.), phenolic acids (ferulic acid, etc.), polyacetylenes, etc.
Properties: Antispasmodic, peripheral vasodilatory, antihypertensive, platelet aggregation inhibitory, antimicrobial, sedative.
Uses: Internally it is used (as an h. p.) for cerebrovascular disease (= a complex condition associated with changes in the brain blood flow), coronary
heart disease (= a condition associated with decreased blood supply to the
heart), to prevent or alleviate angina pectoris (= chest pain due to insufficient blood supply to the heart), and bronchial asthma. Chuan xiong may

be helpful for intermittent claudication (= pain / cramp / weakness in the legs on walking) and Raynaud's disease (= pale or red-blue patchy fingers). **Caution:** Unless advised by a health professional, Chuan xiong should not be taken during pregnancy and lactation. A possible combination with anticoagulants (warfarin, etc.) and / or platelet aggregation inhibitors (aspirin, etc.) should be made only by a health professional. Otherwise, there are no reports of contraindications or side effects when used properly.

References: (9) p. 552; (13) p. 432; (29) p. 70; (41) Vols. 1-7; (42) Vol. 6, p. 563.

LUNGWORT

Other Common Name(s): common lungwort
Botanical Name(s): *Pulmonaria officinalis* L. [Fam.: Boraginaceae]
Aerial part
Constituents: Mucilaginous polysaccharides, minerals (silicic acid, iron, manganese, copper), flavonoids (flavonols), allantoin, tannins (condensed and hydrolyzable t.), phenolic acids (chlorogenic acid, etc.), but no pyrrolizidine alkaloids.
Properties: Demulcent, mild expectorant, emollient, astringent.
Uses: Internally it is used (as a tea, h. p.; usually combined with other herbs) for inflammations of the upper respiratory tract (bronchitis, tracheitis, laryngitis with hoarseness; coughs), gastrointestinal tract (diarrhea, etc., incl. hemorrhoids) and genitourinary tract (cystitis, etc.). Due to its silicic acid content, it has been used as an adjuvant for pulmonary tuberculosis. Silicic acid is recommended for inflammatory changes in the connective tissue of joints, muscles, blood vessels, skin and other organs. Externally it is used (as a wash, wet compress) for wounds.
Caution: There are no reports of contraindications or side effects when used properly.

References: (1) Vol. 6, p. 310; (3) Vol. 6a, p. 972; (6) p. 102; (8) p. 467; (15) p. 173; (17) p. 465; (23) p. 218; (27) p. 264; (37) p. 1141; (46) p. 1156; (47) p. 2238; (51) p. 154; (69) p. 28.

LYCIUM

Other Common Name(s): 1) lycium, barbary wolfberry, wolfberry, matrimony vine 2) lycium, Chinese wolfberry, Chinese boxthorn
Botanical Name(s): 1) *Lycium barbatum* L. 2) *Lycium chinense* Mill. [Fam.: Solanaceae]
Fruit (berries) (Goji berries)
It is used only the ripe fruit.
Constituents: Vitamins (B_1, B_2, C, β-carotene = a provitamin A, niacin), minerals (calcium, phosphor, iron), carotenoids (zeaxanthin palmitate = physalien, β-carotene, etc.), biogenic amines (betaine, choline), polysaccha-

234

rides, amino acids, sugars, and possibly phytosterol derivatives (withanolides), but no tropane alkaloids.

Properties: Tonic, immunomodulant, antioxidant, mild antihyperglycemic.

Uses: <u>Internally</u> it is used (as a tea, h. p.) for fatigue, feeling of weakness, decreased mental and physical performance, erectile dysfunction, vertigo, tinnitus, impaired hearing, impaired vision, and as an adjuvant for diabetes.

Caution: Lycium should be avoided in cases of diarrhea. Manufacturers should evaluate alkaloids (Solanaceae fruit!). Otherwise, there are no reports of contraindications or side effects when used properly.

References: (1) Vol. 5, p. 718; (3) Vol. 5, p. 596; (9) p. 358; (13) p. 432; (18) p. 241; (31) p. 752; (37) p. 845.

LYSIMACHIA

Other Common Name(s): 1) moneywort, creeping charley 2) yellow loosestrife

Botanical Name(s): 1) *Lysimachia nummularia* L. 2) *Lysimachia vulgaris* L. [Fam.: Primulaceae]

<u>**Aerial part**</u>

Constituents: Flavonoids (quercetin, kaempferol, and their glycosides), triterpenoid saponins, tannins (possibly of condensed type), phenolic acids (caffeic acid, etc.), etc.

Properties: Astringent, wound-healing, expectorant, antimicrobial.

Uses: <u>Internally</u> it is used (as a tea, h. p.) for inflammations of the gastrointestinal tract (diarrhea, etc.) and upper respiratory tract (bronchitis, etc.; coughs). <u>Externally</u> it is used (as a wash, poultice) for minor skin inflammations, eczemas, wounds and ulcers, and (as a mouthwash, gargle) for inflammations of the mouth and throat.

Caution: There are no reports of contraindications or side effects when used properly.

References: (1) Vol. 5, p. 728; (3) Vol. 615; (8) p. 349; (24) p. 258; (35) p. 497; (37) p. 847; (47) p. 1810; (51) p. 144; (87) Vol. 2, p. 13.

MADDER

Botanical Name(s): *Rubia tinctorum* L. [Fam.: Rubiaceae]

<u>**Root**</u>

Constituents: Anthranoid pigments (ruberythric acid = alizarin-primveroside, alizarin, rubiadin, lucidin, lucidin-primveroside), iridoids (asperuloside, etc.), pectin, etc.

Properties: Antilithitic (= preventing / relieving urinary stones), antispasmodic, diuretic. Ruberythric acid forms chelates with calcium and magnesium ions, lowers their concentration in urine, and therefore prevents the formation of stones.

Uses: <u>Internally</u> it has been used for the prevention of the urinary stones chiefly composed of calcium oxalate / phosphate. In food industry it has been used as a coloring ingredient.

Caution: The anthranoids of madder (esp. lucidin), in animal tests, have shown mutagenic and carcinogenic effects. In view of this, madder is almost no longer used.

References: (3) Vol. 6b, p. 179; (6) p. 191; (7) p. 246; (8) p. 493; (13) p. 422; (23) p. 360; (37) p. 1203; (47) p. 2353; (51) p. 192.

MAGNOLIA

Botanical Name(s): *Magnolia biondii* Pamp.; *Magnolia denudata* Desr. in Lam.; *Magnolia sprengeri* Pamp.; and some other *Magnolia* spp. [Fam.: Magnoliaceae]

Flower bud (xin yi)

Constituents: Isoquinoline alkaloids (magnoflorine, salicifoline, etc.), lignans (lirioresinol and pinoresinol derivatives, etc.), volatile oil (with 1,8-cineole, eugenol, terpinen-4-ol, citral, etc.), flavonoids (anthocyanins, etc.), etc.

Properties: Antihistaminic, analgesic, local anesthetic, antihypertensive, uterotonic, antifungal, antibacterial, antiviral.

Uses: <u>Internally</u> it is used (as an h. p.) chiefly for allergic rhinitis, also for headaches. <u>Externally</u> it is used (as an ointment) for rhinitis, sinusitis, and eczema, among others.

Caution: Magnolia should not be taken during pregnancy and lactation. Internally should be used only as directed by an experienced practitioner (alkaloid containing herb!).

References: (2) Vol. 3, p. 148; (9) p. 362; (41) Vols. 1-7; (49) Vol. 2, p. 161; (52) p. 468.

MAIDENHAIR FERN

Other Common Name(s): true maidenhair, Venus' hair fern

Botanical Name(s): *Adiantum capillus-veneris* L. [Fam.: Adiantaceae (Polypodiaceae)]

Fern (frond)

Constituents: Tannins (oligomeric proanthocyanidins = OPCs), flavonoids (flavonols), mucilaginous polysaccharides, a bitter principle (a flavanone: naringin), phenolic acids (derivatives of caffeic and coumaric acids), triterpenes (adiantone, etc.), etc.

Properties: Demulcent, antitussive (mucosal protective effect), bitter tonic, astringent. Fronds with roots have also shown antihyperglycemic effect.

Uses: <u>Internally</u> it is used (as a tea, h. p.) for inflammations of the upper respiratory tract (bronchitis, laryngitis with hoarseness; coughs: irritating

236

cough, whooping cough). It is also used as a flavor ingredient in some syrupy drug products.

Caution: There are no reports of contraindications or side effects when used properly.

References: (1) Vol. 4, p. 85; (3) Vol. 2, p. 1102; (10) p. 181; (15) p. 14; (27) p. 72; (35) p. 303; (37) p. 21; (46) p. 222; (49) Vol. 1, p. 370.

MALABAR NUT TREE

Other Common Name(s): adhatoda
Botanical Name(s): *Justicia adhatoda* L. = *Adhatoda vasica* Nees [Fam.: Acanthaceae]
Leaf
Constituents: Quinazoline alkaloids (chiefly vasicine = peganine, bitter taste), volatile oil (unpleasant smelling), minerals, etc.
Properties: Expectorant, antispasmodic (bronchial active).
Uses: Internally it is used (as an h. p.; usually combined with other herbs) for inflammatory and spastic conditions of the upper respiratory tract (bronchitis, bronchial asthma; coughs). Vasicine has served as a model for the development of new expectorants (bromhexin, ambroxol).
Caution: It should be avoided during pregnancy. At higher doses than recommended it causes gastrointestinal irritations (with nausea, vomiting, diarrhea).

References: (1) Vol. 5, p. 595; (3) Vol. 2, p. 595; (8) p. 331; (12) p. 948; (36) p. 491; (37) p. 21.

MALE FERN

Botanical Name(s): *Dryopteris filix-mas* (L.) Schott = *Aspidium filix-mas* (L.) Sw. [Fam.: Aspidiaceae (Polypodiaceae)]
Root (rhizome)
Constituents: Phloroglucinol derivatives (acyl-phloroglucinols: chiefly flavaspidic acid and filicic acid), tannins, fixed oil, sugars, starch, etc.
Properties: Taeniafuge. It paralyzes tapeworms (= *Taenia* spp.) but doesn't kill them. It is also effective against hookworms (*Ancylostoma* spp. and *Necator* spp.), but has no effect against roundworms (= *Ascaris* spp.) and pinworms (= *Oxyuris* spp.)
Uses: Male fern ether soluble extract (= "filicin" = Oleoresin of Male Fern = Aspidium Oleoresin) has been used for tapeworm infestations, but today is largely replaced by synthetic anthelmintics.
Caution: Male fern should not be used in children under 4 years of age, during pregnancy and lactation, in cases of anemia, diabetes, as well as cardiovascular, liver and kidney disorders. Filicin is toxic if absorbed. To expel the paralyzed tapeworms it should be used only saline purgatives, not oils

237

(castor oil, etc.). A concomitant consumption of alcoholic drinks should also be avoided because, like oils, it increases the absorption and the toxicity of male fern extract.

References: (1) Vol. 4, p. 1201; (3) Vol. 4, p. 731; (8) p. 231; (9) p. 49; (36) p. 218; (37) p. 441; (46) p. 582; (49) Vol. 1, p. 363; (65) p. 191; (66) p. 163.

MALLOW

Other Common Name(s): 1) high / common mallow, malva 2) cultivated Mauritania mallow 3) blue / dwarf / common mallow
Botanical Name(s): 1) *Malva sylvestris* L. 2) *Malva sylvestris* L. ssp. *mauritiana* (L.) Asch. et Graeb. 3) *Malva neglecta* Wallr. [Fam.: Malvaceae]
<u>Flower</u> (high m.; cultivated m.), <u>leaf</u> (high m.; dwarf m.)
Constituents: Mucilaginous polysaccharides (rich), flavonoids (in flower: anthocyanins; in leaf: flavones), tannins (small amounts), etc.
Properties: Demulcent, emollient, anti-inflammatory.
Uses: <u>Internally</u> they are used (as a tea, h. p.) for inflammations of the upper respiratory tract (bronchitis, laryngitis with hoarseness; irritating dry coughs), gastrointestinal tract (gastritis, etc., ulcerative colitis), and genitourinary tract (cystitis, etc.). <u>Externally</u> they are used (as a mouthwash, gargle) for inflammations of the mouth and throat, and (as a poultice) for minor skin inflammations and eczemas.
Caution: There are no reports of contraindications or side effects when used properly.

References: (1) Vol. 5, p. 755; (3) Vol. 5, p. 680; (6) pp. 99, 315; (8) p. 353; (12) p. 364; (13) p. 370; (16) p. 68; (17) p. 364; (19) p. 150; (22) p. 118; (23) p. 209; (28) p. 76; (46) p. 913; (47) p. 1825; (48) p. 111; (51) p. 118.

MANACÁ

Botanical Name(s): *Brunfelsia uniflora* (Pohl) D. Don = *Brunfelsia hopeana* (Hook.) Benth. [Fam.: Solanaceae]
<u>Root</u>
Constituents: It is reported to contain coumarins (rich in scopoletin, also aesculetin), furanocoumarins, alkaloids of unknown structure (manacine, brunfelsine, hopeanine), tannins, and starch. It possibly contains saponins.
Properties: Diuretic, anti-inflammatory and analgesic, antibacterial, laxative, emmenagogue. Scopoletin has shown anti-inflammatory, antispasmodic, antibacterial and antifungal effects. Alkaloids, which possibly are of tropane type, may play an important role in the effects.
Uses: <u>Internally</u> it is used as an anti-inflammatory and antidyscratic (= blood purifier; tea, h. p.) for chronic rheumatic complaints and endogenous skin disorders (atopic eczema, itching, syphilitic skin lesions, etc.).

Caution: An absolute contraindication should be pregnancy and lactation. Manacá should be used only as directed by an experienced practitioner. At high doses it is toxic (alkaloid-containing, Solanaceae herb!).

References: (3) Vol. 3, p. 522; (4) Vol. 2, p. 128; (10) p. 182; (31) p. 364; (35) p. 509; (37) p. 240; (41) Vols. 1-7; (61) p. 424; (66) p. 336; (85) p. 945.

MANDRAKE

Other Common Name(s): European mandrake
Botanical Name(s): *Mandragora officinarum* L. [Fam.: Solanaceae]
Root
Constituents: Tropane alkaloids: chiefly scopolamine, also (−)-hyoscia-mine, atropine, belladonnine, cuskohygrine, etc. It contains also coumarins (scopolin, scopoletin), among others.
Properties and Uses: Today it is only incorporated in a few products. Man-drake extract has been used much like belladonna, i. e. as antispasmodic and antisecretory, for peptic ulcers and spastic conditions of the gastrointestinal, upper respiratory and genitourinary tracts.
Caution: Mandrake is toxic and should be used only as directed by a health professional. It should not be taken during pregnancy, and the same contra-indications mentioned for belladonna, henbane and jimson weed apply also to mandragora.

References: (1) Vol. 5, p. 765; (3) Vol. 5, p. 687; (8) p. 354; (36) p. 358; (37) p. 860; (47) p. 1835; (65) p. 309; (71) p. 234.

MANNA

Other Common Name(s): flowering ash
Botanical Name(s): *Fraxinus ornus* L. [Fam.: Oleaceae]
Manna
It is the dried exudation obtained by transverse cuts from the trunk.
Constituents: Chiefly a sugar alcohol (mannitol), sugars (glucose, fruc-tose), mucilaginous polysaccharides, and traces of coumarins and bitter principles.
Properties: Mild laxative (osmotic / bulk laxative), nutrient.
Uses: Internally it is used (as an h. p.) for constipation and conditions that a facilitated defecation is sought (hemorrhoids, during pregnancy, after op-erations in rectum or anal area, etc.). Manna is also recommended for chil-dren and the elderly.
Caution: Manna should not be taken in cases of bowel obstruction. In rare cases it may cause gastrointestinal disturbances (flatulence, bloating, nau-sea). Otherwise, there are no reports of contraindications or side effects when used properly.

References: (1) Vol. 5, p. 196; (3) Vol. 4, p. 1052; (8) p. 269; (19) p. 150; (27) p. 142; (36) p. 182; (37) p. 557; (48) p. 20; (73) p. 743.

MAPLE, SUGAR

Botanical Name(s): *Acer saccharum* Marsh. [Fam.: Aceraceae]
Maple Syrup
Constituents: Chiefly sugars (chiefly sucrose, also fructose, glucose, etc.), also small amounts of organic acids (malic acid, etc.), proteins, and minerals (potassium, etc.).
Properties and Uses: Maple syrup is used as a natural sweetener particularly in baking and cooking.
Caution: Diabetics should not consume maple syrup. Otherwise, there are no reports of contraindications or side effects when used properly.
Note: Other sources of maple syrup are Ashleaf maple: *Acer negundo* L.; red maple: *Acer rubrum* L.; black maple: *Acer nigrum* Michx. f.; etc.
Bark (inner bark)
It is obtained from different *Acer* spp., including producers of maple syrup.
Constituents: Among the possible constituents are, triterpenoid saponins, phenolics (tannins, gallic and ellagic acids, coniferyl and sinapyl aldehydes), a sugar alcohol (polygalitol), a cyclitol (quebrachitol), and allantoin.
Properties: Expectorant, astringent, diuretic, antimicrobial.
Uses: Internally it is used for inflammations (also when minor hemorrhages are present) of the upper respiratory tract (bronchitis, etc.; coughs), gastrointestinal tract (diarrhea, etc.), and genitourinary tract (cystitis, etc.). To enhance the effects in problems of the genitourinary tract, the fluid intake (incl. herbal teas) should be more than 2 liters per day.
Caution: At higher doses than recommended it causes gastrointestinal irritations (with nausea, vomiting). For minor hemorrhages it should be used on professional's advice.

References: (2) Vol. 2, p. 13; (3) Vol. 2, p. 878; (5) Vol. 1, p. 10; (18) p. 188; (31) p. 477; (32) Vol. 3, p. 1716; (37) pp. 8, 45; (41) Vols. 1-7; (42) Vol. 3, p. 49; (44) p. 41; (52) p. 8.

MARCELA

Other Common Name(s): macela, Brazilian chamomile
Botanical Name(s): *Achyrocline satureioides* (Lam.) DC. [Fam.: Asteraceae (Compositae)]
Aerial part, flower
Constituents: (Aerial part): volatile oil (with pinene, p-cymene, etc.), flavonoids (flavonols, methoxy-flavones), water-soluble polysaccharides, phenol glycosides (calleryanin, etc.), phenolic acids (caffeic acid, etc.), α-pyrones (yangonin, etc.), etc.
Properties: Aromatic, bitter tonic, anti-inflammatory, analgesic, antispas-

modic, sedative, mild immunomodulant.

Uses: Internally it is used (as a tea, h. p.) for inflammatory and spastic conditions of the gastrointestinal tract (loss of appetite, impaired digestion, cramps, diarrhea, etc.), upper respiratory tract (spastic bronchitis, bronchial asthma; as a diaphoretic hot tea for the common cold) and genitourinary tract (cystitis, etc.), and for dysmenorrhea (= painful menstruation without pathology). Marcela is also recommended to enhance the effects of antimicrobial therapies and to increase resistance to viral and bacterial infections.

Caution: There are no reports of contraindications or side effects when used properly. Nevertheless, before using it for dysmenorrhea, the gynecologic problem should be judged by a health professional.

References: (1) Vol. 4, p. 61; (3) Vol. 2, p. 896; (5) Vol. 1, p. 15; (6) pp. 262, 270; (18) p. 288; (41) Vols. 1-7; (52) p. 10.

MARIJUANA

Other Common Name(s): cannabis, Indian hemp
Botanical Name(s): *Cannabis sativa* L. ssp. *indica* (Lam.) E. Small et Cronquist = *Cannabis indica* Lam. [Fam.: Cannabaceae]
Aerial part (flowering top of the female plant)
Constituents: A resin that contains cannabinoids, of which the most important are tetrahydrocannabinol (= THC = dronabinol = Δ^9-tetrahydrocannabinol = delta-9-tetrahydrocannabinol = Δ^9-THC) and cannabidiol (= CBD), cannabinol, etc., depending on the origin and chemical type. It also contains volatile oil, flavonoids, choline, trigonelline, etc.
Properties: In regard to its mental and behavioral effects, at low doses, marijuana initially exerts euphoriant effect followed by a sedative effect (with impaired concentration and psychomotor performance). At higher doses as well as in certain persons, predisposed or sensitive to it, it may cause confusion, anxiety, panic, mood changes, and even mild hallucinations. Marijuana also exerts appetite stimulating, muscular relaxings, antispasmodic, analgesic effect for chronic pains, and decreases the intraocular pressure. THC is considered responsible for most of the mentioned effects.
Uses: Marijuana, particularly THC and synthetic cannabinoids, are recently used for the treatment of nausea, vomiting, weight loss caused by chemotherapy and HIV/AIDS, to improve appetite in the same conditions, and for epilepsy, glaucoma, and bronchial asthma.
Caution: Marijuana has not shown addictive effects or to cause abstinence syndrome. Nevertheless, a great concern should be the fact that it may lead to strong addictions. Certainly there are side effects, esp. with a chronic use and / or high doses, but further details are beyond the scope of this book.

References: (1) Vol. 4, p. 640; (3) Vol. 3, p. 652; (11) p. 101; (13) p. 284; (36) p. 525; (37) p. 265; (46) p. 206; (48) p. 445; (49) Vol. 2, p. 96; (65) p. 259; (66) p. 960; (67) p. 476; (83) p. 449; (84) pp. 575, 1110.

241

MARJORAM

Other Common Name(s): sweet marjoram
Botanical Name(s): *Origanum majorana* L. = *Majorana hortensis* Moench [Fam.: Lamiaceae (Labiatae)]
Aerial part
Constituents: Volatile oil (with terpinen-4-ol, α-terpineol, sabinene, terpinenes, etc.), flavonoids (flavones), a phenol glycoside (arbutin), Lamiaceae tannins (rosmarinic acid and other caffeic acid derivatives), bitter principles, triterpenes, phytosterols, etc.
Properties: Aromatic, bitter tonic, antispasmodic, carminative, diuretic, antioxidant, antibacterial, antiviral (against *Herpes simplex*). Marjoram is also mild neurotonic and antidepressant.
Uses: Marjoram is extensively used as a spice in food industry and culinary practice, and it is also beneficial due to its antioxidant effect. Internally it is used (as a tea, h. p.) for inflammatory and spastic conditions of the gastrointestinal tract (impaired digestion, cramps, flatulence, diarrhea), upper respiratory tract (the common cold, spastic bronchitis, bronchial asthma, also as a hot diaphoretic tea) and genitourinary tract (cystitis, urethritis, prostatitis, etc.), and for minor nervous fatigue and headaches. To enhance the effects in problems of the genitourinary tract, the fluid intake (incl. herbal teas) should be more than 2 liters per day. Externally it is used (as an ointment) for cold sores (= herpes simplex), (as a mouthwash, gargle) for inflammations of the mouth and throat, and (as a poultice) for wounds.
Caution: Due to hydroquinone, marjoram should not be applied externally in babies and young children. Otherwise, there are no reports of contraindications or side effects when used properly.

References: (1) Vol. 5, p. 952; (3) Vol. 5, p. 662; (8) p. 392; (9) p. 364; (12) p. 664; (37) p. 1007; (47) p. 1819; (48) p. 530; (51) p. 170.

MARSHMALLOW

Other Common Name(s): althaea, althea
Botanical Name(s): *Althaea officinalis* L. [Fam.: Malvaceae]
Root, leaf, flower
Constituents: Mucilaginous polysaccharides (root is richer, esp. in autumn), flavonoids (leaf, root: flavones; flower: anthocyanins). Root is also rich in starch, pectin and sucrose, and contains an amino acid (asparagine).
Properties: Demulcent, antitussive (mucosal protective effect), emollient. Mucilaginous polysaccharides may exert mild immunomodulant effect.
Uses: Internally it is used (as a tea, h. p.) for inflammatory conditions of the upper respiratory tract (pharyngitis, laryngitis, tracheitis, bronchitis; irritating dry coughs), gastrointestinal tract (gastritis, peptic ulcers, ulcerative colitis, combined with other herbs for irritable bowel syndrome; also as an

242

enema), and genitourinary tract (cystitis, gravel, nonobstructive urinary stones). Externally it is used (as a mouthwash, gargle) for inflammations of the mouth and throat, (as a wet compress, poultice, ointment) for minor skin inflammations, burns, and wounds.

Caution: Marshmallow may impair the absorption of some drugs. In view of this, when taking a vital oral medication, drugs should be taken about one hour apart from marshmallow products. Otherwise, there are no reports of contraindications or side effects when used properly.

References: (1) Vol. 4, p. 233; (3) Vol. 2, p. 1237; (6) pp. 99, 139; (13) p. 368; (14) p. 151; (15) p. 22; (16) p. 65; (17) p. 54; (19) p. 69; (22) p. 118; (23) 208; (27) p. 27; (28) pp. 73, 76; (37) p. 52; (46) p. 51; (47) p. 492; (48) p. 111.

MASTIC TREE

Other Common Name(s): lentisk, mastiche tree
Botanical Name(s): *Pistacia lentiscus* L., preferred var. *chia* DC., but also var. *lentiscus* [Fam.: Anacardiaceae]

Mastic
It is the dried oleoresin that escapes naturally, or after incisions or wounds made to the trunk or larger branches.

Constituents: Resin (with triterpenoid acids and alcohols: masticadienonic acid, oleanolic acid, tirucallol, etc.), volatile oil (with α-pinene, etc.), a bitter principle (possibly oleanolic acid), etc.

Properties: Stomachic, antiulcer (= prevents or helps in healing peptic ulcers; cimetidin-like effect), carminative, diuretic, astringent.

Uses: Internally it is used (as an h. p.) for gastrointestinal disorders (impaired digestion, upper abdominal pains, minor peptic ulcers, diarrhea), and for inflammatory conditions of the genitourinary tract (cystitis, urethritis, leukorrhea). To enhance the effects in problems of the genitourinary tract, the fluid intake (incl. herbal teas) should be more than 2 liters per day. Externally it is used (as a mouthwash combination product) for inflammations of the mouth, and (as a plaster) for wounds. It is also an ingredient in dental temporary fillings, varnishes, alcoholic and non-alcoholic beverages and perfumes, among others.

Caution: There are no reports of contraindications or side effects when used properly.

References: (2) Vol. 3, p. 398; (3) Vol. 6a, p. 727; (11a) p. 143; (27) p. 186; (35) p. 522; (36) p. 290; (37) p. 1089; (49) Vol. 2, p. 308; (52) p. 606; (55) p. 135; (66) p. 339.

MATÉ

Other Common Name(s): Paraguay tea, yerba maté
Botanical Name(s): *Ilex paraguariensis* A. St.-Hil. [Fam.: Aquifoliaceae]
Leaf

243

Constituents: Purine alkaloids (chiefly caffeine; theobromine: ca. ½ of the caffeine content), tannins (caffeic acid derivatives: chlorogenic acid, etc.; etc.), flavonoids, triterpenoid saponins, volatile oil (traces), etc.

Properties: CNS and respiratory stimulant (see COFFEE), increases the contractility of the heart muscle (= positive inotropic effect), increases the rate of the heartbeat (= positive chronotropic effect), diuretic (see CACAO), promotes the breakdown of glycogen into glucose (= glycogenolytic effect), promotes the breakdown of fats into free fatty acids and glycerol (= lipolytic effect). Caffeine is partially combined with phenolic acids therefore its CNS stimulant effects are modified. Theobromine is a mild diuretic and smooth muscle relaxant, and a weak CNS stimulant. Chlorogenic acid has been shown to inhibit the biosynthesis of prostaglandins and leukotrienes, and to exert choleretic, antibacterial and antiviral effects. See COFFEE; CACAO.

Uses: Maté is consumed mainly as a popular stimulant beverage. It is recommended as an invigorator for minor fatigue and feeling of weakness, short-term decreased mental and physical performance and for convalescence as it exerts at the same time bitter tonic effect, among others.

Caution: See COFFEE.

References: (1) Vol. 5, p. 508; (3) Vol. 5, p. 224; (8) p. 321; (13) p. 269; (15) p. 117; (16) p. 205; (17) p. 372; (19) p. 152; (23) p. 316; (31) p. 475; (36) p. 403; (37) p. 697; (48) p. 1083; (49) Vol. 2, p. 319.

MATICO

Other Common Name(s): matico pepper
Botanical Name(s): *Piper angustifolium* Lam. = *Piper elongatum* Vahl [Fam.: Piperaceae]

Leaf

Constituents: Volatile oil (with apiole, dillapiole, asarone, borneol, 1,8-cineole, etc.), a bitter principle (maticin), tannins, resin, etc.

Properties: Aromatic, bitter tonic, diuretic, antibacterial, astringent, hemostatic, wound-healing, and it is claimed to be aphrodisiac.

Uses: Internally it is used (as a tea, h. p.) for inflammations (also when minor hemorrhages are present, but on professional's advice) of the genitourinary tract (cystitis, urethritis, leukorrhea, etc.) and gastrointestinal tract (non-ulcer dyspepsia, diarrhea, ulcerative colitis, etc., incl. hemorrhoids). Matico is extensively used as a spice, and it is beneficial due also to its antioxidant effect. To enhance the effects in problems of the genitourinary tract, the fluid intake (incl. herbal teas) should be more than 2 liters per day. Externally it is used (as a wash, wet compress, poultice) for wounds, ulcers, and hemorrhoids, including cases with minor bleedings.

Caution: It should not be taken during pregnancy and lactation. Otherwise, there are no reports of contraindications or side effects when used properly.

References: (1) Vol. 6, p. 197; (3) Vol. 6a, p. 711; (15) p. 161; (24) p. 454; (35) p. 522; (36) p. 477; (37) p. 1084; (47) p. 1851; (48) p. 862; (66) p. 339.

MAYAPPLE

Other Common Name(s): American mandrake
Botanical Name(s): *Podophyllum peltatum* L. [Fam.: Berberidaceae]
Podophyllin
Podophyllin is the the dried purified extract of the root.
Constituents: Lignans, including podophyllotoxin, α-peltatin, β-peltatin, etc., and some of their glycosides.
Properties: Antiviral (against papillomaviruses) and antimitotic (= inhibits or disrupts a type of cell division) due to podophyllotoxin, and cholagogue (at low doses) and purgative (at high doses) due in large part to peltatins.
Uses: <u>Externally</u> it is used podophyllotoxin (as a paint, ointment) for venereal warts (= genital warts = condylomata acuminata) and common and plantar warts. Semisynthetic derivatives of podophyllotoxin (etoposide, teniposide) are antineoplastic drugs. <u>Internally</u> are still used (podophyllin or mayapple root: in a combination product) for their cholagogue and laxative effects.
Caution: Podophyllin or mayapple root should not be taken during pregnancy and lactation. Podophyllotoxin products should be used only as directed by a health professional. The application should be made on warts, avoiding the adjacent area, because it is very irritating. A longer duration of action may lead to blisters, even tissue necrosis.
Note: Podophyllin is obtained at a higher yield from Himalayan mayapple: *Podophyllum hexandrum* Royle = *Podophyllum emodi* Wall. ex Hook.f. et Thomson, which is richer in podophyllotoxin and contains no peltatins.

References: (3) Vol. 6a, p. 787; (6) pp. 278, 363; (7) p. 287; (8) p. 448; (9) p. 422; (11) p. 137; (12) p. 814; (13) p. 519; (19) p. 85; (22) p. 245; (23) p. 413; (36) p. 422; (37) p. 1096; (46) p. 1121; (47) p. 2177; (48) p. 284.

MEADOWSWEET

Other Common Name(s): queen-of-the-meadow
Botanical Name(s): *Filipendula ulmaria* (L.) Maxim. = *Spiraea ulmaria* L. [Fam.: Rosaceae]
Flower
Constituents: Phenol glycosides (monotropitin, spiraein; aglycones respectivelly salicylic aldehyde, methyl-salicylate), volatile oil (with salicylic aldehyde, etc.), flavonoids (flavonols: quercetin and kaempferol glycosides), tannins (gallotannins, ellagitannins), etc.
Properties: Anti-inflammatory, analgesic, antipyretic, diuretic, mild urinary antiseptic, astringent. Its phenol glycosides are converted (chiefly in the liver) to the active principle, namely salicylic acid, to exert then anti-inflammatory, analgesic and antipyretic effects (see WILLOW).
Uses: <u>Internally</u> it is used (as a tea, h. p.) for minor cases of rheumatic complaints (incl. rheumatoid arthritis), the common cold and feverish states

245

(taken also as a diaphoretic hot tea), and for minor inflammations of the genitourinary tract (cystitis, urethritis, pyelitis, etc.) and gastrointestinal tract (diarrhea, etc.). To enhance the effects in problems of the genitourinary tract, the fluid intake (incl. herbal teas) should be more than 2 liters per day. Externally it is used (as a wet compress, poultice) for minor skin inflammations.

Caution: See WILLOW

References: (1) Vol. 5, p. 148; (3) Vol. 4, p. 997; (6) p. 233; (8) p. 264; (12) p. 858; (14) p. 158; (15) p. 91; (17) p. 565; (19) p. 145; (20) p. 191; (22) p. 201; (27) p. 241; (28) p. 181; (47) p. 2593; (48) p. 251; (51) p. 102.

MELIA

Other Common Name(s): Chinaberry tree, China tree
Botanical Name(s): *Melia azedarach* L. = *Melia toosendan* Siebold et Zucc. [Fam.: Meliaceae]

Bark
Constituents: Tannins (rich), bitter principles (nortriterpenes of limonoid type), phenolic acids (vanillic acid, etc.), saponins, flavonoids, alkaloids, resin, etc.
Properties: Astringent, bitter tonic, antipyretic, anthelmintic.
Uses: Melia bark is chiefly used in traditional medicine. Externally it is used (as a wash, wet compress) for minor skin inflammations, eczema, and ulcers. Internally it is used (as a tea) for intestinal worms (against roundworms = *Ascaris* spp.), and feverish states.
Caution: It should not be taken during pregnancy and lactation. Internally it should be used only as directed by an experienced practitioner.

Leaf
Constituents: Saponins, flavonoids, phenolic acids, carotenoids, alkaloids, etc.
Properties: Stomachic, antispasmodic, laxative, anthelmintic.
Uses: Melia leaf is chiefly used in traditional medicine. Externally it is used (as a wash, wet compress) for minor skin inflammations, eczema, and ulcers. Internally it is used (as a tea, combined with other herbs) for gastrointestinal problems (cramps, constipation, worm infestation).
Caution: See Bark.

References: (3) Vol. 5, p. 753; (27) p. 214; (36) p. 42; (52) p. 487.

MELILOT, YELLOW

Other Common Name(s): yellow sweetclover
Botanical Name(s): *Melilotus officinalis* (L.) Pall. [Fam.: Fabaceae (Leguminosae)]
Aerial part

246

Constituents: Coumarins (coumarin, melilotin, scopoletin, etc.), phenolic acids (ferulic acid, etc.), flavonoids (flavonols), volatile oil, saponins, mucilaginous polysaccharides, tannins, etc.

Properties: Anti-inflammatory, antiexudative, antiedematous, antispasmodic, improves blood and lymphatic circulation.

Uses: Internally it is used (as a standardized product to coumarin content) for peripheral venous disorders (varicose veins in the legs, hemorrhoids, etc.), thrombophlebitis (= inflammation of a vein associated with an attached blood clot / thrombus), postthrombotic syndrome (= symptoms associated with the presence of a blood clot / thrombus in a blood vessel or heart chamber), and lymphatic congestion. Externally it is used (as a wet compress, poultice, ointment, plaster) for bruises, sprains, and boils, and (as a mouthwash, gargle) for inflammations of the mouth and throat.

Caution: It should not be taken during pregnancy and lactation. In rare cases it may cause headache, especially if taken at higher doses than recommended. Internally should be used only products standardized to coumarin.

References: (2) Vol. 3, p. 199; (3) Vol. 5, p. 755; (6) p. 79; (8) p. 364; (16) p. 116; (17) p. 380; (19) p. 217; (23) p. 201; (37) p. 875; (47) p. 1862; (48) p. 269; (51) p. 104.

MELON

Botanical Name(s): *Cucumis melo* L. [Fam.: Cucurbitaceae]
Seed
Constituents: Phytosterols (7-sterols: stigmastenol, α-spinasterol, etc.), fixed oil (with unsaturated fatty acids), amino acids (arginine, phenylalanine, etc.), a protein (globulin), etc.

Properties and Uses: Internally it is used in traditional medicine, mainly as a diuretic. Based on constituents it may be beneficial for early stages of benign prostatic hyperplasia (= BPH), much like pumpkin seed (see PUMPKIN). In traditional veterinary medicine it is used for intestinal worms (roundworms = *Ascaris* spp.; tapeworms = *Taenia* spp.) in cats.

Caution: There are no reports of contraindications or side effects when used properly.

References: (1) Vol. 4, p. 1065; (3) Vol. 4, p. 358; (36) p. 494; (52) p. 231; (57) p. 245.

MEZEREON

Other Common Name(s): 1) mezereon 2) spurge flax 3) spurge laurel
Botanical Name(s): 1) *Daphne mezereum* L. 2) *Daphne gnidium* L. 3) *Daphne laureola* L. [Fam.: Thymeleaceae]
Bark (mezereon bark)
It is the dried bark obtained from mezereon, spurge flax and spurge laurel.

Constituents: Coumarins (daphnetin, umbelliferone, and their glycosides), flavonoids, phenol glycosides (daphnoside, etc.), lignans (lariciresinol, etc.), diterpenes (daphnane type: daphnetoxin, etc.), etc.

Properties: (Externally): Rubefacient, counterirritant, analgesic. (Internally): At low doses it exerts laxative and diuretic effects, while at higher doses it is a strong purgative. Some diterpenes of daphnane type have shown antileukemic and antitumoral effects, but they are very toxic.

Uses: Externally it has been used (as a liniment, ointment combination product) for rheumatic pains. In traditional medicine it has also been applied on growths. Internally it has been used as an antidyscratic (= blood purifier; combined with other herbs) for syphilis, atopic eczema (= chronic eczema of internal origin) and chronic rheumatic complaints, and constipation and intestinal worms, among others.

Caution: Mezereon is very toxic and not for self-treatment. It is no longer used internally. When taken internally, it has caused irritations of the kidneys (with nephritis) and gastrointestinal tract (with gastroenteritis, vomiting). An experienced practitioner should supervise external applications as it may cause blisters if applied in higher concentrations or left on the painful site longer than advised.

References: (2) Vol. 2, p. 500; (3) Vol. 4, p. 443; (31) p. 645; (37) p. 386; (47) p. 1903; (48) p. 655; (65) p. 138; (66) p. 342.

MILK THISTLE

Other Common Name(s): Mary's thistle
Botanical Name(s): *Silybum marianum* (L.) Gaertn. = *Carduus marianus* L. [Fam.: Asteraceae (Compositae)]
Fruit (commonly called seed)
Constituents: Flavanolignans (collectively referred to as silymarin: silybin = silybinin, silydianin, silychristin, etc.), a flavanonol (taxifolin: structural basis of flavanolignans), flavonols (quercetin, kaempferol), flavones (apigenin, chrysoeriol), lignans (coniferyl alcohol dimers), lipids (fixed oil, phytosterols), biogenic amines (tyramine, betaine, etc.), proteins, etc.

Properties: Protects liver cells from damaging effects of toxic substances, promotes regeneration of liver tissue, antioxidant, anti-inflammatory, mild cholagogue. Its main liver-active constituent is silymarin, with its most active component silybin (= silybinin). To the overall effect of the herb surely contribute other flavonoids, lignans, and biogenic amines.

Uses: Internally it is used (silymarin, purified silybin, dried extract standardized to silymarin / silybin) for liver damage (caused by toxins, alcohol abuse, drugs, etc.), chronic hepatitis, fatty liver, and as an adjuvant for cirrhosis; (powdered fruit as a tea, combined with other herbs, combination products with standardized extract) for inflammations of the gastrointestinal and biliary tracts (with loss of appetite, impaired digestion, nausea, flatu-

248

lence, constipation, hemorrhoids). It has also been used for minor cases of hypotension (= low blood pressure; tyramine is an indirect-acting sympathomimetic, see CEREUS, NIGHT-BLOOMING). Externally it is used (as a wet compress) for varicose ulcers (= ulcus cruris) and bleeding hemorrhoids. Tyramine is a topical hemostatic.

Caution: In rare cases it may exert mild laxative effect. Otherwise, there are no reports of contraindications or side effects when used properly.

References: (2) Vol. 3, p. 549; (3) Vol. 6b, p. 398; (6) p. 140; (7) p. 236; (8) p. 519; (12) p. 863; (12a) p. 681; (13) p. 314; (16) p. 140; (17) p. 126; (19) pp. 151, 209; (22) p. 76; (23) p. 119; (28) pp. 143, 152; (47) p. 830; (48) p. 288; (51) p. 221; (65) p. 387.

MILKWEED

Other Common Name(s): common milkweed
Botanical Name(s): *Asclepias syriaca* L. = *Asclepias cornuti* Decne. [Fam.: Asclepiadaceae]
Root (rhizome)
Constituents: Cardiac glycosides (chiefly syrioside), alkaloids (nicotine), bitter principles (possibly steroidal ester-glycosides), etc.
Properties: Cardiotonic, diuretic. Syrioside has shown digitalis-like effect, but milder than digitoxin. See DIGITALIS.
Uses: Milkweed is chiefly used in traditional medicine. Internally it is used (as a tea; at low doses) for dropsy and asthma (possibly, both caused by heart failure), gravel, to check excessive hemorrhage following childbirth, and for venereal diseases and rheumatic complaints, among others. Externally it is used (as a poultice, paint: fresh root, milky juice) for warts (common w., plantar w.).
Caution: See MILKWEED, BUTTERFLY.

References: (2) Vol. 2, p. 196; (3) Vol. 3, p. 284; (25) p. 154; (42) Vol. 3, p. 202; (44) p. 108; (52) p. 79.

MILKWEED, BUTTERFLY

Other Common Name(s): butterfly weed
Botanical Name(s): *Asclepias tuberosa* L. [Fam.: Asclepiadaceae]
Root (rhizome) (pleurisy root)
Constituents: Cardiac glycosides (glucofrugoside, frugoside, etc.), mucilaginous polysaccharides, bitter principles (possibly steroidal ester-glycosides), tannins (gallotannins). Its glycosidic mixture has been formerly designated as asclepiadin.
Properties: Cardiotonic (digitalis-like effect; see DIGITALIS), expectorant, estrogen-like, uterotonic. The mentioned effects vary depending on doses.
Uses: Butterfly milkweed is chiefly used in traditional medicine. Internally it is used (as a tea; at low doses) for cardiac insufficiency, respiratory com-

plaints (bronchitis, influenza, pleurisy, pneumonia), and to check excessive hemorrhage following childbirth. Externally it is used (as a poultice) for bruises and swellings.

Caution: Butterfly milkweed is a toxic herb and not for self-treatment. Unless advised by a health professional, it should not be taken during pregnancy and lactation. At high doses, it causes vomiting and diarrhea, which are also signs of an intoxication from cardiac glycosides.

References: (2) Vol. 2, p. 197; (3) Vol. 3, p. 284; (15) p. 35; (18) p. 253; (25) p. 136; (29) p. 17; (44) p. 109; (46) p. 111; (47) p. 627; (52) p. 79; (66) p. 163.

MISTLETOE, AMERICAN

Botanical Name(s): *Phoradendron leucarpum* (Raf.) Reveal et M.C. Johnst. = *Phoradendron serotinum* (Raf.) M.C. Johnst. = *Phoradendron flavescens* Nutt. ex Engelm [Fam.: Viscaceae (Loranthaceae)]
Aerial part
Constituents: A toxic protein, namely phoratoxin, which is similar to viscotoxin of European mistletoe, etc. It also contains biogenic amines (tyramine, phenylethylamine).

Properties: Phoratoxin, when injected (iv) into animals, has been shown to slow heartbeat, lower blood pressure, and to weaken the heart muscle contractility (= negative inotropic effect). Tyramine and phenylethylamine are indirect-acting sympathomimetics, which when taken orally are mainly inactivated by monoamine oxidase. When found unchanged in the bloodstream, in small concentrations they increase the contractility of the heart muscle (= positive inotropic effect). Phenylethylamine is also a skin irritant, which explains at least in part the contact dermatitis sometimes caused by mistletoe.

Uses: American mistletoe is chiefly used in traditional medicine. Internally it is used (as a tea) for epilepsy, to hasten labor or cause abortion, and to check the hemorrhage following childbirth, among others.

Caution: It should not be taken during pregnancy and lactation. American mistletoe should be used only as directed by an experienced practitioner. It may cause contact dermatitis. See also CEREUS, NIGHT-BLOOMING.

References: (3) Vol. 6a, p. 622; (5) Vol. 1, p. 826; (12a) p. 449; (21) p. 257; (25) p. 296; (29) p. 85; (31) pp. 81, 83; (44) p. 393.

MISTLETOE, EUROPEAN

Botanical Name(s): *Viscum album* L. [Fam.: Viscaceae (Loranthaceae)]
Aerial part
Constituents: Polypeptides (viscotoxins), glycoproteins (lectins), water-soluble polysaccharides, lignans (syringaresinol, eleutheroside E), a phenol glycoside (syringin), flavonoids, biogenic amines (tyramine, β-phenylethylamine, acetylcholine, choline, etc.), etc.

250

Properties: (Products for parenteral use): Cytotoxic and immunomodulant, attributed to viscotoxins, lectins and water-soluble polysaccharides. (Extract, powder, tea, for oral use): Antihypertensive, which may be due at least in part to polypeptides, lignans and flavonoids. It is not yet known the complex role of biogenic amines, although they are mostly destroyed before reaching the bloodstream.

Uses: Parenterally it is used as a palliative treatment (after radical operations, with chemotherapy and radiotherapy) for certain malignant tumors. Orally it is used as an adjuvant (h. p.; usually combined with other herbs) for hypertension and complaints associated with it (vertigo, headache, etc.).

Caution: European mistletoe should not be taken during pregnancy. Products for parenteral use may cause severe allergic reactions, fever, headache, angina pectoris and orthostatic circulatory problems. In view of this, parenteral administrations should be supervised by a health professional. With oral administration at normal doses there are no side effects, besides allergic reactions in rare cases. Nevertheless, it should be used only products of a known host plant as it plays an important role in the constituents and effects of mistletoe. Mistletoe fruits are highly toxic therefore they should not exceed a standard limit.

References: (1) Vol. 6, p. 1160; (3) Vol. 6c, p. 492; (6) pp. 58, 280; (8) p. 590; (13) p. 555; (15) p. 235; (17) p. 628; (22) p. 247; (23) p. 191; (28) p. 146; (46) p. 1760; (47) p. 2833; (48) p. 218; (71) p. 234.

MOSS, ICELAND

Botanical Name(s): *Cetraria islandica* (L.) Ach. = *Lobaria islandica* Hoffm. [Fam.: Parmeliaceae]

Iceland moss is lichen (= a symbiotic association of a fungus with an alga) but commonly called moss.

Thallus (= a complete plant body, which is not differentiated into root, stem and leaves)

Constituents: Depsidones (so-called lichenic acids: cetraric acid, etc.; bitter tasting), dibenzofurans (usnic acid, etc.), polysaccharides (D-glucans = D-glucose polymers: the water-insoluble lichenin and water-soluble isolichenin; and galactomannans), volatile oil, etc.

Properties: Demulcent, antitussive (mucosal protective effect), emollient, antibacterial (against *Staphylococcus* spp., *Streptococcus* spp., *Mycobacterium tuberculosis*, *Bacillus subtilis*), anti-inflammatory, bitter tonic, antiemetic, mild immunomodulant. Lichenic acids and usnic acid are phenolic compounds and account for most of the effects, except demulcent / emollient and antitussive effects, which are due to mucilaginous polysaccharides. The immunomodulating effect is in large part due to water-soluble polysaccharides and partly due to bitter lichenic acids.

Uses: Internally it is used (as a tea, h. p.) for inflammations of the upper respiratory tract (laryngitis, pharyngitis, tracheitis, bronchitis; irritating dry coughs; also as a lozenge) and gastrointestinal tract (loss of appetite, vomiting, minor diarrhea), beneficial for minor fatigue and convalescence. In traditional medicine it is also used for morning sickness. In pharmaceutical practice it is also used to modify the taste of certain drug products. Externally it is used (as a wash, wet compress, poultice) for minor skin inflammations and wounds.

Caution: Due to lichenic acids, in rare cases it may cause contact skin irritations. Otherwise, there are no reports of contraindications or side effects when used properly (incl. internal use).

References: (1) Vol. 4, p. 791; (3) Vol. 3, p. 824; (5) Vol. 2, p. 142; (6) pp. 108, 116; (8) p. 140; (16) p. 67; (17) p. 343; (19) p. 114; (22) p. 118; (23) pp. 66, 212; (36) pp. 31, 217, 475; (37) p. 299; (46) p. 817; (49) Vol. 1, p. 359; (51) p. 233.

MOSS, LUNGWORT

Other Common Name(s): lungmoss, lungwort lichen
Botanical Name(s): *Lobaria pulmonaria* (L.) Hoffm. = *Sticta pulmonaria* (L.) Biroli [Fam.: Lobariaceae (Stictaceae)]
Lungmoss is lichen (= a symbiotic association of a fungus with an alga) but commonly it is called moss.
Thallus (= a complete plant body, which is not differentiated into root, stem and leaves)
Constituents: Depsidones (so-called lichenic acids: stictic acid, etc.; bitter tasting), mucilaginous polysaccharides, phytosterols (5-sterols: ergosterol, fucosterol), fatty acids, proteins, etc.
Properties: Demulcent, antitussive (mucosal protective effect), emollient, bitter tonic, antibacterial. The effects are milder than Iceland moss.
Uses: Internally it is used (as a tea, h. p.) for inflammations of the upper respiratory tract (laryngitis, pharyngitis, tracheitis, bronchitis, etc.). Externally it is used (as a wet compress, poultice) for minor skin inflammations and wounds.
Caution: Due to lichenic acids, in rare cases it may cause contact skin irritations. Otherwise, there are no reports of contraindications or side effects when used properly.

References: (3) Vol. 5, p. 550; (5) Vol. 2, p. 149; (10) p. 178; (15) p. 133; (23) p. 213; (36) p. 477; (37) p. 837; (47) p. 2614; (49) Vol. 1, p. 360; (87) Vol. 1, p. 47.

MOSS, OAK

Botanical Name(s): *Evernia prunastri* (L.) Ach. [Fam.: Usneaceae]
Oak moss is lichen (= a symbiotic association of a fungus with an alga) but commonly called moss.
Thallus (= a complete plant body, which is not differentiated into root, stem and leaves)

Constituents: Depsides (open-ring lichenic acids: evernic acid, etc.), dibenzofurans (usnic acid, etc.), volatile oil (with orcin derivatives, also thujone, borneol, 1,8-cineole, geraniol, vanillin, etc.), polysaccharides, resin, wax, etc.

Properties: Aromatic, antibacterial.

Uses: Oak moss is chiefly used as a fixative in perfumery. It is also used for the industrial isolation of usnic acid and evernic acid, both phenolic compounds with antibacterial effect (against *Staphylococcus* spp., *Streptococcus* spp., etc.). They are incorporated in combination products used chiefly externally (as ointment, spray, powder) for inflammations of the mucous membranes and the skin (infected wounds, boils, etc.), but also internally for inflammations of the upper respiratory and gastrointestinal tracts.

Caution: Due to lichenic acids, it may cause contact skin irritations. Otherwise, there are no reports of contraindications or side effects when used properly.

References: (3) Vol. 4, p. 893; (5) Vol. 3, p. 146; (31) p. 1251; (37) p. 1430; (49) Vol. 1, p. 362.

MOSSY STONECROP

Other Common Name(s): wall grass, wall pepper
Botanical Name(s): *Sedum acre* L. [Fam.: Crassulaceae]
Aerial part
Constituents: Piperidine alkaloids (sedamine, sedacrine, etc.), flavonoids (isorhamnetin, its glycosides, etc.), tannins, polysaccharides (mucilaginous p., gum), 4-hydroxy-3-methoxy-phenylethyl alcohol, organic acids, etc.

Properties: Antispasmodic, diuretic, mild counterirritant, wound-healing.

Uses: Internally it is used (as a tea, h. p.; combined with other herbs) for minor cases of hypertension and for the prevention of arteriosclerosis. Externally it is used (as a wash, wet compress, poultice) for wounds, ulcers and lichen planus (= a skin itching condition), (as a poultice, paint: fresh herb, juice) for warts (common w., plantar w.), and (as a mouthwash, gargle) for inflammations of the mouth and throat.

Caution: It should not be taken in cases of inflammations of the gastrointestinal and genitourinary tracts. Otherwise, there are no reports of contraindications or side effects when used properly.

References: (1) Vol. 6, p. 651; (3) Vol. 6b, p. 349; (24) p. 454; (36) p. 772; (37) p. 1251; (47) p. 2512; (51) p. 94.

MOTHERWORT

Botanical Name(s): *Leonurus cardiaca* L. [Fam.: Lamiaceae (Labiatae)]
Aerial part
Constituents: Iridoids (ajugoside = leonuride, etc.), diterpenes (leocardin,

253

etc.), triterpenes (ursolic acid, etc.), phenolic acids (caffeic acid derivatives), flavonoids (chiefly flavonols; also methoxy-flavones: genkwanin), proline-betaines (stachydrine, betonicine), phenylethanoid glycosides (acteoside = verbascoside, etc.), tannins, etc., but no cardiac glycosides and true alkaloids.

Properties: Slows an elevated rate of the heartbeat (= negative chronotropic effect), sedative, antihypertensive, astringent. The mentioned effects are mild.

Uses: Internally it is used (as a tea, h. p.; usually combined with other herbs) for minor nervous cardiac disorders (tachycardia = rapid heartbeat, etc.) and hypertension, which are often associated with hyperthyroidism (= Basedow's disease), menopausal syndrome, premenstrual syndrome and menstrual complaints.

Caution: There are no reports of contraindications or side effects when used properly.

References: (1) Vol. 5, p. 647; (3) Vol. 5, p. 483; (8) p. 340; (12) pp. 437, 504; (14) p. 161; (15) p. 129; (16) p. 99; (17) p. 338; (19) p. 104; (20) p. 197; (23) p. 151; (46) p. 810; (47) p. 1738; (51) p. 164; (86) Vol. 1, p. 86.

MOUNTAIN ASH, AMERICAN

Botanical Name(s): *Sorbus americana* Marsh. = *Pyrus americana* (Marsh.) DC. [Fam.: Rosaceae]

Fruit (ripe)

Constituents: There are no reports available.

Properties and Uses: It is chiefly used in traditional medicine.

Internally it is used for scurvy, to aid digestion, and for intestinal worms.

Caution: There are no reports of contraindications or side effects when used properly.

Bark (inner bark)

Constituents: There are no reports available.

Properties: It is claimed to be bitter tonic, antipyretic and antiseptic.

Uses: It is chiefly used in traditional medicine. Internally it is used (as a tea) for minor fatigue, feverish states and colds, and venereal diseases, among others.

Caution: There are no reports of contraindications or side effects when used properly.

References: (3) Vol. 6b, p. 475; (25) p. 276; (44) p. 538.

MOUNTAIN ASH, EUROPEAN

Botanical Name(s): *Sorbus aucuparia* L. = *Pyrus aucuparia* (L.) Gaertn. [Fam.: Rosaceae]

254

Fruit (ripe)

Constituents: Vitamin C, parasorbic acid and sugars (sorbose, etc.), a sugar alcohol (sorbitol), pectin, tannins, organic acids (malic and tartaric acids, etc.), carotenoids, flavonoids, cyanogenic glycosides (chiefly in seeds).

Properties: (Depending on preparation): Astringent, mild diuretic, laxative. Parasorbic acid is considered responsible for the diuretic and laxative effects. By boiling it is destroyed.

Uses: Internally it is used (as a decoction, or by boiling down to a purée) for diarrhea; (fresh fruit) as a laxative for constipation and as a vitamin C supplement. Externally it is used (as a gargle) for sore throat and hoarseness.

Caution: Parasorbic acid is irritating to the mucous membranes (gastrointestinal, genitourinary, nose, eyes). Therefore, consumption of great amounts of fresh fruit and contact with nose or eyes should be avoided. Otherwise, there are no reports of contraindications or side effects when used properly.

References: (1) Vol. 6, p. 766; (3) Vol. 6b, p. 473; (24) p. 109; (37) p. 1283; (47) p. 2577; (86) Vol. 2, p. 112; (87) Vol. 1, p. 186.

MOUNTAIN AVENS

Other Common Name(s): white dryad
Botanical Name(s): *Dryas octopetala* L. [Fam.: Rosaceae]
Aerial part
Constituents: Tannins (proanthocyanidins), flavonoids (flavonols, 8-methoxy-flavonols), triterpenoid pseudosaponins (tormentoside = diglucoside of tormentillic acid), etc.

Properties: Astringent, mild anti-inflammatory.

Uses: Internally it is used (as a tea, h. p.) for inflammations of the gastrointestinal tract (gastritis, diarrhea, etc., incl. hemorrhoids; also when minor hemorrhages are present, but on professional's advice). It is also used as a substitute for black tea, under the name of Kaisertee or Schweizertee, which is justifiable as it contains proanthocyanidins and flavonoids, and at the same time lacks toxic constituents. Externally it is used (as a mouthwash, gargle) for inflammations of the mouth and throat, and (as a wash, wet compress, poultice) for minor skin inflammations, wounds and ulcers.

Caution: There are no reports of contraindications or side effects when used properly.

References: (1) Vol. 4, p. 1197; (3) Vol. 4, p. 730; (41) Vols. 1-7; (52) p. 265.

MOUNTAIN LAUREL

Other Common Name(s): American laurel, kalmia
Botanical Name(s): *Kalmia latifolia* L. [Fam.: Ericaceae]

Leaf

Constituents: Diterpenoid polyphenols of grayanotoxin type (chiefly acetylandromedol = andromedotoxin = grayanotoxin I, etc.; toxic!; cf. RHODO-DENDRON), flavonoids (chiefly dihydro-chalcones: phloridzin, etc.), a phenol glycoside (arbutin), and it possibly contains tannins, among others.

Properties: Kalmia is reported to be narcotic and astringent. Andromedotoxin at low doses has been shown to increase the heart contractile force and lower blood pressure, and at high doses to exert aconite-like effects (drugged state, convulsions, cardiac arrest). Phloridzin causes glucosuria.

Uses: Andromedotoxin is incorporated in some products used for hypertension (cf. RHODODENDRON). Kalmia is chiefly used in traditional medicine. Externally it is used for Tinea capitis (= fungal infection of the scalp), psoriasis, syphilitic skin rashes, and rheumatic pains. Internally it has been used (as a tea) for diarrhea.

Caution: Kalmia is a toxic herb and not for self-treatment. Medicines containing andromedotoxin should be used only as directed by a health professional. See: RHODODENDRON.

Note: Sheep laurel: *Kalmia angustifolia* L. is considered an adulterant of mountain laurel and is even more toxic.

References: (1) Vol. 5, p. 608; (8) p. 332; (12) p. 501; (13) p. 415; (36) p. 45; (37) pp. 11, 752; (41) Vols. 1-7; (44) p. 292; (47) p. 1685.

MOUSE-EAR

Other Common Name(s): mouse-ear, hawkweed
Botanical Name(s): *Hieracium pilosella* L. = *Pilosella officinarum* C.H. et F.W. Schultz, [Fam.: Asteraceae (Compositae)]

Aerial part

Constituents: Flavonoids (flavones: luteolin, luteolin-glucoside), coumarins (umbelliferone and its glucoside), phenolic acids (caffeic and chlorogenic acids), tannins, bitter principles, mucilaginous polysaccharides, etc.

Properties: Mild diuretic, anti-inflammatory, antispasmodic, astringent, antibacterial, and it is claimed to be choleretic and cholagogic. The antibacterial effect may be due to luteolin and umbelliferone.

Uses: Internally it is used (as a tea, h. p.) for inflammations (also when minor hemorrhages are present) of the genitourinary tract (cystitis, urethritis, pyelitis, etc., gravel, nonobstructive urinary stones; with proteinuria, uremia), gastrointestinal tract (diarrhea, ulcerative colitis, etc.), upper respiratory tract (bronchitis, etc.), and hepatobiliary tract. To enhance the effects in problems of the genitourinary tract, the fluid intake (incl. herbal teas) should be more than 2 liters per day. Externally it is used (as a mouthwash, gargle) for inflammations of the mouth and throat, and (as a wet compress, poultice) for minor skin inflammations and wounds.

Caution: There are no reports of contraindications or side effects when used

256

properly. For minor hemorrhages it should be used on professional's advice.

References: (3) Vol. 5, p. 81; (10) p. 194; (15) p. 158; (28) p. 72; (31) pp. 365, 404; (35) p. 384; (47) p. 1553; (51) p. 224; (87) Vol. 2, p. 231.

MUDAR

Other Common Name(s): 1) mudar, madar, giant milkweed, giant swallowwort 2) mudar, madar, swallowwort
Botanical Name(s): 1) *Calotropis gigantea* (L.) W.T. Aiton 2) *Calotropis procera* (Aiton) W.T. Aiton [Fam.: Asclepiadaceae]
Root bark
Constituents: Cardiac glycosides (calotropin, calactin, uscharidin, etc.), triterpenes (amyrins, taraxasterols), phytosterols, etc.
Properties: It has been attributed ipecac-like effects, i. e. expectorant (at low doses) and emetic (at high doses). Its cardiac glycosides exert digitalis-like effect (see DIGITALIS). Calotropin has shown antitumoral effect (against human epidermoid carcinoma cells of nasopharynx).
Uses: It is used almost only in traditional medicine. Internally it is used for epilepsy, convulsions an hysteria, for leprosy, elephantiasis and syphilis, and for gastrointestinal complaints (incl. diarrhea), among others. Externally it is used (as a paint: milky juice) for growths, tumors, warts (common w., plantar w.), boils, and rheumatic pains, among others.
Caution: Mudar is toxic and not for self-treatment. The emetic effect (at high doses) may be a sign of intoxication with cardiac glycosides. Mudar should be used only as directed by an experienced practitioner.

References: (1) Vol. 4, p. 621; (3) Vol. 3, p. 617; (37) p. 260; (41) Vols. 1-7.

MUGWORT

Botanical Name(s): *Artemisia vulgaris* L. [Fam.: Asteraceae (Compositae)]
Aerial part
Constituents: Volatile oil (with 1,8-cineole, camphor, linalool or thujone as its major components; depending on the origin), bitter principles (sesquiterpene lactones: psilostachyin, etc.), coumarins, flavonoids, polyacetylenes, phytosterols, carotenoids, glycoproteins, etc.
Properties: Aromatic, bitter tonic, antimicrobial, mild choleretic, antispasmodic.
Uses: Mugwort is chiefly used as a flavor ingredient in herbal vinegars, seasonings and beverages. Internally it is used (as a tea, h. p.) for loss of appetite and nonulcer dyspepsia (with flatulence, burping, heartburn, minor cramps, etc.).
Caution: At higher doses than recommended it causes gastrointestinal irritations (with nausea, vomiting, diarrhea). Due to sesquiterpene lactones it

257

may cause allergic contact dermatitis to persons hypersensitive to other Asteraceae plants (e. g. arnica, chamomile, feverfew, ragweed, tansy, yarrow) that contain them. Otherwise, there are no reports of contraindications and side effects when used properly.

References: (1) Vol. 4, p. 373; (3) Vol. 3, p. 265; (15) p. 33; (17) p. 83; (37) p. 135; (46) p. 105; (47) p. 597; (51) p. 212.

MUIRA PUAMA

Other Common Name(s): potency wood
Botanical Name(s): *Ptychopetalum olacoides* Benth.; *Ptychopetalum uncinatum* Anselmino [Fam.: Olacaceae]
Wood (barked stem wood)
Constituents: Esters of saturated fatty acids (chiefly behenic acid: C_{20}) with triterpenoid alcohols (chiefly lupeol) and phytosterols (5-sterols: β-sitosterol, etc.), volatile oil (with α-pinene, etc.), tannins, alkaloids, etc.
Properties: Tonic (reported to be CNS stimulant, sympathomimetic), astringent, and it is claimed to be aphrodisiac.
Uses: Internally it is used (as a tea, h. p.; usually combined with other herbs) for fatigue, feeling of weakness, diarrhea, and for low sexual drive and erectile dysfunction. Based on reported effects, it may be beneficial for minor cases of hypotension (= low blood pressure), especially when associated with minor fatigue.
Caution: Considering the possible presence of alkaloids and the already reported effects, it is best used on experienced practitioner's advice. Muira puama should be avoided at least in cases of hypertension. A combination with ephedra and / or caffeine or caffeine rich herbs / drinks (coffee, guaraná, tea, mate, cola, etc.) may result in overstimulation of the nervous system. In view of this such combinations should be made only by health professionals.

References: (1) Vol. 6, p. 307; (3) Vol. 6a, p. 969; (6) p. 293; (8) p. 466; (15) p. 132; (42) Vol. 5, p. 230; (46) p. 971.

MULBERRY

Other Common Name(s): 1) black mulberry 2) white mulberry
Botanical Name(s): 1) *Morus nigra* L. 2) *Morus alba* L. [Fam.: Moraceae]
Fresh fruit (black mulberry is preferred)
Constituents: (Black mulberry): Sugars (invert sugar, sucrose), pectin, organic acids (malic and citric acids), vitamin C, flavonoids (anthocyanins, flavonols), minerals, etc.
Properties: Mild laxative, nutrient, acidulous, refrigerant, antimicrobial.
Uses: Internally it is used (usually as mulberry syrup) for minor constipation and feverish states, and as a flavor and coloring ingredient in syrupy medi-
258

cines. Externally it is used (as a mouthwash, gargle) for inflammations of the mouth and throat.

Caution: There are no reports of contraindications or side effects when used properly. In cases of gastrointestinal ulcers, consumption of mulberries in excessive amounts should be avoided.

Leaf (white mulberry)

Constituents: Flavonoids (rich in rutin), organic acids, amino acids, vitamins (complex B), etc.

Properties: It is claimed to exert mild antihyperglycemic effect.

Uses: Internally it is used as an adjuvant (tea, h. p.) for diabetes.

Caution: There are no reports of contraindications or side effects when used properly.

References: (3) Vol. 5, p. 897; (10) p. 195; (27) p. 148; (35) p. 558; (37) p. 924; (46) p. 644; (47) p. 1927; (51) p. 248.

MULLEIN

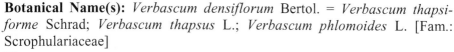

Botanical Name(s): *Verbascum densiflorum* Bertol. = *Verbascum thapsiforme* Schrad; *Verbascum thapsus* L.; *Verbascum phlomoides* L. [Fam.: Scrophulariaceae]

Flower

Constituents: Triterpenoid saponins (verbascosaponin, etc.), mucilaginous polysaccharides, flavonoids (rutin, etc.), iridoids (aucubin, etc.), phenylethanoid glycosides (verbascoside = acteoside, etc.), etc.

Properties: Expectorant, demulcent, antitussive (mucosal protective effect), emollient, anti-inflammatory, antimicrobial, diuretic. It is expectorant due in large part to saponins, demulcent, antitussive and emollient due to mucilage, diuretic due in large part to flavonoids, and anti-inflammatory due in large part to verbascoside (by inhibiting the biosynthesis of leukotrienes) and flavonoids. Aucubin and other iridoids exert also antimicrobial effect.

Uses: Internally it is used (as a tea, h. p.) for inflammations of the upper respiratory tract (bronchitis, tracheitis, laryngitis with hoarseness, etc.; coughs: irritating dry cough, due to thickened bronchial secretion, whooping cough), as an adjuvant for bronchial asthma, and as a diaphoretic hot tea for the common cold. Mullein is also recommended for children and the elderly. Externally it is used the same as leaf.

Caution: There are no reports of contraindications or side effects when used properly.

Leaf

Constituents: Mucilaginous polysaccharides, iridoids, saponins, etc.

Properties: Emollient, wound-healing, demulcent, expectorant.

Uses: Externally it is used (as a poultice) for minor skin inflammations, bruises, wounds, ulcers and hemorrhoids. Internally it is used (as a tea, h. p.) for inflammations of the upper respiratory tract.

Caution: There are no reports of contraindications or side effects when used properly.

References: (2) Vol. 3, p. 759; (3) Vol. 6c, p. 417; p. 582; (12) p. 448; (13) p. 316; (15) p. 226; (16) p. 65; (17) p. 608; (19) p. 248; (22) p. 119; (23) p. 210; (27) p. 326; (47) p. 2789; (51) p. 184.

MUSTARD

Other Common Name(s): 1) black mustard 2) brown / Indian / Chinese mustard
Botanical Name(s): 1) *Brassica nigra* (L.) W. D. J. Koch 2) *Brassica juncea* (L.) Czernov [Fam.: Brassicaceae (Cruciferae)]
Seed
Constituents: Glucosinolates (sinigrin = allyl-glucosinolate, etc.; mainly in the intact seed; cf. HORSERADISH), a bitter principle (sinapine), mucilaginous polysaccharides, fixed oil, proteins, enzymes, etc. The chief constituent of the distilled mustard oil is allyl-isothiocyanate (see Properties).
Properties: Rubefacient, counterirritant. Under the action of enzymes (when the seed is crushed and comes into contact with moisture and lukewarm temperature) sinigrin liberates the volatile allyl-isothiocyanate, responsible for the pungent flavor and the mentioned effects.
Uses: Externally it is used (as a plaster) for inflammations of the upper respiratory tract (bronchitis, etc.), and (as a plaster, poultice, liniment) for rheumatic pains. White mustard acts milder and is safer (see MUSTARD, WHITE).
Caution: It should not be taken in cases of varicose veins and severe circulatory disorders. Follow carefully the manufacturer's instructions as it may cause blisters if left on the painful site longer than advised, and even necrosis if used concentrated products.

References: (1) Vol. 4, p. 544; Vol. 6, p. 705; (3) Vol. 3, p. 496; (6) p. 129; (8) p. 106; (9) p. 379; (13) p. 149; (17) p. 558; (22) p. 205; (47) p. 2554; (48) p. 202; (51) p. 86.

MUSTARD, GARLIC

Other Common Name(s): hedge garlic
Botanical Name(s): *Alliaria petiolata* (M. Bieb.) Cavara et Grande = *Erysimum alliaria* L. = *Sisymbrium alliaria* (L.) Scop. [Fam.: Brassicaceae (Cruciferae)]
Whole plant (with root, fresh)
Constituents: Glucosinolates (chiefly sinigrin = allyl-glucosinolate; cf. MUSTARD; HORSERADISH), vitamins (A, C), enzymes, etc. Under the action of myrosinase (see MUSTARD) sinigrin liberates the volatile allyl-isothiocyanate, responsible for the pungent flavor and which is the main constituent of the distilled oil.

Properties: Antibacterial, stomachic, diuretic, antioxidant.
Uses: Internally it is used (as a tea, h. p.) for inflammations of the upper respiratory and gastrointestinal tracts, and as an antidyscratic (= blood purifier) for atopic eczema (= chronic eczema of internal origin) and chronic rheumatic complaints. It is also used as a spicy salad (usually as an additive), with beneficial effects on the digestive system and as a natural supplement of vitamins. Externally it is used (as a wash, wet compress, poultice) for infected wounds, ulcers, and (as a poultice) for minor rheumatic pains.
Caution: See CRESS, GARDEN; MUSTARD, HEDGE.

References: (1) Vol. 4, p. 180; (3) Vol. 2, p. 1209; (5) Vol. 1, p. 1002; (28) pp. 199, 120; (35) p. 571.

MUSTARD, HEDGE

Other Common Name(s): bank cress
Botanical Name(s): *Sisymbrium officinale* (L.) Scop. = *Erysimum officinale* L. [Fam.: Brassicaceae (Cruciferae)]
Leaf (fresh)
Constituents: Glucosinolates (sinigrin = allyl-glucosinolate, etc.; mainly in the intact fresh material; cf. HORSERADISH; MUSTARD; MUSTARD, GARLIC), mucilaginous polysaccharides, volatile oil (with allyl-isothiocyanate, etc.; mainly in the processed / dried material), vitamin C, enzymes, flavonoids, etc. Flowering top contains cardiac glycosides (!).
Properties: Expectorant (upper respiratory secretagogue effect), antispasmodic, antibacterial, diuretic. Isothiocyanates, liberated from glucosinolates, are responsible for most of the mentioned effects.
Uses: Internally it is used (as a tea, h. p.) for pharyngitis, laryngitis (even hoarseness with loss of voice), bronchitis, and minor cases of bronchial asthma. Topically it is used (as a lozenge) for the same conditions.
Caution: For the upper respiratory problems only leaves should be used because flowering tops (especially seeds) contain higher amounts of cardiac glycosides. Otherwise, there are no reports of contraindications or side effects when used properly.

References: (1) Vol. 6, p. 718; (3) Vol. 6b, p. 417; (10) p. 140; (27) p. 119; (35) p. 570; (37) p. 1274; (46) p. 558; (48) p. 203; (51) p. 92.

MUSTARD, WHITE

Other Common Name(s): yellow mustard
Botanical Name(s): *Sinapis alba* L. = *Brassica alba* Rabenh. [Fam.: Brassicaceae (Cruciferae)]
Seed
Constituents: Glucosinolates (chiefly sinalbin = p-hydroxybenzyl-glucosi-

nolate), a bitter principle (sinapine), digestible proteins, phytosterols, fixed oil, mucilaginous polysaccharides, enzymes, etc. Under the action of my-rosinase sinalbin liberates the non volatile p-hydroxybenzyl isothiocyanate, which gives to the seeds and their products a milder and retaining pungent flavor, compared to the black and brown mustards (see MUSTARD).

Properties: Stomachic, antibacterial, rubefacient, counterirritant.

Uses: White mustard is an important ingredient in prepared mustard, used widely as an appetizer, with antioxidant effects. Internally it is used (as a tea, h. p.) for inflammations of the upper respiratory tract (bronchitis, the common cold, etc.). Externally it is used (as a poultice) for inflammations of the respiratory tract (bronchitis, the common cold, etc.) and rheumatic pains.

Caution: It may cause allergic reactions if hypersensitive to white mustard. It should not be consumed in large amounts as it may cause irritations of the gastrointestinal tract, and should be avoided in severe kidney disorders and peptic ulcers. See CRESS, GARDEN; MUSTARD.

References: (1) Vol. 6, p. 705; (3) Vol. 6b, p. 411; (9) p. 379; (13) p. 149; (19) p. 206; (29) p. 108; (37) p. 1272; (47) p. 2556.

MYROBALAN, BELLERIC

Other Common Name(s): bedda nut tree
Botanical Name(s): *Terminalia bellerica* (Gaertn.) Roxb. = *Myrobalanus bellerica* Gaertn. [Fam.: Combretaceae]
Fruit (belleric myrobalan, bedda nut)
Constituents: Tannins (rich in ellagitannins), sugars (glucose, fructose, etc.), triterpenoid saponins (possibly belleric acid and its derivatives), and a blue pigment. Seed contains fixed oil rich in unsaturated fatty acids.
Properties: (Ripe fruit): Bitter tonic, antipyretic, choleretic, astringent. (Half-ripe fruit): Laxative.
Uses: Internally it is used (as a tea, h. p.: ripe fruit, without seed) for loss of appetite and nonulcer dyspepsia, feverish states, and diarrhea; (half-ripe fruit) for constipation. Externally it is used (as a mouthwash, gargle) for in-flammations of the mouth and throat, and (as a wash, wet compress) for skin inflammations, eczema and ulcers. It is widely used in tanning industry.
Caution: Avoid doses higher than recommended. Seeds are reported to ex-ert narcotic effects. In view of this, fruits deprived of seeds should be used only.

References: (1) Vol. 6, p. 916; (3) Vol. 6c, p. 40; (41) Vols. 1-7.

MYROBALAN, CHEBULIC

Other Common Name(s): black myrobalan, true myrobalan
Botanical Name(s): *Terminalia chebula* Retz. [Fam.: Combretaceae]

Fruit (ripe fruit)
Constituents: Tannins (rich in hydrolyzable t.: terchebulin, corilagin, chebulagic acid, etc.), sugars, organic acids (incl. shikimic acid), free amino acids (rich in proline, arginine, asparagine), and it is reported to contain sennoside A. Seed contains fixed oil rich in unsaturated fatty acids.
Properties: Astringent, mild laxative, antibacterial. Chebulagic acid has shown liver protective effect.
Uses: Black myrobalan is chiefly used in tanning industry. Externally it is used (as a mouthwash, gargle) for inflammations of the mouth and throat, and (as a wash) for minor skin inflammations, eczema, wounds and ulcers. Internally it is used (as a tea, h. p.; at low doses) for diarrhea.
Caution: It should not be taken during pregnancy and lactation as shikimic acid has been shown to be mutagenic. Avoid doses higher than recommended.

References: (1) Vol. 6, p. 920; (3) Vol. 6c, p. 37; (31) pp. 32, 524; (37) p. 1355.

MYRRH

Other Common Name(s): myrrh tree
Botanical Name(s): *Commiphora molmol* Engl.; *Commiphora myrrha* (Nees) Engl.; *Commiphora africana* (A. Rich.) Engl.; *Commiphora erythrea* (Ehreb.) Engl.; *Commiphora madacascariensis* Jacq. = *Commiphora abyssinica* (O.Berg) Engl.; *Commiphora schimperi* (O.Berg) Engl. [Fam.: Burseraceae]

Myrrh
It is the hardened gum-oleoresin that exudes naturally or is obtained by incisions made to the bark.
Constituents: Volatile oil (with ethanol-soluble sesquiterpenes), gum (ethanol-insoluble; mainly water-soluble), and resin (with resin acids: commiphoric acids; ethanol-soluble).
Properties: Antimicrobial, analgesic, anti-inflammatory, astringent, wound-healing.
Uses: Externally it is used (as a paint, diluted powder) for gingivitis (= inflammations of the gums), denture sores and canker sores, (as a mouthwash, gargle) for inflammations of the mouth and throat, and (as a paint) for minor wounds and ulcers. Internally it is chiefly used in traditional medicine for inflammatory conditions of the gastrointestinal and upper respiratory tracts.
Caution: It may cause a temporary burning, after paint with the undiluted tincture, and allergic contact dermatitis to persons hypersensitive to it. Internally it should not be used during pregnancy and lactation. Otherwise, there are no reports of contraindications or side effects when used properly.

References: (1) Vol. 4, p. 963; (3) Vol. 4, p. 256; (6) p. 116; (9) p. 382; (11) p. 103; (12) p. 746; (13) p. 138; (14) p. 163; (15) p. 72; (16) p. 90; (17) p. 400; (19) p. 162; (36) p. 289; (48) p. 581.

MYRTLE

Other Common Name(s): wax myrtle
Botanical Name(s): *Myrtus communis* L. [Fam.: Myrtaceae]
Leaf
Constituents: Volatile oil (with 1,8-cineole, limonene, α-pinene, etc.), tannins (hydrolyzable and condensed t.), flavonoids (flavonols, etc.), phloroglucinols (myrtucommulones), etc.
Properties: Astringent, antimicrobial, expectorant (bronchial secretagogue effect). The astringent effect is due to tannins. The rest of the effects are due in large part to cineole. Cf. EUCALYPTUS; CAJUPUT
Uses: Internally it is used (as a tea, h. p.) for inflammations of the upper respiratory tract (the common cold, bronchitis, tracheitis, pharyngitis, laryngitis, sinusitis; coughs due to thickened bronchial secretion), also those of the gastrointestinal tract (diarrhea, etc., incl. hemorrhoids) and genitourinary tract (cystitis, prostatitis, etc.). To enhance the effects in problems of the genitourinary tract, the fluid intake (incl. herbal teas) should be more than 2 liters per day. Externally it is used (as a vaginal irrigation / sitz bath / wash) for leukorrhea and vulvovaginitis, (as a partial bath) for tired and sweating feet, and (as a mouthwash, chewing) for bad breath.
Caution: See EUCALYPTUS.
Myrtol
Myrtol is obtained by fractional distillation (160°-180° C) from myrtle oil (= volatile oil of leaf).
Constituents: Chiefly 1,8-cineole, also limonene, α-pinene, etc.
Properties: Antimicrobial, expectorant (bronchial secretagogue effect).
Uses: Internally it is used for inflammations of the upper respiratory tract (bronchitis, sinusitis, etc.; coughs).
Caution: See EUCALYPTUS.

References: (1) Vol. 5, p. 904; (3) Vol. 5, p. 938; (8) p. 378; (12) p. 726; (27) p. 228; (47) p. 1956; (49) Vol. 2, p. 447; (72) nr. 23062.

NARAS

Botanical Name(s): *Acanthosicyos horridus* Welw. ex Benth et Hook. f. [Fam.: Cucurbitaceae]
Naras oil
It is the fixed oil obtained from the seeds.
Constituents: Chiefly glycerides (fatty acids component: chiefly oleic and linoleic acids), etc.
Properties: Emollient, demulcent, nutrient.
Uses: It is used in cosmetics the same as almond oil, and as edible oil.
Caution: There are no reports of contraindications or side effects when used properly.

Seed

When boiled in water and then dried, seeds gain an almond-like taste. They are consumed as butter pits and in the production of pastries.

References: (1) Vol. 4, p. 44; (5) Vol. 1, p. 10; (52) p. 7.

NEEM

Other Common Name(s): bead tree, margosa
Botanical Name(s): *Azadirachta indica* A. Juss. = *Melia azadirachta* L. [Fam.: Meliaceae]
Bark, Leaf
Constituents: Bitter principles (nortriterpenes of limonoid type: azadirachtin, etc.), flavonoids (flavonols: quercetin, etc.), tannins, etc.
Properties: Antibacterial, antifungal, insecticidal, antihyperglycemic, bitter tonic, febrifuge, antimalarial, anthelmintic, astringent. The mentioned effects are due in large part to nortriterpenes and tannins. Azadirachtin has shown potent insect antifeedant effect, while it is safe for humans.
Uses: Internally it is used (as a tea, h. p.) for feverish states and chronic mallaria, intestinal worms, non-ulcer dyspepsia, and diabetes. Externally it is used (as a wash) for wounds and ulcers, (as a vaginal irrigation / sitz bath / wash) for vulvovaginitis, (as a wash, paste) for pediculosis (= infestation with lice), (as a paint) for gingivitis (= inflammations of the gums), and for fungal skin infections. Neem products (rich in azadirachtin) are used as insect-repellents and insecticides.
Caution: It should not be taken during pregnancy and lactation. At higher doses than recommended it causes gastrointestinal irritations (with nausea, vomiting, diarrhea).
Note: Neem seed oil is used externally for rheumatic pains and skin parasites, among others.

References: (3) Vol. 3, p. 107; (12) p. 98; (13) p. 38; (31) p. 730; (41) Vols. 1-7; (42) Vol. 5, p. 60, 65, 68; (48) p. 765; (52) p. 91.

NETTLE

Other Common Name(s): 1) stinging nettle, nettle 2) dwarf nettle
Botanical Name(s): 1) *Urtica dioica* L. 2) *Urtica urens* L. [Fam.: Urticaceae]
Leaf
Constituents: Flavonoids (flavonols), minerals (potassium, silicic acid, calcium), coumarins (scopoletin), phenolic acids (chlorogenic acid, etc.; dwarf n.: also caffeoyl-malic acid), phytosterols (5-sterols: β-sitosterol, etc.), biogenic amines (histamine, acetylcholine, serotonin), chlorophylls, carotenoids, etc.

265

Properties: Anti-inflammatory, diuretic, local anesthetic, antidiarrheal, hemostatic. The effects are mild. The anti-inflammatory effect is due in large part to caffeoyl-malic acid and other related phenolic acid derivatives, which have been shown to inhibit the biosynthesis of prostaglandins and leukotrienes. The diuretic effect is due in large part to potassium salts.

Uses: Internally it is used as an anti-inflammatory and antidyscratic (= blood purifier; tea, h. p.) for rheumatic complaints (incl. rheumatoid arthritis) and chronic skin disorders, and as a flushing-out treatment (= herbal tea or product + liquids: more than 2 liters per day; sometimes combined with a medication) for inflammations of the genitourinary tract (cystitis, etc.), urinary gravel and nonobstructive stones and to prevent relapsing urinary infections / gravel / stones. It is also used (as a tea, h. p.) for inflammations of the gastrointestinal tract (diarrhea, ulcerative colitis, etc., incl. hemorrhoids; also when minor hemorrhages are present, but on professional's advice). Externally it is used (as an alcoholic liniment, prepared with fresh herb) for rheumatic and neuralgic pains (incl. sciatica), and (as a wet cotton, drops, irrigation with the fresh juice) for nosebleed.

Caution: There are no reports of contraindications or side effects when used properly. Nevertheless, a flushing-out treatment is contraindicated in cases of obstructive urinary stones, edema due to impaired heart or kidney function and kidney inflammations (here can be used on health professional's advice to enhance the effects of an antimicrobial therapy).

Root

Constituents: Phytosterols (5-sterols: β-sitosterol, β-sitosterolin = β-sitosterol-glucoside, etc.), coumarins (scopoletin, etc.), lignans (neo-olivil, etc.), a lectin (UDA = Urtica dioica agglutinin), polysaccharides (incl. water-soluble p.), triterpenes (oleanolic acid, etc.), minerals (silicic acid, etc.), ceramides (= amides of fatty acids), etc.

Properties: Nettle root extract has been shown to inhibit the biosynthesis of DHT (= dihydrotestosterone, one of the main causes of a BPH) in the prostatic tissue as well as its binding to the receptors, with antiproliferative effect (= inhibition of prostatic cell division and growth). The effect is due in large part to phytosterols. UDA and water-soluble polysaccharides account for the anti-inflammatory and immunomodulating effects. Scopoletin has shown anti-inflammatory, antispasmodic and antibacterial effects, among others. To the overall effect may contribute also lignans, triterpenes and silicic acid, among others.

Uses: Internally it is used (as a standardized product) for micturition problems associated with early stages of benign prostatic hyperplasia (= BPH: stages I, II). Rational treatments with nettle root standardized extract have resulted in an increase of urinary volume and flow, decrease of frequency of urination and decrease of residual urine. Externally it is used (as a hair rinse: diluted herbal vinegar) for hair loss.

266

Caution: Before using nettle root products for BPH, the prostate problem should be judged by a health professional. Nettle root products should be standardized to sterols. In rare cases it may cause a mild gastrointestinal discomfort. Otherwise, there are no reports of contraindications or side effects when used properly.

References: (2) Vol. 3, p. 711; (3) Vol. 6c, p. 360; (6) p. 185; (7) p. 253; (8) p. 570; (13) p. 425; (14) p. 166; (15) p. 224; (16) pp. 47, 152; (17) pp. 590, 596; (19) pp. 53, 54; (22) p. 105; (23) pp. 265, 274; (31) p. 364; (46) p. 1056; (47) p. 2746; (48) p. 756; (49) Vol. 2, p. 96.

NETTLE, WHITE

Other Common Name(s): dead nettle
Botanical Name(s): *Lamium album* L. [Fam.: Lamiaceae (Labiatae)]
Flower, aerial part
Constituents: Mucilaginous polysaccharides, triterpenoid saponins, iridoids (lamalbide, etc.), phenolic acids (chlorogenic acid, etc.), phenylethanoid glycosides (lamalboside, acteoside = verbascoside), flavonoids (flavonols), tannins, biogenic amines (histamine, tyramine), and volatile oil (traces).
Properties: Demulcent, expectorant, anti-inflammatory, bitter tonic, diuretic, astringent, antipruritic. Mucilage and saponins account for the demulcent and expectorant effects. The anti-inflammatory effect is due to flavonoids, phenylethanoids, iridoids and phenolic acids. Its bitter tonic effect is due to iridoids.
Uses: Internally it is used (as a tea, h. p.) for inflammations of the upper respiratory tract (bronchitis, etc.; coughs), gastrointestinal tract (gastritis, heartburn, diarrhea, etc., incl. hemorrhoids) and genitourinary tract (cystitis, urethritis, leukorrhea, etc.), and as an anti-inflammatory and antidyscratic (= depurative) for atopic eczema (= chronic eczema of internal origin) and chronic rheumatic complaints. Externally it is used (as a wet compress, poultice) for minor skin inflammations, itching and burns, (as a mouthwash, gargle) for inflammations of the mouth and throat, and (as a vaginal irrigation / sitz bath / wash) for leukorrhea.
Caution: There are no reports of contraindications or side effects when used properly.

References: (2) Vol. 3, p. 26; (3) Vol. 5, p. 441; (6) p. 316; (8) p. 334; (16) pp. 27, 69; (17) p. 331; (19) p. 223; (23) p. 376; (47) p. 1705; (48) p. 608; (51) p. 164.

NEW JERSEY TEA

Other Common Name(s): red root, Jersey tea
Botanical Name(s): *Ceanothus americanus* L. [Fam.: Rhamnaceae]
Leaf
Constituents: Flavonoids (flavonols: quercetin and rutin, kaempferol, etc.;

anthocyanins: cyanidin and delphinidin glycosides), tannins (possibly condensed proanthocyanidins), etc.

Properties: Astringent, antioxidant.

Uses: New Jersey tea is chiefly used as a safe substitute of black tea, beneficial due to its antioxidant effect. Internally it is used (as a tea, h. p.) for minor diarrhea. Externally it is used (as a mouthwash, gargle) for inflammations of the mouth and throat.

Caution: There are no reports of contraindications or side effects when used properly.

Root bark

Constituents: Minor peptide alkaloids (ceanothines, americine, etc.), tannins (hydrolyzable t.), phlobaphenes, organic acids (malonic and malic acids, etc.), phenolic acids (vanillic and syringic acids), etc.

Properties: Astringent, antispasmodic, antimicrobial.

Uses: Internally it is used (as a tea, h. p.) for minor inflammatory and spastic conditions of the gastrointestinal tract (diarrhea, stomachache) and upper respiratory tract (the common cold, spastic bronchitis, bronchial asthma; minor whooping cough). Externally it is used (as a mouthwash, gargle) for inflammations of the mouth and throat, (as a vaginal irrigation / sitz bath / wash) for leukorrhea, and (as a partial bath) for injured and sweating feet.

Caution: When used internally, an experienced practitioner should direct it. It should not be taken during pregnancy and lactation.

References: (1) Vol. 4, p. 746; (3) Vol. 3, p. 778; (25) p. 248; (31) p. 239; (35) p. 673; (44) p. 144; (47) p. 867.

NORI

Botanical Name(s): *Porphyra tenera* Kjellman [Fam.: Bangiaceae]; Class: Rhodophyceae (red algae).

Alga

Constituents: A polysaccharide (with galactose, -sulfate), proteins (with amino acids: glutamic acid, etc.), vitamins (rich in β-carotene = a provitamin A, also B_1, B_2, B_6, niacin, C, folic acid, B_{12}, choline), lipids (phosphatides), minerals (iodine, calcium, sodium, phosphor, iron), volatile oil, etc.

Properties and Uses: Nori is chiefly used as tonic seafood. It is also beneficial for minor cases of endemic goiter (= enlargement of thyroid gland due to iodine deficiency).

Caution: Nori should not be taken in cases of hyperthyroidism (= Basedow's disease). For long-term consumptions, a health professional should be consulted. Manufacturers should evaluate iodine content and advice accordingly.

References: (3) Vol. 6a, p. 840; (5) Vol. 2, p. 90.

268

NUT GRASS

Other Common Name(s): cyperus
Botanical Name(s): *Cyperus rotundus* L. [Fam.: Cyperaceae]
Root (tuberous rhizome)
Constituents: It is reported to contain volatile oil (with sesquiterpenes), triterpenes, flavonoids (possibly flavonols), organic acids, a bitter principle, carbohydrates (sugars, starch, pectin), and alkaloids (possibly of indole type). It possibly contains tannins (condensed t.) and silicic acid.
Properties: Diuretic, demulcent, astringent, carminative, bitter tonic. Nut grass is also reported to exert emmenagogue and galactagogue effects.
Uses: Internally it is used (usually combined with other herbs) as a flushing-out treatment (= herbal tea or product + liquids: more than 2 liters per day; sometimes combined with a medication) for inflammations of the genitourinary tract (cystitis, etc.), urinary gravel and nonobstructive stones, to prevent relapsing urinary infections / gravel / stones, and (as a tea, h. p.) for loss of appetite and nonulcer dyspepsia (with flatulence, minor diarrhea) and feverish states.
Caution: Unless advised by a health professional, it should not be taken during pregnancy and lactation. Manufacturers should run tests for alkaloids and cardiac glycosides. A flushing-out treatment is contraindicated in cases of obstructive urinary stones, edema due to impaired heart or kidney function and kidney inflammations (here can be used on health professional's advice to enhance the effects of an antimicrobial therapy).

References: (3) Vol. 4, p. 422; (5) Vol. 1, p. 384; (18) p. 325; (41) Vols. 1-7; (52) p. 239.

NUTMEG

Botanical Name(s): *Myristica fragrans* Houtt. = *Myristica moschata* Thunb. [Fam.: Myristicaceae]
Seed (nutmeg)
Constituents: Volatile oil (chiefly with monoterpenes: camphene, pinenes, geraniol; also phenylpropanoids: myristicin, elemicin, etc.), fixed oil, starch, proteins, a triterpenoid saponin, phytosterols, etc.
Properties: Aromatic, stomachic, carminative, antispasmodic, anti-inflammatory, antibacterial (against *Salmonella paratyphi*, *Staphylococcus aureus*, etc.). At low doses nutmeg exerts mild antidepressive effect (by inhibiting monoamine oxidase = MAO) and amphetamine-like CNS stimulant effect, which are due to metabolites of myristicin and elemicin.
Uses: Nutmeg is widely used as a spice in culinary practice and is an important flavor ingredient in food industry. Internally it is used (as a tea, h. p.) for nonulcer dyspepsia (with flatulence, bloating, cramps, nausea, etc.) and inflammations of the gastrointestinal tract (diarrhea). In traditional medicine it is also used (at small doses) to improve mood and mental per-

formance. Externally it is used (as an ointment, liniment: with nutmeg oil) for inflammations of the upper respiratory tract (the common cold, etc.), and rheumatic pains.

Caution: There are no reports of contraindications or side effects when used properly (incl. as a spice in small amounts). Nevertheless, nutmeg should not be taken during pregnancy and lactation. It should not be combined with MAOI antidepressant drugs (e. g. phenelzine) or herbs (e. g. St. John's wort) as it may potentiate their effect. At high doses (more than 5 g) it causes headache, drowsiness, confusion, etc., even hallucinations.

Mace (aril, outer cover of nutmeg)
It is richer in volatile oil than the seed. Its volatile oil contains similar constituents, but myristicin is in higher concentrations. Mace is used the same as nutmeg.

References: (1) Vol. 5, p. 867; (3) Vol. 5, p. 920; (8) p. 375; (9) p. 385; (11) p. 97; (12) p. 715; (13) p. 144; (15) p. 147; (29) p. 77; (48) p. 567.

NUX-VOMICA

Other Common Name(s): poison-nut tree, strychnine tree
Botanical Name(s): *Strychnos nux-vomica* L. [Fam.: Loganiaceae]
Seed
Constituents: Indole alkaloids (strychnine, brucine, etc.), fixed oil, triterpenes, phytosterols, etc.
Properties: (At low doses): Bitter tonic (increases secretions of exocrine glands of digestive tract), general tonic (enhances reflexes, the perception of sensory stimuli, and the tonus of smooth and skeletal musculature). The effects are due in large part to strychnine, a stimulant of the central nervous system (esp. of the medulla oblongata and the spinal cord).
Uses: Internally it is used (tincture: mainly in a combination product, at low doses) for loss of appetite and nonulcer dyspepsia (with sluggish bowels), and short-term fatigue. Strychnine has been used as an antidote to poisonings by barbiturates and other sedative-hypnotics, but due to its toxicity and as there are available other drug alternatives it is no longer used for this.
Caution: Nux-vomica should be used on health professional's advice. It should not be used in infants and in cases of severe liver disorders (cumulative effect!). In rare cases, even at low doses, it may cause abnormal increase of the gastric secretion, and reflexes. At high doses, it causes abnormal increase of reflexes, and restlessness. Toxic doses result in spasms of skeletal musculature, tetanic convulsions, respiratory paralysis, and death.

References: (1) Vol. 6, p. 828; (3) Vol. 6b, p. 598; (6) p. 292; (8) p. 537; (11) p. 171; (12) p. 1040; (13) p. 261; (23) p. 316; (36) p. 391; (46) p. 984; (47) p. 1985; (48) p. 1013.

OAK

Other Common Name(s): 1) English oak 2) sessile oak
Botanical Name(s): 1) *Quercus robur* L. 2) *Quercus petraea* (Matt.) Liebl. [Fam.: Fagaceae]
Bark (from the young branches)
Constituents: Tannins (chiefly oligomeric proanthocyanidins = OPCs; rich), flavonoids (flavonols: quercetin; flavan-3-ols: catechins), triterpenes, phytosterols (5-sterols: β-sitosterol, etc.), etc.
Properties: Astringent, hemostatic, antimicrobial, anti-inflammatory, wound-healing. The effects are due in large part to tannins, but also flavonoids contribute to the overall effects.
Uses: Externally it is used (as a mouthwash, gargle) for inflammations of the mouth and throat, (as a wash, partial bath, wet compress) for chilblains, sweating feet, wounds, weeping eczema, (as a vaginal irrigation / sitz bath / wash) for leukorrhea and vulvovaginitis, (as a wet compress, partial bath, enema) for hemorrhoids, (as a wet compress) for sore nipples, and (as a cotton swab, drops, irrigation with the tea) for nosebleed. Internally it is used (as a tea, h. p.) for inflammations of the gastrointestinal tract (diarrhea, ulcerative colitis, etc., incl. hemorrhoids; also when minor hemorrhages are present, but on professional's advice).
Caution: There are no reports of contraindications or side effects when used properly.

References: (1) Vol. 6, p. 341; (3) Vol. 6a, p. 1005; (6) pp. 336, 361; (7) p. 213; (12) p. 884; (13) p. 339; (15) p. 175; (16) pp. 24, 81, 148; (17) p. 472; (19) p. 71; (23) pp. 95, 329; (27) p. 277; (37) p. 1158; (47) p. 2269; (48) p. 388; (51) p. 246.

OAK, GALL

Other Common Name(s): Aleppo oak, Asian holly oak
Botanical Name(s): *Quercus infectoria* G. Olivier [Fam.: Fagaceae]
Gall (nutgall, Aleppo gall)
Constituents: Tannic acid (= tannin: a mixture of hexa- and hepta-galloyl-glucose; very rich), gallic acid, ellagic acid, sugars, starch, gum, resin, volatile oil (small amounts).
Properties: Astringent, hemostatic.
Uses: Galls are chiefly used as a natural source in the production of tannic acid. Externally it is used (as a paint) for gingivitis (= inflammations of the gums) and chilblains, (as a mouthwash, gargle) for inflammations of the mouth and throat, and (as an ointment) for minor skin inflammations, eczema and hemorrhoids, among others. Internally it is used (as a suppository combination product) for hemorrhoids. Raw tannic acid is used in leather industry.
Caution: It should not be applied to a large area when the skin is damaged. Internally should be used only products standardized to tannin content.

271

Chinese gall (Japanese gall, sumac gall)
It is formed on Chinese sumac, nutgall tree: *Rhus chinensis* Mill. [Fam.: Anacardiaceae]. Tannic acid produced from them consists of octa- and nona-galloyl-glucose. Chinese gall is chiefly used in the production of gallic acid.

References: (1) Vol. 6, p. 337; (3) Vol. 6a, p. 1015; (9) p. 485; (11) p. 142; (12) p. 879; (13) p. 338; (36) pp. 228, 495; (37) p. 570; (48) p. 388.

OAT

Botanical Name(s): *Avena sativa* L. [Fam.: Poaceae (Gramineae)]
Oat (oat grain)
Constituents: Carbohydrates (chiefly starch, also cellulose and water-soluble polysaccharides), proteins (incl. gluten), lipids (fixed oil, phytosterols), minerals (silicic acid, etc.), vitamins (esp. B complex), steroidal saponins (avenacosides), avenein (= vanillin-glucoside), etc.
Properties: Nutrient, tonic, demulcent, emollient, cholesterol reducing. Water-soluble polysaccharides may account for the cholesterol reducing effect, same as mucilage of psyllium (see PSYLLIUM). To this effect may contribute steroidal saponins (see FENUGREEK). Water-soluble polysaccharides may also exert mild immunomodulating effect.
Uses: Internally it is used as a nutrient and as a dietary aid for convalescence, minor fatigue, high cholesterol and triglycerides, and for inflammations of the gastrointestinal tract (gastritis, peptic ulcers, diarrhea) and genitourinary tract. Externally it is used (as a poultice, partial bath) for minor skin inflammations.
Caution: Oat should not be consumed by persons that have shown gluten intolerance. Otherwise, there are no reports of contraindications or side effects when used properly.

Aerial part
Constituents: Minerals (rich in silicic acid, iron and zinc), flavonoids (chiefly flavones: vitexin, apigenin, etc.), steroidal saponins (avenacosides), carbohydrates (chiefly glucose polymers), etc.
Properties: Tonic, sedative, diuretic, emollient, anti-inflammatory.
Uses: Internally it is used (as an h. p.; usually combined with other herbs) for minor fatigue, insomnia, loss of appetite, high cholesterol, and rheumatic complaints. Externally it is used (as a partial bath) for minor skin inflammations and rheumatic pains.
Caution: There are no reports of contraindications or side effects when used properly.

References: (1) Vol. 4, p. 438; (3) Vol. 3, p. 342; (8) p. 94; (13) p. 402; (16) p. 30; (17) p. 92; (25) p. 146; (27) p. 45; (35) p. 597; (37) p. 166; (47) p. 649; (51) p. 48.

OKRA

Botanical Name(s): *Abelmoschus esculentus* (L.) Moench = *Hibiscus esculentus* L. [Fam.: Malvaceae]

Fruit (unripe, fresh)

Constituents: Mucilaginous polysaccharides, proteins, volatile oil (in seeds, with musk-like aroma), etc.

Properties: Demulcent, diuretic, antihyperglycemic, emollient.

Uses: Internally it is used as an adjuvant for inflammations and ulcerations of the gastrointestinal tract (gastritis, peptic ulcers, etc.), minor inflammations of the genitourinary tract (cystitis, etc.), and diabetes. Externally it is used (as a poultice) for minor skin inflammations. Okra fruits are extensively used as a vegetable, beneficial due also to the mentioned effects.

Caution: In rare cases it may cause contact dermatitis. Otherwise, there are no reports of contraindications or side effects when used properly.

Seed is traditionally roasted and used as a coffee substitute (Gombo coffee).

Root is rich in mucilaginous polysaccharides and has been used as a substitute for marshmallow root.

References: (1) Vol. 4, p. 4; (3) Vol. 5, p. 80; (37) p. 1; (52) p. 1.

OLEANDER

Botanical Name(s): *Nerium oleander* L. [Fam.: Apocynaceae]

Leaf

Constituents: Cardiac glycosides (oleandrin, etc., with aglycone oleandrigenin = 16-acetyl-gitoxigenin), flavonoids (flavonols), a polysaccharide, etc.

Properties: Digitalis-like cardiotonic. Compared to digitalis it acts quicker, less intensive, less cumulative, and is a strong diuretic. See DIGITALIS.

Uses: Internally it is used (as a standardized combination product, only combined with lily-of-the-valley or squill, but not digitalis) for early stages of heart failure.

Caution: Oleander is toxic and not for self-treatment. It is used only as directed by a health professional. Oleander products should be standardized to the cardiac glycosides content. See DIGITALIS.

References: (2) Vol. 3, p. 240; (3) Vol. 6a, p. 179; (7) p. 110; (8) p. 382; (12a) p. 575; (13) p. 191; (36) p. 318; (46) p. 996; (48) p. 749.

OLIVE

Botanical Name(s): *Olea europaea* L. [Fam.: Oleaceae]

Leaf

Constituents: Bitter principles (a seco-iridoid: oleuropein = oleuropeoside; oleanolic acid), triterpenes (oleanolic and crataegolic acids), a phenylethanoid glycoside (acteoside = verbascoside), a biogenic amine (choline), fla-

273

vonoids (flavones, flavonols), tannins (hydrolyzable t.), phytosterols, squalene, etc.

Properties: Peripheral vasodilatory, antispasmodic, antihypertensive, antiarrhythmic, diuretic, antihyperglycemic, cholesterol and triglyceride reducing, antipyretic, antioxidant. The effects are mild. Oleuropein has shown peripheral vasodilatory, antihypertensive and antiarrhythmic effects. As with other bitter seco-iridoids, oleuropein exerts immunomodulating effect (see GENTIAN). It may act in synergism with squalene, which has shown antibacterial and immunomodulating effects. Acteoside has been shown to be anti-inflammatory (by inhibit the biosynthesis of leukotrienes) and liver protective.

Uses: Internally it is used (the standardized extract, often combined with other herbs) as an adjuvant for minor cases of hypertension and diabetes, and as a preventive for arteriosclerosis and coronary heart disease (= a condition associated with decreased blood supply to the heart). In traditional medicine it is also used for feverish states and rheumatic complaints (incl. rheumatoid arthritis). Based on the traditional uses and the effects of constituents, it may be beneficial as a mild immunostimulant for common and relapsing bacterial and viral infections. Oleuropein is an unstable glycoside therefore extracts are mostly prepared from fresh leaves.

Caution: Olive leaf is best used as a standardized product to oleuropein. At higher doses than recommended it may cause gastrointestinal irritations (with nausea, vomiting). Otherwise, there are no reports of contraindications or side effects when used properly.

Olive oil
It is the fixed oil obtained by cold expression from the ripe fruits.

Constituents: Chiefly glycerides (fatty acids component: chiefly oleic acid, also palmitic and linoleic acids), also phytosterols (5-sterols: β-sitosterol, etc.), squalene, etc.

Properties: Nutrient, demulcent, emollient, cholagogue, mild laxative. Squalene has shown antibacterial, immunomodulant and antitumoral effects. Olive oil has been shown to increase levels of HDL due in large part to oleic acid, a monounsaturated fatty acid.

Uses: Internally it is used for complaints of the biliary tract (inflammations, nonobstructive gallstones, sluggish gallbladder) and gastrointestinal tract (hyperacidity, flatulence, gastrointestinal ulcers, constipation), among others. A regular consumption (with salads, etc.) has been shown to be beneficial by modifying blood cholesterol levels (it increases levels of HDL) and by improving immune response. Externally it is used (as a liniment, ointment, soap, oil) for minor burns, skin irritations due to psoriasis and eczematous crusts, (as a warm enema) to soften hardened stools, and as massage oil. It is also used as a solvent for fat-soluble drugs.

Caution: For problems of the biliary tract, olive oil should be used on health professional's advice. When applied externally, in rare cases it may cause skin allergic reactions. Otherwise, there are no reports of contraindications or side effects when used properly.

References: (1) Vol. 5, p. 936; (3) Vol. 6a, p. 306; (6) p. 58; (8) p. 387; (12) p. 254; (13) pp. 386, 418; (23) p. 193; (27) p. 238; (28) p. 145; (31) pp. 576, 744; (37) p. 994; (46) p. 1012; (48) pp. 143, 602; (49) Vol. 3, p. 27; (65) p. 102; (72) nr.16006.

ONION

Botanical Name(s): *Allium cepa* L. [Fam.: Liliaceae (Alliaceae)]
Bulb
Constituents: Sulfur compounds (based on cysteine sulfoxide: homologues of alliin of garlic, and peptides), flavonoids (quercetin, in yellow and red sorts), phenolic acids (brown yellow shells are very rich in protocatechuic acid), carbohydrates (fructose polymers, sugar alcohols, sucrose), adenosine, etc.
Properties: Antibacterial, anti-inflammatory, wound-healing, antasthmatic, mild antihypertensive, diuretic, cholesterol and triglyceride reducing, platelet aggregation inhibitory, antioxidant, antihyperglycemic. Most of the effects are attributed to sulfur-containing compounds. Flavonoids contribute to the diuretic and antioxidant effects, while protocatechuic acid has shown liver protective, anti-inflammatory, and antifungal effects, among others.
Uses: Internally it is used (as an h. p., fresh onion) for inflammatory and spastic conditions of the upper respiratory tract (the common cold, bronchitis, bronchial asthma; coughs), gastrointestinal tract (loss of appetite, flatulence, minor cramps), as an adjuvant for hypertension and diabetes, and for the prevention of high cholesterol and triglycerides and arteriosclerosis. Externally it is used (as an ointment, poultice) for bruises, sprains, boils, insect bites, and (as a liniment) for hair loss.
Caution: There are no reports of contraindications or side effects when used or consumed properly.

References: (1) Vol. 4, p. 184; (3) Vol. 2, p. 1213; (6) pp. 67, 110, 364; (7) p. 137; (8) p. 33; (9) p. 391; (13) p. 154; (24) p. 369; (27) p. 94; (31) p. 461; (37) p. 45; (47) p. 880; (48) p. 209; (59) p. 5.

ORANGE, BITTER

Botanical Name(s): *Citrus × aurantium* L. [Fam.: Rutaceae]
Peel (most of the white layer removed)
Constituents: Volatile oil (with limonene, etc.), bitter principles (flavanone neohesperidosides: neohesperidin, naringin; if white layer is present, nortriterpenes of limonoid type), flavonoids (hesperidin, rutin, etc.), etc.
Properties: Aromatic, bitter tonic, mild antispasmodic.
Uses: Internally it is used (as a tea, h. p.) for loss of appetite and nonulcer dyspepsia (with flatulence, etc.), and as a flavor ingredient in drug products.

Caution: When handling the herb avoid contact with skin and then exposure to strong sunrays as it may cause phototoxic skin irritations, due to its high limonene content.

Fruit (unripe)

Constituents: Bitter principles (peel: flavanone neohesperidosides; seeds: nortriterpenes), volatile oil (with linalyl acetate, etc.), organic acids (citric and malic acids), pectin, tannins, etc.

Properties and Uses: Almost the same as peel.

Caution: It doesn't seem to cause photosensitization.

References: (3) Vol. 4, p. 83; (6) pp. 133, 134, 290; (7) p. 189; (8) p. 169; (12) p. 676; (13) p. 166; (17) pp. 88, 89; (19) p. 181; (27) p. 36; (29) p. 32; (37) p. 337; (46) p. 95; (47) p. 642; (49) Vol. 2, p. 296.

OREGANO

Other Common Name(s): "European Oregano" (here: Greek Oregano, known as such; Turkish Oregano, known as such)

Botanical Name(s): *Origanum vulgare* L. ssp. *viride* (Boiss.) Hayek = *Origanum heracleoticum* L.; *Origanum vulgare* L. ssp. *hirtum* (Link) Ietswaart = *Origanum heracleoticum* auct. non L.; other *Origanum vulgare* L. ssp.; *Origanum onites* L.; [Fam.: Lamiaceae (Labiatae)]

Aerial part

It is the dried and rubbed aerial part of spicy *Origanum* spp. with volatile oil rich in carvacrol.

Constituents: Volatile oil (see Oregano oil; pungent taste), a bitter principle (a flavanone neohesperidoside: naringin), flavonoids, Lamiaceae tannins (rosmarinic acid and other caffeic acid derivatives), phenolic acids (vanillic acid, syringic acid, Lamiaceae tannins), etc.

Properties: Aromatic, antibacterial, antifungal, expectorant, antispasmodic, choleretic, carminative, anti-inflammatory, antioxidant, diuretic. The mentioned properties are due in large part to the volatile oil with its constituents and phenolic acids. Rosmarinic acid and other related phenolic acid derivatives have been shown to inhibit the biosynthesis of prostaglandins and leukotrienes (this explains its anti-inflammatory effect) and exert choleretic, antibacterial, and antiviral effects.

Uses: Oregano is chiefly used as a spice in culinary practice and food industry. Internally it is used (as a tea, h. p.) for inflammatory and spastic conditions of the upper respiratory tract (bronchitis, laryngitis, pharyngitis, minor bronchial asthma; coughs due to thickened bronchial secretion), gastrointestinal tract (flatulence, minor cramps, diarrhea), genitourinary and hepatobiliary tracts, and as a diaphoretic hot tea for the common cold. To enhance the effects in problems of the genitourinary tract, the fluid intake (incl. herbal teas) should be more than 2 liters per day. Externally it is used (as a mouthwash, gargle) for inflammations of the mouth and throat, (as an ointment) for wounds, and (as a partial bath) for rheumatic pains.

276

Caution: There are no reports of contraindications or side effects when used properly. Nevertheless, a consumption of excessive amounts should be avoided during pregnancy and lactation and in cases of biliary obstruction.

Oregano oil

It is the volatile oil obtained by steam distillation from the aerial part.

Constituents: Carvacrol as its major constituent, also γ-terpinene, p-cymene, thymol, and other terpenes (chiefly monoterpenes).

Properties: Aromatic, antiseptic, etc., much like aerial part (q. v.).

Uses: Oregano oil is used internally (a few drops on sugar, in capsules) and externally (in a combination product) for almost the same conditions as the herb.

Caution: Oregano oil causes skin irritation therefore an application of the undiluted oil should be avoided.

References: (1) Vol. 5, p. 959; (3) Vol. 6a, p. 332; (9) p. 398; (29) p. 80; (37) p. 1008; (47) p. 2036; (48) p. 539; (51) p. 170.

OREGANO, MEXICAN

Other Common Name(s): Mexican sage
Botanical Name(s): *Lippia graveolens* Kunth. [Fam.: Verbenaceae]
Aerial part
Constituents: Volatile oil (with carvacrol, thymol, p-cymene, 1,8-cineole, etc.), bitter principles (iridoids; a flavanone neohesperidoside: naringin, in higher concentrations than oregano), flavonoids, naphthoquinones (lapachenole, etc.), etc.
Properties: Aromatic, bitter tonic, antimicrobial, etc., much like oregano (= "European Oregano"; see OREGANO), and it is reported to exert emmenagogic and antifertility effects. Compared to "European Oregano" it is bitterer and less pungent. Lapachenole has been shown to be carcinogenic and may account for the reported antifertility effect.
Uses: Mexican oregano is chiefly used as a spice. In traditional medicine it is used as a natural remedy for birth control.
Caution: It should not be taken during pregnancy. It may cause contact allergic reactions, due in large part to naphthoquinones. See also OREGANO.

References: (1) Vol. 5, p. 688; (9) p. 398; (31) pp. 381, 545; (52) p. 449.

OREGON GRAPE

Other Common Name(s): holly-leaf barberry, mountain grape, Oregon grapeholly, Oregon barberry
Botanical Name(s): *Mahonia aquifolium* (Pursh) Nutt. = *Berberis aquifolium* Pursh [Fam.: Berberidaceae]
Root (adventitious root), **bark**

Constituents, Properties, Uses, and Caution: Much like European barberry. See BARBERRY. Externally it is used (as an ointment that contains its tincture) for psoriasis and common acne (= acne vulgaris), and (as a vaginal irrigation / sitz bath / wash / suppository) for vulvovaginitis.

Berry (ripe)
Constituents, Properties, Uses, and Caution: Much like European barberry. See BARBERRY.

References: (1) Vol. 5, p. 746; (6) p. 351; (15) p. 40; (19) p. 861; (29) p. 73; (44) p. 328; (68) p. 18; (71) p. 282; (72) nr. 31273.

ORRIS

Botanical Name(s): *Iris germanica* L.; *Iris germanica* L. var. *florentina* = *Iris florentina* auct.; *Iris pallida* Lam. [Fam.: Iridaceae]
Root (peeled rhizome)
Constituents: Volatile oil (with irones, etc.), mucilaginous polysaccharides, tannins, triterpenes, xanthones, phytosterols (5-sterols: β-sitosterol, etc.), flavonoids (isoflavones, etc.), phenolic acids, starch (rich), wax, etc.
Properties: Aromatic, mild expectorant, demulcent, antidiarrheal, diuretic.
Uses: Internally it is used (as a tea, h. p.) for inflammations of the upper respiratory tract (bronchitis, etc.; coughs) and gastrointestinal tract (diarrhea, vomiting). Orris is widely used as a fragrance and fixative ingredient in perfumery. It is also used as a flavor ingredient in some oral hygiene products (toothpastes, lozenges for bad breath, etc.) and liqueurs and bitters.
Caution: There are no reports of contraindications or side effects when used properly.

References: (2) Vol. 2, p. 875; (3) Vol. 5, p. 275; (8) p. 325; (12) p. 616; (15) p. 119; (17) p. 316; (27) p. 169; (28) p. 79; (36) p. 327; (37) p. 730; (41) Vols. 1-7; (46) p. 773; (49) Vol. 2, p. 76.

OSHA

Other Common Name(s): Porter's lovage
Botanical Name(s): *Ligusticum porteri* J.M. Coult. et Rose [Fam.: Apiaceae (Umbelliferae)]
Root
Constituents: Alkyl-phthalides (diligustilide, riligustilide), normally, steam-distilling. Other possible constituents are coumarins, furanocoumarins, polyacetylenes, and phenolic acids (cf. DONG QUAI; LOVAGE-s).
Properties: Antispasmodic, expectorant, bitter tonic, antibacterial. The antispasmodic effect may be due to alkyl-phthalides. Both diligustilide and riligustilide are dimers of ligustilide, which has shown strong antispasmodic effect (see DONG QUAI; LOVAGE).
Uses: Internally it is used (as a tea, h. p.) for inflammatory and spastic conditions of the upper respiratory tract (bronchitis, pharyngitis, minor bron-

278

chial asthma, etc.; coughs), genitourinary tract (primary dysmenorrhea, etc.), and gastrointestinal tract (heartburn, flatulence, bloating, nausea, vomiting, cramps). <u>Externally</u> it is used (as a gargle) for sore throat.

Caution: Osha is best avoided during pregnancy and lactation. It possibly contains phototoxic linear furanocoumarins as its active constituents. In Apiaceae, the alkaloids are seldom found, but some *Ligusticum* spp. is reported to contain them. Manufacturers should evaluate furanocoumarins and alkaloids, and then advise accordingly.

References: (18) p. 273; (29) p. 70; (41) Vols. 1-7; (42) Vol. 6, p. 585; (44) p. 306; (48) p. 519; (52) p. 444.

OSWEGO TEA

Other Common Name(s): Oswego beebalm, scarlet beebalm, scarlet monarda
Botanical Name(s): *Monarda didyma* L. [Fam.: Lamiaceae (Labiatae)]
Aerial part
Constituents: Volatile oil (chiefly with phenols: thymol, carvacrol, thymohydroquinone; also linalool, limonene, etc.), flavonoids (chiefly flavonols: quercetin glycosides, incl. rutin, hyperin, quercitrin; methoxy-flavones: genkwanin and its glycosides; flavanones: isosakuranetin and naringenin glycosides; anthocyanins), triterpenes (ursolic acid, etc.), phytosterols (5-sterols: β-sitosterol, etc.), bitter principles (ursolic acid, possibly diterpenoid lactones), Lamiaceae tannins (rosmarinic acid and other caffeic acid derivatives), etc.
Properties: Aromatic, bitter tonic, antispasmodic, carminative, diuretic, anti-inflammatory, antimicrobial, expectorant, astringent, antioxidant.
Uses: <u>Internally</u> it is used as a caffeine-free, pleasant-tasting, and antioxidant tea substitute. It is beneficial for loss of appetite and nonulcer dyspepsia (with flatulence, minor cramps, minor diarrhea), the common cold and feverish states (taken as a diaphoretic hot tea), and for mild inflammatory and spastic conditions of the genitourinary tract.
Caution: There are no reports of contraindications or side effects when used properly. Nevertheless, Oswego tea is best avoided during pregnancy and lactation.

References: (3) Vol. 5, p. 880; (25) p. 162; (29) p. 76; (37) p. 918; (44) p. 346; (52) p. 505; (57) p. 539.

PAPAYA

Botanical Name(s): *Carica papaya* L. [Fam.: Caricaceae]
Papain (raw papain = papayotin)
Raw papain is the dried juice that flows after shallow incisions made to the full-grown but unripe fruit of papaya.

Constituents: Chiefly enzymes (papain, chymopapains, etc.).
Properties: Proteolytic (= splits proteins).
Uses: Internally it is used as a digestant (usually combined with other enzymes) for dyspeptic disorders (with impaired digestion of proteinic foods) chiefly associated with impaired external secretion of pancreas. It is also used as an adjuvant to prevent edemas after surgeries or traumatic injuries (esp. in the nasal and paranasal cavities) and for thrombophlebitis (= inflammation of a vein associated with an attached blood clot / thrombus). In food industry it is used as a meat tenderizer. Externally it is used as an ingredient in some dental / oral hygiene products.
Caution: It should not be taken during pregnancy and in cases of clotting disorders. A possible combination of papain products with anticoagulants (warfarin, etc.) and / or platelet aggregation inhibitors (aspirin, etc.) should be made only by a health professional. Papain may cause contact dermatitis and irritations of the respiratory tract (if the powder is inhaled). Papain products should contain papain standardized to its proteolytic activity.

References: (2) Vol. 2, p. 291; (3) Vol. 3, p. 711; (11) p. 190; (13) p. 442; (19) p. 168; (21) p. 279; (23) p. 390; (37) pp. 279, 1024; (47) p. 842; (48) p. 221; (67) p. 846.

PARSLEY

Botanical Name(s): *Petroselinum crispum* (Mill.) Nyman ex A.W. Hill = *Petroselinum sativum* Hoffm. [Fam.: Apiaceae (Umbelliferae)]
Aerial part, root
Constituents: Volatile oil (with apiole, myristicin, etc.; the aerial part is richer), flavonoids (flavones: apiin, etc.; the aerial part is richer), furanocoumarins (higher concentrations in root), polyacetylenes (in root only), etc.
Properties: Diuretic, antispasmodic, carminative, emmenagogue, mild uterotonic. The effects are due in large part to the volatile oil and flavonoids. Apiole has shown antispasmodic, vasodilatory and emmenagogic effects. Myristicin has shown antispasmodic and MAO (= monoamine oxidase) inhibitory effects. Flavonoids contribute mainly to the diuretic effect.
Uses: Internally it is chiefly used (usually combined with other herbs) as a flushing-out treatment (= herbal tea or product + liquids: more than 2 liters per day; sometimes combined with a medication) for inflammations of the genitourinary tract (cystitis, etc.), urinary gravel and nonobstructive stones and to prevent relapsing urinary infections / gravel / stones. It is also used (as a tea, h. p.) for primary dysmenorrhea (= painful menstruation without pathology) and secondary amenorrhea and oligomenorrhea (= ceased / infrequent / scanty menstruation without pathology), as an antidyscratic (= depurative) for chronic rheumatic complaints, and (combined with other herbs) for minor inflammatory and spastic conditions of the gastrointestinal and biliary tracts (flatulence, intestinal cramps, nonobstructive gallstones).

Externally it is used (as a poultice with fresh leaves) applied on breast to stop the secretion of milk in nursing mothers, (as a poultice) for insect bites, and (as a mouthwash, chewing) for bad breath.

Caution: Parsley should not be taken during pregnancy. Unless advised by a health professional, parsley should not be taken during lactation. Before using it for gynecologic disorders, the problem should be judged by a health professional. When handling the herb avoid contact with skin, and when taking its products (esp. root products) avoid exposure to strong sunrays as it may cause phototoxic skin irritations. A flushing-out treatment is contra-indicated in cases of obstructive urinary stones, edema due to impaired heart or kidney function and kidney inflammations (here can be used on health professional's advice to enhance the effects of an antimicrobial therapy).

References: (1) Vol. 6, p. 105; (3) Vol. 6a, p. 542; (6) p. 183; (8) p. 417; (13) p. 128; (14) p. 168; (15) p. 154; (16) p. 163; (17) p. 432; (19) p. 175; (20) p. 203; (22) p. 92; (23) p. 255; (27) p. 267; (29) p. 84; (31) p. 484; (47) p. 2089; (48) p. 519; (51) p. 128.

PARSLEY PIERT

Other Common Name(s): parsley breakstone
Botanical Name(s): *Aphanes arvensis* L. = *Alchemilla arvensis* (L.) Scop. [Fam.: Rosaceae]
Aerial part
Constituents: No reports are available. It possibly contains similar con-stituents of a better-known species, namely *Alchemilla xanthochlora*. See LADY'S MANTLE.
Properties: Diuretic, demulcent, astringent, wound-healing.
Uses: Internally it is used (as a tea, h. p.; usually combined with other herbs) for inflammations (also when minor hemorrhages are present) of the geni-tourinary tract (cystitis, urethritis, urinary gravel and nonobstructive stoness; menorrhagia / hypermenorrhea = prolonged / heavy menstruation) and gas-trointestinal tract (diarrhea, ulcerative colitis, etc., incl. hemorrhoids). To enhance the effects in problems of the genitourinary tract, the fluid intake (incl. herbal teas) should be more than 2 liters per day. Externally it is used (as a wet compress, poultice) for minor skin inflammations and wounds.
Caution: For minor hemorrhages and gynecologic disorders it should be used on health professional's advice. Otherwise, there are no reports of con-traindications or side effects when used properly.

References: (3) Vol. 3, p. 117; (10) p. 209; (15) p. 27; (18) p. 168; (20) p. 205; (35) p. 615; (45) p. 167; (52) p. 60.

PARTRIDGE BERRY

Other Common Name(s): squawvine
Botanical Name(s): *Mitchella repens* L. [Fam.: Rubiaceae]

281

Aerial part

Constituents: Largely unknown. It has been reported to contain glycosides, tannins and mucilage. There are also controversial reports on alkaloids. Possibly among the reported glycosides are iridoids and triterpenoid saponins. Tannins may be of condensed type (incl. proanthocyanidins).

Properties: Emmenagogue, uterotonic, mild oxytocic, hemostatic, diuretic, astringent, demulcent.

Uses: Internally it is used (as a tea, h. p.) for secondary amenorrhea and oligomenorrhea (= ceased / infrequent / scanty menstruation without pathology), menorrhagia / hypermenorrhea (= prolonged / heavy menstruation), postpartum hemorrhage (= h. following childbirth), as an adjuvant for metrorrhagia (= nonmenstrual uterine bleeding), and a hypotonic uterus in general. It is also used for inflammations (also when minor hemorrhages are present) of the genitourinary tract (cystitis, etc.), and gastrointestinal tract (diarrhea, etc., incl. hemorrhoids). Externally it is used (as a wet compress, poultice) for small cuts and wounds.

Caution: Partridge berry is not an herb for self-treatment. It should be used only as directed by a health professional. Depending on doses and pregnancy stage, it may support a pregnancy or induce labor / abortion. Manufacturers should evaluate the reported alkaloids.

References: (3) Vol. 5, p. 871; (15) p. 146; (18) p. 248; (25) p. 26; (32) Vol. 3, p. 1322; (35) p. 766; (36) pp. 47, 477; (44) p. 345; (45) p. 234; (47) p. 1920; (52) p. 503; (57) p. 537; (71) p. 10.

PASSIONFLOWER

Other Common Name(s): apricot vine, maypop, wild passionflower
Botanical Name(s): *Passiflora incarnata* L. [Fam.: Passifloraceae]
Aerial part
Constituents: Flavonoids (flavones: chiefly apigenin-C-glycosides, incl. isovitexin, vitexin, schaftoside, etc.; etc.), a γ-pyrone derivative (maltol = laricinic acid), coumarins, volatile oil (traces), indole alkaloids (harman, etc.; traces or absent), glycoproteins, phenolic acids, cyanogenic glycosides, etc.

Properties: Sedative, anxiolytic (GABA-mimetic effect), antispasmodic, mild muscle relaxant. The effects are due in large part to C-glycosylflavones and maltol, both γ-pyrone derivatives (flavonoids are benzo γ-pyrone derivatives), and possibly indole alkaloids (although in traces) and coumarins.

Uses: Internally it is used (as an h. p., tea; usually combined with other herbs) for nervousness, anxiety, insomnia, and nervous cardiac disorders (tachycardia = rapid heartbeat). Passionflower may be beneficial for primary dysmenorrhea (= painful menstruation without pathology), mild withdrawal syndromes (after stopping a prolonged use of alcohol or benzodiazepines), minor cases of chorea (= a nervous disorder with involuntary jerky movements mainly of limbs and face), and as an adjuvant for epilepsy.

282

Caution: There are no reports of contraindications or side effects when used properly. A possible combination of passionflower with sedative, hypnotic, and antidepressant drugs should be made only by a health professional.

References: (1) Vol. 6, p. 35; (3) Vol. 6a, p. 473; (6) p. 215; (7) p. 90; (8) p. 408; (12) p. 862; (13) p. 419; (14) p. 171; (16) p. 182; (17) p. 419; (19) p. 172; (20) p. 206; (22) p. 159; (41) Vols. 1-7; (46) p. 1080; (47) p. 2070; (48) p. 331; (66) p. 372.

PATCHOULY

Botanical Name(s): *Pogostemon cablin* (Blanco) Benth. = *Pogostemon patchouly* Pellet. [Fam.: Lamiaceae (Labiatae)]
Leaf
Constituents: Volatile oil (see Patchouly oil), tannins, etc.
Properties: Aromatic, antibacterial, antispasmodic, mild astringent, and it is claimed to be aphrodisiac.
Uses: Internally it is used (as a tea, h. p.; usually combined with other herbs) for inflammations of the upper respiratory tract (the common cold, bronchitis; coughs) and gastrointestinal tract (nausea, vomiting, minor cramps, diarrhea), and as an adjuvant for headaches. Externally it is used (as a mouthwash, gargle) for inflammations of the mouth and throat, and (as a mouthwash) for bad breath.
Caution: There are no reports of contraindications or side effects when used properly.
Patchouly oil
It is the volatile oil obtained by steam distillation from the partly fermented leaves.
Constituents: Chiefly patchouly alcohol (= patchouly camphor), norpatchoulenol, dhelwangine (= pogostone), eugenol, benzaldehyde, cinnamic aldehyde, etc.
Properties: Aromatic, insect-repellent.
Uses: Patchouly oil is chiefly used as a fragrance ingredient in cosmetics and perfumery. It is also used as an insect-repellent.
Caution: There are no reports of contraindications or side effects when used properly.

References: (3) Vol. 6a, p. 796; (9) p. 411; (29) p. 89; (37) p. 1097; (41) Vols. 1-7; (45) p. 250; (48) p. 548; (52) p. 616.

PAU D'ARCO

Other Common Name(s): lapacho
Botanical Name(s): *Tabebuia impetiginosa* (Mart. ex DC.) Standl. = *Tabebuia avellanedae* Lorentz ex Griseb. [Fam.: Bignoniaceae]
Bark (inner bark)

Constituents: Naphthoquinones (lapachol, lapachone, xyloidone, etc.; heartwood is much richer), phenolic acids (veratric acid, etc.), tannins, coumarins, flavonoids, saponins, etc.

Properties: Antibacterial (against some *Bacillus* spp., *S. aureus*, etc.), antifungal (against *Candida* spp.), immunomodulant, astringent, anti-inflammatory. Lapachol has been shown to inhibit certain tumors.

Uses: Internally it is used (as a tea, h. p.) for inflammations of the upper respiratory tract (the common cold, bronchitis, etc.), gastrointestinal tract (gastritis, diarrhea, etc.) and genitourinary tract (cystitis, urethritis, prostatitis, etc.), and for feverish states. To enhance the effects in problems of the genitourinary tract, the fluid intake (incl. herbal teas) should be more than 2 liters per day. In traditional medicine it is also used for certain tumors and leukemia. Externally it is used (as a wash, wet compress) for minor skin inflammations, fungal infections, eczema, wounds and ulcers, (as a poultice, ointment) for boils, and (as a vaginal irrigation / sitz bath / wash) for vulvovaginitis.

Caution: Powdered herb may cause allergic irritations of the skin and the upper respiratory tract. Otherwise, there are no reports of contraindications or side effects when used properly.

References: (1) Vol. 6, p. 883; (3) Vol. 6c, p. 29; (6) p. 284; (21) p. 287; (31) p. 501; (37) p. 1341; (41) Vols. 1-7; (48) p. 415; (52) p. 776; (89) p. 220.

PEACH

Botanical Name(s): *Prunus persica* (L.) Batsch = *Amygdalus persica* L. [Fam.: Rosaceae]

Peach oil (= persic oil)
It is the fixed oil, not the volatile oil, obtained by cold expression from the seeds.

Constituents: Chiefly glycerides (fatty acids component: chiefly oleic acid, also linoleic, palmitic and stearic acids), etc.

Properties: Emollient, demulcent, mild laxative.

Uses: Peach oil is used the same as almond oil (see ALMOND).
Externally it is used for chapped hands and as an ingredient in cold creams and lipsticks. Internally it is used for minor constipation.

Caution: Peach oil should not be taken in cases of bowel obstruction. Otherwise, there are no reports of contraindications or side effects when used properly. See also ALMOND.

Leaf

Constituents: A cyanogenic glycoside (amygdalin), phenolic acids, phytosterols, triterpenes, tannins, hydrocarbons, etc.

Properties: Antitussive (cough suppressant effect), sedative, diuretic.

Uses: Internally it is sometimes used as a substitute of cherry laurel (see CHERRY LAUREL).

284

Caution: Peach leaf should not be taken during pregnancy and lactation. See CHERRY LAUREL.

References: (3) Vol. 6a, p. 949; (5) Vol. 1, p. 881; (11) p. 73; (35) p. 619; (37) p. 189.

PEANUT

Botanical Name(s): *Arachis hypogaea* L. [Fam.: Fabaceae (Leguminosae)]
Peanut oil (= arachis oil)
It is the fixed oil obtained by expression from the seeds.
Constituents: Chiefly glycerides (fatty acids component: chiefly oleic, linoleic and palmitic acids), vitamin E (rich), etc. Peanut oil of South America is richer in linoleic acid (an omega-6 fatty acid).
Properties: Nutrient, demulcent, emollient.
Uses: Externally it is used for crusty head and dried skin in babies. Internally it is used (as a warm enema) to soften the hardened stools. In pharmaceutical industry peanut oil is used in the production of oils and liniments and as a vehicle of fat-soluble drugs.
Caution: It should not be used for acute and weeping skin irritations.

References: (1) Vol. 4, p. 316; (3) Vol. 3, p. 166; (8) p. 64; (11) pp. 69, 71; (12) p. 253; (13) p. 387; (48) p. 139.

PELLITORY, SPANISH

Other Common Name(s): longwort, mayweed, Roman pyrethrum
Botanical Name(s): *Anacyclus pyrethrum* (L.) Link [Fam.: Asteraceae (Compositae)]
Root
Constituents: Pungent principles (chiefly isobutylamides: pellitorin, anacyclin, etc., similar to those found in *Echinacea*), lignans (sesamin, etc.), minerals (manganese, zinc, copper, etc.), inulin, tannins, etc.
Properties: Rubefacient, local anesthetic, pungent sialagogue (= increases the flow of saliva), stomachic, and possibly antimicrobial.
Its main active constituents are considered isobutylamides.
Uses: Externally it is used (as a cotton swab with tincture) for toothache, (as a mouthwash, gargle, chewing) for aching inflammations of the mouth and throat, dry mouth and loss of voice, (as a wet compress, poultice) for headache, and (as a poultice) for neuralgic and rheumatic pains. Internally it is used (as a tea, h. p.) for nonulcer dyspepsia (with sluggish bowels).
Caution: Spanish pellitory should not be taken during pregnancy and lactation. At higher doses than recommended it causes gastrointestinal irritations (with nausea, vomiting, colics, diarrhea), headache, even stupor. Avoid contact with the eyes or the inhalation of powdered root (irritant!)

References: (2) Vol. 2, p. 76; (3) Vol. 3, p. 68; (35) p. 621; (41) Vols. 1-7; (46) p. 2251; (52) p. 47; (66) p. 409.

PELLITORY-OF-THE-WALL

Other Common Name(s): upright pellitory
Botanical Name(s): *Parietaria officinalis* L. [Fam.: Urticaceae]
Aerial part
Constituents: Flavonoids (flavonols), minerals (potassium), mucilage, tannins, bitter principles (possibly flavanone neohesperidosides), etc.
Properties: Diuretic, demulcent, emollient, astringent, wound-healing. Flavonoids and potassium account for the diuretic effect. The demulcent and emollient effects are due to mucilaginous polysaccharides. Tannins are astringent and account in large part for the wound-healing effect.
Uses: Internally it is used (usually combined with other herbs) as a flushing-out treatment (= herbal tea or product + liquids: more than 2 liters per day; sometimes combined with a medication) for inflammations of the genitourinary tract (cystitis, etc.), urinary gravel and nonobstructive stones, to prevent relapsing urinary infections / gravel / stones, and as an antidyscratic (= depurative; tea, h. p.) for chronic rheumatic complaints. Externally it is used (as a poultice) for minor skin inflammations, wounds, ulcers, sore nipples, and hemorrhoids.
Caution: There are no reports of contraindications or side effects when used properly. Nevertheless, a flushing-out treatment is contraindicated in cases of obstructive urinary stones, edema due to impaired heart or kidney function and kidney inflammations (here can be used on health professional's advice to enhance the effects of an antimicrobial therapy).

References: (3) Vol. 6a, p. 464; (8) p. 407; (15) p. 153; (27) p. 249; (28) p. 161; (29) p. 82; (35) p. 624; (46) p. 1078; (47) p. 2062; (49) Vol. 2, p. 95.

PENNYROYAL, AMERICAN

Botanical Name(s): *Hedeoma pulegioides* (L.) Pers. [Fam.: Lamiaceae (Labiatae)]
Aerial part
Constituents: Volatile oil (see American pennyroyal oil), flavonoids (diosmin, etc.), tannins, organic acids, etc.
Properties: Stomachic, carminative, antispasmodic, emmenagogue, insect-repellent.
Uses: Internally it is used (at low doses, as a tea, h. p.) for nonulcer dyspepsia (with flatulence, minor cramps, minor diarrhea), primary dysmenorrhea (= painful menstruation without pathology), secondary amenorrhea and oligomenorrhea (= ceased / infrequent / scanty menstruation without pathology), and as a diaphoretic hot tea for the common cold and feverish states.
Caution: It should not be used during pregnancy and lactation as well as in infants and young children. Before using it for gynecologic disorders, the problem should be judged by a health professional.

286

American pennyroyal oil

It is the volatile oil obtained by steam distillation from the aerial part.

Constituents: Chiefly pulegone (normally, much less than European pennyroyal), menthone, isomenthone, etc.

Properties: Aromatic, insect-repellent.

Uses: It is chiefly used as a fragrance ingredient in perfume and soap industries. Diluted in alcohol and sprayed on floor, it is used as a flea repellent.

Caution: Normally, it contains much less pulegone than the European pennyroyal. Nevertheless, internally it should be used only if the pulegone content is known and on health professional's advice.

References: (3) Vol. 5, p. 20; (5) Vol. 1, p. 564; (25) p. 190; (29) p. 60; (37) p. 645; (44) p. 256; (48) p. 547.

PENNYROYAL, EUROPEAN

Botanical Name(s): *Mentha pulegium* L. [Fam.: Lamiaceae (Labiatae)]

Aerial part

Constituents: Volatile oil (see European pennyroyal oil), flavonoids (diosmin, etc.), tannins, etc.

Properties: Carminative, antispasmodic, emmenagogue, insect-repellent.

Uses: Internally it is used (as a tea, h. p.; usually combined with other herbs) for nonulcer dyspepsia (with flatulence, minor cramps, etc.), primary dysmenorrhea (= painful menstruation without pathology), secondary amenorrhea and oligomenorrhea (= ceased / infrequent / scanty menstruation without pathology), and as a diaphoretic hot tea for the common cold and feverish states.

Caution: It should not be used during pregnancy and lactation as well as in infants and children. Before using it for dysmenorrhea, the gynecologic problem should be judged by a health professional. At higher doses than recommended it can be toxic (see European pennyroyal oil).

European pennyroyal oil

It is the volatile oil obtained by steam distillation from the aerial part.

Constituents: Depending on chemotype, it contains as its chief constituent, pulegone, piperitenone, or piperitone.

Properties: Aromatic, antifungal, insect-repellent.

Uses: It is an ingredient in many oral hygiene products. Pulegone is used for the semisynthetic production of menthol.

Caution: European pennyroyal oil is hepatotoxic due to its high pulegone content. In view of this, it should not be used internally. When taken at high doses, it has caused choking, vomiting, elevated blood pressure, and death due to respiratory failure.

References: (1) Vol. 5, p. 839; (3) Vol. 5, p. 775; (12a) p. 701; (15) p. 143; (20) p. 208; (29) p. 75; (37) p. 879; (47) p. 1880; (48) p. 547; (51) p. 174.

PEONY, CHINESE

Other Common Name(s): fragrant peony
Botanical Name(s): *Paeonia lactiflora* Pall. = *Paeonia albiflora* Pall. = *Paeonia edulis* Salisb. [Fam.: Paeoniaceae]
Root (white peony root; bai shao)
Fresh root (without rootlets) before being dried in the sun is boiled for a short while and peeled, or firstly peeled, boiled and then dried.
Constituents: Monoterpenoid glycosides (paeoniflorin, albiflorin, etc.), acetophenones (paeonol, etc.), tannins (gallotannins), volatile oil (with benzoic acid, etc.), phytosterols (5-sterols: β-sitosterol, etc.), carbohydrates (starch, sucrose, also water-soluble polysaccharides: paeonans), etc.
Properties: Anti-inflammatory, analgesic, antispasmodic, sedative, vasodilatory, platelet aggregation inhibitory, cholesterol and triglyceride reducing, immunomodulant, antioxidant, liver protective, antihyperglycemic, antibacterial, astringent. It is also reported to lower elevated levels of androgens in females. Most important constituents are considered paeoniflorin, paeonol, gallotannins, and their derivatives formed with processing.
Uses: Internally it is used (as an h. p., tea) for inflammatory conditions (rheumatoid arthritis, atopic eczema = eczema of internal origin, hepatitis), spastic conditions of the genitourinary tract (primary dysmenorrhea = painful menstruation without pathology), headaches, cerebrovascular disease (= a complex condition associated with changes in the brain blood flow), impaired mental performance (incl. cognitive function), vertigo (= a type of dizziness), and secondary amenorrhea and oligomenorrhea (= ceased / infrequent / scanty menstruation without pathology). It may be beneficial for common acne (= acne vulgaris). Externally it is used for skin inflammations, wounds and burns.
Caution: It should not be taken during pregnancy. Otherwise, there are no reports of contraindications or side effects when used properly.
Note: Red peony root is derived from the same species or from *Paeonia veitchii* Lynch, but it is not peeled before drying. It contains similar constituents and is used much like white peony root.

References: (1) Vol. 6, p. 3; (3) Vol. 6a, p. 383; (9) p. 545; (31) pp. 470, 547; (36) p. 509; (41) Vols. 1-7; (42) Vol. 5, p. 259; (48) p. 478; (53) p. 200; (59) p. 195.

PEONY, EUROPEAN

Botanical Name(s): *Paeonia officinalis* L. emend. Willd. s. l.; *Paeonia mascula* (L.) Mill. s. l. = *Paeonia corallina* Retz. [Fam.: Paeoniaceae]
Flower (petals)
Constituents: Flavonoids (anthocyanins: paeonin = paeonidin-3, 5-diglucoside, in the red variety; flavonols: kaempferol glycosides), tannins (hydrolyzable t.), mucilaginous polysaccharides, etc.
Properties: Astringent, anti-inflammatory, emollient. The effects are mild.

Uses: Internally it is used as a safe coloring ingredient in herbal teas to enhance their appearance. Externally it is used (as a wash, wet compress, poultice) for minor skin inflammations, ulcers, anal fissures, and hemorrhoids. **Caution:** Internally, it is used only as a coloring ingredient in herbal teas. When used alone, at high doses it has caused gastrointestinal irritations (with vomiting, diarrhea).

Root

Constituents: Monoterpenoid glycosides (chiefly paeoniflorin; less than Chinese peony; no albiflorin), carbohydrates (starch, sucrose; more than Chinese peony), tannins (gallotannins; less than Chinese peony), volatile oil, etc.

Properties and Uses: Much like Chinese peony (see PEONY, CHINESE).
Caution: See PEONY, CHINESE.

References: (1) Vol. 6, p. 7; (3) Vol. 6a, p. 384; (8) p. 397; (10) p. 212; (17) p. 417; (18) p. 200; (31) p. 547; (41) Vols. 1-7; (42) Vol. 5, p. 259.

PEONY, TREE

Other Common Name(s): mountain peony
Botanical Name(s): *Paeonia suffruticosa* Andrews = *Paeonia moutan* Sims = *Paeonia arborea* Donn [Fam.: Paeoniaceae]
Root bark (= mu dan, mu dan pi, moutan)
Constituents: Acetophenones (free paeonol, paeonol glycosides, etc.), monoterpenoid glycosides (chiefly paeoniflorin), tannins (gallotannins), phytosterols (possibly 5-sterols), volatile oil, carbohydrates (starch), etc.
Properties: Anti-inflammatory, analgesic, antipyretic, antispasmodic and platelet aggregation inhibitory, possibly by inhibiting cyclooxygenase, antihypertensive, mainly by inhibiting ACE (= angiotensin converting enzyme), antihistaminic, sedative, antihyperglycemic, antibacterial, astringent. Most of the effects are attributed to paeonol and paeoniflorin.
Uses: Internally it is used (as a tea, h. p.) for inflammatory conditions (also when allergic components are present) of the skin (atopic eczema = chronic eczema of internal origin, urticaria), upper respiratory tract (rhinitis, sinusitis, the common cold, flu) and gastrointestinal tract (gastroenteritis, appendicitis), primary dysmenorrhea (= painful menstruation without pathology), for abdominal / arthritic / post-traumatic pains, as an adjuvant for minor hypertension, and as a preventive for arteriosclerosis. Externally it is used (as a mouthwash, paint) for gingivitis (= inflammations of the gums), and (as a lotion, cream) for minor skin inflammations and allergic conditions.
Caution: Unless advised by a health professional, it should not be taken during pregnancy and lactation. Otherwise, there are no reports of contraindications or side effects when used properly.

References: (1) Vol. 6, p. 9; (3) Vol. 6a, p. 385; (9) p. 544; (31) pp. 470, 547; (36) p. 507; (41) Vols. 1-7; (42) Vol. 5, p. 260; (48) p. 478; (53) p. 207.

PEPPER

Botanical Name(s): *Piper nigrum* L. [Fam.: Piperaceae]
Fruit (black pepper)
Constituents: Pungent principles (amides: chiefly piperine, also the pungent and bitter chavicine, etc.), volatile oil (with sabinene, limonene, caryophyllene, pinenes, etc.), phenolic acids, polysaccharides, fixed oil, etc.
Properties: Aromatic, digestive secretagogue (increases secretions of the mouth, stomach, and liver), anti-inflammatory (NSAID-like effect, by inhibiting the biosynthesis of prostaglandins), antimicrobial, antioxidant, tonic, rubefacient, local anesthetic. Pungent principles and the volatile oil account for most of the effects.
Uses: Black pepper is chiefly used as a spice in culinary practice, beneficial for loss of appetite and nonulcer dyspepsia (with stomachache, flatulence, sluggish bowels, etc.), and for inflammations of the upper respiratory tract (bronchitis, etc.; coughs; also as a diaphoretic hot tea). Its consumption in moderate amounts is beneficial due to its antioxidant and tonic effects. Externally it is used (as an ointment, liniment) for neuralgic and rheumatic pains, and (as a cotton swab with tincture) for toothache.
Caution: There are no reports of side effects when used in moderate amounts as a spice. Black pepper should be avoided for prolonged periods in cases of liver problems and inflammations of the gastrointestinal tract.

References: (1) Vol. 6, p. 213; (3) Vol. 6a, p. 697; (8) p. 441; (9) p. 415; (12a) p. 281; (13) p. 147; (27) p. 254; (31) p. 252; (37) p. 1086; (48) p. 861; (49) Vol. 2, p. 110.

PEPPER TREE, BRAZILIAN

Botanical Name(s): *Schinus terebinthifolius* Raddi [Fam.: Anacardiaceae]
Fruit (Christmasberry, pink pepper)
Constituents: Phenols (cardanols, cardol), phenolic acids (gallic acid, etc.), flavonoids (a biflavone: amentoflavone; etc.), triterpenes (masticadienonic acid derivatives), volatile oil (with limonene, α- and β-phellandrene, etc.), fixed oil, etc. Depending on the origin, its volatile oil may contain 3-carene in variable amounts.
Properties: Antimicrobial, anti-inflammatory, astringent. Cardanol and cardol have been shown to be inhibitors of some tumors.
Uses: Brazilian pepper is chiefly used in traditional medicine. Externally it is used (as a wash, wet compress) for wounds and ulcers and (as a poultice) for growths.
Caution: It may irritate the skin and respiratory and gastrointestinal tracts. This is due to phenols, which are closely related to urushiols of poison ivy (q. v.), and 3-carene oxidation products (when 3-carene is present).

References: (1) Vol. 6, p. 634; (3) Vol. 6b, p. 317; (29) p. 104; (31) p. 456; (41) Vols. 1-7; (52) p. 702; (57) p. 753.

290

PEPPER TREE, PERUVIAN

Other Common Name(s): California pepper tree, molle
Botanical Name(s): *Schinus molle* L. [Fam.: Anacardiaceae]
Fruit (California pepper, molle seed)
Constituents: Volatile oil (with limonene, α- and β-phellandrene, etc.), triterpenes (masticadienonic acid derivatives), fixed oil, tannins, etc.
Properties: Aromatic, bitter tonic, diuretic, laxative, local anesthetic.
Uses: California pepper is chiefly used as a spice, beneficial for loss of appetite and nonulcer dyspepsia (with sluggish bowels, minor constipation). Internally it is also used (as a tea, h. p.) for minor inflammations of the upper respiratory tract (bronchitis, etc.; coughs), and genitourinary tract (cystitis, urethritis, etc.). Externally it is used (as a liniment) for rheumatic and neuralgic pains.
Caution: It should not be taken during pregnancy and lactation, in cases of obstructive urinary stones, edema due to impaired heart or kidney function and kidney inflammations. Consumption of large amounts causes gastrointestinal irritations (with nausea, vomiting, diarrhea). Otherwise, there are no reports of contraindications or side effects when used and consumed properly.
Leaf
Constituents: Volatile oil, gum-resin, tannins, flavonoids, fatty acids, phytosterols, etc.
Properties: Diuretic, antimicrobial, astringent, local anesthetic. Its effects are milder than the fruit.
Uses: Internally it is used (as a tea, h. p.) for inflammations of the genitourinary tract (cystitis, etc.) and upper respiratory tract (bronchitis, etc.; coughs), and to induce diuresis when this is advisable. To enhance the effects in problems of the genitourinary tract, the fluid intake (incl. herbal teas) should be more than 2 liters per day. Externally it is used (as a gargle, mouthwash) for inflammations and ulcerations of the mouth, (as a vaginal irrigation / sitz bath / wash) for leukorrhea and vulvovaginitis, and (as a poultice, wet compress) for wounds, rheumatic and neuralgic pains (incl. sciatica).
Caution: See Fruit.

References: (1) Vol. 6, p. 627; (3) Vol. 6b, p. 317; (29) p. 104; (41) Vols. 1-7; (52) p. 705; (57) p. 753.

PEPPERMINT

Botanical Name(s): *Mentha × piperita* L. [Fam.: Lamiaceae (Labiatae)]
Leaf
Constituents: Volatile oil (see Peppermint oil), Lamiaceae tannins (rosmarinic acid and other caffeic acid derivatives), triterpenes (ursolic and

oleanolic acids; both bitter tasting), flavonoids (eriocitrin, etc.), coumarins (aesculetin, etc.), biogenic amines (choline, betaine), etc.

Properties: Antispasmodic, choleretic, cholagogue, stomachic, carminative, mild astringent, antimicrobial. Due to Lamiaceae tannins, triterpenes, etc., leaf acts somehow different to the oil. It is mild stomachic and astringent, and compared to the oil its antispasmodic and cholagogic effects are milder. Rosmarinic acid and related caffeic acid derivatives have been shown to inhibit the biosynthesis of leukotrienes and prostaglandins, and to exert choleretic, antibacterial and antiviral effects.

Uses: Internally it is used (as a tea, h. p.) for impaired digestion and spastic complaints of the gastrointestinal tract (nausea, vomiting, flatulence, minor cramps, irritable bowel syndrome) and biliary tract (minor cramps, nonobstructive gallstones), and complaints following a cholecystectomy (often combined with celandine, turmeric, etc.). It is an important ingredient in many herbal teas used for different conditions (gastrointestinal, hepatobiliary, nervous, etc.). Externally it is used (as a mouthwash, chewing) for bad breath.

Caution: Peppermint should not be taken in cases of biliary obstruction. In cases of nonobstructive gallstones it can be used but only on health professional's advice. Otherwise, there are no reports of contraindications or side effects when used properly.

Peppermint oil

It is the volatile oil obtained by steam distillation from the fresh aerial part.

Constituents: Chiefly menthol (free and esterified), menthone, 1,8-cineole, menthofuran, neomenthol, isomenthone, limonene, pinenes, pulegone, etc.

Properties: Aromatic, antispasmodic, carminative, cholagogue, antibacterial, cooling and local anesthetic.

Uses: Internally it is used (a few drops in a glass of water; in capsule / dragée) for spastic complaints of the gastrointestinal tract (flatulence, bloating, burping, irritable bowel syndrome), biliary tract (cramps, nonobstructive gallstones), and as an adjuvant for the common cold. Externally it is used (as an ointment, cream, liniment, application of a few drops) for inflammations of the upper respiratory tract (the common cold; coughs), neuralgic pains (incl. headaches), muscular pains, sprains, itching, and (as a mouthwash: a few drops in a glass of water; combination products) for the oral hygiene. Peppermint oil is extensively used as a flavor ingredient in pharmaceutical and food products.

Caution: Peppermint oil should not be taken in cases of biliary obstruction and severe liver disorders. In cases of nonobstructive gallstones it can be used but only on health professional's advice. Otherwise, there are no reports of contraindications or side effects when used properly.

References: (1) Vol. 5, p. 828; (3) Vol. 5, p. 767; (8) p. 368; (12) pp. 689, 735; (13) p. 100; (14) p. 174; (16) pp. 127, 143; (17) p. 391; (19) pp. 176, 177; (23) p. 49; (46) p. 937; (47) p. 1872; (48) p. 532.

PERIWINKLE, LESSER

Botanical Name(s): *Vinca minor* L. [Fam.: Apocynaceae]
Leaf
Constituents: Indole alkaloids (vincamine, etc.), triterpenes (ursolic acid, etc.), an iridoid (loganic acid), phytosterols, phenolic acids, flavonoids, etc.
Properties: Vincamine exerts mild antihypertensive, sedative and antispasmodic effects, and increases cerebral blood flow.
Uses: Internally is used (vincamine, extracts standardized to vincamine) for cerebrovascular disease (= a complex condition associated with changes in the brain blood flow), minor hypertension, Ménière's disease (= a sudden attack, with violent dizziness, nausea and vomiting, ringing in the ear), and vascular retinopathy associated with hypertension. Externally it is used leaf (as a gargle) for sore throat, (as a wash, wet compress, poultice) for minor skin inflammations, eczema, milk crust and wounds.
Caution: Vincamine or extracts standardized to the vincamine content are used only as directed by health professionals. They should not be taken in cases of intracranial hypertension, cerebral tumors, retinal hemorrhage, during pregnancy, and should not be combined with potassium depleting diuretics (e. g. hydrochlorthiazide) or laxatives (e. g. Senna) and antiarrhythmic drugs (e. g. quinidine).

References: (1) Vol. 6, p. 1127; (3) Vol. 6c, p. 446; (6) p. 51; (8) p. 586; (12a) p. 548; (13) p. 258; (23) p. 181; (37) p. 1451; (47) p. 2812; (48) p. 1023; (51) p. 150; (72) nr. 36079; (73) p. 1236.

PERIWINKLE, MADAGASCAR

Botanical Name(s): *Catharanthus roseus* (L.) G. Don. = *Vinca rosea* L. [Fam.: Apocynaceae]
Leaf, root
Constituents: Indole alkaloids (chiefly vindoline), and the more interesting group of bisindole type (vinblastine, vincristine, etc.). It also contains vincamine (see PERIWINKLE, LESSER), among many others.
Properties: Vinblastine and vincristine are antineoplastic drugs, inhibitors of mitosis (a type of cell division). Vindoline has shown antihyperglycemic effect.
Uses: Leaf and root are not used as such but for the extraction of alkaloids. Vinblastine is used for Hodgkin's disease, choriocarcinoma, malign lymphoma, testicular tumors, breast cancer, etc. Vincristine is used for acute leukemia, malign lymphoma, lymphosarcoma, reticulosarcoma, etc.
Caution: Vinblastine and vincristine are prescription drugs, used only as directed by a health professional. Further details are beyond the scope of this book.

References: (3) Vol. 3, p. 771; (6) p. 278; (8) p. 127; (11) p. 170; (12) p. 1036; (13) p. 257; (48) p. 1016.

PERUVIAN BALSAM TREE

Botanical Name(s): *Myroxylon balsamum* (L.) Harms var. *pereirae* (Royle) Harms [Fam.: Fabaceae (Leguminosae)]

Peruvian balsam (balsam-of-Peru)

It is a pathological exudate of the exposed wood.

Constituents: Cinnamein (a mixture: esters of benzoic and cinnamic acids with benzyl alcohol), resin (esters of the same acids with peruresinotannol), free benzoic and cinnamic acids, and some nerolidol, vanillin, etc.

Properties: Aromatic, antimicrobial, wound-healing, mild local anesthetic, antiparasitic (against *Sarcoptes scabiei*).

Uses: Externally it is used (as an ointment, liniment, etc.) for minor wounds, ulcers (incl. varicose ulcers = ulcus cruris), burns, bruises, hemorrhoids, cracks, and scabies (= the itch). Internally it is used (as an inhalation combination product) for inflammations of the upper respiratory tract, and (as a suppository combination product) for hemorrhoids. It is an important ingredient in cosmetics and perfumery.

Caution: In some hypersensitive individuals it may cause skin allergic reactions. In view of this, before applying, the product should be tried on a small skin area. Unless advised by a health professional, Peruvian balsam should not be used for more than one week.

References: (1) Vol. 5, p. 894; (3) Vol. 5, p. 928; (6) pp. 336, 348; (8) p. 376; (9) p. 65; (11) p. 104; (13) p. 136; (16) p. 33; (19) p. 173; (36) p. 183; (37) p. 176; (46) p. 122; (48) p. 254; (49) Vol. 2, p. 383.

PICHI

Other Common Name(s): fabiana

Botanical Name(s): *Fabiana imbricata* Ruiz. et Pav. [Fam.: Solanaceae]

Leaf and twig

Constituents: A quinoline alkaloid (fabianine), coumarins (fabiatrin, scopoletin, etc.), sugars (mannoheptulose, xylose), sugar alcohols (arabitol, mannitol, perseitol), acetophenones (acetovanillone = apocynin, etc.), anthranoids (erythroglaucin, physcion), minerals (rich in magnesium), phytosterols, volatile oil, tannins, etc.

Properties: Diuretic, anthelmintic (against *Distomum hepaticum*).

Uses: Internally it is used (as a tea, h. p.) chiefly for inflammations of the genitourinary tract (cystitis, urethritis, urinary incontinence) and gravel and nonobstructive urinary stones (also when minor hemorrhages are present, but on professional's advice). In veterinary medicine it is used for liver fluke disease. To enhance the effects in problems of the genitourinary tract, the fluid intake (incl. herbal teas) should be more than 2 liters per day.

Caution: Pichi should not be taken in cases of obstructive urinary stones and kidney inflammations (here can be used on health professional's advice to enhance the effects of an antimicrobial therapy).

294

References: (3) Vol. 4, p. 904; (5) Vol. 1, p. 492; (10) p. 215; (35) p. 632; (37) p. 511; (41) Vols. 1-7; (52) p. 302; (66) p. 390.

PICRORHIZA

Other Common Name(s): katuka, katukarohini, kutaki, kutki
Botanical Name(s): *Picrorhiza kurroa* Royle ex Benth. [Fam.: Scrophulariaceae]
Root (rhizome)
Constituents: Iridoids (catalpol derivatives: picrosides I-III, kutkoside), bitter principles (cucurbitacins, iridoids), acetophenones (chiefly androsin = apocynin- or acetovanillone-glucoside; picein, etc.), etc.
Properties: Bitter tonic, choleretic, liver protective, laxative, antiviral (against hepatitis B virus), antibacterial, anti-inflammatory, antispasmodic, immunomodulant. Iridoids account for most of the effects. Cucurbitacins exert laxative effect. Some acetophenones have shown inhibitory effect on platelet aggregation and biosynthesis of prostaglandins and leukotrienes.
Uses: Internally it is used (as a tea, h. p.) for loss of appetite and nonulcer dyspepsia (with flatulence, nausea, minor constipation), liver disorders (chronic hepatitis, adjuvant for cirrhosis), and for inflammatory and spastic conditions of the upper respiratory tract (bronchitis, bronchial asthma).
Caution: Picrorhiza products are best standardized to picrosides and kutkoside. Unless advised by a health professional, picrorhiza should not be taken during pregnancy and lactation. Doses higher than recommended my cause gastrointestinal irritations (with vomiting, diarrhea). Otherwise, there are no reports of contraindications or side effects when used properly.

References: (2) Vol. 3, p. 387; (3) Vol. 6a, p. 655; (6) p. 146; (13) p. 420; (18) p. 339; (31) p. 466; (36) p. 437; (37) p. 1076; (41) Vols. 1-7; (45) p. 246; (52) p. 596.

PILEWORT

Other Common Name(s): lesser celandine
Botanical Name(s): *Ranunculus ficaria* L. = *Ficaria ranunculoides* Roth [Fam.: Ranunculaceae]
Aerial part
Constituents: (Fresh herb): protoanemonin (an unstable compound); (dried herb): anemonin (= protoanemonin dimer); and (fresh or dried): saponins, tannins, etc.
Properties: (Fresh herb): Counterirritant / vesicant (depending on concentration), analgesic. (Dried herb): Antimicrobial, astringent, demulcent, diuretic. Anemonin is non-toxic and has shown antimicrobial effect. Protoanemonin is toxic and a strong local irritant (cf. PULSATILLA).
Uses: Externally it is used (as an ointment: fresh herb) for hemorrhoids. Internally it is used (only dried!; as a tea, h. p.; combined with other herbs) for

hemorrhoids and as an antidyscratic (= blood purifier) for atopic eczema (= chronic eczema of internal origin) and chronic rheumatic complaints.

Caution: Internally should be used only dried herb and as directed by an experienced practitioner. Even dried, pilewort should not be taken during pregnancy as it may still contain protoanemonin (teratogenic, abortifacient!; cf. PULSATILLA). Fresh herb should be handled with care (see Properties), even when used externally. If taken internally, fresh herb (also dried herb at higher doses than recommended) causes strong gastrointestinal irritations (with vomiting, diarrhea), etc.

References: (3) Vol. 6b, p. 12; (10) p. 215; (15) p. 176; (35) p. 179; (37) p. 1169; (46) p. 276; (47) p. 2284; (48) p. 747.

PINE

Other Common Name(s): 1) slash pine 2) Aleppo pine 3) giant pine 4) dwarf / mountain / mugo pine 5) European / black pine 6) longleaf pine 7) maritime / cluster pine 8) big pine 9) Eastern / white pine 10) Scotch pine

Botanical Name(s): 1) *Pinus elliotii* Engelmann 2) *Pinus halepensis* Miller 3) *Pinus lambertiana* Douglas 4) *Pinus mugo* Turra 5) *Pinus nigra* Arnold 6) *Pinus palustris* Mil 7) *Pinus pinaster* Aiton = *Pinus maritima* Poir 8) *Pinus ponderosa* Douglas ex P. et C. Laws. 9) *Pinus strobus* L. 10) *Pinus sylvestris* L.; etc. [Fam.: Pinaceae]

Pine needle oil

It is the volatile oil obtained by steam distillation from the fresh needles and twigs of dwarf pine: *P. mugo* Turra and subspecies, or Scotch pine: *P. sylvestris* L.

Constituents: The oil obtained from dwarf pine contains chiefly α- and β-phellandrene, also bornyl acetate, α- and β-pinene, etc. The oil obtained from Scotch pine contains chiefly α-pinene, also β-phellandrene, 3-carene, etc.

Properties: Rubefacient, antimicrobial, expectorant.

Uses: Externally it is used (as a liniment, cream, ointment) for inflammations of the upper respiratory tract (bronchitis, tracheitis, etc.; coughs) and rheumatic and neuralgic pains. Internally it is used (as an inhalation) for inflammations of the upper respiratory tract (bronchitis, tracheitis, etc.; coughs).

Caution: See Oil of turpentine.

Pine bud

It is the dried bud of Scotch pine.

Constituents: Volatile oil (with bornyl acetate, α- and β-pinene), a bitter principle (pinipicrin), organic acids (quinic acid, etc.), flavonoids, an acetophenone (picein), sugars (fructose, etc.), sugar alcohols, etc.

Properties: Mild expectorant, antiseptic, tonic (claimed to be blood circulation stimulant).

Uses: Internally it is used (as a tea, h. p.) for inflammations of the upper respiratory tract (the common cold, etc., also as a diaphoretic hot tea). Externally it is used (as a liniment, ointment) for minor neuralgic pains.

Caution: There are no reports of contraindications or side effects when used properly.

Turpentine

It is the crude oleoresin (commonly referred to as balsam) obtained mainly from species 1, 6, 7, 10, also 2 and 5, etc.

Constituents: Volatile oil (see Oil of turpentine) and a resin (see Colophony).

Properties: Rubefacient, counterirritant, antimicrobial.

Uses: Externally it is used (as a plaster, ointment) for rheumatic and neuralgic pains, for which oil of turpentine is preferred. Turpentine is chiefly used in the production of the oil of turpentine and colophony.

Caution: See Oil of turpentine.

Oil of turpentine (rectified)

From turpentine is distilled the oil of turpentine, which after a treatment with alkali undergoes another distillation (temp. 155-162° C) to yield the rectified oil of turpentine.

Constituents: Chiefly α- and β-pinene, also limonene and 3-carene (its oxidation products are skin and mucosal irritants!). In longleaf pine, 3-carene is found in lower concentrations, hence preferred.

Properties: Rubefacient, counterirritant, antimicrobial.

Uses: Externally it is used (as a plaster, ointment, liniment) for rheumatic and neuralgic pains, (as an ointment, inhalation) for inflammations of the upper respiratory tract (chronic bronchitis, etc.). As an important source of α- and β-pinene, oil of turpentine is used in chemical industry in the production of camphor, fragrances and other terpenoids.

Caution: It may cause allergic reactions, especially when employing the oil that has been stored for a prolonged period or unprotected from oxygen, light, moisture and warm temperature. Avoid applications on a large skin area because it may be harmful to kidneys and CNS. It should not be used (inhaled) in cases of acute inflammations of the upper respiratory tract, bronchial asthma, and whooping cough.

Colophony (colophony resin, rosin)

It is the hardened resin obtained by straining the residue of turpentine, after distilling the oil of turpentine.

Constituents: Chiefly resin acids (diterpenes: abietic acid, etc., or pimaric acid, etc.; depending on the origin, age, etc.), hydrocarbons (collectively referred to as resene), volatile oil (traces).

Properties: Counterirritant, antibacterial. The effects are mild.

Uses: Externally it is used (light-colored and transparent colophony, in plasters and ointments) for rheumatic and neuralgic pains. Colophony is chiefly used in varnish, cosmetic and perfume industries.

Caution: It may cause contact allergic reactions.

Pine tar

It is obtained by destructive distillation (without access of air) from pine-wood (trunk, twig, root). With Pinaceae-tar is to be understood a tar produced as above, from pines (*Pinus* spp.), but also other Pinaceae (spruces: *Picea* spp., and larches: *Larix* spp.).

Constituents: Phenols (phenol, cresols, methyl cresols, pyrocatechol, guaiacol, etc.), hydrocarbons (benzene, toluene, xylenes, naphthalene, etc.), organic acids (acetic acid, resin acids, etc.), etc.

Properties: Antimicrobial, keratolytic, anti-eczematous, antipruritic, antiparasitic (against *Sarcoptes scabiei*).

Uses: Externally it is used (as an ointment, lotion, paint, partial bath) for chronic eczema and psoriasis, lichen planus (= a skin itching condition), and scabies (= the itch).

Caution: Pine tar products should not be used in acute cases. Partial baths containing a pine tar product as an additive may cause blackheads and folliculitis. Therefore, they should be applied based on advice and monitored by a health professional.

References: (1) Vol. 6, p. 158; (3) Vol. 6a, p. 677; (5) Vol. 2, p. 211; (8) p. 432; (9) pp. 419, 502; (11) pp. 100, 102; (12) pp. 718, 733; (13) p. 115; (36) pp. 223, 268; (37) p. 1082; (46) pp. 1104, 1107; (47) p. 2135; (48) p. 582; (51) p. 238.

PINEAPPLE

Botanical Name(s): *Ananas comosus* (L.) Merr. = *Ananas ananas* (L.) Voss = *Bromelia ananas* L. = *Bromelia comosus* L. [Fam.: Bromeliaceae]

Fruit (fresh)

Constituents: Organic acids (citric acid, etc.), sugars (sucrose, invert sugar), enzymes (collectively referred to as bromelain: bromelain A, B, etc.; unripe fruit is richer), vitamins (C, B_1, B_2, niacinamide), aromatic compounds, flavonoids (a cyanidin glycoside), phenolic acids (caffeic acid, etc.), etc.

Properties: Refrigerant, digestant (mild proteolytic effect; see bromelain), and mild diuretic and laxative.

Uses: Internally it is used (fresh juice, raw) for feverish and thirsty states and as a mild digestant for dyspeptic disorders (with minor constipation).

Caution: See Bromelain.

Bromelain (raw bromelain)

It is a mixture of proteolytic enzymes (bromelain A, B, etc.), which is obtained from the fresh fruit. The "stem" of the fruit is richer.

Properties: Proteolytic (= splits proteins), platelet aggregation inhibitory, anticoagulant, anti-inflammatory, antiexudative and antiedematous.

Uses: Internally it is used as a digestant (usually combined with other enzymes) for dyspeptic disorders (with impaired digestion of proteinic foods) chiefly associated with impaired external secretion of pancreas, (as an en-

teric coated product, also combined with other enzymes) to prevent edemas after surgeries or traumatic injuries (esp. in the nasal and paranasal cavities), for bruises, thrombophlebitis, and as an adjuvant for rheumatic complaints (incl. rheumatoid arthritis). In food industry it is used as a meat tenderizer.
Caution: Bromelain should not be taken during pregnancy and in cases of clotting disorders. It may increase the effects of antibiotics (tetracycline, etc.), anticoagulants (warfarin, etc.) and platelet aggregation inhibitors (aspirin, etc.). In view of this, a possible combination with them should be made only by a health professional. In rare cases it may cause allergic reactions (after intake or skin contact) and gastrointestinal irritations (with diarrhea). Bromelain products should contain bromelain standardized to its proteolytic activity.

References: (1) Vol. 4, p. 272; (3) Vol. 3, p. 73; (6) p. 242; (7) p. 292; (8) p. 54; (13) p. 442; (19) p. 56; (23) p. 390; (27) p. 30; (37) p. 235; (48) p. 223; (67) p. 846; (91) pp. 128, 129.

PIPSISSEWA

Other Common Name(s): prince's pine
Botanical Name(s): *Chimaphila umbellata* (L.) W.P.C. Barton = *Pirola umbellata* L. [Fam.: Pyrolaceae]
Aerial part
Constituents: Phenol glycosides (arbutin = hydroquinone-glucoside, etc.), naphthoquinones (chimaphilin, etc.), tannins (condensed and hydrolyzable t.), flavonoids (flavonols), triterpenes (taraxasterol, ursolic acid), phytosterols, etc.
Properties: Antibacterial (also urinary active), antifungal, bitter tonic, stomachic, mild immunomodulant, astringent, mild diuretic. The urinary antiseptic effect is due to hydroquinone (liberated from arbutin) and chimaphilin. Chimaphilin, at normal doses, found in pipsissewa preparations, has been shown to stimulate phagocytosis. This justifies at least in part the traditional use for different inflammatory conditions (incl. scrofula).
Uses: Internally it is used (as a tea, h. p.) for inflammations of the genitourinary tract (cystitis, urethritis, prostatitis, pyelonephritis) and upper respiratory tract (bronchitis, the common cold, etc.), and for loss of appetite and nonulcer dyspepsia. To enhance the effects in the urinary tract, urine should be slightly alkaline (this can be achieved by consuming a diet rich in vegetables and / or taking about a teaspoonful per day of baking soda) and the fluid intake (incl. herbal teas) should be more than 2 liters per day. Pipsissewa extract is also used as a flavor ingredient in some beverages (root beer, etc.). Externally it is used (as a wash, wet compress) for minor skin inflammations and wounds, and (as a poultice) for swellings. Poultices prepared with fresh plant material exert rubefacient and counterirritant effects and are used for rheumatic pains.

Caution: See UVA-URSI. Due to chimaphilin, it may cause skin allergic reactions (especially fresh plant). Due to hydroquinone, pipsissewa should not be applied externally in babies and young children.

References: (1) Vol. 4, p. 849; (3) Vol. 3, p. 852; (9) p. 421; (27) p. 87; (31) p. 494; (44) p. 157; (46) p. 287; (47) p. 942; (51) p. 142; (66) p. 213.

PLANTAIN

Other Common Name(s): 1) English / narrow-leaf plantain, ribgrass, ribwort 2) broad-leaf / greater plantain 3) hoary plantain
Botanical Name(s): 1) *Plantago lanceolata* L. 2) *Plantago major* L. 3) *Plantago media* L. [Fam.: Plantaginaceae]
Leaf
Constituents: Iridoids (aucubin = aucubigenin-glucoside, catalpol, etc.), mucilaginous polysaccharides, phenylethanoid glycosides (acteoside = verbascoside, etc.), phenolic acids (incl. caffeic acid derivatives), flavonoids (flavones), tannins, minerals (silicic acid, zinc, potassium), a saponin, coumarins, etc. English plantain is richer in aucubin.
Properties: Antibacterial, anti-inflammatory, astringent, emollient, wound-healing, demulcent, liver protective, mild immunomodulant. Aucubin has shown anti-inflammatory, liver protective, laxative, and diuretic effects, while aucubigenin has shown antibacterial and antitumoral effects. Acteoside has shown anti-inflammatory (by inhibiting the biosynthesis of leukotrienes) and liver protective effects, which are enhanced by phenolic acids. Mucilages are emollient and demulcent. Tannins are astringent and contribute to the wound-healing and anti-inflammatory effects.
Uses: Internally it is used (as a tea, h. p.) for inflammations (also when minor hemorrhages are present) particularly of the upper respiratory tract (the common cold, bronchitis, etc.; irritating dry coughs), also gastrointestinal (diarrhea, hemorrhoids, etc.; also as a small enema for ulcerative colitis) and genitourinary tracts (cystitis, etc.). To enhance the effects in problems of the genitourinary tract, the fluid intake (incl. herbal teas) should be more than 2 liters per day. Externally it is used (as a wash, wet compress, poultice; also prepared with fresh leaves) for minor skin inflammations, wounds, boils, insect bites, poison ivy dermatitis, hemorrhoids, (as a mouthwash) for inflammations of the mouth, and (as a wet cotton, drops, irrigation with the fresh juice or tea) for nosebleed. In traditional medicine poultices are also prepared with fresh leaves and used for wounds, and boils. This is well justifiable due to the antibacterial effect of aucubigenin and the astringent and wound-healing effects of tannins.
Caution: In rare cases it may cause contact allergic reactions. For cases with minor hemorrhages it should be used only on professional's advice. Otherwise, there are no reports of contraindications or side effects when used properly.

300

References: (1) Vol. 6, p. 224; (3) Vol. 6a, p. 747; (6) pp. 99, 116; (8) p. 446; (12) p. 446; (13) p. 369; (16) p. 68; (17) p. 443; (19) p. 215; (20) p. 210; (22) p. 119; (23) p. 402; (31) pp. 488, 572; (37) p. 1091; (46) p. 1100; (47) p. 2159; (48) p. 110; (51) p. 188.

PLATYCODON

Other Common Name(s): balloon flower, Chinese / Japanese bellflower
Botanical Name(s): *Platycodon grandiflorum* (Jacq.) A. DC. [Fam.: Campanulaceae]

Root

Constituents: Triterpenoid saponins (platycodins A-C, etc.), volatile oil (pungent taste), phytosterols (7-sterols: α-spinasterol, etc.; 5-sterols: stigmastenol, etc.), triterpenes (betulin, etc.), alkaloids (in traces), etc.

Properties: Anti-inflammatory (cortisone-like effect), expectorant, antispasmodic (atropine-like effect), analgesic, antiulcer (= prevents or helps in healing peptic ulcers), sedative, antibacterial (against *S. aureus*, *M. tuberculosis*, *E. coli*, *Shigella* spp., etc.), cholesterol and triglyceride reducing. Most of the effects are attributed to platycodins, but phytosterols and other triterpenes surely contribute to the overall effect.

Uses: Internally it is used (as a tea, h. p.) for inflammations of the upper respiratory tract (spastic bronchitis, pharyngitis, laryngitis with hoarseness, bronchial asthma; dry coughs) and gastrointestinal tract (gastritis, incl. peptic ulcers; diarrhea, etc.; possibly for irritable bowel syndrome), and as an adjuvant for high cholesterol and triglycerides. Due also to 7-sterols (see PUMPKIN) it may be beneficial for early stages of benign prostatic hyperplasia (= BPH).

Caution: Platycodon should not be taken during pregnancy and it is best to avoid it during lactation. Alcoholic drinks may interact with platycodon. A possible combination of platycodon with sedative, hypnotic and antidepressant drugs should be made only by a health professional. Otherwise, there are no reports of contraindications or side effects when used properly.

References: (1) Vol. 6, p. 239; (3) Vol. 6a, p. 765; (5) Vol. 3, p. 474; (29) p. 88; (36) p. 509; (41) Vols. 1-7; (52) p. 612; (53) p. 155; (59) p. 213.

POISON IVY

Botanical Name(s): *Toxicodendron radicans* (L.) Kuntze [Fam.: Anacardiaceae]

Leaf

Constituents: Phenolic compounds (as catechol derivatives) collectively referred to as urushiols (including urushiol), which are contained in the milky juice. It also contains tannins (including gallic acid), flavonoids (flavonols),

301

gum and resin, among others.

Properties: Urushiols are very strong contact allergenic compounds. Even 1 µg (one thousandths of a milligram) may cause severe inflammations to persons hypersensitive to them.

Uses: Poison ivy is used only in Homeopathy.

Herbal remedies for poison ivy dermatitis: There are a number of herbs recommended, as a poultice prepared with the fresh plant material or as a wet compress, to alleviate or cure it. Among them, jewelweed (*Impatiens capensis* Meerb. = *Impatiens fulva* Nutt.; *Impatiens pallida* Nutt.; Fam.: Balsaminaceae) seems to be one of the most efficacious. See also BEDSTRAW; GRINDELIA; PLANTAIN.

References: (1) Vol. 6, p. 458; (3) Vol. 6b, p. 124; (22) p. 214; (37) p. 1390; (58) p. 123; (66) p. 804.

POKE

Other Common Name(s): pokeweed

Botanical Name(s): *Phytolacca americana* L. = *Phytolacca decandra* L. [Fam.: Phytolaccaceae]

Root

Constituents: Triterpenoid saponins (phytolaccosides), lectins, histamine (in high concentrations), GABA (= gamma-aminobutyrric acid), minerals (potassium), phytosterols, starch, sucrose, etc.

Properties: Poke root saponins have shown anti-inflammatory and antiedematous effects.

Uses: Internally it has been used for chronic rheumatic complaints (incl. rheumatoid arthritis) and atopic eczema (= chronic eczema of internal origin) but due to its toxicity is obsolete. Products that contain isolated and standardized saponins could be more acceptable. Externally it is used (as a poultice) for bruises, sprains and swellings, and (as a wash, wet compress) for eczema and bacterial and fungal skin infections.

Caution: Poke root is not for self-treatment. Due in large part to lectins, histamine and GABA, poke root is very toxic. Symptoms of intoxication are nausea, vomiting, abdominal cramps, watery diarrhea, weakness, bronchial spasms, tachycardia (= rapid heartbeat) and lowered blood pressure, among others. Poke root should not be taken during pregnancy and lactation.

References: (2) Vol. 3, p. 361; (3) Vol. 6a, p. 644; (13) p. 420; (20) p. 215; (21) p. 297; (29) p. 85; (44) p. 397; (46) p. 608; (47) p. 2115; (66) p. 389; (71) p. 234.

POLYPODY

Other Common Name(s): brake fern, rock brake

Botanical Name(s): *Polypodium vulgare* L. [Fam.: Polypodiaceae]

Root (rhizome)

Constituents: Steroidal saponins (osladin, polypodosaponin, etc.), phytosterols (ecdysteroids: polypodins A and B, etc.), tannins (condensed t.), a bitter principle, starch, fixed oil, resin, etc. Osladin has a very sweet taste. It is ca. 3,000 times sweeter than sucrose.

Properties: Cholagogue, laxative, expectorant.

Uses: Internally it is used (as a tea, h. p.) for minor hepatobiliary problems (with impaired bile flow) and problems associated with it (impaired digestion, minor constipation), and for inflammations of the upper respiratory tract (bronchitis, etc.; coughs).

Caution: There are no reports of contraindications or side effects when used properly. Nevertheless, polypody is best avoided during pregnancy and lactation.

References: (3) Vol. 6a, p. 823; (8) p. 453; (10) p. 221; (13) p. 171; (27) p. 264; (28) p. 107; (35) p. 307; (37) p. 1006; (47) p. 2198; (51) p. 232.

POPLAR

Other Common Name(s): 1) black poplar, balm-of-Gilead 2) balsam poplar, balm-of-Gilead 3) white poplar, quaking aspen

Botanical Name(s): 1) *Populus nigra* L. 2) *Populus balsamifera* L. ssp. *balsamifera* = *Populus candicans* Aiton. = *Populus tacamahaca* Mill. 3) *Populus tremuloides* Michx. [Fam.: Salicaceae]

Bud

It is the leaf bud obtained from species 1 and 2, and more seldom from other *Populus* spp.

Constituents: Volatile oil (with α- and β-caryophyllene, etc.), flavonoids (flavones, flavonols, flavanones, etc.), phenol glycosides (salicin, populin), phenolic acids (caffeic acid derivatives, gallic acid), etc.

Properties: Anti-inflammatory and analgesic, antimicrobial, wound-healing, expectorant. The NSAID-like anti-inflammatory and analgesic effects are due in large part to phenol glycosides (see WILLOW). To the anti-inflammatory effect surely contribute flavonoids and phenolic acids.

Uses: Externally it is used (as an ointment, poultice) for minor skin inflammations, burns, itching, hemorrhoids, rheumatic pains, and (as a gargle) for inflammations of the throat. Internally it is used (as an h. p., tea) for inflammations of the genitourinary tract (cystitis, urethritis, prostatitis, urinary incontinence), micturition problems associated with early stages of benign prostatic hyperplasia (= BPH), for inflammations of the upper respiratory tract (bronchitis, laryngitis, etc.; coughs) and gastrointestinal tract (incl. hemorrhoids), and for minor rheumatic complaints (incl. rheumatoid arthritis). To enhance the effects in problems of the genitourinary tract, the fluid intake (incl. herbal teas) should be more than 2 liters per day.

Caution: In rare cases it may cause skin allergic reactions. Otherwise, there are no reports of contraindications or side effects when used properly.

303

Bark
It consists of the dried bark of twigs of white poplar or quaking aspen.
Constituents: Phenol glycosides (salicin, populin, salicortin, salireposide, etc.), tannins, etc. The content of phenol glycosides in quaking aspen bark is lower than in some willows, but it is possible to be higher than in white willow bark.
Properties: See WILLOW. While from salicin, populin and salicortin in our body is produced salicylic acid, from salireposide is produced gentisic acid (= 5-hydroxy-salicylic acid), which is as effective as salicylic acid.
Uses and Caution: See WILLOW.

References: (3) Vol. 6a, pp. 834, 837; (8) p. 455; (9) p. 58; (14) p. 27; (15) pp. 103, 168; (19) pp. 169, 170; (23) p. 266; (24) p. 456; (27) p. 261; (28) p. 199; (29) p. 90; (37) p. 1110; (47) p. 2207.

POPPY, CALIFORNIA

Botanical Name(s): *Eschscholtzia californica* A. Cham. [Fam.: Papaveraceae]
Aerial part
Constituents: Isoquinoline alkaloids (chiefly californidine, also eschscholtzine, allocryptopine, protopine, sanguinarine, chelerythrine, etc.), flavonoids (rutin, etc.), carotenoids, etc.
Properties: Sedative, antispasmodic, mild analgesic.
Uses: Internally it is used (as an h. p., tea; usually combined with other herbs) for nervousness, anxiety, insomnia, and for mild spastic conditions of the gastrointestinal, hepatobiliary, respiratory and genitourinary tracts.
Caution: It should not be taken during pregnancy because allocryptopine and possibly other alkaloids exert oxytocic effect. Alcoholic drinks may interact with California poppy. A possible combination of California poppy with sedative, hypnotic, and antidepressant drugs should be made only by a health professional. Otherwise, there are no reports of contraindications or side effects when used properly.

References: (1) Vol. 5, p. 111; (3) Vol. 4, p. 831; (8) p. 253; (13) p. 234; (23) p. 300; (29) p. 49; (31) p. 192; (37) p. 484; (44) p. 228; (48) p. 918.

POPPY, FIELD

Other Common Name(s): corn poppy, red poppy
Botanical Name(s): *Papaver rhoeas* L. [Fam.: Papaveraceae]
Petal
Constituents: Rhoeadan alkaloids (chiefly rhoeadine = tetrahydrobenzazepin, also isorhoeadine, rhoeagenine, etc.), flavonoids (anthocyanins: mecocyanin, cyanin), mucilaginous polysaccharides, etc.
Properties: Sedative, antitussive (possibly cough suppressant effect), demulcent. The effects are mild.

304

Uses: Internally it is used (as a tea, h. p.; combined with other herbs) for minor nervous disorders (nervousness, insomnia, cardiac arrhythmias) and minor inflammations of the upper respiratory tract (laryngitis with hoarseness, etc.; irritating dry coughs). It is particularly recommended for children and the elderly. It is also used as a coloring ingredient in herbal teas to enhance their appearance.

Caution: There are no reports of contraindications or side effects when used properly.

References: (2) Vol. 3, p. 287; (3) Vol. 6a, p. 444; (17) p. 497; (27) p. 248; (28) p. 218; (35) p. 651; (37) p. 1024; (46) p. 1074; (48) p. 919; (49) Vol. 2, p. 206.

POPPY, OPIUM

Other Common Name(s): poppyseed poppy
Botanical Name(s): *Papaver somniferum* L. [Fam.: Papaveraceae]
Opium
It is the dried juice obtained by incisions made to the unripe capsules.

Constituents: Isoquinoline alkaloids of morphinan group (chiefly morphine, also codeine, thebaine, etc.) and benzylisoquinoline group (chiefly noscapine = narcotine, also papaverine, narceine, etc.), also sugars, mucilaginous polysaccharides, resin, etc.

Properties: In general, opium acts much like morphine, with some differences due to an existing partial synergism and antagonism between the alkaloids. Morphine (at normal doses) is analgesic (typical narcotic analgesic), sedative, euphoriant, hypnotic, suppressant of the gastrointestinal and bronchial secretions, suppressant of cough (milder than codeine) and respiration, causes constipation (stronger than codeine), and (at high doses) exerts narcotic effect. Codeine is antitussive (stronger than morphine; by suppressing the medullary cough center) and analgesic (milder than morphine), and has been shown to be much less prone to habit forming than morphine. Papaverine is antispasmodic. Noscapine, like codeine, is antitussive and potentiates the analgesic effect of morphine.

Uses: Opium and opium poppy straw are used for the isolation of the alkaloids. Opium phytopharmaceuticals (titrated opium powder, extract, tincture, etc.) are used for the symptomatic treatment of acute diarrhea and seldom for coughs and pains.

Caution: Opium is a prescription drug. Opium and morphine, and to a lesser extent codeine, besides the usual side effects (constipation, delayed emptying of the urinary bladder and gallbladder, etc.), with a chronic intake develop tolerance and dependence, and due to respiratory depression (less intensive with opium, due to the presence of noscapine and thebaine) toxic doses result in respiratory paralysis. Other details are beyond the scope of this book.

References: (2) Vol. 3, p. 289; (3) Vol. 6a, p. 404; (6) p. 355; (11) p. 163; (12) p. 994; (13) p. 229; (23)

p. 96; (37) pp. 610, 1024; (46) p. 1064; (48) p. 929.

POTATO

Botanical Name(s): *Solanum tuberosum* L. [Fam.: Solanaceae]
Fresh juice
Fresh juice is prepared preferably from the red skin variety.
Constituents: Glycoalkaloids (= glycosidic steroidal alkaloids: α-chaconine, α-solanine; very small amounts), carbohydrates (chiefly starch, some mucilaginous polysaccharides), vitamin C, etc.
Properties: Relieves spasms and decreases hyperacidity of the stomach, demulcent. Potato glycoalkaloids have shown parasympatholytic activity (belladonna-like or atropine-like effect; see BELLADONNA). The demulcent effect is due to mucilaginous polysaccharides and starch.
Uses: Internally it is used (as a standardized product, also combined with other herbs) mainly for stomach complaints such as gastritis with hyperacidity. It has also been used for pharyngitis and laryngitis (possibly those cases caused by a gastro-esophageal reflux, with symptoms of heartburn).
Caution: It should not be taken during pregnancy and lactation. It is best used as a standardized product to alkaloids content. The germinated potatoes or those with green spots should not be used as they contain much higher concentrations of alkaloids.
Note: Potato is a valuable potassium supplement.

References: (1) Vol. 6, p. 746; (3) Vol. 6b, p. 442; (8) p. 526; (23) p. 76; (37) p. 1277; (47) p. 2566.

PRICKLY ASH, SOUTHERN

Other Common Name(s): Hercule's club
Botanical Name(s): *Zanthoxylum clava-herculis* L. = *Zanthoxylum macrophyllum* Nutt. [Fam.: Rutaceae]
Bark (= toothache bark)
Constituents: Pungent principles (amides: chiefly herclavin, also neoherculin, etc., similar to those found in *Echinacea*), lignans (asarinin, sesamin), benzophenathridine alkaloids (chelerythrine, nitidine, etc.), etc.
Properties: Counterirritant, local anesthetic, anti-inflammatory and antirheumatic, bitter tonic, circulatory stimulant, antimicrobial.
Uses: Externally it is used (as a pasty mass applied to the tooth, cotton swab, or by chewing the bark) for toothache, (as a gargle) for sore throat and chronic laryngitis, (as a lotion, ointment, poultice) for neuralgic and rheumatic pains, and (as a wash, wet compress) for minor skin inflammations. Internally it is used (as a tea, h. p.) for rheumatic complaints (incl. rheumatoid arthritis) and conditions associated with an impaired peripheral blood circulation (incl. intermittent claudication = pain / cramp / weakness in the legs on walking, and Raynaud's disease = pale or red-blue patchy fin-

gers / toes). It is also used (as a tea, h. p.) for inflammations of the gastrointestinal tract (impaired digestion, flatulence, cramps, diarrhea), upper respiratory tract (the common cold, etc.; coughs; also as a diaphoretic hot tea) and genitourinary tract (cystitis, urethritis, etc.). To enhance the effects in problems of the genitourinary tract, the fluid intake (incl. herbal teas) should be more than 2 liters per day.

Caution: Southern prickly ash should not be taken during pregnancy and lactation, and higher doses then recommended should be avoided. It is best used as directed by an experienced practitioner.

Note: Bark of **northern prickly ash**: *Zanthoxylum americanum* Mill. is stated to exert the same effects and in traditional medicine it is used the same as southern prickly ash. However, there are no reports that it contains pungent amides, which play an important role in the overall effect. Northern prickly ash is reported to contain coumarins (pyranocoumarins of xanthyletin type), benzophenathridine alkaloids, and a phenylethylamine derivative (candicine) with nicotine-like effect.

References: (2) Vol. 3, p. 825; (3) Vol. 6c, p. 548; (9) p. 46; (14) p. 177; (15) p. 237; (20) p. 220; (25) p. 238; (31) p. 311; (41) Vols. 1-7; (44) p. 609; (45) p. 151; (52) p. 881.

PSYLLIUM

Other Common Name(s): 1) plantago arenaria, French / Spanish psyllium
2) Indian plantain, Indian psyllium, ispaghula
Botanical Name(s): 1) *Plantago arenaria* Waldst. et Kit. = *Plantago psyllium* L. 2) *Plantago ovata* Forssk. = *Plantago ispaghula* Roxb. [Fam.: Plantaginaceae]
Seed (psyllium), **seed husk** (ispaghula husk)
Seed is obtained from both species and is usually known as psyllium. In trade, seed obtained from the second species is also known as ispaghula. Husk is obtained from the second species.
Constituents: (Seed): Mucilaginous polysaccharides (localized in the seed coat or husk), fixed oil (with glycerides of linoleic and oleic acids), proteins, sugars, triterpenes, iridoids (aucubin, etc.), alkaloids (traces), etc.
Properties: Bulk laxative, antidiarrheal, demulcent, emollient, anti-inflammatory, mild cholesterol and triglyceride reducing. Mucilages are not absorbed from the gastrointestinal tract. There, they absorb water, swell and increase the bulk, and soften the consistency of stools, due to which results a facilitated defecation. By retaining the fluids, so decreasing bowel discharges and irritations, they exert antidiarrheal effect. Mucilages may bind dietary cholesterol and the available bile salts, and increase their fecal excretion. Then the liver to synthesize biliary acids will utilize the excessive LDL-cholesterol.
Uses: Internally it is used for constipation and conditions that a facilitated defecation is sought (hemorrhoids, during pregnancy, after operations in the

rectum or anal area, etc.), for diarrhea, irritable bowel syndrome, Crohn's disease, and as an adjuvant for high cholesterol and triglycerides. Externally it is used (as a wet compress, lotion with mucilage) for minor skin inflammations, and (as a poultice) for boils and carbuncles, among others.

Caution: It should not be swallowed dry but taken short after mixing the recommended amount with a glass of water or other fluid and followed by taking another portion of fluid. It should not be taken in cases of intestinal obstructions or spastic conditions. It may impair the absorption of some drugs. In view of this, when taking a vital oral medication, drugs should be taken about one hour apart from psyllium.

References: (1) Vol. 6, p. 222; (3) Vol. 6a, p. 754; (6) p. 156; (8) p. 443; (12) p. 366; (13) p. 370; (16) p. 144; (17) p. 463; (19) pp. 82, 111; (20) p. 173; (29) p. 87; (37) p. 1091; (48) p. 106; (59) p. 202.

PULSATILLA

Other Common Name(s): 1) European Pasqueflower, pulsatilla 2) meadow Pasqueflower, pulsatilla, windflower
Botanical Name(s): 1) *Pulsatilla vulgaris* Mill. = *Anemone pulsatilla* L. 2) *Pulsatilla pratensis* (L.) Mill. = *Anemone pratensis* L. [Fam.: Ranunculaceae]
Aerial part
Constituents: (Dried herb): Anemonin (= protoanemonin dimer); (fresh herb): protoanemonin (an unstable compound); and (fresh or dried): tannins, flavonoids, saponins, organic acids, etc.
Properties: (Dried herb): Antimicrobial, antispasmodic, diuretic, sedative. (Fresh herb): Counterirritant / vesicant (depending on concentration) and analgesic. Anemonin is non-toxic and has shown antimicrobial effect. Protoanemonin is toxic and a strong local irritant.
Uses: Pulsatilla is chiefly used in traditional medicine. Internally it is used (only dried!; as a tea) for inflammatory and spastic conditions of the genitourinary, hepatobiliary, gastrointestinal, and upper respiratory tracts. To enhance the effects in problems of the genitourinary tract, the fluid intake (incl. herbal teas) should be more than 2 liters per day. Externally it is used (as poultice, liniment: fresh herb) for rheumatic and neuralgic pains, and (as wash, wet compress: dried herb) for bacterial and fungal skin infections.
Caution: Internally should be used only dried herb and as directed by an experienced practitioner. Even dried, pulsatilla should not be taken during pregnancy as it may still contain protoanemonin (teratogenic, abortifacient!). Fresh herb should be handled with care (see Properties), even when used externally. If taken internally, fresh herb (also dried herb at higher doses than recommended) causes strong gastrointestinal irritations (with vomiting, diarrhea), etc.

References: (1) Vol. 6, p. 321; (3) Vol. 6a, p. 975; (14) p. 179; (15) p. 173; (20) p. 222; (27) p. 274; (46) p. 1158; (47) p. 2243; (48) p. 747; (49) Vol. 2, p. 152.

PULSATILLA, CHINESE

Botanical Name(s): *Pulsatilla chinensis* (Bunge) Regel = *Anemone chinensis* Bunge; and closely related species [Fam.: Ranunculaceae]
Root (dried)
Constituents: Anemonin (= protoanemonin dimer), triterpenoid saponins, tannins, etc. Fresh root contains the unstable protoanemonin (a non-glycosidic monomer), which on drying or boiling is transformed into a dimeric compound (anemonin; cf. PULSATILLA).
Properties: (Dried root): Antibacterial, antifungal, antiprotozoal (against *Entamoeba* spp., *Trichomonas* spp.). Anemonin is non-toxic but protoanemonin, which is found in fresh root, is toxic and a strong local irritant.
Uses: Internally it is used (dried root; as a tea, h. p.) for infections of the gastrointestinal tract (diarrhea, amebic dysentery, possibly hepatic amebiasis), genitourinary tract (caused by *Trichomonas vaginalis*), and upper respiratory tract. To enhance the effects in problems of the genitourinary tract, the fluid intake (incl. herbal teas) should be more than 2 liters per day. Externally it is used (as a vaginal irrigation / sitz bath / wash: dried root) for vulvovaginitis (caused by *Trichomonas vaginalis*), and (as a wash, wet compress: dried root) for bacterial and fungal skin infections
Caution: Internally should be used only dried herb and as directed by an experienced practitioner. Even dried, Chinese pulsatilla should not be taken during pregnancy as it may still contain protoanemonin (teratogenic, abortifacient!; cf. PULSATILLA). Fresh root should be handled with care (see Properties), even when used externally. If taken internally, fresh root (also dried root at higher doses than recommended) causes strong gastrointestinal irritations (with vomiting, diarrhea), etc.

References: (1) Vol. 6, p. 315; (41) Vols. 1-7; (42) Vol. 6, p. 47; (45) p. 257; (48) p. 747.

PUMPKIN

Botanical Name(s): *Cucurbita pepo* L. [Fam.: Cucurbitaceae]
Seed
Constituents: Phytosterols (rich in 7-sterols: α-spinasterol, α-spinasterol-glucoside, etc.; also 5-sterols: clerosterol, etc.), fixed oil (with linoleic acid, etc.; β- and γ-tocopherol), minerals (rich in selenium), amino acids (incl. cucurbitine), etc. Free sterols and tocopherols are contained in the fixed oil.
Properties: Pumpkin seed extract has been shown to inhibit the biosynthesis of DHT (= dihydrotestosterone, one of the main causes of a BPH) in the prostatic tissue as well as its binding to the receptors. It also has shown anti-inflammatory, antioxidant, antibacterial, diuretic and bladder tonic effects. Its main active constituents are considered 7-sterols. Tocopherols, selenium and linoleic acid (an omega-6 fatty acid) contribute synergistically to the antioxidant, anti-inflammatory and bladder tonic effects. Pumpkin seed exerts

also anthelmintic effect, which is attributed to cucurbitine.
Uses: Internally it is used (as a standardized product, raw seed) for micturition problems associated with early stages of benign prostatic hyperplasia (=
BPH: stages I and II) and for irritable bladder (with urinary incontinence)
and childhood enuresis. Rational treatments with pumpkin standardized
products have resulted in a decrease or disappearance of difficulties in starting the urination, increase of urine flow, and decrease of frequency of urination and residual urine. It is also used for intestinal worms (tapeworms =
Taenia spp.; roundworms = *Ascaris* spp.). Due to phytosterols and high concentrations of linoleic acid, seeds may be beneficial for high cholesterol.
Caution: Before using pumpkin seed products for BPH, the prostate problem should be judged by a health professional. Pumpkin seed is best used as
a standardized product to sterols content. Otherwise, there are no reports of
contraindications or side effects when used properly.

References: (1) Vol. 4, p. 1073; (3) Vol. 4, p. 360; (6) pp. 194, 197; (7) p. 254; (8) p. 201; (16) p. 154;
(17) p. 178; (19) p. 135; (23) pp. 115, 264; (37) p. 371; (47) p. 1140; (48) p. 758.

PYGEUM

Other Common Name(s): African plum
Botanical Name(s): *Prunus africana* (Hook. f.) Kalkman = *Pygeum africanum* Hook. f. [Fam.: Rosaceae]
Bark (trunk bark)
Constituents: Phytosterols (5-sterols: β-sitosteol, β-sitosterolin = β-sitos-
teol-glucoside, β-sitosterone, etc.), fatty acids, triterpenoids (oleanolic acid,
saponins), ferulic acid esters (docosyl-ferulate, tetracosyl-ferulate), free long
chain aliphatic alcohols (C_{22}: docosyl alcohol = *n*-docosanol; C_{24}: tetracosyl
alcohol = *n*-tetracosanol), cyanogenic glycosides, etc.
Properties: Pygeum africanum extract (= PAE) has shown anti-inflammatory effect by inhibiting the biosynthesis of prostaglandins, and antiandro-
genic effect by competitively inhibiting the biosynthesis of androgens, with
prostatic antiproliferative effects (= inhibition of prostate cells division and
growth). Its most important active constituents are considered phytosterols
and other triterpenes, fatty acids and ferulic acid esters.
Uses: Internally it is used (PAE: mainly in a combination product) for micturition problems associated with benign prostatic hyperplasia (= BPH). Rational treatments with PAE have resulted in a decrease of difficulties in
starting the urination, increase of urinary volume and flow, decrease of frequency of urination and residual urine. PAE has also shown to increase
prostatic secretions so it may be beneficial for some types of male infertility.
Caution: Before using pygeum products for BPH, the prostate problem
should be judged by a health professional. Pygeum products should contain
PAE standardized to sterols and other triterpenes (expressed as β-sitosterol)
and aliphatic alcohols (expressed as *n*-docosanol). In rare cases it may cause

310

a temporary stomach upset. Otherwise, there are no reports of contraindications or side effects when used properly.

References: (3) Vol. 6a, p. 954; (5) Vol. 3, p. 503; (6) p. 198; (22) p. 106; (36) p. 516; (37) p. 1136; (41) Vols. 1-7; (48) p. 161; (68) p. 189; (89) p. 286.

PYRETHRUM

Other Common Name(s): 1) Dalmatian insect flower 2) Caucasian insect flower, Persian insect flower
Botanical Name(s): 1) *Chrysanthemum cinerariifolium* (Trev.) Vis. = *Pyrethrum cinerariifolium* Trev. 2) *Chrysanthemum coccineum* Willd.; *Chrysanthemum marschallii* Aschers [Fam.: Asteraceae (Compositae)]
Flower
Constituents: Pyrethrins (a mixture of pyrethrins I and II, cinerins I and II, and jasmolins I and II). They are esters of keto-alcohols (pyrethrolone, cinerolone, jasmolone) with mono or dicarboxylic acids (series I: chrysanthemic acid; series II: pyrethric acid), etc.
Properties: Pyrethrum is a contact poison (more precisely, neurotoxic) for cold-blooded animals (insects, etc.). From pyrethrins, the more active is pyrethrin I, followed by pyrethrin II.
Uses: Powder and especially spray products with active principles dissolved in organic solvents are used as insecticides or insect-repellents for most of household insects. As pyrethrins are unstable, the synthetic analogs, the so-called pyrethroids are more preferred.
Caution: With normal spraying amounts pyrethrins do not cause untoward effects as they have a low toxicity for mammalians. Only if taken orally in high concentrations they can be harmful to humans and other mammalians.

References: (3) Vol. 3, p. 895; (8) p. 150; (13) p. 36; (36) p. 534; (37) p. 328; (46) p. 410; (48) p. 613.

QUASSIA

Other Common Name(s): 1) Surinam quassia, quassia 2) Jamaica quassia, bitterwood
Botanical Name(s): 1) *Quassia amara* L. 2) *Picrasma excelsa* (Sw.) Planch. = *Quassia excelsa* Sw.[Fam.: Simaroubaceae; both species]
Stem-wood
Constituents: Bitter principles (nortriterpenes of quassinoids type: quassin, neoquassin, etc.), coumarins (scopoletin), etc., but no tannins.
Properties: Bitter tonic. Quassin has shown antipyretic, anthelmintic, and insecticidal effects. Nortriterpenes of quassinoid type have shown antiprotozoal (esp. against *Entamoeba* spp., but also *Plasmodium* spp.), antiviral, antibacterial, and anthelmintic effects.
Uses: Internally it is used (as an h. p., tea) chiefly for loss of appetite and

nonulcer dyspepsia (with fullness, nausea, vomiting, atonic diarrhea) and convalescence. It traditional medicine it is also used as an enema for intestinal worms (against pinworms = *Oxyuris* spp.). In bitter tonic mixtures quassia is often preferred to other bitter botanicals because it doesn't contain tannins. Quassin is often used as a substitute of quinine in the production of bitters. Externally it has been used in traditional medicine for head lice (= pediculosis capitis) and proven effective. Nevertheless, it is no longer used for this purpose because there are other drug alternatives available.

Caution: It should not be taken during pregnancy. At higher doses than recommended it causes gastrointestinal irritations (with nausea, vomiting, diarrhea). Otherwise, there are no reports of contraindications or side effects when used properly.

References: (2) Vol. 3, pp. 379, 433; (3) Vol. 6a, pp. 652, 1000, (6) pp. 133, 134; (7) p. 186; (8) p. 470; (9) p. 430; (12) pp. 98, 520; (13) p. 166; (17) p. 468; (20) p. 223; (31) p. 728; (46) p. 1165; (47) p. 2259; (48) p. 765; (49) Vol. 2, p. 305; (66) p. 410.

QUEBRACHO, WHITE

Other Common Name(s): quebracho
Botanical Name(s): *Aspidosperma quebracho-blanco* Schlecht. [Fam.: Apocynaceae]
Bark (white quebracho)
Constituents: Indole alkaloids (chiefly aspidospermine and quebrachine = yohimbine, etc.), triterpenes, tannins, a cyclitol (quebrachitol), etc.
Properties: Respiratory stimulant, expectorant, aphrodisiac. Aspidospermine has shown respiratory stimulant effect. The mild aphrodisiac effect is due to yohimbine (see YOHIMBE).
Uses: Internally it is used (as an h. p., tea; combined with other herbs) for respiratory disorders (the common cold, bronchitis, bronchial asthma, pulmonary emphysema; coughs). It is also used for erectile dysfunction.
Caution: It should be used only as directed by an experienced practitioner as it contains potential alkaloids. At higher doses than recommended it causes gastrointestinal irritations (with nausea, vomiting).

References: (1) Vol. 4, p. 401; (3) Vol. 3, p. 294; (8) p. 86; (17) p. 470; (31) pp. 161, 164; (46) p. 1170; (47) p. 2264.

QUILLAJA

Other Common Name(s): soap tree
Botanical Name(s): *Quillaja saponaria* Molina [Fam.: Rosaceae]
Bark (soap bark) (bark of the trunk without cork)
Constituents: Triterpenoid saponins (quillaja saponin-21 = QS-21, etc., very rich; with aglycone: quillaic acid; cf. SOAPWORT, RED), tannins, sugars, starch, calcium oxalate (high concentrations), etc.

312

Properties: Expectorant, astringent, cholesterol reducing. The effects, except astringent, are due to saponins. QS-21 has shown immunomodulant effect.

Uses: Soap bark extract and isolated saponin are chiefly used as foaming ingredients in alcoholic and non-alcoholic beverages, and as foaming ingredients and detergents in shampoos, mouthwashes and toothpastes, among others. Externally it is used (as a wash) for scalp problems (dandruff, hair loss), (as a partial bath) for athlete's foot, and (as a wet compress) for bruises. Internally it is seldom used (combined with other herbs) for inflammations of the upper respiratory tract (chronic bronchitis, etc.; coughs). The isolated genuine saponin (Q-21) is used as an immunostimulant.

Caution: It should not be taken in cases of gastrointestinal ulcers. At higher doses than recommended it causes gastrointestinal irritations (with cramps, nausea, vomiting, diarrhea). As it is rich in saponins, avoid contact with eyes or inhalation of powdered bark as it irritates the mucous membranes.

References: (2) Vol. 3, p. 434; (3) Vol. 6a, p. 1015; (9) p. 432; (12) p. 550; (13) p. 208; (15) p. 175; (17) p. 476; (37) p. 1159; (46) p. 1184; (47) p. 2278; (48) p. 710; (49) Vol. 2, p. 423; (66) p. 411.

QUINCE

Botanical Name(s): *Cydonia oblonga* Mill. = *Cydonia vulgaris* Pers. [Fam.: Rosaceae]

Seed

Constituents: Mucilaginous polysaccharides (very rich), a cyanogenic glycoside (amygdalin), an enzyme (emulsin), fixed oil, minerals, tannins, etc.

Properties: Emollient, demulcent

Uses: Externally it is used (as a poultice, mucilage, fat-free ointment) for minor burns and ulcers, minor skin inflammations and chaps (hands, lips, nipples), and in cosmetics in the production of hair-fixing lotions and fat-free face lotions. Internally it is used (as a mucilage) for inflammations of the gastrointestinal tract (minor diarrhea, etc.)

Caution: When preparing the mucilage seeds should not be crushed because the enzyme (emulsin) will come into contact with amygdalin, which will liberate hydrocyanic acid (toxic!).

Fruit (ripe)

Constituents: Pectin, sugars, organic acids (malic acid, etc.), vitamin C, some tannins, flavonoids (leucoanthocyanidins), volatile oil, etc.

Properties: Demulcent, mild astringent, antidiarrheal, aromatic.

Uses: Internally it is used (as a decoction, or by boiling down to a purée) for minor diarrhea. Externally it is used (as a mouthwash, gargle) for inflammations of the mouth and throat. In culinary practice and food industry ripe quince fruit is used in the production of jellies and preserves.

Caution: There are no reports of contraindications or side effects when used properly.

References: (2) Vol. 2, p. 482; (3) Vol. 4, p. 406; (12a) p. 131; (27) p. 102; (36) p. 216; (37) p. 380; (48) p. 118; (49) Vol. 2, p. 422; (66) p. 261.

QUINCE, FLOWERING

Other Common Name(s): Chinese quince, Japanese quince
Botanical Name(s): *Chaenomeles speciosa* (Sweet) Nakai = *Chaenomeles lagenaria* (Loisel.) Koidz. [Fam.: Rosaceae]
Fruit (ripe, dried)
Constituents: A sugar alcohol (sorbitol; possibly rich), organic acids (citric, malic and tartaric acids), and vitamin C. It possibly contains pectin, small amounts of tannins (proanthocyanidins), and pseudosaponins.
Properties: Stomachic, cholagogue, laxative, mild astringent, diuretic, demulcent.
Uses: Internally it is used (as a tea, h. p.) for loss of appetite and nonulcer dyspepsia (with flatulence, nausea), and minor constipation, which are often associated with impaired bile flow. It is also used for morning sickness, and as an antidyscratic (= blood purifier) for chronic rheumatic complaints. It is recommended as a dietetic aid to diabetics (sorbitol, is transformed in the liver into fructose, then converted to glycogen without the need of insulin).
Caution: There are no reports of contraindications or side effects when used properly.

References: (1) Vol. 4, p. 796; (36) p. 508; (37) p. 1283; (52) p. 174; (73) p. 1121.

RADISH, BLACK

Botanical Name(s): *Raphanus sativus* L. var. *niger* (Miller) S. Kerner [Fam.: Brassicaceae (Cruciferae)]
Root (fresh)
Constituents: Glucosinolates (glucoraphanin = 4-methylthio-3-butenyl-glucosinolate; mainly in the intact fresh material), vitamin C, enzymes, etc.
Properties: Cholagogue, gastrointestinal tonic (increases secretions and motility of the upper gastrointestinal tract), antimicrobial, expectorant (bronchial secretagogue effect), diuretic. If fresh root is crushed, processed, or dried, glucosinolates (under the action of enzymes) liberate isothiocyanates (4-methylthio-3-butenyl-isothiocyanate, etc.), which are responsible for the mild pungent flavor and most of the mentioned effects.
Uses: Internally it is used (fresh root, freshly prepared juice) for nonulcer dyspepsia (with flatulence, sluggish bowels, minor constipation, headache) associated with impaired bile flow, and for inflammatory conditions of the upper respiratory tract (bronchitis, etc.; coughs due to thickened secretion).
Caution: See CRESS, GARDEN.

References: (1) Vol. 6, p. 356; (3) Vol. 6b, p. 16; (6) p. 148; (8) p. 473; (16) p. 132; (19) p. 187; (23) p. 134; (24) p. 268; (27) p. 283; (28) p. 108; (37) p. 1169; (48) p. 203; (51) p. 86.

RASPBERRY

Botanical Name(s): *Rubus idaeus* L. [Fam.: Rosaceae]

Leaf

Constituents: Tannins (gallotannins, ellagitannins), flavonoids (rutin, etc.), organic acids (succinic and lactic acids), some vitamin C, etc.

Properties: Astringent, antispasmodic. The effects are mild.

Uses: Internally it is used (as a tea, h. p.) for diarrhea and primary dysmenorrhea (= painful menstruation without pathology). If fresh leaves undergo fermentation before drying, they gain a flavor, which makes them suitable as a caffeine-free herbal tea. Externally it is used (as a mouthwash, gargle) for inflammations of the mouth and throat, and (as a wash, wet compress) for minor skin inflammations, wounds, ulcers and hemorrhoids.

Caution: There are no reports of contraindications or side effects when used properly.

Fruit

Constituents: Organic acids (chiefly citric acid), sugars, flavonoids (anthocyanins), pectin, volatile oil, etc.

Properties: Acidulous, refrigerant.

Uses: Raspberry tea is used as a refreshing drink for feverish and thirsty states. Raspberry syrup, which is prepared from fresh fruits, is used in pharmaceutical practice in flavoring drug products.

Caution: There are no reports of contraindications or side effects when used properly.

References: (3) Vol. 6b, p. 186; (17) p. 512; (20) p. 226; (27) p. 175; (37) p. 1204; (46) p. 801; (66) p. 419.

RAUWOLFIA

Other Common Name(s): Indian snakeroot

Botanical Name(s): *Rauvolfia serpentina* (L.) Benth. ex Kurz [Fam.: Apocynaceae]

Root

Constituents: Indole alkaloids (localized chiefly in root-bark) of yohimbine type (reserpine, rescinnamine, deserpidine, yohimbine, etc.), raubasine type (raubasine, serpentine, etc.) and ajmaline type (ajmaline, etc.), starch, etc.

Properties: The root or the whole extract exerts at the same time antihypertensive and sedative effects, due in large part to reserpine, rescinnamine and deserpidine. Serpentine exerts antihypertensive effect, while ajmaline exerts antiarrhythmic effect.

Uses: Internally it is used (titrated extract, seldom powdered root) chiefly for hypertension, but also for anxiety and sinus tachycardia (= rapid heartbeat) associated with elevated tension of sympathetic nervous system and catecholamines drive. Reserpine is still used, but only as an antihypertensive

315

and not as a sedative.

Caution: Rauwolfia and reserpine are used only by prescription. They should not be taken in cases of depressive states, peptic ulcers, pheochromocytoma, and during pregnancy and lactation. Further details are beyond the scope of this book.

<u>Note</u>: For the industrial isolation of alkaloids are also used other *Rauvolfia* spp. such as *R. vomitoria* Afz. and *R. tetraphylla* L., among others.

References: (1) Vol. 6, p. 363; (3) Vol. 6b, p. 19; (8) p. 474; (11) p. 167; (12) p. 1031; (13) p. 253; (17) p. 482; (19) p. 186; (37) p. 1170; (46) p. 1207; (48) p. 1025; (59) p. 221; (67) p. 484, 608.

RED CLOVER

Botanical Name(s): *Trifolium pratense* L. [Fam.: Fabaceae (Leguminosae)]

<u>Flower</u> (flower head)

Constituents: Flavonoids (very rich in isoflavones: formononetin, biochanin A, daidzein, genistein), coumestans (= coumarono-coumarins: coumestrol, etc.), clovamides (= amides of caffeic acid with dopa), volatile oil (with methyl salicylate, etc.), phytosterols, etc.

Properties: Estrogen-like, antioxidant, antitumoral, antispasmodic, expectorant, anti-inflammatory, wound-healing. Isoflavones and coumestrol are plant constituents with estrogen-like effect (= phytoestrogens; coumestrol acts much stronger), whose metabolites have been shown to inhibit binding of stronger estrogens (e. g. estradiol) to their receptors therefore regarded as antiestrogens. Depending on the hormone imbalance stage (when estrogens level is lower than expected) they may exert proestrogenic effects. Cf. ALFALFA; KUDZU; SOY. Dopa (= dihydroxy-phenylalanine) is a precursor of catecholamines (epinephrine, norepinephrine) and melanin.

Uses: <u>Internally</u> it is used (concentrated extract standardized to the isoflavones content; isolated isoflavones) as a supplement of phytoestrogens, to alleviate menopausal syndrome (= hot flashes, sweating, tachycardia, insomnia, emotional instability, depressive mood, fatigue, decreased vaginal lubrication, etc.), and to prevent postmenopausal problems (osteoporosis, high cholesterol and triglycerides, breast and uterine cancer, etc.) and prostate cancer. As a tea or liquid extract it is used for inflammations of the upper respiratory tract. It is also used as an antidyscratic (= blood purifier) and anti-inflammatory (tea, h. p.) for atopic eczema (= chronic eczema of internal origin) and chronic rheumatic complaints. <u>Externally</u> it is used (as a wash, compress, poultice) for chronic skin diseases (psoriasis, eczema, etc.).

Caution: There are no reports of contraindications or side effects when used properly but, as with other herbs with estrogen-like effect, red clover should not be taken in cases of estrogen receptor-positive (ER+) tumors. During pregnancy and lactation it can be used on health professional's advice.

References: (1) Vol. 6, p. 992; (3) Vol. 6c, p. 265; (9) p. 177; (14) p. 183; (15) p. 215; (20) p. 227; (29) p. 117; (31) p. 415; (41) Vols. 1-7; (47) p. 2723; (48) p. 349.

REHMANNIA

Botanical Name(s): *Rehmannia glutinosa* Libosch. ex Fisch. et Mey. [Fam.: Scrophulariaceae]
Root (raw tuber, dried)
Constituents: Bitter principles (iridoids: catalpol, also ajugol, rehmanniosides, etc.), phenylethanoid glycosides (acteoside = verbascoside, also purpureaside C, echinacoside, etc.), sugars (stachyose, also sucrose, galactose, etc.), water-soluble polysaccharides, amino acids, phytosterols, etc.
Properties: Bitter tonic, anti-inflammatory, antipyretic, antibacterial, liver protective, antioxidant, laxative, diuretic. Iridoids have shown bitter tonic, choleretic, liver protective, laxative, diuretic, anti-inflammatory, antibacterial, antiviral, antifungal, and immunomodulant effects, among others. Acteoside and other phenylethanoid glycosides have been shown to be anti-inflammatory (by inhibiting the biosynthesis of leukotrienes), liver protective, and antioxidant. Water-soluble polysaccharides have shown immunomodulant effect. An important role possibly plays also galactose, which in rehmannia is found free, or as a component of stachyose, water-soluble polysaccharides and galactosides.
Uses: Internally it is used (as a tea, h. p.) for loss of appetite and nonulcer dyspepsia (with sluggish bowels, minor constipation), inflammations of the liver (chronic hepatitis) and genitourinary tract, feverish states, minor fatigue, and convalescence. It is also used as an antidyscratic (= blood purifier) and anti-inflammatory (tea, h. p.) for chronic rheumatic complaints and atopic eczema (= chronic eczema of internal origin). To enhance the effects in problems of the genitourinary tract, the fluid intake (incl. herbal teas) should be more than 2 liters per day. Externally it is used for minor skin inflammations.
Caution: There are no reports of contraindications or side effects when used properly. Nevertheless, it is best to avoid it during pregnancy and lactation. At higher doses than recommended it may cause gastrointestinal irritations (with nausea, vomiting, diarrhea).

References: (1) Vol. 6, p. 384; (5) Vol. 3, p. 509; (9) p. 435; (13) p. 434; (31) pp. 472, 569; (37) p. 1174; (41) Vols. 1-7; (45) p. 123; (53) p. 127.

RESTHARROW

Other Common Name(s): cammock, spiny restharrow
Botanical Name(s): *Ononis campestris* Koch et Ziz = *Ononis spinosa* L. [Fam.: Fabaceae (Leguminosae)]
Root
Constituents: Flavonoids (isoflavones: formononetin, ononin, etc. and closely related pterocarpanes: trifolirhizin, etc.), triterpenes (α-onocerin = onocol, etc.), phenolic acids (caffeic acid, etc.), tannins, phytosterols, etc.

Properties: Diuretic, anti-inflammatory.

Uses: Internally it is used (usually combined with other herbs) as a flushing-out treatment (= herbal tea or product + liquids: more than 2 liters per day; sometimes combined with a medication) for inflammations of the genitourinary tract (cystitis, etc.), urinary gravel and nonobstructive stones, to prevent relapsing urinary infections / gravel / stones, and as an anti-inflammatory and antidyscratic = blood purifier; tea, h. p.) for atopic eczema (= chronic eczema of internal origin) and chronic rheumatic complaints. Externally it is used (as a mouthwash) for inflammations of the mouth.

Caution: There are no reports of contraindications or side effects when used properly. Nevertheless, a flushing-out treatment is contraindicated in cases of obstructive urinary stones, edema due to impaired heart or kidney function and kidney inflammations (here can be used on health professional's advice to enhance the effects of an antimicrobial therapy).

References: (2) Vol. 3, p. 265; (3) Vol. 6a, p. 312; (6) pp. 184, 353, 360; (8) p. 389; (13) p. 317; (16) p. 161; (17) p. 410; (19) p. 101; (23) p. 256; (27) p. 35; (46) p. 1023; (47) p. 2021; (51) p. 256.

RHATANY

Other Common Name(s): Peruvian krameria, Peruvian rhatany
Botanical Name(s): *Krameria lappacea* (Dombey) Burdet et B.B. Simpson = *Krameria triandra* Ruiz et Pav. [Fam.: Krameriaceae]
Root
Constituents: Tannins (proanthocyanidins; rich), phlobaphenes (rhatany red or krameria red), lignans, starch (rich), calcium oxalate, etc.
Properties: Astringent, hemostatic, antimicrobial.
Uses: Externally it is used (as a mouthwash, gargle, paint) for inflammations of the mouth and throat (incl. canker sore), (as a wet compress) for minor cuts, wounds and sore nipples, and (as an ointment) for hemorrhoids. Internally it is used (as a tea, h. p.; at low doses) for diarrhea and inflammations of the gastrointestinal tract, and (as a suppository) for hemorrhoids.
Caution: A topical application of concentrated solutions (tincture, esp. liquid extract) may cause irritation. Internal applications should be limited to a few days. Otherwise, there are no reports of contraindications or side effects when used properly.

References: (1) Vol. 5, p. 615; (3) Vol. 5, p. 409; (6) p. 116; (8) p. 333; (12) p. 882; (13) p. 340; (14) p. 185; (15) p. 124; (16) p. 83; (17) p. 479; (22) p. 226; (27) p. 285; (28) p. 124; (29) p. 66; (36) p. 229; (46) p. 1204; (47) p. 2292; (48) p. 391.

RHODIOLA

Other Common Name(s): arctic rose, king's crown, snowdownrose
Botanical Name(s): *Rhodiola rosea* L. = *Sedum rosea* (L.) Scop. [Fam.: Crassulaceae]

Root (arctic root, golden root, rose root)
Constituents: Phenylpropanoid glycosides (rosavins: rosavin, etc.; agly-cone: cinnamyl alcohol), a phenylethanoid glycoside (salidroside = rhodi-oloside; aglycone: tyrosol), flavonoids (catechins, flavonols), tannins (hy-drolyzable t., also proanthocyanidins), phenolic acids (caffeic acid deriva-tives, etc.), volatile oil (with geraniol, etc.), etc. Tyrosol = salidrosol = 2-(4-hydroxyphenyl) ethanol = p-hydroxyphenethyl alcohol, is also found free.
Properties: Adaptogenic, tonic, antidepressant, antioxidant, liver protective, astringent. Rhodiola has been shown to improve physical and mental per-formance (incl. cognitive function) and mood, and is a cardiovascular stimu-lant, among others. Through oxidation (chiefly in the liver), cinnamyl alco-hol is converted to cinnamic aldehyde, an indirect-acting sympathomimetic (ephedra-like effect, cf. EPHEDRA). Tyrosol (= p-tyrosol) is closely related to tyramine, an indirect-acting sympathomimetic (cf. CEREUS, NIGHT-BLOOMING). It is antioxidant and liver protective due to flavonoids, phe-nylpropanoid glycosides and phenolic acids. Cinnamic acid, normally an ox-idation product of cinnamic aldehyde, has also shown cytostatic effect against certain tumors (cf. CINNAMON).
Uses: Internally it is used (as an h. p.) chiefly for mental and physical fa-tigue, depressive mood, and minor cases of hypotension (= low blood pres-sure) and headaches associated with exhaustion. Healthy individuals use it, as directed by experienced practitioners, to increase mental and physical performance. It is also used for hemorrhoids (also when minor hemorrhages are present, but on professional's advice). Externally it is used (as a mouth-wash, gargle) for inflammations of the mouth and throat.
Caution: Rhodiola products should be standardized to rosavins (as rosavin) and salidroside content. They should not be used in nervousness, sleep dis-orders, hypertension, and should not be taken late afternoon and in the even-ing. They should not be used for more than 6 weeks, except on professional advice up to 12 weeks. A possible combination with cardioactive herbs (lily-of-the-valley, etc.) or caffeine rich herbs / drinks (coffee, cola, guaraná, ma-té, tea) should be made only by health professionals. MAOI antidepressant drugs or herbs (e. g. phenelzine, St. John's wort) should not be used with rhodiola as they may cause a risky increase of its ephedra-like effects.

References: (1) Vol. 4, p. 890; (3) Vol. 6b, p. 351; (5) Vol. 1, p. 986; (18) p. 164; (41) Vols. 1-7; (52) p. 712; (57) p. 762; (65) p. 387; (86) Vol. 1, p. 132; (87) Vol. 1, p. 179; (93) p. 33.

RHODODENDRON

Other Common Name(s): yellow-flowered rhododendron
Botanical Name(s): *Rhododendron aureum* Georgi = *Rhododendron chry-santhum* Pallas [Fam.: Ericaceae]
Leafy stem
Constituents: Diterpenoid polyphenols of grayanotoxin type (acetylandro-

medol = andromedotoxin = grayanotoxin I, etc.; toxic!; cf. MOUNTAIN LAUREL), a phenol glycoside (arbutin), a bitter principle (an aromatic alcohol glycoside: rhododendrin), flavonoids (flavonols), triterpenes (oleanolic acid, etc.), volatile oil, tannins, etc.

Properties: Antihypertensive, antipyretic, antimicrobial, astringent, diuretic. Andromedotoxin exerts antihypertensive effect and increases the contractility of the heart muscle (see MOUNTAIN LAUREL).

Uses: Internally it is used (the herb, andromedotoxin: only in a combination product) for hypertension. The herb has also been used for feverish states, inflammations of the gastrointestinal tract, and rheumatic complaints.

Caution: Rhododendron is toxic and not for self-treatment. Products that contain rhododendron or andromedotoxin should be used only as directed by a health professional. At higher doses than recommended rhododendron and andromedotoxin cause nausea, vomiting, diarrhea, convulsions and death due to respiratory and cardiac arrest. Rhododendron is also a topical irritant.

References: (1) Vol. 6, p. 441; (3) Vol. 6b, p. 117; (6) p. 58; (8) p. 485; (12a) p. 180; (23) p. 193; (31) p. 547; (37) p. 1188; (47) p. 2307; (51) p. 268.

RHUBARB, CHINESE

Other Common Name(s): Turkey rhubarb
Botanical Name(s): *Rheum palmatum* L.; *Rheum officinale* Baill. [Fam.: Polygonaceae]

Root

Constituents: Anthranoids (glycosides of anthraquinones and dianthrones, and free anthraquinones), tannins (gallotannins, also proanthocyanidins), starch, calcium oxalate, etc.

Properties: (At low doses): Stomachic, astringent. (At high doses): Laxative (large intestine stimulant laxative; see SENNA).

Uses: Internally it is used (as a tea, h. p.; at small doses; mainly combined with other herbs) for nonulcer dyspepsia, minor diarrhea and hepatobiliary disorders, and (as a tea, h. p.; at higher doses; mainly combined with other herbs) for constipation. Externally it is used (as a paint, gel) for inflammations of the oral cavity (gingivitis, stomatitis, etc.).

Caution: See SENNA. Chinese rhubarb should not be taken in cases of bowel and gallbladder obstructions, and in cases of a known history of oxalate kidney stones. In cases of nonobstructive gallstones it can be used but only on health professional's advice. Fresh root and non-cured freshly dried root cause griping effect. To minimize griping effect, Chinese rhubarb root is best stored for at least 1 year.

Note: Root of monk's / mountain rhubarb (*Rumex alpinus* L.) serves as a good substitute for Chinese rhubarb, esp. for problems of the oral cavity.

References: (1) Vol. 6, p. 418; (3) Vol. 6b, p. 96; (6) p. 116; (7) p. 229; (8) p. 481; (12) p. 921; (13) p. 294; (14) p. 188; (17) p. 492; (19) p. 188; (22) p. 61; (23) p. 101; (46) p. 1186; (48) p. 437; (59) p. 231.

ROOIBOS

Botanical Name(s): *Aspalathus linearis* (Burm. f.) R. Dahlgren [Fam.: Fabaceae (Leguminosae)]

Aerial part

With rooibos tea or red bush tea, here, is to be undersood leaves and fine twigs, firstly fermented, then dried.

Constituents: Flavonoids (very ich; flavones: luteolin-C-glucosides; flavonols: quercetin glycosides; chalcones: esp. rich in aspalathin, a dihydrochalcone), phenolic acids, volatile oil (with guaiacol, etc.), tannins (gallotannins), vitamin C, minerals (K, Mg, Mn, Cu, Fe, etc.), etc.

Properties and Uses: Rooibos tea is used as a caffeine-free refreshing beverage, valued for its safety, low tannins content, and its antioxidant effect (due in large part to flavonoids).

Caution: There are no contraindications or side effects when used properly.

References: (1) Vol. 4, p. 394; (3) Vol. 3, p. 289; (21) p. 313; (37) p. 148; (41) Vols. 1-7; (48) p. 342; (52) p. 81.

ROSE

Other Common Name(s): 1) hip roses: a) dog rose, wild dog rose b) wild rose; 2) cultivated roses: a) cabbage rose b) French / red rose

Botanical Name(s): 1) a) *Rosa canina* L. b) *Rosa pendulina* L. 2) a) *Rosa centifolia* L. b) *Rosa gallica* L. [Fam.: Rosaceae]

Rose hip

Rose hip is a pseudofruit that consists of the pulpy receptacle with "seeds" (real fruits, as achenes contained within the pulpy receptacle), obtained from the hip roses such as dog rose and wild rose.

Constituents: Vitamin C, organic acids (malic and citric acids), flavonoids (chiefly flavonols: quercetin, rutin, kaempferol), pectin, sugars (invert sugar, etc.), tannins (proanthocyanidins), carotenoids (carotenes, lutein, etc.), etc.

Properties: The same as vitamin C. The effects of vitamin C are enhanced by flavonols with their antioxidant and "vitamin P"-like effect (= help in normalizing an increased microvascular permeability and fragility). Rose hips exert mild stomachic, laxative and diuretic effects. The diuretic effect is attributed in large part to the "seeds".

Used: Internally it is used as a natural supplement of vitamin C and as a refreshing drink, beneficial for feverish states and complaints of the gastrointestinal tract (impaired digestion, minor constipation). It is incorporated in different diuretic teas.

Caution: When preparing a tea, it should be well filtered to avoid possible irritations caused by the hairs. Otherwise, there are no reports of contraindications or side effects when used properly.

Rose petal

It is obtained from the cultivated roses.

Constituents: Volatile oil (see Rose oil), tannins (chiefly condensed t.), flavonoids (anthocyanins, flavonols), organic acids (quinic acid, etc.), etc.

Properties: Aromatic, astringent, anti-inflammatory.

Uses: Externally it is used (as a mouthwash, gargle, paint) for inflammations of the mouth and throat.

Caution: There are no reports of contraindications or side effects when used properly.

Rose oil

It is the volatile oil obtained by steam distillation from fresh flowers.

Constituents: Chiefly geraniol, also citronellol, nerol, and the special and highly aromatic 2-phenylethanol, among others. The oils obtained by extraction contain higher concentrations of 2-phenylethanol.

Properties: Aromatic, mild antimicrobial.

Uses: Its is an important fragrance and flavor ingredient used in perfume, food, and pharmaceutical industries.

Caution: There are no reports of contraindications or side effects when used properly.

References: (2) Vol. 3, p. 445; (3) Vol. 6b, p. 161; (8) p. 489; (9) p. 441; (17) p. 502; (19) p. 192; (36) p. 263; (37) p. 1197; (46) pp. 1360, 1363; (47) pp. 2334, 2341; (48) p. 394; (49) Vol. 2, p. 420; (51) p. 261.

ROSEMARY

Botanical Name(s): *Rosmarinus officinalis* L. [Fam.: Lamiaceae (Labiatae)]

Leaf

Constituents: Volatile oil (see Rosemary oil), bitter principles (diterpenoid lactones: carnosol = picrosalvin, carnosolic acid, etc.), Lamiaceae tannins (rosmarinic acid and other caffeic acid derivatives), flavonoids (flavones: luteolin, etc.), triterpenes (oleanolic acid, ursolic acid, etc.), salicylates, etc.

Properties: Bitter tonic, antioxidant, choleretic, cholagogue, anti-inflammatory, mild neurocirculatory stimulant, antimicrobial, mild cholesterol and triglyceride reducing, diuretic, emmenagogue. The bitter tonic and antioxidant effects are due in large part to carnosol and carnosolic acid. Rosmarinic acid and related caffeic acid derivatives have been shown to inhibit the biosynthesis of leukotrienes and prostaglandins, and to exert choleretic, antibacterial and antiviral effects. The effects of rosemary leaf in the hepatobiliary tract (incl. mild cholesterol and triglyceride reducing effects) are due in large part to caffeic acid derivatives. To these effects contribute also carnosol, carnosolic acid, and luteolin (esp. as cholesterol and triglyceride reducer, also anti-inflammatory).

Uses: Rosemary is widely used as a spice and it is also beneficial due to its antioxidant effect. Internally it is used (as a tea, h. p.) for loss of appetite and nonulcer dyspepsia, especially when associated with minor hepatobili-

322

ary disorders. Rosemary is also used for minor cases of hypotension (= low blood pressure), fatigue and convalescence. Externally it is used (as a wash, wet compress) for wounds and eczema, (as a partial / full bath) for rheumatic pains and neurocirculatory (= nervous and circulatory systems) weakness, and (as a mouthwash, chewing) for bad breath.

Caution: There are no reports of contraindications or side effects when used properly. Nevertheless, higher doses than recommended as well as consumption in excessive amounts should be avoided during pregnancy.

Rosemary oil

It is the volatile oil obtained by steam distillation preferably from leaves, but also leafy stalks are used.

Constituents: 1,8-Cineole (= eucalyptol), borneol, α-pinene, camphene, camphor, linalool, etc., with differences depending on origin and harvest.

Properties: Mild rubefacient and counterirritant, antimicrobial, antifungal, antiviral.

Uses: Rosemary oil is an important ingredient in cosmetics, perfumery and food industry. Externally it is used (as a solution, liniment, ointment, partial / full bath) for rheumatic complaints and neurocirculatory (= nervous and circulatory systems) weakness, (as a liniment) for hair loss, and (in a full bath) for its relaxing and tonic effects. Internally it is used (a few drops on sugar) almost the same as leaf.

Caution: It should not be taken during pregnancy. In rare cases it may cause skin allergic reactions.

References: (1) Vol. 6, p. 490; (3) Vol. 6b, p. 172; (6) p. 60; (8) p. 490; (9) p. 446; (12) pp. 754, 785; (13) p. 111; (16) p. 128; (17) p. 506; (19) p. 192; (20) p. 229; (23) p. 195; (37) p. 1199; (46) p. 1365; (47) p. 2346; (48) p. 249.

RUDBECKIA

Other Common Name(s): 1) orange coneflower 2) black-eyed Susan 3) brown-eyed Susan, cutleaf coneflower

Botanical Name(s): 1) *Rudbeckia fulgida* Ait. var. *speciosa* (Wender.) Perdue = *Rudbeckia speciosa* Wender. 2) *Rudbeckia hirta* L. 3) *Rudbeckia laciniata* L. [Fam.: Asteraceae (Compositae)]

Root

Constituents: Volatile oil, polyacetylenes (1,2-dithian-alkynes: thiarubrines A, B, etc.), water-soluble polysaccharides (methylglucurono-xylans), sesquiterpene lactones, phytosterols, triterpenes, etc. As a member of Heliantheae tribe it may contain benzofurans.

Properties: Antibacterial, antifungal, antiviral, immunomodulant, diuretic, bitter tonic, anthelmintic. Thiarubrines have shown antibacterial, antifungal, antiviral, and anthelmintic (against roundworms = *Ascaris* spp. and pinworms = *Oxyuris* spp.) effects. The immunomodulating effect (orange cone flower acts stronger) is due in large part to water-soluble polysaccharides,

323

enhanced by bitter sesquiterpenoid lactones. Benzofurans, if present, exert antibacterial effect.

Uses: <u>Internally</u> it is used (as a tea, h. p.) for inflammations (especially cases of relapsing nature) of the genitourinary tract (cystitis, urethritis, prostatitis) and upper respiratory tract (the common cold, bronchitis, etc.; also as a diaphoretic hot tea for feverish states), and for loss of appetite, nonulcer dyspepsia, and intestinal worms (roundworms, pinworms). To enhance the effects in problems of the genitourinary tract, the fluid intake (incl. herbal teas) should be more than 2 liters per day. <u>Externally</u> it is used (as a wash, wet compress) for minor skin inflammations, wounds and ulcers.

Caution: Rudbeckia should not be taken during pregnancy and lactation. Due to sesquiterpene lactones it may cause allergic contact dermatitis to persons hypersensitive to other Asteraceae plants (e. g. arnica, chamomile, feverfew, ragweed, tansy, yarrow) that contain them. The toxic unsaturated pyrrolizidine alkaloids (= UPAs) are found only in a few species of Heliantheae tribe. Nevertheless, manufacturers should evaluate them and consider their limits. For dosage limits of UPAs see COLTSFOOT. Normally, it should not be taken for more than 8 weeks without a break for 2-3 weeks. See ECHINACEA; BETA GLUCANS.

References: (1) Vol. 6, p. 504; (3) Vol. 6b, p. 190; (18) p. 283; (25) p. 126; (31) pp. 51, 388; (41) Vols. 1-7; (44) p. 494; (52) p. 680; (57) p. 724.

RUE

Botanical Name(s): *Ruta graveolens* L. [Fam.: Rutaceae]
Aerial part
Constituents: Furanocoumarins (bergaptene, psoralene, etc.), coumarins (coumarin, etc.), flavonoids (rutin, etc.), volatile oil (with methyl-*n*-nonyl-ketone, etc.), alkaloids (quinoline, furoquinoline and acridone types), etc.
Properties: Antispasmodic, emmenagogue, mild sedative, anti-inflammatory, stomachic, rubefacient, counterirritant.
Uses: <u>Internally</u> it is used (as a tea, h. p.; only combined with other herbs) for primary dysmenorrhea (= painful menstruation without pathology), secondary amenorrhea and oligomenorrhea (= ceased / infrequent / scanty menstruation without pathology), and minor intestinal cramps. <u>Externally</u> it is used (as a wet compress) for bruises, sprains, neuralgic and rheumatic pains.
Caution: Rue (esp. distilled oil) is toxic therefore it should be used only as directed by an experienced practitioner. It should not be taken during pregnancy (oxytocic / abortifacient!, abused at high doses with fatal results) and lactation. Before using it for gynecologic disorders, the problem should be judged by a health professional. Besides the phototoxic reactions, which may happen even at normal doses after exposure to strong sunrays, at high doses it causes severe gastrointestinal irritation, liver and kidney damage, mental confusion, and tachycardia, among others.

References: (1) Vol. 6, p. 509; (3) Vol. 6b, p. 204; (6) p. 306; (8) p. 498; (9) p. 451; (15) p. 183; (23) pp. 202, 366; (24) p. 266; (27) p. 296; (37) p. 1206; (46) p. 1372; (47) p. 2372; (51) p. 112; (66) p. 419.

RUPTUREWORT

Other Common Name(s): 1) smooth rupturewort 2) hairy rupturewort
Botanical Name(s): 1) *Herniaria glabra* L. 2) *Herniaria hirsuta* L. [Fam.: Caryophyllaceae]
Aerial part
Constituents: Triterpenoid saponins (herniaria-saponins), flavonoids (flavonols), coumarins (herniarin, umbelliferone, etc.), tannins, volatile oil, etc.
Properties: Diuretic, antispasmodic, urinary antiseptic, expectorant, astringent. The effects are mild. Besides the diuretic and expectorant effects of saponins and diuretic and antispasmodic effects of flavonoids, here contribute also coumarins with their antibacterial and antifungal effects.
Uses: Internally it is used (as a tea, h. p.; usually combined with other herbs) for inflammatory and spastic conditions of the genitourinary tract (cystitis, urethritis, pyelitis, etc., gravel, nonobstructive urinary stones; with proteinuria) and upper respiratory tract (bronchitis, etc.; coughs), and as an antidyscratic (= blood purifier) for chronic skin disorders (incl. psoriasis). To enhance the effects in problems of the genitourinary tract, the fluid intake (incl. herbal teas) should be more than 2 liters per day.
Caution: There are no reports of contraindications or side effects when used properly.

References: (3) Vol. 5, p. 54; (6) p. 184; (8) p. 306; (13) p. 218; (17) p. 294; (23) pp. 251, 336; (31) pp. 359, 365; (37) p. 655; (47) p. 1547; (49) Vol. 2, p. 135; (51) p. 70.

SAFFLOWER

Botanical Name(s): *Carthamus tinctorius* L. [Fam.: Asteraceae (Compositae)]
Flower
Constituents: Pigments, as flavonoids (glycosidic chalcones: yellow carthamin, red carthamone; a glycosidic flavanone: colorless neocarthamin), which predominate according to the variety. It also contains lignans and polysaccharides, among others.
Properties: Anti-inflammatory, platelet aggregation inhibitory, immunomodulant. Flavonoids account at least in part for the anti-inflammatory effect. Lignans have shown anti-inflammatory, liver protective, immunomodulant, and antimicrobial effects. Water-soluble polysaccharides have shown immunomodulant effect.
Uses: Internally it is used (as an h. p., tea) for inflammations of the upper respiratory tract (bronchitis; coughs) and as an adjuvant for cardiovascular disorders in general. In traditional medicine it is also used for dysmenorrhea

325

(= painful menstruation), and secondary amenorrhea and oligomenorrhea (= ceased / infrequent / scanty menstruation without pathology). Safflower is also used as a red / yellow / orange coloring ingredient, often incorporated in herbal teas. Externally it is used (as a wash, wet compress, poultice) for bruises, wounds and ulcers, and (as a liniment) for hair loss. As a coloring ingredient it is also incorporated in products for external applications.

Caution: There are no reports of contraindications or side effects when used properly. Nevertheless, before using it for gynecologic disorders, the problem should be judged by a health professional.

Safflower oil
It is the fixed oil obtained from the seeds.

Constituents: Chiefly glycerides (fatty acids component: chiefly linoleic acid, which is an omega-6 fatty acid, etc.), phytosterols (5-sterols: β-sitosterol, etc.), α-tocopherol, etc.

Properties: Cholesterol reducing, emollient. The cholesterol reducing effect is due in large part to linoleic acid, but β-sitosterol may also play an important role (see HYPOXIS ROOPERI).

Uses: Internally it is used as a dietary aid (also as a salad / cooking oil) to prevent and reduce high cholesterol. Externally it is used as an ingredient in skin care products.

Caution: There are no reports of contraindications or side effects when used properly.

References: (3) Vol. 3, p. 725; (8) p. 118; (9) p. 551; (10) p. 239; (11) p. 73; (12) pp. 262, 822; (13) p. 389; (36) p. 508; (37) p. 283; (45) p. 181; (48) p. 151.

SAFFRON

Other Common Name(s): Spanish saffron, true saffron
Botanical Name(s): *Crocus sativus* L. [Fam.: Iridaceae]
Stigma
Constituents: Yellow pigments (carotenoids: chiefly crocin, and related derivatives, etc.), a bitter principle (picrocrocin = safranal-glucoside), volatile oil (with safranal), fixed oil, triterpenes, carbohydrates (pentosans, pectin, starch), etc.

Properties: Stomachic, antispasmodic, emmenagogue, sedative, antidepressant, antioxidant.

Uses: In food and pharmaceutical industry it is used as a flavor and coloring ingredient. Internally it has been used (as a tea, h. p.) for primary dysmenorrhea (= painful menstruation without pathology), and recently for mild to moderate depression.

Caution: There are no reports of contraindications or side effects when consumed in moderate amounts as a flavor ingredient. Before using saffron for dysmenorrhea, the gynecologic problem should be judged by a health professional. At high doses, it causes irritations of the gastrointestinal and genitourinary tracts. It has been abused (at high doses) to induce abortion and often has resulted in heavy intoxications. Saffron is not to be confused with safflower, obtained from *Carthamus tinctorius* L. (see SAFFLOWER).

References: (2) Vol. 2, p. 437; (3) Vol. 4, p. 336; (8) p. 199; (12) p. 615; (13) p. 110; (17) p. 175; (28) p. 172; (36) p. 457; (37) p. 368; (46) p. 1800; (47) p. 1122; (48) p. 777; (66) p. 256.

SAGE

Other Common Name(s): garden sage, common sage, Dalmatian sage
Botanical Name(s): *Salvia officinalis* L. [Fam.: Lamiaceae (Labiatae)]
Leaf
Constituents: Volatile oil (see Sage oil), Lamiaceae tannins (rosmarinic acid and other caffeic acid derivatives), flavonoids (flavones, flavonols), bitter principles (diterpenoid lactones: carnosol = picrosalvin, carnosolic acid, etc.), triterpenes (ursolic acid, etc.), etc.
Properties: Aromatic, stomachic, antibacterial, antifungal, antiviral (against *Herpes* spp.), astringent, anti-inflammatory, antioxidant, antihidrotic (= sweat-inhibiting). The antibacterial and antifungal effects are due in large part to thujone and 1,8-cineole (see Sage oil). Lamiaceae tannins account for the anti-herpes and mild astringent effects, and contribute as antioxidants. Flavonoids contribute chiefly as anti-inflammatory and antioxidants.
Uses: Sage is extensively used as a spice in culinary practice and food industry, especially for meat products. Externally it is used (as a mouthwash, gargle, paint) for inflammations of the mouth and throat, denture sores and canker sores, and (as a mouthwash, chewing) for bad breath. Internally it is used (as a tea, h. p.) for nonulcer dyspepsia (with flatulence, minor diarrhea) and inflammations of the upper respiratory tract (the common cold, pharyngitis, laryngitis, tracheitis, bronchitis; coughs). Sage is also used to check excessive sweating and the secretion of milk in nursing mothers.
Caution: Sage should not be taken during pregnancy. To check milk secretion and excessive sweating sage should be used based on health professional's advice. Alcoholic extracts are much richer in essential oil and β-thujone (see Sage oil) therefore they should not be taken at higher doses than recommended. Otherwise, there are no reports of side effects when consumed as a spice in moderate amounts and taken at recommended doses (for max. 4 weeks).
Sage oil
It is the volatile oil obtained by steam distillation from the flowering tops.
Constituents: Chiefly α-thujone and β-thujone, also camphor, 1,8-cineole, borneol, etc.
Properties: Aromatic, antibacterial, antifungal, antihidrotic (= sweat-inhibiting).
Uses: Sage oil is used in food industry much like sage leaf. It is a fragrance ingredient in many oral hygiene products, and is also used in cosmetics and

perfumery. <u>Internally</u> it is used (as a few drops dose) to check excessive sweating.

Caution: Ingestion of sage oil at high doses may cause severe intoxicating effect in the CNS (epileptiform seizures) due to the neurotoxic effects of β-thujone (cf. TANSY; THUJA; WORMWOOD).

References: (1) Vol. 6, p. 547; (3) Vol. 6b, p. 241; (6) pp. 115, 362; (8) p. 503; (9) p. 457; (12) pp. 740, 782; (13) p. 104; (17) p. 521; (19) p. 197; (20) p. 231; (22) p. 227; (28) pp. 158, 173; (46) p. 1409; (47) p. 2400; (48) p. 540; (51) p. 166.

SAGE, CHINESE

Other Common Name(s): Chinese salvia, red-root sage
Botanical Name(s): *Salvia miltiorrhiza* Bunge [Fam.: Lamiaceae (Labiatae)]
<u>Root</u> (dan shen, tan shen)
Constituents: Diterpenes (tanshinones and related compounds), phenolic acid derivatives (lithospermic acid B = salvianolic acid B, rosmarinic acid) and closely related compounds, namely pyrocatechol derivatives (danshensu = 3,4-dihydroxyphenyl lactic acid, salvianolic acids, protocatechuic aldehyde, etc.), etc.
Properties: Platelet aggregation inhibitory, antioxidant, anti-inflammatory (possibly with antiallergic effect), liver protective, antimicrobial, mild sedative. Dan shen products, standardized to tanshinones content, have been shown to decrease blood stasis and improve peripheral blood flow (incl. cerebral blood flow, coronary blood flow). Dan shen has been shown to reduce voluntary alcohol intake. To the overall effect surely contribute phenolic acid derivatives and closely related compounds.
Uses: <u>Internally</u> it is used as an adjuvant (tea, h. p.) for cerebrovascular disease (= a complex condition associated with impaired blood flow in the brain), coronary heart disease (= a condition associated with decreased blood supply to the heart), and inflammations of the liver (chronic hepatitis) and skin (boils, carbuncles, etc.). Dan shen is also used for primary dysmenorrhea (= painful menstruation without pathology) and secondary amenorrhea and oligomenorrhea (= ceased / infrequent / scanty menstruation without pathology), and may be helpful for intermittent claudication (= pain / cramp / weakness in the legs on walking) and alcoholism.
Caution: Before using it for gynecologic disorders, the problem should be judged by a health professional. A possible combination of dan shen products with anticoagulants (warfarin, etc.) and / or platelet aggregation inhibitors (aspirin, etc.) should be made only by a health professional. Otherwise, there are no reports of contraindications or side effects when used properly.
Note: It is not to be confused with Red Ginseng (see GINSENG).

References: (1) Vol. 6, p. 544; (3) Vol. 6b, p. 252; (13) p. 435; (41) Vols. 1-7; (45) p. 129; (48) p. 241; (53) p. 122; (68) p. 65.

SAGE, GREEK

Other Common Name(s): Turkish sage, three-lobe sage
Botanical Name(s): *Salvia triloba* L. f. = *Salvia fruticosa* Mill. [Fam.: Lamiaceae (Labiatae)]
Leaf
Constituents: Volatile oil (with 1,8-cineole, also camphor, thujone, etc.), Lamiaceae tannins (rosmarinic acid and other caffeic acid derivatives), flavonoids (flavones, methoxy-flavones), a bitter principle (a diterpenoid lactone: carnosol), triterpenes (ursolic acid, oleanolic acid), etc.
Properties: Aromatic, stomachic, antibacterial, antifungal, antioxidant, anti-inflammatory. Cf. SAGE.
Uses: It is chiefly used as a spice much like garden sage (see SAGE), with which is sometimes mixed or is found as an adulterant. Compared to garden sage, it has a eucalyptus-like flavor (essential oil contains about eight times less thujone, about 5 times more cineole; leaves contain less carnosol). Externally it is used (as a mouthwash, gargle) for inflammations of the mouth and throat, and (as a mouthwash, chewing) for bad breath. Internally it is used (as a tea, h. p.) for minor inflammations of the upper respiratory tract (the common cold, bronchitis, etc.; coughs). For problems of the upper respiratory tract Greek / Turkish sage should be preferred to the garden / Dalmatian sage.
Caution: Greek / Turkish sage, due to its lower thujones content, is less toxic than garden sage. For caution, due to its high cineole content, see EUCALYPTUS. Otherwise, there are no reports of side effects when used properly and when consumed as a spice in moderate amounts.

References: (1) Vol. 6, p. 568; (3) Vol. 6b, p. 249; (12) p. 740; (13) p. 104; (16) p. 85; (17) p. 525; (20) p. 231; (46) p. 1414.

SAGE, SPANISH

Botanical Name(s): *Salvia lavandulifolia* Vahl. [Fam.: Lamiaceae (Labiatae)]
Leaf (Spanish sage leaf)
Constituents: Volatile oil (see Spanish sage oil), Lamiaceae tannins (rosmarinic acid and other caffeic acid derivatives), flavonoids (flavones), etc., but no carnosol.
Properties and Uses: Spanish sage is chiefly used for the distillation of the volatile oil (see Spanish sage oil).
Spanish sage oil
It is the volatile oil obtained by steam distillation from the leaf.
Constituents: Camphor and 1,8-cineole as its major constituents, but almost no thujone.
Properties: Aromatic, antibacterial, antifungal.

Uses: Spanish sage oil is used as a fragrance ingredient in cosmetics and perfumery, adding to the product its antibacterial and antifungal effects. It is also used in food industry as a flavor ingredient in some alcoholic bitters and nonalcoholic beverages, among others.
Caution: There are no reports of contraindications or side effects when used properly.

References: (1) Vol. 6, p. 541; (9) p. 457; (13) p. 105; (46) p. 1414; (52) p. 691.

SALEP

Botanical Name(s): *Orchis* spp.: *O. mascula* L.; *O. morio* L.; *O. militaris* L.; etc.; *Anacamptis pyramidalis* L. Rich.; *Platanthera bifolia* L. Rich. [Fam.: Orchidaceae]
Root (tuber)
Constituents: Mucilage (a glucomannan; very rich), starch (rich), proteins (rich), fats (small amounts), minerals (potassium, calcium), etc.
Properties: Demulcent, nutrient, suspending.
Uses: Internally it is used (as a tea, h. p.) for inflammations of the gastrointestinal tract (diarrhea, etc.) and as a nutrient during convalescence, particularly in children and the elderly. Due to mucilage it is also beneficial for high cholesterol (see PSYLLIUM). In the Middle East and Balkans it is used much like arrowroot (cf. ARROWROOT). The prepared mucilage of salep can also be employed as a suspending agent in the preparation of suspensions.
Caution: Salep may impair the absorption of some drugs. In view of this, when taking a vital oral medication, drugs should be taken about one hour apart from salep products. Otherwise, there are no reports of contraindications or side effects when used properly.

References: (2) Vol. 3, p. 271; (3) Vol. 6a, p. 325; (8) p. 391; (10) p. 241; (12) p. 309; (13) p. 374; (24) p. 194; (35) p. 602; (37) p. 1005; (87) Vol. 2, p. 248.

SALSIFY, SPANISH

Other Common Name(s): black salsify, viper's grass
Botanical Name(s): *Scorzonera hispanica* L. [Fam.: Asteraceae (Compositae)]
Root
Constituents: Inulin, sugars, a phenol glycoside (coniferin), trigonelline (= nicotinic acid N-methyl-betaine), amino acids (histidine, arginine, etc.), enzymes (protease, etc.), triterpenes (taraxasterol, etc.), etc.
Properties: Stomachic, laxative, diuretic. The effects are mild.
Uses: Fresh root is chiefly used as a salad, with beneficial effects on the gastrointestinal and genitourinary tracts. It is also used as an antidyscratic (=

blood purifier; fresh root, tea, h. p.) for chronic rheumatic complaints and atopic eczema (= chronic eczema of internal origin).

Caution: There are no reports of contraindications or side effects when used properly.

References: (3) Vol. 6b, p. 335; (27) p. 310; (37) p. 1247; (87) Vol. 2, p. 231.

SAMPHIRE

Other Common Name(s): sea fennel, sea samphire, rock fennel, rock samphire
Botanical Name(s): *Crithmum maritimum* L. [Fam.: Apiaceae (Umbelliferae)]
<u>Aerial part</u>
Constituents: Vitamin C, polyacetylenes (falcarinone derivatives), flavonoids (diosmin, etc.), volatile oil (with dillapiole, thymol methyl ether, limonene, sabinene, etc.), furanocoumarins, minerals (Zn, Fe, Mg, I, etc.), etc.
Properties: Stomachic, diuretic, anti-inflammatory, antimicrobial, antioxidant. The effects are mild. Diosmin and other flavonoids, together with vitamin C, contribute to the anti-inflammatory, antioxidant and diuretic effects. Many open chain polyacetylenes (falcarinone, etc.) are considered natural antibiotics. The presence of iodine may explain, at least in part, the traditional use to control overweight.
Uses: <u>Internally</u> it is used (usually fresh, also as a tea) for its pleasant salty and spicy taste, and as a natural supplement of vitamin C and flavonoids, with beneficial effects as antioxidant. Its beneficial effects on the gastrointestinal and genitourinary tracts are due also to the antimicrobial properties. In traditional medicine samphire is also used to control overweight.
Caution: Samphire should not be consumed in excessive amounts during pregnancy. Due to furanocoumarins, when handling the herb avoid contact with skin and when taking its products avoid exposure to strong sunrays, as it may cause phototoxic skin irritations. Manufacturers should evaluate iodine content and advice accordingly. Otherwise, there are no reports of contraindications or side effects when used properly.

References: (5) Vol. 1, p. 358; (10) p. 241; (31) pp. 49, 396; (35) p. 709; (41) Vols. 1-7; (42) Vol. 6, pp. 569, 575; (52) p. 227; (57) p. 239.

SANDALWOOD

Other Common Name(s): East Indian sandalwood, white / yellow sandalwood, white / yellow saunders
Botanical Name(s): *Santalum album* Rumph. [Fam.: Santalaceae]
<u>Sandalwood</u> (East Indian sandalwood, white / yellow sandalwood, white / yellow saunders). It is consists of dried heartwood.

331

Constituents: Volatile oil (see East Indian sandalwood oil), phenolic compounds (sinapic, coniferyl and syringic aldehydes, vanillin), phytosterols, triterpenes, tannins, resin, calcium oxalate, etc.

Properties: Antibacterial, diuretic, antispasmodic. The effects are attributed in large part to the volatile oil and santalols, but phenolic compounds may also play an important role.

Uses: Internally it is used (as a tea, h. p.; usually combined with other herbs) for inflammations of the genitourinary tract (cystitis, urethritis, prostatitis, leukorrhea), upper respiratory tract (chronic bronchitis, the common cold, etc.), and gastrointestinal tract (diarrhea, etc.). To enhance the effects in problems of the genitourinary tract, the fluid intake (incl. herbal teas) should be more than 2 liters per day. Externally it is used (as a wet compress, poultice, h.p.) for minor skin inflammations.

Caution: Sandalwood should not be taken during pregnancy and lactation, and in cases of impaired renal function. At higher doses than recommended it causes gastrointestinal irritations (with vomiting, nausea). It should not be taken for more than 6 weeks as it may damage kidney tissue.

East Indian santalwood oil (= white / yellow sandalwood oil, white / yellow saunders oil)
It is the volatile oil obtained by steam distillation from the heartwood chips.

Constituents: Chiefly cis-α-santalol and cis-β-santalol, also other sesquiterpenes.

Properties and Uses: East Indian sandalwood oil is chiefly used in perfumery.

Caution: It should not be used internally as it has been shown to irritate the kidneys and gastrointestinal tract.

References: (1) Vol. 6, p. 600; (3) Vol. 6b, p. 275; (6) p. 189; (8) p. 510; (9) p. 460; (10) p. 242; (12a) p. 694; (19) p. 198; (36) p. 288; (37) p. 1222; (41) Vols. 1-7; (47) p. 2438.

SANDARAC TREE

Botanical Name(s): *Tetraclinis articulata* (Vahl.) Masters = *Callitris quadrivalvis* Vent. = *Thuja articulata* Vahl. [Fam.: Cupressaceae]

Sandarac
It is the hardened oleoresin (commonly referred to as sandarac resin or sandarac gum) that exudes naturally from the stem.

Constituents: Chiefly resin (with diterpenoid acids: sandaracopimaric acid, etc.), volatile oil (with pinenes, thymoquinone, etc.), bitter principles (possibly diterpenes), etc.

Properties: Counterirritant, antimicrobial, antipyretic.

Uses: Externally it is used (as a plaster, etc.) for rheumatic pains, and in dentistry for temporary fillings. Internally it is used (as an h. p.) for diarrhea and feverish states. Sandarac is also used as an ingredient in cosmetics, paints, varnishes, and incenses.

Caution: Internally, it should be used on experienced practitioner's advice. Otherwise, there are no reports of contraindications or side effects when used properly.

References: (2) Vol. 3, p. 654; (3) Vol. 3, p. 609; (4) Vol. 2, p. 629; (36) p. 291; (37) p. 1359; (41) Vols. 1-7; (42) Vol. 1, pp. 352, 366; (49) Vol. 1, p. 393.

SANICLE, EUROPEAN

Other Common Name(s): wood sanicle
Botanical Name(s): *Sanicula europaea* L. [Fam.: Apiaceae (Umbelliferae)]
Aerial part
Constituents: Esterified triterpenoid saponins (esters of saniculosides), Lamiaceae tannins (rosmarinic acid and other caffeic acid derivatives), flavonoids (flavonols), organic acids, sugars, volatile oil, etc.
Properties: Expectorant, antimicrobial, astringent, diuretic. Saponins account for most of the effects, except astringent. Rosmarinic acid and related caffeic acid derivatives exert astringent, choleretic, antibacterial and antiviral effects. They also exert anti-inflammatory effect by inhibiting the biosynthesis of leukotrienes and prostaglandins.
Uses: Internally it is used (as a tea, h. p.) for inflammations (also when minor hemorrhages are present, but on professional's advice) of the upper respiratory tract (bronchitis, tracheitis, laryngitis, etc.; minor coughs due to thickened bronchial secretion), gastrointestinal tract (diarrhea, ulcerative colitis, etc., incl. hemorrhoids), and genitourinary tract (cystitis, urethritis, pyelitis). To enhance the effects in problems of the genitourinary tract, the fluid intake (incl. herbal teas) should be more than 2 liters per day. Externally it is used (as a mouthwash, gargle) for inflammations of the mouth and throat, and (as a wash, wet compress, poultice) for minor skin inflammations, wounds, ulcers, hemorrhoids and eczema.
Caution: There are no reports of contraindications or side effects when used properly.

References: (1) Vol. 6, p. 595; (3) Vol. 6b, 271; (8) p. 509; (19) p. 199; (24) p. 278; (35) p. 711; (37) p. 1222; (41) Vols. 1-7; (47) p. 2433; (51) p. 124.

SANICLE, MARYLAND

Other Common Name(s): black sanicle, black snakeroot
Botanical Name(s): *Sanicula marilandica* L. [Fam.: Apiaceae (Umbelliferae)]
Root
Constituents: Not well known. It is reported to contain triterpenoid saponins, volatile oil and resin.
Properties and Uses: Maryland sanicle is chiefly used in traditional medi-

cine. Internally it is used (as a tea, h. p.) for inflammations of the genitourinary tract, rheumatic and feverish states, and constipation, among others. Externally it is used (as a wash, poultice) for minor skin inflammations and ulcers, among others.

Caution: There are no reports of contraindications or side effects when used properly.

References: (1) Vol. 6, p. 598; (3) Vol. 6b, p. 274; (25) p. 62; (35) p. 712; (44) p. 517.

SANTOLINA

Other Common Name(s): garden cypress, lavender cotton
Botanical Name(s): *Santolina chamaecyparissus* L. [Fam.: Asteraceae (Compositae)]
Aerial part
Constituents: Volatile oil (with monoterpenes: artemisia ketone, santolinatriene, pinenes, etc.; sesquiterpenes), flavonoids (flavonols: patuletin, etc.; flavones: luteolin, etc.; and their glycosides), phenolic acids (caffeic and vanillic acids), tannins (condensed t.), coumarins, phytosterols, etc.
Properties: Anthelmintic, stomachic, antispasmodic, anti-inflammatory, astringent, emmenagogue, insecticidal.
Uses: Santolina is chiefly used as a moth repellent and in traditional medicine. Internally it is used for intestinal worms, loss of appetite and nonulcer dyspepsia (with flatulence, minor cramps), and for primary dysmenorrhea (= painful menstruation without pathology). Externally it is used (as a mouthwash) for inflammations of the mouth, (as a vaginal irrigation / sitz bath / wash) for vulvovaginitis, and (as a wash, wet compress, poultice) for skin inflammations. Santolina is also used as an insect-repellent.
Caution: Santolina should be used only as directed by an experienced practitioner. Before using it for dysmenorrhea, the gynecologic problem should be judged by a health professional.

References: (3) Vol. 6b, p. 279; (27) p. 307; (35) p. 473; (41) Vols. 1-7.

SARSAPARILLA

Other Common Name(s): 1) Mexican sarsaparilla 2) Honduran / Jamaican sarsaparilla 3) Ecuadorian sarsaparilla
Botanical Name(s): 1) *Smilax aristolochiifolia* Mill. 2) *Smilax regelii* Killip et C.V. Morton = *Smilax officinalis* Kunth 3) *Smilax febrifuga* Kunth; and other *Smilax* spp. [Fam.: Smilacaceae]
Root
Constituents: Steroidal saponins (with aglycones: sarsapogenin, smilagenin), phytosterols (5-sterols: β-sitosterol, etc.), phenolic acid derivatives, minerals (esp. potassium), starch (rich) and resin.

Properties: Diuretic, anti-inflammatory, liver protective, stomachic, anti-fungal, mild cholesterol reducing. Steroidal saponins account in large part for the diuretic, anti-inflammatory, antifungal and cholesterol reducing (see FENUGREEK) effects. Phytosterols contribute to the anti-inflammatory and cholesterol reducing effects (see HYPOXIS ROOPERI). Phenolic acids account for the liver protective effect and contribute to the anti-inflammatory effect (see ROSEMARY). Potassium salts exert diuretic effect.

Uses: Internally it is chiefly used as an anti-inflammatory and antidyscratic (= blood purifier; tea, h. p.) for chronic endogenous skin disorders (atopic eczema, psoriasis, itching, leprotic or syphilitic skin lesions, etc.) and chronic rheumatic complaints, and as an adjuvant for high cholesterol. It is also used as a foaming and flavor ingredient in root beer.

Caution: Doses higher than recommended should be avoided during pregnancy. At high doses, it may cause gastrointestinal irritations (with nausea, vomiting, diarrhea) and genitourinary tract (damage of kidney tissue). As with other herbs rich in saponins, it can influence the absorption and / or excretion of some drugs. In view of this, when taking a vital oral medication, drugs should be ingested about one hour apart from sarsaparilla.

References: (1) Vol. 6, p. 723; (3) Vol. 6b, p. 425; (6) p. 239; (8) p. 523; (9) p. 462; (12) p. 564; (14) p. 194; (15) p. 197; (20) p. 233; (22) p. 241; (23) p. 336; (31) p. 689; (37) p. 1275; (46) p. 1406; (66) p. 433; (71) p. 234.

SASSAFRAS

Botanical Name(s): *Sassafras albidum* (Nutt.) Nees. = *Sassafras officinale* T. Nees et C.H. Ebern [Fam.: Lauraceae]

Root bark

Constituents: Volatile oil (with safrole, also pinenes, phellandrene, eugenol, etc.), aporphine alkaloids (boldine, etc.), lignans, tannins, phytosterols, resin, polysaccharides (gum, mucilage, starch), etc.

Properties: Aromatic, diuretic, antimicrobial, carminative. There are reports for carcinogenic and hepatotoxic effects, due in large part to safrole.

Uses: Internally it has been used (usually combined with sarsaparilla, guaiacum) as an antidyscratic (= blood purifier) for chronic rheumatic complaints and atopic eczema (chronic eczema of internal origin), among others.

Caution: Due to the risk of carcinogenic and hepatotoxic effects, sassafras should not be taken for any medicinal purpose, particularly during pregnancy and lactation.

Note: Sassafras oil, obtained by steam distillation from the underground parts of the tree, has been used as a fragrance ingredient, and applied externally (as a paint, liniment) has been used for rheumatic pains, among others. Due to its toxicity it is no longer used.

References: (1) Vol. 6, p. 610; (3) Vol. 6b, p. 292; (9) p. 463; (20) p. 235; (22) p. 242; (37) p. 1227; (46) p. 1437; (47) p. 2457; (48) p. 552; (66) p. 434.

SAUNDERS, RED

Other Common Name(s): red sandalwood
Botanical Name(s): *Pterocarpus santalinus* L. f. [Fam.: Fabaceae (Papilionaceae)]
Wood (red saunders, red sandalwood)
It is the cut and dried heartwood.
Constituents: Red pigments (benzoxanthenones: santalins A, B, etc.), flavonoids (pterocarpanes: pterocarpin, etc.; neoflavonoids), stilbenoids (pterostilbene, etc.), phenolic acids (gallic acid), volatile oil, triterpenes, etc.
Properties: Astringent, antifungal, antibacterial (against *Helicobacter pylori*), diuretic, mild antihyperglycemic.
Uses: Red saunders is chiefly used as a red coloring ingredient in drug products, liqueurs, and meat products, among others. Internally it has been used as an adjuvant (tea, h. p.) for inflammations and ulcerations of the gastrointestinal tract (diarrhea, peptic ulcers, etc.) and minor cases of diabetes, and as an antidyscratic (= blood purifier; tea, h. p.) for chronic skin disorders. Externally it has been used for minor cuts and wounds, and fungal skin infections, among others.
Caution: There are no reports of contraindications or side effects when used properly. As its pigments are water-insoluble, there is no reason to incorporate it in herbal mixtures. Red saunders is found as an adulterant of saffron (!).

References: (2) Vol. 3, p. 419; (3) Vol. 6a, p. 965; (8) p. 465; (17) p. 533; (36) p. 497; (37) p. 1140; (41) Vols. 1-7; (66) p. 431.

SAVIN

Other Common Name(s): sabine
Botanical Name(s): *Juniperus sabina* L. [Fam.: Cupressaceae]
Tops
Constituents: Volatile oil (with sabinyl acetate, sabinol, sabinene, etc.), lignans (podophyllotoxin derivatives), sesquiterpenes, diterpenes, coumarins, etc.
Properties: Antiviral (against papillomaviruses), rubefacient, counterirritant, emmenagogue, uterotonic. The effects are due in large part to the volatile oil. The antiviral effect is due to podophyllotoxin derivatives.
Uses: Externally it is used (as an ointment, paint) much like mayapple (see MAYAPPLE) chiefly for genital warts (= venereal warts = condylomata acuminata), but also other warts (common w., plantar w.). It is also used (as a liniment, ointment combination product) for neuralgic pains, rheumatic pains, and hair loss.
Caution: Savin is toxic and not for self-treatment. The applications should be supervised by a health professional. The product should be applied on

warts, avoiding the adjacent area. A longer duration of action may lead to blisters, even tissue necrosis (see also MAYAPPLE). It is no longer used internally because even at normal doses it causes irritations of the genitourinary tract. It has been taken at large doses to induce abortion, often with fatal results.

References: (1) Vol. 5, p. 582; (3) Vol. 5, p. 341; (5) Vol. 2, p. 203; (8) p. 330; (31) p. 566; (37) p. 741; (41) Vols. 1-7; (46) p. 1386; (47) p. 2388; (49) Vol. 1, p. 387; (66) p. 420.

SAVORY

Other Common Name(s): 1) summer savory 2) winter savory
Botanical Name(s): 1) *Satureja hortensis* L. 2) *Satureja montana* L. [Fam.: Lamiaceae (Labiatae)]
Aerial part (chiefly leaves with tender stems)
Constituents: Volatile oil (with carvacrol, also γ-terpinene, p-cymene, etc.), Lamiaceae tannins (rosmarinic acid and other caffeic acid derivatives), triterpenes (ursolic acid, oleanolic acid), flavonoids, phytosterols, etc.
Properties: Aromatic, stomachic, antibacterial, antifungal, antispasmodic, carminative, antioxidant, diuretic, astringent. Winter savory acts stronger. The stomachic effect is due to bitter triterpenes and phenolic acids. Rosmarinic acid and related caffeic acid derivatives have been shown to inhibit the biosynthesis of leukotrienes and prostaglandins, and to exert choleretic, antibacterial and antiviral effects.
Uses: Savory is chiefly used in culinary practice and food industry as a spice and flavor ingredient particularly in meat and vegetable products. Internally it is used (as a tea, h. p.) for minor inflammatory and spastic conditions of the gastrointestinal tract (diarrhea, nausea, flatulence, cramps), upper respiratory tract (the common cold, bronchitis, etc.; coughs), also genitourinary and hepatobiliary tracts. Externally it is used (as a mouthwash) for bacterial and fungal infections of the mouth.
Caution: During pregnancy it may be used only in moderate amounts as a spice but not for the mentioned indications. Otherwise, there are no reports of contraindications or side effects when used properly.

References: (2) Vol. 3, p. 520; (3) Vol. 6b, p. 295; (8) p. 513; (9) p. 465; (12) p. 782; (20) p. 256; (29) p. 104; (35) p. 718; (37) p. 1226; (47) p. 2462; (48) p. 540; (51) p. 168.

SAW PALMETTO

Other Common Name(s): sabal palm
Botanical Name(s): *Serenoa repens* (W. Bartram) Small = *Sabal serrulata* (Michx.) Schult. f. = *Serenoa serrulata* (Michx.) Hook. F. Ex B. D. Jacks. [Fam.: Arecaceae (Palmae)]
Fruit (berry) (saw palmetto = sabal)

Constituents: Lipids, water-soluble polysaccharides, flavonoids, invert sugar, etc. Among lipids are, fatty acids (chiefly saturated: lauric and myristic acids, etc.), which are found chiefly free and partly as esters with long chain aliphatic alcohols and glycerol, and phytosterols (5-sterols: β-sitosterol, β-sitosterolin = β-sitosterol-glucoside, esterified β-sitosterol).

Properties: Saw palmetto extract has been shown to inhibit the conversion of testosterone to dihydrotestosterone (= DHT, a stronger androgen, the main cause of BPH) as well as their binding to the receptors in the prostatic tissue, with antiproliferative effect (= inhibition of prostatic cell division and growth). The effect is achieved without influencing blood levels of androgens, so without lowering the sexual drive (= loss of libido). Other effects that it exerts in the prostate are, anti-inflammatory, antiedematous and antispasmodic, mainly by inhibiting the biosynthesis of prostaglandins and leukotrienes.

Uses: Internally it is used (as an h. p. rich in free fatty acids and sterols) for micturition problems associated with early stages of benign prostatic hyperplasia (= BPH: stages I and II). Rational treatments with saw palmetto fat-soluble extract (rich in free fatty acids and sterols) have resulted in a decrease or disappearance of difficulties in starting the urination, increase of urine flow, and decrease of frequency of urination and residual urine.

Caution: Before using saw palmetto products for BPH, the prostate problem should be judged by a health professional. Saw palmetto products should be rich in free fatty acids and sterols. Often they are standardized to the free fatty acids content. In rare cases it may cause stomach upset. Otherwise, there are no reports of contraindications or side effects when used properly.

References: (1) Vol. 6, p. 680; (3) Vol. 6b, p. 370; (6) p. 198; (7) p. 251; (8) p. 517; (9) p. 467; (13) p. 423; (20) p. 237; (22) p. 103; (26) p. 217; (37) p. 1257; (48) p. 162; (66) p. 420; (68) p. 202.

SAXIFRAGE, BURNET

Other Common Name(s): 1) greater burnet saxifrage 2) lesser burnet saxifrage

Botanical Name(s): 1) *Pimpinella major* (L.) Huds. 2) *Pimpinella saxifraga* L. [Fam.: Apiaceae (Umbelliferae)]

Root

Constituents: Volatile oil (with esters of isoeugenol, etc.), coumarins and furanocoumarins (small amounts), phenolic acids (caffeic acid, etc.), saponins, polyacetylenes, phytosterols, etc.

Properties: Expectorant (bronchial secretagogue effect), diuretic, mild antispasmodic, stomachic, emmenagogue, antimicrobial.

Uses: Internally it is used (as a tea, h. p.) for inflammatory and spastic conditions of the upper respiratory tract (the common cold, pharyngitis, laryngitis with hoarseness, tracheitis, spastic bronchitis, bronchial asthma;

338

coughs due to thickened bronchial secretion) and genitourinary tract (cystitis, etc., gravel, nonobstructive urinary stones), nonulcer dyspepsia (with minor cramps, bloating), primary dysmenorrhea (= painful menstruation without pathology), and as an antidyscratic (= blood purifier) for chronic rheumatic complaints. To enhance the effects in problems of the genitourinary tract, the fluid intake (incl. herbal teas) should be more than 2 liters per day. It is also used as a flavor ingredient in liqueur / liquor industry. Externally it is used (as a gargle, mouthwash) for inflammations of the mouth and throat, and (as a wash, wet compress) for minor wounds.

Caution: There are no reports of contraindications or side effects when used properly. Nevertheless, before using it for dysmenorrhea, the gynecologic problem should be judged by a health professional.

References: (1) Vol. 6, p. 147; (3) Vol. 6a, p. 667; (8) p. 431; (13) p. 327; (16) p. 60; (17) p. 440; (19) p. 45; (23) p. 216; (24) p. 84; (27) p. 331; (47) p. 2128; (51) p. 130.

SCAMMONY, MEXICAN

Other Common Name(s): Orizaba jalap
Botanical Name(s): *Ipomoea orizabensis* (Pellet.) Led. ex Steud. [Fam.: Convolvulaceae]
Root (tuber), **resin**
Mexican scammony resin is the dried purified extract of the tuber.
Constituents: Tuber contains resin, glycoretins, phytosterols, etc. Resin consists of glycoretins (chiefly scammonin = orizabin, also α-scammonin), which are ester glycosides (see: JALAP).
Properties: Drastic purgative (resin is much stronger).
Uses: Internally it is used (as an h. p.; only combined with other herbs) for habitual constipation (cf. JALAP).
Caution: Mexican scamony should be used only as directed by an experienced practitioner. It should not be taken during pregnancy and lactation and in cases of inflammations of the gastrointestinal tract.

References: (1) Vol. 5, p. 540; (3) Vol. 5, p. 264; (8) p. 324; (12a) p. 66; (13) p. 302; (36) p. 291; (37) p. 729; (48) p. 180.

SCHISANDRA

Other Common Name(s): Chinese schisandra
Botanical Name(s): *Schisandra chinensis* (Turcz.) Baill.; *Schisandra sphenanthera* Rehd. et Wils. [Fam.: Schisandraceae]
Fruit
Constituents: Lignans (schisandrins, schisandrols, schisantherins, gomisins), phytosterols (5-sterols: β-sitosterol, etc.), organic acids (citric and malic acids), vitamins (A, C, E), sugars, pectin, volatile oil, etc.

Properties: Protects liver cells from damaging effects of toxic substances, promotes regeneration of liver tissue, immunomodulant (chiefly by increasing lymphocyte count), neurotonic, antioxidant, and antimicrobial effects, among others. Most of the effects are attributed to lignans.

Uses: Internally it is used (as tea, h. p.) for liver disorders (chronic hepatitis, adjuvant for cirrhosis), minor fatigue and feeling of weakness, decreased mental and physical performance, convalescence, low sexual drive, erectile dysfunction, for inflammations of the gastrointestinal tract (diarrhea, etc.), respiratory tract (bronchitis, etc.; coughs), genitourinary tract (cystitis, urinary incontinence, etc.) and the skin (eczema, etc.), and for decreased immune response in general.

Caution: Normally, it should be used for 1-3 months. Before a possible resuming a break is necessary. In rare cases it may cause stomach upset or skin allergic reactions. Otherwise, there are no reports of contraindications or side effects when used properly.

References: (1) Vol. 6, p. 641; (3) Vol. 6b, p. 318; (6) p. 146; (9) p. 469; (22) p. 79; (36) p. 438; (41) Vols. 1-7; (45) p. 132; (53) p. 146; (86) Vol. 1, p. 132.

SCHISANDRA, JAPANESE

Other Common Name(s): Japanese kadsura
Botanical Name(s): *Kadsura japonica* (L.) Dunal = *Schisandra japonica* (L.) Baill. [Fam.: Schisandraceae]
Fruit
Constituents: Lignans (kadsurarin, esters of binankadsurin A), volatile oil (with germacrene C, δ-elemen-9-ol, etc.), phytosterols (kadsuric acid, etc.), etc.

Properties and Uses: It is reported to have similar values of Chinese schisandra (see SCHISANDRA, CHINESE), which often adulterates.
Caution: See SCHISANDRA, CHINESE.

References: (1) Vol. 5, p. 606; (41) Vols. 1-7; (42) Vol. 6, p. 340; (52) p. 413.

SCOPOLIA

Other Common Name(s): Russian belladonna, Japanese belladonna
Botanical Name(s): *Scopolia carniolica* Jacq. [Fam.: Solanaceae]
Root
Constituents: Tropane alkaloids: chiefly (−)-hyosciamine, also (−)-scopolamine, atropine = (±)-hyosciamine, cuskohygrine, etc.; coumarins (scopoletin and its glucoside); phenolic acids (chlorogenic acid, etc.); etc.

Properties: Due to the parasympatholytic activity of hyosciamine / atropine, scopolia exerts antispasmodic and antisecretory effects, among others. Cf. BELLADONNA; HENBANE.

340

Uses: Today scopolia is chiefly used for the industrial production of alkaloids. It is still found in some standardized combination products used for spastic conditions of the gastrointestinal and genitourinary tracts. It has also been used for Parkinson's disease (= a chronic neurologic disorder, with muscular weakness and tremor, sluggish movement and abnormal gait).
Caution: Scopolia is toxic and not for self-treatment. It should be used only as directed by a health professional. The same cautions mentioned for belladonna, henbane, mandrake and stramonium apply also to scopolia. See BELLADONNA.

References: (3) Vol. 331; (6) p. 195; (8) p. 514; (12a) p. 514; (13) p. 241; (19) p. 96; (36) p. 358; (48) p. 806.

SCOTCH BROOM

Other Common Name(s): scoparium
Botanical Name(s): *Cytisus scoparius* (L.) Link. = *Spartium scoparium* L. = *Sarothamnus scoparius* (L.) Wimm. ex W.D.J. Koch [Fam.: Fabaceae (Leguminosae)]
Aerial part
Constituents: Quinolizidine alkaloids (chiefly sparteine, also α-isosparteine, etc.), biogenic amines (tyramine, etc.; mainly in flower), flavonoids (flavone-C-glycosides: scoparoside; flavonols; mainly in flower), etc. Sparteine and related alkaloids are steam distilling liquids.
Properties: Cardio-sedative (= normalizes a "nervous heart") and mild coronary dilator due in large part to sparteine, mild cardiotonic due in large part to tyramine (see CEREUS, NIGHT-BLOOMING), diuretic due in large part to flavonoids (esp. scoparoside), and increases the tonus and contractions of the uterus (= uterotonic and oxytocic) due in large part to sparteine.
Uses: Internally it is used (as a standardized product) for cardiac arrhythmias (esp. tachycardia = rapid heartbeat) and minor cases of cardiovascular insufficiency (with edemas, hypotension = low blood pressure, angina pectoris = chest pain due to insufficient blood supply to the heart). It has also been used for postpartum hemorrhage (= h. following childbirth), menorrhagia / hypermenorrhea (= prolonged / heavy menstruation) but is obsolete.
Caution: Scotch broom should be used only as directed by a health professional. It should not be used in cases of hypertension. Unless advised by a health professional, it should not be taken during pregnancy and lactation. A concomitant use with MAOI antidepressant drugs (e. g. phenelzine) or herbs (e. g. St. John's wort) and certain antihypertensive drugs (reserpine, guanethidine) should be avoided as it may lead to synergistic effect. Otherwise, there are no reports of contraindications or side effects when used properly. See also CEREUS, NIGHT-BLOOMING.

References: (1) Vol. 4, p. 1126; (3) Vol. 4, p. 430; (6) pp. 48, 60; (11a) p. 463; (13) p. 276; (15) p. 191; (17) p. 539; (20) p. 50; (23) pp. 183, 373; (28) p. 137; (46) p. 668; (48) p. 851.

SEA BUCKTHORN

Botanical Name(s): *Hippophae rhamnoides* L. [Fam.: Elaeagnaceae]

Fruit

Constituents: Vitamins (rich in vitamin C, also B_1, E, "P" = flavonols, folic acid, provitamin A = carotene), organic acids (malic acid, etc.), carotenoids (carotenes, lutein = xanthophyll, etc.), sugar alcohols (mannitol, etc.), flavonoids (flavonols, anthocyanins), fixed oil (chiefly in seeds), etc.

Properties: Same as vitamin C, antitumoral, acidulous, refrigerant.

Uses: Internally it is used as a natural supplement of vitamins, particularly vitamin C, and as a valuable antioxidant. Juices, drinks and other products produced usually with fresh sea buckthorn berries, are chiefly used for feverish and thirsty states.

Caution: There are no reports of contraindications or side effects when used properly.

Sea buckthorn oil

It is the fixed oil contained mainly in seeds, and it is obtained by cold expression from the fruits.

Constituents: Glycerides (fatty acids component: linoleic, linolenic, and oleic acids), vitamin E, carotenoids, phytosterols, etc.

Properties: Emollient, vulnerary, demulcent, liver protective, antiulcer, platelet aggregation inhibitory.

Uses: Externally it is used for minor wounds and burns, and to protect the skin and enhance healing of injuries caused by exposure to sunrays or roentgen rays. Internally it is used as an adjuvant for peptic ulcers.

Caution: There are no reports of contraindications or side effects when used properly.

References: (2) Vol. 2, p. 849; (3) Vol. 5, p. 84; (8) p. 308; (12a) p. 149; (24) p. 276; (37) p. 664; (51) p. 266; (52) p. 375; (86) Vol. 2, p. 110; (87) Vol. 2, p. 183.

SEA LAVENDER

Botanical Name(s): *Limonium gerberi* Soldano = *Statice latifolia* Sm.; *Limonium vulgare* Mill. = *Statice limonium* L.; *Limonium carolinianum* (Walt.) Britt.; and other *Limonium* spp. (= *Statice* spp.): [Fam.: Plumbaginaceae]

Root

Constituents: Tannins (rich in condensed and hydrolyzable t.), flavonoids (chiefly flavonols), organic acids, etc.

Properties: Astringent, anti-inflammatory, hemostatic.

Uses: Internally it is used (as a tea, h. p.) for inflammations (also when minor hemorrhages are present) of the gastrointestinal tract (diarrhea, etc., incl. hemorrhoids), and genitourinary and respiratory tracts. Externally it is used (as a mouthwash, gargle, paint) for inflammations of the mouth and throat, inflamed and bleeding gums, (as a wash, wet compress, poultice) for ulcers and hemorrhoids, and (as a vaginal irrigation / sitz bath / wash) for leukorrhea. For minor hemorrhages it should be used on professional's advice. **Caution:** There are no reports of contraindications or side effects when used properly. At higher doses than recommended it may cause gastrointestinal irritations (with nausea, vomiting).

References: (3) Vol. 5, p. 511; (5) Vol. 1, p. 653; (18) p. 145; (31) p. 505; (35) p. 474; (36) p. 46; (41) Vols. 1-7; (42) Vol. 5, p. 345; (44) p. 307; (52) p. 446.

SENEGA

Other Common Name(s): Seneca snakeroot, senega snakeroot
Botanical Name(s): *Polygala senega* L. [Fam.: Polygalaceae]
Root (Seneca snakeroot, senega snakeroot)
Constituents: Triterpenoid saponins (senegin, etc.), phenol glycosides (aglycone: methyl salicylate), volatile oil (with methyl salicylate, etc.), xanthones, lipids, sugars, etc.
Properties: (At low doses): Expectorant (bronchial secretagogue effect), diuretic, anti-inflammatory (possibly NSAID-like). (At high doses): Emetic.
Uses: Internally it is used (as a tea, h. p.) for inflammations of the upper respiratory tract (bronchitis, etc.; coughs due to thickened bronchial secretion), as an adjuvant for emphysema and bronchial asthma and other conditions of the upper respiratory tract, when bronchial secretions need to become more fluid. It is also used as an anti-inflammatory and antidyscratic (= blood purifier) for chronic rheumatic complaints.
Caution: It should not be taken during pregnancy and lactation, in cases of inflammations of the gastrointestinal tract (ulcers, gastritis, diarrhea, ulcerative colitis) and internal bleedings (respiratory, gastrointestinal). At higher doses than recommended it causes gastrointestinal irritations (with nausea, vomiting, diarrhea).
Note: With **polygala root** is to be understood the root derived from other closely related *Polygala* spp. including *P. tenuifolia* Willd. and *P. sibirica* L., among others. They resemble very much in constituents and effects and are used interchangeably as Seneca snakeroot.

References: (3) Vol. 6a, p. 802; (6) p. 101; (8) p. 451; (14) p. 196; (15) p. 195; (17) p. 450; (19) p. 206; (20) p. 241; (22) p. 124; (28) p. 79; (46) p. 1143; (47) p. 2531; (48) p. 699.

SENNA

Botanical Name(s): *Cassia angustifolia* Vahl; *Cassia senna* L. = *Cassia acutifolia* Delile [Fam.: Fabaceae (Caesalpiniaceae)]
Leaf, pod
Constituents: Anthranoids (chiefly dianthrone glycosides: sennosides A-D, etc.; also anthraquinone derivatives: glycosidic and free), bitter principles,

343

mucilaginous polysaccharides, flavonoids, naphthalene glycosides, etc.

Properties: Laxative (large intestine stimulant laxative). Under the attack of large intestine flora anthranoid glycosides are hydrolyzed and then, with other available free anthraquinones, are reduced to the active anthrones. They inhibit the absorption of electrolytes and water from the colon and increase the secretion of electrolytes and water into intestine. This results in increased peristalsis and discharge of soft stools.

Uses: Internally it is used (as a tea, h. p.) for constipation (atonic, not spastic) and conditions in which facilitated defecation is sought such as hemorrhoids, anal fissure, after operations in rectum or anal area, etc.

Caution: Senna may cause abdominal griping when used as a tea. This is less intensive when used products with purified and standardized extracts. It should not be taken during pregnancy, lactation, menstruation, in cases of bowel obstruction, and inflammatory gastrointestinal disorders (ulcerative colitis, Crohn's disease, appendicitis). Unless advised by a health professional, it should not be used in children under 12 years. It is best used as a standardized product and for a short period (maximum 8-10 days). Its chronic use or abuse may cause electrolyte imbalance, especially potassium deficiency, which is very risky particularly when combined with cardiac glycosides.

References: (1) Vol. 4, p. 701; (3) Vol. 3, p. 738; (6) p. 165; (8) p. 121; (9) p. 472; (11) p. 54; (12) p. 910; (13) p. 299; (14) p. 199; (17) p. 546; (19) p. 207; (22) p. 60; (23) p. 100; (36) p. 235; (46) p. 1512; (48) p. 427; (59) pp. 241, 250; (68) p. 208.

SHEPHERD'S PURSE

Botanical Name(s): *Capsella bursa-pastoris* (L.) Medik. [Fam.: Brassicaceae (Cruciferae)]

Aerial part

Constituents: A peptide, non-protein amino acids, flavonoids (flavones: luteolin, scolymoside, diosmin, etc.), choline derivatives (sinapine = sinapic acid choline ester; acetylcholine), minerals (potassium, calcium), phenolic acids (caffeic acid derivatives), etc.

Properties: Mild uterotonic (ergot-like effect) and hemostatic, anti-inflammatory. Its mild uterotonic effect is attributed to a peptide, but to the overall effect may contribute also other constituents (flavonoids, etc.).

Uses: Internally it is used (as a tea, h. p.) for menorrhagia / hypermenorrhea (= prolonged / heavy menstruation), postpartum hemorrhage (= h. following childbirth), as an adjuvant for metrorrhagia (= nonmenstrual uterine bleeding), and for inflammations (also when minor hemorrhages are present) of the genitourinary tract (cystitis, etc., gravel, nonobstructive stones), gastrointestinal tract (diarrhea, ulcerative colitis, etc., incl. hemorrhoids) and upper respiratory tract (minor nosebleed, etc.). Externally it is used (as a poultice, wet compress) for minor cuts and wounds, (as a wet cotton, drops, irri-

344

gation with the fresh juice or tea) for nosebleed, and (as a mouthwash) for inflammations of the mouth.
Caution: Unless advised by a health professional, shepherd's purse should not be taken during pregnancy. For any kind of hemorrhage it should be used on health professional's advice. Otherwise, there are no reports of contraindications or side effects when used properly.

References: (1) Vol. 4, p. 656; (3) Vol. 3, p. 666; (6) p. 314; (7) p. 273; (8) p. 112; (12b) p. 151; (15) p. 46; (16) p. 31; (17) p. 113; (19) p. 105; (20) p. 245; (23) p. 373; (24) p. 166; (28) p. 169; (37) p. 267; (41) Vols. 1-7; (46) p. 224; (47) p. 745; (51) p. 88.

SILVERWEED

Botanical Name(s): *Argentina anserina* (L.) Rydb. = *Potentilla anserina* L. = *Potentilla argentia* Huds. [Fam.: Rosaceae]
Aerial part
Constituents: Tannins (gallotannins, ellagitannins), flavonoids (flavonols, anthocyanins), phenolic acids (caffeic acid, etc.), a biogenic amine (choline), phytosterols, coumarins, etc.
Properties: Astringent, anti-inflammatory, mild antispasmodic / tonic (uterine active).
Uses: Internally it is used (as a tea, h. p.) for inflammations of the gastrointestinal tract (diarrhea, ulcerative colitis, etc., incl. hemorrhoids; also when minor hemorrhages are present), and for primary dysmenorrhea (= painful menstruation without pathology). Externally it is used (as a mouthwash, gargle, paint) for inflammations of the mouth and throat, gingivitis (= inflammations of the gums), denture sore, and (as a wash, wet compress, poultice) for minor skin inflammations, eczema, wounds and ulcers.
Caution: There are no reports of contraindications or side effects when used properly. Nevertheless, before using it for dysmenorrhea and any kind of hemorrhage, the problem should be judged by a health professional.

References: (1) Vol. 6, p. 255; (3) Vol. 6a, p. 845; (6) p. 306; (7) p. 273; (8) p. 457; (16) pp. 82, 170; (17) p. 72; (19) p. 86; (23) pp. 53, 365; (37) p. 1113; (46) p. 2212; (51) p. 98.

SIMARUBA

Other Common Name(s): simarouba, bitter damson, mountain damson
Botanical Name(s): *Simarouba amara* Aubl. = *Quassia simaruba* L. f. [Fam.: Simaroubaceae]
Root bark (simaruba bark, Orinoco bark)
Constituents: Bitter principles (nortriterpenes of quassinoid type: simarubin, etc.), tannins (rich), volatile oil, indole alkaloids (5-hydroxycanthin-6-one, etc.), fats, resin, etc.
Properties: Bitter tonic, astringent, antiprotozoal, antipyretic. Nortriterpenes of quassinoid type (incl. simarubin) have shown antiprotozoal (esp.

against *Entamoeba* spp., but also *Plasmodium* spp.), antiviral, antibacterial and anthelmintic effects. Canthin-6-one, a closely related compound of the mentioned alkaloid and which is found in Chinese Tree-of-Heaven (see TREE-OF-HEAVEN, CHINESE) has shown antibacterial effect.

Uses: Internally it is used (as a tea, h. p.) for loss of appetite, diarrhea, amebic dysentery and feverish states.

Caution: It should not be taken during pregnancy and lactation. At higher doses than recommended it causes gastrointestinal irritations (with nausea, vomiting, diarrhea).

References: (3) Vol. 6b, p. 406; (5) Vol. 1, p. 895; (10) p. 251; (27) p. 318; (31) pp. 168, 728; (35) p. 741; (37) p. 1271; (41) Vols. 1-7; (49) Vol. 2, p. 306; (52) p. 725.

SKULLCAP

Other Common Name(s): blue skullcap, scullcap
Botanical Name(s): *Scutellaria lateriflora* L. [Fam.: Lamiaceae (Labiatae)]
Aerial part
Constituents: Bitter principles (iridoids), flavonoids (flavones: scutellarein glycosides, etc.; etc.), Lamiaceae tannins (rosmarinic acid and other caffeic acid derivatives), volatile oil, resin, etc.
Properties: Bitter tonic, stomachic, sedative, antispasmodic, astringent, aromatic. The effects are mild.
Uses: Internally it is used (as a tea, h. p.; often combined with other herbs) for loss of appetite and nonulcer dyspepsia (with minor cramps), convalescence, minor cases of nervous fatigue, anxiety and insomnia, and as a diaphoretic hot tea for feverish states. As there are reports of mild uterine antispasmodic effect, it may be helpful for dysmenorrhea (= painful menstruation without pathology).
Caution: There are no reports of contraindications or side effects when used properly. Skullcap has been found adulterated with germander, a hepatotoxic herb (see GERMANDER). In view of this, only experienced practitioners should handle it and manufacturers should run tests accordingly.

References: (3) Vol. 6b, p. 340; (10) p. 247; (15) p. 193; (20) p. 239; (25) p. 211; (31) pp. 392, 572; (35) p. 724; (45) p. 134; (47) p. 2498; (48) p. 651; (65) p. 406; (66) p. 437; (68) p. 207.

SKULLCAP, BAIKAL

Other Common Name(s): Chinese skullcap
Botanical Name(s): *Scutellaria baicalensis* Georgi = *Scutellaria macrantha* Fisch. [Fam.: Lamiaceae (Labiatae)]
Root
Constituents: Bitter principles (iridoids: catalpol, etc.), flavonoids (rich in flavones: baicalein, scutellarein, wogonin, and their glycosides), Lamiaceae tannins (rosmarinic acid and other caffeic acid derivatives), phytosterols,

volatile oil, etc.

Properties: Bitter tonic, anti-inflammatory, antiallergic, antispasmodic, antioxidant, liver protective, antibacterial, diuretic, astringent. Iridoids have shown bitter tonic, choleretic, liver protective, laxative, diuretic, anti-inflammatory, antibacterial, antiviral, antifungal and immunomodulant effects, among others. Baikal skullcap flavones have shown anti-inflammatory, antiallergic, antispasmodic and platelet aggregation inhibitory effects by inhibiting the biosynthesis of leukotrienes and prostaglandins.

Uses: Internally it is used (as a tea, h. p.) for inflammatory and spastic conditions of the gastrointestinal tract (loss of appetite, impaired digestion, diarrhea, etc.), liver (chronic hepatitis), upper respiratory tract (spastic bronchitis, the common cold, bronchial asthma) and genitourinary tract (cystitis, etc.). It is also used as an adjuvant for cardiovascular disorders in general. To enhance the effects in problems of the genitourinary tract, the fluid intake (incl. herbal teas) should be more than 2 liters per day.

Caution: There are no reports of contraindications or side effects when used properly.

References: (3) Vol. 6b, p. 339; (10) p. 247; (13) p. 436; (15) p. 193; (20) p. 239; (31) pp. 392, 414; (41) Vols. 1-7; (45) p. 133; (48) p. 651; (53) p. 33.

SKUNK CABBAGE

Botanical Name(s): *Symplocarpus foetidus* (L.) Salisb. ex Nutt. = *Dracontium foetidum* L. [Fam.: Araceae]

Root (rhizome and root)

Constituents: Resin, pungent principles, saponins, calcium oxalate (high concentration) and starch (rich). It possibly contains mucilaginous polysaccharides, cyanogenic glycosides, and phytosterols. The reported pungent principles possibly are 5-alkyl or 5-alkenyl-resorcinol derivatives.

Properties: Expectorant, antispasmodic, mild sedative, rubefacient.

Uses: Skunk cabbage is chiefly used in traditional medicine. Internally it is used (as a tea, h. p.) for inflammatory and spastic conditions of the upper respiratory tract (spastic bronchitis, etc., bronchial asthma; coughs due to thickened bronchial secretion), and epilepsy. Externally it is used (as a wet compress, poultice) for rheumatic pains.

Caution: Most plants of Araceae family are toxic, partly due to cyanogenic glycosides, which liberate hydrocyanic acid. In view of this, skunk cabbage should be used based on an experienced practitioner's advice. It should not be taken during pregnancy and lactation, in gastrointestinal ulcers, cardiovascular problems, and in cases of a known history of oxalate kidney stones. At higher doses than recommended it may cause gastrointestinal irritations (with nausea, vomiting). Fresh material may cause contact skin irritations.

References: (3) Vol. 6b, p. 710; (15) p. 203; (18) p. 299; (20) p. 247; (25) p. 229; (35) p. 742; (37) p. 1337; (42) Vol. 2, pp. 77, 78; (44) p. 548.

SLIPPERY ELM

Botanical Name(s): *Ulmus rubra* Muhl. = *Ulmus fulva* Michx. [Fam.: Ulmaceae]
Bark (inner bark)
Constituents: Mucilaginous polysaccharides (very rich), starch, tannins, phytosterols (5-sterols: β-sitosterol, etc.), minerals, etc. Slippery elm mucilage consists chiefly of galactose.
Properties: Demulcent, antitussive (mucosal protective effect), mild bulk laxative, nutritive, emollient. The mucilaginous polysaccharides account for most of the effects. They may also exert mild immunomodulant effect.
Uses: Internally it is used (as a tea, h. p.) for inflammations of the upper respiratory tract (laryngitis, pharyngitis, tracheitis, bronchitis; irritating dry coughs; also as a lozenge) and inflammatory and ulcerative conditions of the gastrointestinal tract (esophagitis, gastritis, heartburn, peptic ulcers, irritable bowel syndrome, changes in bowel movements; also as an enema). It is also used for inflammations of the genitourinary tract (cystitis, gravel, nonobstructive urinary stones) and as an ingredient in convalescent foods. Externally it is used (as a mouthwash, gargle) for inflammations of the mouth and throat, and (as a poultice) for boils, minor wound and burns.
Caution: Slippery elm may impair the absorption of some drugs. In view of this, when taking a vital oral medication, drugs should be taken about one hour apart from slippery elm products. Otherwise, there are no reports of contraindications or side effects when used properly.

References: (1) Vol. 6, p. 1027; (3) Vol. 6c, p. 340; (14) p. 204; (15) p. 222; (20) p. 248; (22) p. 119; (44) p. 577; (52) p. 827; (66) p. 493; (68) p. 212.

SLOE

Other Common Name(s): blackthorn
Botanical Name(s): *Prunus spinosa* L. [Fam.: Rosaceae]
Flower
Constituents: Flavonoids (chiefly kaempferol glycosides), coumarins, and a cyanogenic glycoside (amygdalin; only in fresh flowers).
Properties: Diuretic, laxative. The effects are mild. The diuretic effect is due in large part to kaempferol glycosides.
Uses: Internally it is used (as a tea, h. p.) for minor inflammations of the upper respiratory tract (the common cold, etc., chiefly as a diaphoretic hot tea) and gastrointestinal tract (minor constipation), and as an antidyscratic (= blood purifier) for atopic eczema (= chronic eczema of internal origin) and chronic rheumatic complaints.
Caution: There are no reports of contraindications or side effects when used properly.
Fruit (ripe)

348

Constituents: Organic acids, sugars, pectin, tannins (proanthocyanidins), a cyanogenic glycoside (amygdalin, only in seeds!), etc.
Properties: Astringent.
Uses: <u>Externally</u> it is used (as a mouthwash, gargle) for inflammations of the mouth and throat.
Caution: There are no reports of contraindications or side effects when used properly.

References: (3) Vol. 6a, p. 952; (8) p. 464; (16) p. 86; (17) p. 460; (19) p. 201; (37) p. 1136; (41) Vols. 1-7; (47) p. 2230; (51) p. 255.

SNAKEROOT, VIRGINIA

Other Common Name(s): serpentaria
Botanical Name(s): *Aristolochia serpentaria* L. [Fam.: Aristolochiaceae]
Root
Constituents: Volatile oil (with borneol, etc.), aristolochic acids (aristolochic acid I, etc.), aristolactams (cyclic amides of aristolochic acids), phytosterols (5-sterols: β-sitosterol, β-sitosterolin = β-sitosterol-glucoside), tannins, sugars, starch, etc.
Properties: Bitter tonic, antispasmodic, antibacterial. The effects are attributed in large part to aristolochic acids. Aristolactams are the in vitro- or / and in vivo-transformed products of aristolochic acids. They have shown mutagenic and carcinogenic effects.
Uses: <u>Internally</u> it has been used for dyspeptic complaints and spastic conditions of the gastrointestinal tract, common cold and feverish states, among others. <u>Externally</u> it is used (as a gargle) for sore throat, (as a wash) for infected wounds, and (as a poultice) for insect bites.
Caution: Virginia snakeroot should not be used internally, especially during pregnancy and lactation (see Properties). Cf. BIRTHWORT; GINGER CANADIAN WILD.

References: (2) Vol. 2, p. 179; (3) Vol. 3, p. 208; (12) p. 1248; (25) p. 224; (29) p. 14; (31) p. 117; (35) pp. 104, 744; (37) p. 128; (41) Vols. 1-7; (44) p. 91.

SOAPWORT, RED

Other Common Name(s): soapwort, soapweed
Botanical Name(s): *Saponaria officinalis* L. [Fam.: Caryophyllaceae]
Root (soap root, soapwort root, red soap root)
Constituents: Triterpenoid saponins (saponasides A, D; with aglycone: quillaic acid; cf. QUILLAJA), sugars, gum, etc.
Properties: Expectorant, diuretic, mild laxative, mild cholagogue, cholesterol reducing, anti-inflammatory, antimicrobial. The effects are due in large part to saponins. Soapwort exerts anti-inflammatory effect by inhibiting the biosynthesis of prostaglandins.

349

Uses: <u>Internally</u> it is used (as a tea, h. p.) chiefly for inflammations of the upper respiratory tract (bronchitis, etc.; coughs due to thickened bronchial secretion), also genitourinary and hepatobiliary tracts, as an antidyscratic (= blood purifier) for atopic eczema (= chronic eczema of internal origin) and chronic rheumatic complaints, and (combined with other herbs) for high cholesterol. <u>Externally</u> it is used (as a wash, mouthwash) for fungal infections of the skin and mouth.

Caution: It should not be taken in cases of gastrointestinal ulcers. At higher doses than recommended it causes gastrointestinal irritations (with cramps, nausea, vomiting, diarrhea). As it is rich in saponins, avoid contact with eyes or inhalation of powdered root as it irritates the mucous membranes. Otherwise, there are no reports of contraindications or side effects when used properly.

References: (2) Vol. 3, p. 512; (3) Vol. 6b, p. 283; (6) p. 101; (8) p. 511; (13) p. 210; (17) p. 535; (19) p. 204; (23) p. 217; (24) p. 300; (27) p. 308; (35) p. 748; (46) p. 1432; (47) p. 2444; (48) p. 713; (51) p. 68.

SOAPWORT, WHITE

Botanical Name(s): *Gypsophila paniculata* L., and some other *Gypsophila* spp. [Fam.: Caryophyllaceae]

<u>**Root**</u> (white soapwort root, white soap root)

Constituents: Triterpenoid saponins (chiefly gypsoside A; with aglycone: gypsogenin; richer than soapwort), sugars, triterpenoid acids, phytosterols, etc.

Properties: Expectorant, cholesterol reducing, anti-inflammatory, antimicrobial.

Uses: <u>Internally</u> it is used (as an h. p.) for inflammations of the upper respiratory tract (bronchitis, etc.; coughs due to thickened bronchial secretion), much like soapwort (q. v.). White saponin (= saponinum album) or Gypsophylla saponin is a purified and standardized extract obtained from white soapwort root and some other *Gypsophila* spp., including *G. arrostii* Guss., *G. struthium* Loefl. and *G. fastigiata* L. It is an ingredient in cough products.

Caution: See SOAPWORT, RED.

References: (1) Vol. 5, p. 357; (3) Vol. 4, p. 1223; (5) Vol. 1, p. 556; (12a) p. 207; (13) p. 210; (37) p. 630; (48) p. 713.

SOLOMON'S SEAL, AROMATIC

Other Common Name(s): fragrant Solomon's seal

Botanical Name(s): *Polygonatum odoratum* (Mill.) Druce = *Polygonatum officinale* All. [Fam.: Liliaceae]

<u>**Root**</u> (rhizome)

350

Constituents: Steroidal saponins (with sapogenin: diosgenin; cf. YAM, WILD), mucilaginous polysaccharides, a non-protein amino acid (L-azetidine-2-carboxylic acid), allantoin, a "glucokinin", etc.

Properties: Emollient, wound-healing, demulcent, diuretic, mild antibacterial, mild antihyperglycemic. Most of the effects are attributed to saponins. L-azetidine-2-carboxylic acid has shown mild antibacterial effect. Allantoin has shown wound-healing effect. "Glucokinin" is a coined name. It tells that among the known or unknown constituents of a botanical, there is a constituent with antihyperglycemic effect.

Uses: <u>Externally</u> it is used (as a poultice) for minor skin inflammations, bruises, panaris (= felon), and hemorrhoids. <u>Internally</u> it is used (as a tea, h. p.) for minor inflammations of the gastrointestinal tract (diarrhea, gastroenteritis), genitourinary tract (cystitis, etc.) and upper respiratory tract (bronchitis, pharyngitis, etc.), and as an adjuvant for diabetes. Due to steroidal saponins it may be beneficial for high cholesterol (see FENUGREEK).

Caution: There are no reports of contraindications or side effects when used properly. At higher doses than recommended it may cause gastrointestinal irritations (with nausea, vomiting).

References: (1) Vol. 6, p. 243; (3) Vol. 6a, p. 811; (5) Vol. 1, p. 862; (27) p. 317; (31) p. 65; (37) pp. 45, 600; (41) Vols. 1-7; (42) Vol. 2, p. 339; (47) p. 2187; (51) p. 56.

SORREL

Other Common Name(s): 1) sheep sorrel, sour grass 2) garden / common sorrel
Botanical Name(s): 1) *Rumex acetosella* L. 2) *Rumex acetosa* L. [Fam.: Polygonaceae]
Aerial part
Constituents: Potassium hydrogenoxalate (KHC_2O_4, very soluble!), calcium oxalate, oxalic acid, tartaric acid, vitamin C, anthranoids, tannins, flavonoids (hyperin, rutin), etc.

Properties and Uses: Sorrel is chiefly used as a salad. In traditional medicine it is used as a refrigerant and as an antidyscratic (= blood purifier) particularly for atopic eczema (= chronic eczema of internal origin).

Caution: It should not be taken or consumed in cases of a known history of oxalate kidney stones. Beside this, oxalic acid and potassium oxalate are toxic as they bind calcium ions into the insoluble calcium oxalate, and as a result serum calcium level decreases. Lethal doses of oxalic acid (5-13 g) lead to severe gastroenteritis (with vomiting and diarrhea), kidney damages, convulsions, and death due to cardiac arrest. A maximal dose for oxalic acid has been considered 0.3 gram (single dose) and 1 gram (daily dose). Based on these facts, sorrel should be used with caution, or best avoided. To satisfy the traditional use, one step could be the evaluation of the oxalate content for an area and then, based on the results to allow the consumption.

351

References: (3) Vol. 6b, p. 196; (4) Vol. 1, p. 184; (10) p. 250; (25) p. 214; (35) p. 754; (37) pp. 1013, 1205; (44) p. 495; (65) p. 802; (85) p. 320.

SOUTHERNWOOD

Other Common Name(s): lad's love
Botanical Name(s): *Artemisia abrotanum* L. [Fam.: Asteraceae (Compositae)]
Aerial part
Constituents: Volatile oil (with 1,8-cineole, etc.), bitter principles (sesquiterpene lactones), phenolic acids, coumarins, flavonoids, an alkaloid (abrotanine), etc.
Properties: Aromatic, bitter tonic, mild choleretic, diuretic, antimicrobial.
Uses: Internally it is used (as a tea, h. p.) for loss of appetite and nonulcer dyspepsia (with fullness, bloating, etc.) associated with impaired bile secretion, and for inflammations of the gastrointestinal tract (with diarrhea), genitourinary tract (cystitis, etc.) and upper respiratory tract (bronchitis, etc.). In traditional practice and food industry southernwood is used as a flavor ingredient much like mugwort, incorporating it in herbal vinegars, seasonings, and beverages. Externally it is used (as a poultice) for wounds.
Caution: See MUGWORT.

References: (1) Vol. 4, p. 358; (3) Vol. 3, p. 267; (5) Vol. 1, p. 122; (6) p. 147; (8) p. 76; (15) p. 31; (27) p. 13; (35) p. 754; (36) p. 475; (37) p. 135; (47) p. 357; (51) p. 211.

SOY

Botanical Name(s): *Glycine max* (L.) Merr.; *Glycine soja* Sieb et Zucc. [Fam.: Fabaceae (Leguminosae)]
Seed (soybean)
Constituents: Lipids (fixed oil, fatty acids, phosphatides, tocopherols, phytosterols, squalene), proteins (rich in globulins), carbohydrates (rich in galactose), flavonoids (isoflavones: daidzein, genistein, their glycosides, daidzin, genistin, etc.), triterpenoid saponins (bitter tasting), etc.
Properties: Nutrient, cholesterol and triglyceride reducing, liver protective (see Soy lecithin), estrogen-like, antioxidant. **Isoflavones** (cf. RED CLOVER) are plant constituents of estrogen-like effects (= phytoestrogens), whose metabolites have been shown to inhibit binding of stronger estrogens (e. g. estradiol) to their receptors therefore they are considered antiestrogens. There are also reports that, depending on the hormone imbalance stage (when estrogens level is lower than expected) they may exert proestrogenic effect. Most of them also exert antifungal effect and influence positively in reducing high cholesterol and triglycerides. Genistein has been shown to inhibit protein tyrosine kinase of EGFR (= epidermal growth factor receptor) in tumor cells. Genistin is about 6-7 times stronger than daidzin.

352

Uses: <u>Internally</u> it is used as a nutrient and invigorator, beneficial for high cholesterol and triglycerides, chronic liver disorders (fatty liver, liver damage), and as a natural supplement of phytoestrogens (here isoflavones). Soy products standardized to isoflavones or the isolated soy isoflavones are used to alleviate menopausal syndrome (= hot flashes, sweating, tachycardia, insomnia, emotional instability, depressive mood, fatigue, decreased vaginal lubrication, etc.), and to prevent postmenopausal problems (osteoporosis, high cholesterol, breast and uterine cancer, etc.) and prostate cancer.

Caution: In rare cases it may cause gastrointestinal disturbances (pains, frequent stools). Consumption of excessive amount of soybeans interferes with the oral absorption of thyroxin. In view of this, thyroxin-containing products should be ingested about one hour apart from soybean products. As with other herbs of estrogen-like effects, soy should not be taken in cases of estrogen receptor-positive (ER+) tumors.

Note: Sprouts are richer in coumestrol, the strongest phytoestrogens known.

Soy lecithin

Constituents: Raw soy lecithin contains phosphatides (chiefly phosphatidylcholine = **lecithin**, also phosphatidylethanolamine = colamine-cephalin and phosphatidylinositol), fixed oil, phytosterols, tocopherols, carbohydrates, etc.

Properties: Cholesterol and triglyceride reducing, liver protective, general tonic. Rational treatments with soy lecithin have been shown to help in normalizing plasma levels of HDL and LDL cholesterols as well as transaminases (GOT and GPT). The effects are attributed to its components, namely linoleic acid (an omega-6 fatty acid), phosphoric acid, and choline and ethanolamine (both biogenic amines), which play important roles in the metabolisms.

Uses: <u>Internally</u> it is used (the extract enriched in lecithin) for minor cases of high cholesterol, as a preventive for arteriosclerosis and gallstones, for liver disorders (fatty liver, liver damage, chronic hepatitis) and complaints associated with them (loss of appetite, impaired digestion, etc.). Due to its general tonic effect, it is also advisable as an adjuvant for chronic ailments.

Caution: There are no reports of contraindications or side effects when used properly (orally, recommended dose).

Soybean oil

It is the refined fixed oil obtained by expression from the ripe seeds.

Constituents: Chiefly glycerides (fatty acids component: chiefly linolenic and linoleic acids, considered essential fatty acids = EFAs), phytosterols (5-sterols: β-sitosterol, campesterol, etc.), tocopherols, free fatty acids, etc.

Properties and Uses: <u>Internally</u> it is used as a nutrient and rich supplement of unsaturated fatty acids. <u>Externally</u> it is used as an ingredient in ointments, creams, and liniments.

Caution: There are no reports of contraindications or side effects when used

properly.

References: (1) Vol. 5, p. 300; (3) Vol. 4, p. 1154; (6) p. 145; (7) p. 240; (11) p. 71; (12) pp. 262, 271, 1256; (13) p. 389; (16) p. 111; (19) p. 211; (37) pp. 608, 817; (48) pp. 147, 350; (67) p. 393; (68) p. 213; (70) p. 149; (71) p. 37; (75) p. 236.

SPEARMINT

Botanical Name(s): *Mentha spicata* L. = *Mentha viridis* L. [Fam.: Lamiaceae (Labiatae)]

Leaf
Constituents: Volatile oil (see Spearmint oil), Lamiaceae tannins (rosmarinic acid and other caffeic acid derivatives), bitter principles, flavonoids, etc.
Properties: Aromatic, bitter tonic, choleretic, antispasmodic, carminative, mild antiseptic.
Uses: Internally it is used (as a tea, h. p.) for loss of appetite and nonulcer dyspepsia (with flatulence, nausea, minor cramps, etc.), and as an adjuvant for diarrhea. Externally it is used (as a mouthwash, chewing) for bad breath.

Spearmint oil
It is the volatile oil obtained by steam distillation from the fresh aerial part.
Constituents: Chiefly carvone, also limonene, etc., and the ester acetate of dihydrocuminic alcohol (responsible for the aroma), but no menthol.
Properties: Antispasmodic, carminative, antiseptic.
Uses: Internally it is used (as an inhalation combination product) for colds, (drops on sugar) for colds, flatulence, nausea and gastrointestinal cramps. It is an important flavor ingredient in chewing gum and oral hygiene products.
Caution: In rare cases it may cause contact allergic reactions. Otherwise, there are no reports of contraindications or side effects when used properly.

References: (1) Vol. 5, p. 842; (3) Vol. 5, p. 773; (12) p. 740; (13) p. 103; (17) p. 388; (31) pp. 558, 562; (48) p. 537.

SPEEDWELL

Other Common Name(s): common speedwell
Botanical Name(s): *Veronica officinalis* L. [Fam.: Plantaginaceae]
Aerial part
Constituents: Bitter principles (iridoids: catalpol, catalpol esters, etc.), triterpenoid saponins, tannins, flavonoids, phenolic acids (chlorogenic acid, caffeic acid), etc.
Properties: Bitter tonic, expectorant, astringent, diuretic. The effects are mild.
Uses: Internally it is used (as a tea, h. p.) for loss of appetite and nonulcer dyspepsia (with fullness, minor diarrhea), minor inflammations of the upper respiratory tract (bronchitis, laryngitis with hoarseness, etc.; coughs due to

354

thickened bronchial secretion) and genitourinary tract (cystitis, etc.), and as an antidyscratic (= blood purifier) for chronic rheumatic complaints and atopic eczema (= chronic eczema of internal origin). Externally it is used (as a mouthwash, gargle) for inflammations of the mouth and throat, and (as a wash, wet compress, partial bath) for minor wounds, ulcers and chronic skin diseases.
Caution: There are no reports of contraindications or side effects when used properly.

References: (1) Vol. 6, p. 1118; (3) Vol. 6c, p. 429; (6) p. 102; (8) p. 584; (17) p. 614; (24) p. 121; (27) p. 337; (35) p. 758; (47) p. 2802; (51) p. 186.

SPIGELIA

Other Common Name(s): Indian pink, pinkroot, woodland pinkroot, wormgrass
Botanical Name(s): *Spigelia marilandica* (L.) L. [Fam.: Loganiaceae]
Root
Constituents: According to old reports it contains a toxic alkaloid (spigeline), a bitter acrid resin, and tannins. Possibly, bitter principles are seco-iridoids. Spigeline is reported to be steam distilling, like nicotine and coniine.
Properties: Bitter tonic, antipyretic, anthelmintic. Possibly, the mentioned effects are due to seco-iridoids and spigeline. Spigeline acts similar to pelletierine of pomegranate bark.
Uses: Spigelia is chiefly used in traditional medicine. Internally it is used (as a tea; at low doses) for feverish states and (as a tea; at higher doses, followed by a purgative) for intestinal worms (roundworms = *Ascaris* spp.).
Caution: It should not be taken during pregnancy and lactation. Spigelia should be used supervised by an experienced practitioner. At higher doses than recommended it causes toxic effects on the nervous and cardiovascular systems.

References: (1) Vol. 6, p. 775; (5) Vol. 1, p. 1023; (18) p. 240; (25) p. 148; (29) p. 109; (35) p. 637; (37) p. 1294; (42) Vol. 4, p. 418; (44) p. 541; (52) p. 745; (58) p. 172; (65) p. 192; (66) p. 470.

SPIKENARD

Other Common Name(s): American spikenard
Botanical Name(s): *Aralia racemosa* L. [Fam.: Araliaceae]
Root
Constituents: Volatile oil, triterpenoid saponins, diterpenes (pimarenes, etc.), polyacetylenes (falcarinone, etc.), starch, pectin, tannins, resin, etc.
Properties: Expectorant, antimicrobial, diuretic, mild astringent. Saponins may account in large part for the expectorant effect. Falcarinone and other open chain polyacetylenes are considered natural antibiotics. The diuretic effect may be due to saponins and volatile oil.

Uses: <u>Internally</u> it is used (as a tea, h. p.) for inflammations of the upper respiratory tract (bronchitis, etc.; coughs due to thickened bronchial secretion; as an adjuvant for bronchial asthma), genitourinary tract (cystitis, etc.) and gastrointestinal tract (diarrhea, etc.), and as an antidyscratic (= blood purifier) for atopic eczema (= chronic eczema of internal origin) and chronic rheumatic complaints. To enhance the effects in problems of the genitourinary tract, the fluid intake (incl. herbal teas) should be more than 2 liters per day. <u>Externally</u> it is used (as a poultice) for cuts, wounds, and boils.

Caution: It should not be taken during pregnancy and lactation. Otherwise, there are no reports of contraindications or side effects when used properly.

References: (1) Vol. 4, p. 323; (3) Vol. 3, p. 169; (10) p. 256; (25) p. 63; (29) p. 12; (31) p. 49; (35) p. 760; (37) p. 125; (44) p. 82.

SPILANTHES

Other Common Name(s): pará cress, toothache plant
Botanical Name(s): *Spilanthes oleracea* L.; *Spilanthes acmella* (L.) L. [Fam.: Asteraceae (Compositae)]
<u>Aerial part</u> (leaf, flowering top)
Constituents: Pungent principles (isobutylamides: spilanthol, etc.), volatile oil, tannins, resin, a biogenic amine (choline), phytosterols, etc.
Properties: Anti-inflammatory, local anesthetic, astringent, antibacterial, antifungal, diuretic. Spilanthol has shown anti-inflammatory, local anesthetic, antibacterial, antifungal and insecticidal effects.
Uses: <u>Externally</u> it is used (as a mouthwash, paint) for inflammations of the oral cavity (esp. gingivitis = inflammation of the gums), (as a cotton swab) for toothache, (as a gel, ointment, spray; prepared with standardized extracts) for bruises, sprains, insect bites, rheumatic and muscular pains, and minor wounds. <u>Internally</u> it is used as an adjuvant (tea, h. p.) for inflammations of the genitourinary tract (cystitis, urethritis, prostatitis) and chronic rheumatic complaints. To enhance the effects in problems of the genitourinary tract, the fluid intake (incl. herbal teas) should be more than 2 liters per day.
Caution: Spilanthes products should not be applied in amounts larger than recommended as it may cause skin irritations. Otherwise, there are no reports of contraindications or side effects when used properly.

References: (3) Vol. 6b, p. 494; (5) Vol. 1, p. 1024; (8) p. 531; (37) p. 1294; (52) p. 745; (57) p. 801; (72) nr. 05406.

SPINACH

Botanical Name(s): *Spinacia oleracea* L. [Fam.: Chenopodiaceae]
<u>Leaf</u>

356

Constituents: A biogenic amine (betaine), triterpenoid saponins, oxalic acid, vitamins (β-carotene = a provitamin A, vit. B_1, B_2, B_6, C, D, K_1, folic acid), phytosterols, phosphatides (lecithin), etc.

Properties and Uses: Its consumption is encouraged also as a digestive stimulant (due to betaine, triterpenoid saponins, phosphatides, vitamins). It may be beneficial for cases of anemia, due to its digestive stimulant effects, but not to the iron content. In the past, due to mistaken results, spinach was considered rich in iron.

Caution: There are no reports of contraindications or side effects when consuming spinach as a food.

References: (3) Vol. 6b, p. 496; (5) Vol. 2, p. 1024; (8) p. 532; (12a) p. 207; (37) p. 1294.

SPONGE GOURD

Botanical Name(s): *Luffa operculata* (L.) Cogn. = *Momordica operculata* L. [Fam.: Cucurbitaceae]

Fruit

Constituents: Bitter principles (cucurbitacins), triterpenoid saponins, glycoproteins, etc.

Properties: Laxative, diuretic.

Uses: Sponge gourd is toxic. Internally it is used in traditional medicine, as a laxative and diuretic tea.

Caution: It should not be taken during pregnancy, lactation and in cases of gastrointestinal ulcers. Sponge gourd should be used only as directed by an experienced practitioner.

Bath sponge

Natives prepare it mainly from luffa or loofah: *Luffa aegyptica* Mill. as it doesn't contain the bitter and toxic cucurbitacins. Also sponge gourd is processed and used for this purpose.

References: (1) Vol. 5, p. 713; (3) Vol. 5, p. 586; (31) p. 724; (37) p. 844; (41) Vols. 1-7; (48) p. 220.

SPURGE, PILL-BEARING

Other Common Name(s): asthma herb, garden euphorbia

Botanical Name(s): *Chamaesyce hirta* (L.) Millsp. = *Euphorbia hirta* L. = *Euphorbia pilulifera* auct. non L. [Fam.: Euphorbiaceae]

Aerial part

Constituents: Tannins (ellagitannins: euphorbins), phenolic acids, flavonoids (flavonols: quercetin, etc.), diterpenes (phorbol derivatives, etc.), triterpenes, a biogenic amine (choline), phytosterols, hydrocarbons, organic acids (including shikimic acid), etc.

Properties: Anti-inflammatory, analgesic, antispasmodic, antiallergic, antiprotozoal (against *Entamoeba histolytica*, causative for amebic dysentery), antibacterial (against *Shigella flexneri* and other causatives for bacillary dysentery, *E. coli, S. aureus*, etc.), anthelmintic (against hookworms = *Ancylostoma* spp.), mild astringent, galactagogue.

Uses: Internally it is used (only dried herb!; as a tea, h. p.) for inflammatory and spastic conditions of the upper respiratory tract (hay fever, pharyngitis, laryngitis, bronchitis, bronchial asthma, etc.; spastic dry coughs), gastrointestinal tract (diarrhea, amebic dysentery, cramps; also when minor hemorrhages are present, but on professional's advice) and genitourinary tract (cystitis, urethritis, etc.), for hookworm infestation, and to promote the secretion of milk in nursing mothers. To enhance the effects in problems of the genitourinary tract, the fluid intake (incl. herbal teas) should be more than 2 liters per day. Externally it is used (as a poultice: dried herb, in moderate amounts) for minor cuts, wounds and minor skin inflammations, and (as a paint: fresh juice) for warts (common w., plantar w.).

Caution: Only the dried aerial part is used. Pill-bearing spurge should not be taken during pregnancy and for prolonged period. As a galactagogue, to promote the secretion of milk, it should be used on health professional's advice. At higher doses than recommended it causes gastrointestinal irritations (with nausea, vomiting). Avoid contact of milky juice with the skin and mucous membranes.

References: (2) Vol. 2, p. 633; (3) Vol. 4, p. 877; (9) p. 234; (15) p. 88; (20) p. 109; (27) p. 124; (41) Vols. 1-7; (52) p. 175.

SQUILL

Other Common Name(s): sea onion
Botanical Name(s): *Urginea maritima* (L.) Baker = *Drimia maritima* (L.) Stearn = *Scilla maritima* L. [Fam.: Hyacinthaceae (Liliaceae)]
Bulb (white variety: inner scales, cut and dried)
Constituents: Cardiac glycosides (chiefly scillaren A, also glucoscillaren A, proscillaridin A, etc.; aglycone: scillarenin), mucilaginous polysaccharides (very rich), flavonoids, etc.
Properties: Cardiotonic, diuretic. See DIGITALIS. Compared to digitalis, squill acts milder, is less cumulative, and exerts stronger diuretic effect.
Uses: Internally it is used (as a standardized product) for heart failure in early stages (stages I and II, according to NYHA).
Caution: Squill is toxic and not for self-treatment. It is used only as directed by a health professional. Squill products should be standardized to the cardiac glycosides content. See DIGITALIS.
Note: Red squill is the red variety of the mentioned species. It contains scilliroside, a glycoside with aglycone scillirosidin, which accounts for the rodenticide action. It is not used in medicine, but only as a rat poison.

References: (1) Vol. 6, p. 1037; (3) Vol. 6b, p. 326; (11) p. 120; (12) p. 596; (13) p. 192; (14) p. 205; (16) p. 98; (19) p. 156; (23) p. 167; (36) p. 319; (46) p. 1440; (48) p. 742; (49) Vol. 2, p. 46.

ST. JOHN'S WORT

Botanical Name(s): *Hypericum perforatum* L. [Fam.: Clusiaceae (Hypericaceae)]

Flowering top

Constituents: Flavonoids (flavonols: hyperin, rutin, and other quercetin glycosides; biflavones: I3, II8-biapigenin and amentoflavone = I3', II8-biapigenin), naphthodianthrones (hypericin, pseudohypericin, etc.), phloroglucinol derivatives (hyperforin, etc.), xanthone derivatives (norathyriol = 1,3,6,7-tetrahydroxyxanthone, etc.), tannins (condensed t., including oligomeric proanthocyanidins = OPCs), volatile oil, etc.

Properties: Antidepressant, mild sedative, anti-inflammatory, antibacterial, antiviral, astringent, wound-healing. The antidepressant and sedative effects of St. John's wort extract are due in large part to its TCA-like action (TCA = tetracyclic antidepressants such as imipramin) by blocking the neural uptake of serotonin, norepinephrine and dopamine, partly due to MAO (= monoamine oxidase) and COMT (= catechol-O-methyltransferase) inhibitory actions, and due to the interaction with GABA (= gamma aminobutyrric acid) receptors. For the antidepressant effect it has been considered responsible hypericin but recently this is attributed to other important constituents such as hyperforin, flavonoids (esp. biflavones), and xanthones. The overall effect seems to be due to an *in vivo* synergism of these compounds. Hypericin, as a photosensitizer contributes in utilizing better the sunlight and then adjusting melatonin levels. Most of the extracts are still standardized to hypericin. This doesn't mean that they do not contain the other mentioned active constituents.

Uses: Internally it is used (as a standardized product) for mild to moderate depression (also in young and school children), nervous exhaustion, anxiety, insomnia and childhood enuresis, and (as a tea, h. p.) for inflammations of the gastrointestinal tract (gastritis, diarrhea, ulcerative colitis, incl. hemorrhoids; also when minor hemorrhages are present, but on professional's advice) and genitourinary tract (cystitis, prostatitis, irritable urinary passages, childhood enuresis), and neuralgic pains (sciatica, trigeminal pains, etc.). In traditional medicine it is also used for stuttering and inflammations of the hepatobiliary and upper respiratory tracts. Externally it is used (as a liniment: St. John's wort oil) for wounds, burns, ulcers (incl. varicose ulcers), bruises, hemorrhoids, neuralgic and rheumatic pains, and herpes zoster.

Caution: St. John's wort should not be taken in cases of severe depressive states. It is best to take a standardized product. The effects are expected in 3-6 weeks. Normally, it should not be combined with antidepressant drugs. Any comedication should be monitored. A possible combination with sedative and hypnotic drugs should be made only by a health professional. It should not be combined with immunosuppresants. In rare cases it may cause minor and temporary gastrointestinal discomfort. Phototoxic reactions may occur after exposure to sunrays but only if higher doses than recommended

359

have been taken, particularly by fair skinned persons.

References: (1) Vol. 5, p. 475; (3) Vol. 5, p. 214; (6) p. 217; (7) p. 55; (8) p. 315; (9) p. 310; (12) p. 924; (13) p. 413; (16) p. 187; (17) p. 309; (19) p. 115; (20) p. 250; (22) p. 166; (23) pp. 261, 304; (46) p. 755; (47) p. 1587; (48) p. 439; (51) p. 120; (67) p. 471; (91) p. 74.

STAVESACRE

Other Common Name(s): lousewort, licebane
Botanical Name(s): *Delphinium staphisagria* L. [Fam.: Ranunculaceae]
Seed (= louse seed)
Constituents: Diterpenoid alkaloids (chiefly delphinine*, also staphisagrine), lipids (fixed oil, phytosterols), etc. *) Delphinine is not to be confused with delphinin, which is an anthocyanin.
Properties: Pediculicide, but extremely toxic!
Uses: Externally it has been used (as an ointment, lotion) against pediculosis (= infestation with lice) and for neuralgic and rheumatic pains.
Caution: Delphinine acts very similar to aconitine therefore stavesacre is extremely toxic (see ACONITE). Stavesacre products should be used as directed by an experienced practitioner. They should not be ingested or absorbed. Products should not be applied on injured or inflamed skin and any contact with the eyes or other mucous membranes should be avoided. They may cause skin irritations, especially if left on the infested site longer than advised.

References: (3) Vol. 4, p. 481; (10) p. 258; (31) p. 148; (35) p. 770; (37) p. 391; (47) p. 2603; (49) Vol. 2, p. 144; (65) p. 487; (66) p. 471.

STEPHANIA

Botanical Name(s): *Stephania tetrandra* S. Moore [Fam.: Menispermaceae]
Root
Constituents: Alkaloids, chiefly of bisbenzylisoquinoline type, particularly (+)-tetrandrine, etc., but also protoberberine type.
Properties: Anti-inflammatory, analgesic, antipyretic. Tetrandrine has shown anti-inflammatory, analgesic, antipyretic, tuberculostatic, and calcium antagonistic effects, among others. Its quaternary derivatives have shown curare-like effect, i. e. nondepolarizing muscle relaxant effect.
Uses: Internally it is used (as an h. p., tea) for neuralgic and rheumatic pains (incl. arthritic pains).
Caution: Stephania root should be handled by experienced practitioners and used as directed by them. It has been found adulterated with roots of *Aristolochia fangchi* (rich in toxic aristolochic acids; cf. BIRTHWORT). Therefore, manufacturers should run tests accordingly.

References: (3) Vol. 6b, p. 532; (12) p. 1319; (13) p. 437; (31) p. 219; (41) Vols. 1-7; (42) Vol. 5, p. 430; (48) p. 921; (52) p. 754; (67) p. 244.

STERCULIA

Other Common Name(s): karaya
Botanical Name(s): *Sterculia urens* Roxb., and other *Sterculia* spp. [Fam.: Sterculiaceae]
Gum (sterculia gum, karaya gum, Indian tragacanth)
It exudes naturally or from the incision / tapping made to the trunk, and then is air-dried.
Constituents: Chiefly a polysaccharide (an acetylated heteropolysaccharide), also free acetic acid, minerals, tannins and amino acids (aspartic acid, etc.), but no starch.
Properties: Bulk laxative, demulcent. In the gastrointestinal tract it swells to several times its volume, and is not digested but excreted as such.
Uses: Internally it is used (as granulated sterculia) for chronic constipation, irritable bowel syndrome, diarrhea, and as an aid to a weight-loss diet. In cosmetics it is widely used as a suspending, emulsifying and thickening ingredient in the production of lotions and creams, among others.
Caution: Sterculia products should be mixed with enough liquid before and then followed with enough liquid after ingestion. They should not be taken before going to bed. In rare cases it may cause allergic reactions or gastrointestinal discomfort. Otherwise, there are no reports of contraindications or side effects when used properly.

References: (1) Vol. 6, p. 776; (3) Vol. 6b, p. 533; (8) p. 533; (9) p. 328; (11) p. 43; (12) p. 355; (36) p. 213; (37) p. 1305; (48) p. 91; (49) Vol. 2, p. 265; (74) p. 384.

STEVIA

Botanical Name(s): *Stevia rebaudiana* (Bertoni) Bertoni = *Eupatorium rebaudianum* Bertoni [Fam.: Asteraceae (Compositae)]
Leaf
Properties: Diterpenoid glycosides account for the sweet taste. Stevioside has been shown to be 200-300 times sweeter than sucrose, to reduce postprandial blood glucose levels in cases of type 2 diabetes, and to exert mild antihypertensive effect.
Uses: Internally it is used (leaf powder, whole extract, enriched extract, stevioside) as a calorie-free sweetener, taste modifier, and as an adjuvant for diabetes.
Caution: Stevia may contain sesquiterpene lactones. If so, it may cause contact dermatitis to persons hypersensitive to other Asteraceae plants (e. g. arnica, chamomile, feverfew, ragweed, tansy, yarrow) that contain them. Manufacturers should evaluate them and advice accordingly. Otherwise, there are no reports of contraindications or side effects when used properly.

References: (1) Vol. 6, p. 788; (3) Vol. 6b, p. 537; (8) p. 534; (9) p. 478; (12) p. 502; (13) p. 170; (29) p. 110; (37) p. 1308; (41) Vols. 1-7; (48) p. 653.

STILLINGIA

Other Common Name(s): queen's delight, queen's root, yaw root
Botanical Name(s): *Stillingia sylvatica* Garden ex L. [Fam.: Euphorbiaceae]

Root

Constituents: Diterpenoid esters (designated as stillingia factors: S1, etc.), tannins, volatile oil, an acrid resin, fixed oil, starch, etc.

Properties: (At low doses): Expectorant (bronchial secretagogue effect), digestive secretagogue (increases secretions of the mouth, stomach, and liver), diuretic, and possibly antibacterial. (At high doses): Laxative, emetic. S6 (= gnidilatidin) has shown antileukemic effect.

Uses: Internally it is used (as a tea, h. p.; at low doses) for inflammations of the upper respiratory tract (laryngitis, bronchitis, etc.; coughs due to thickened bronchial secretion), gastrointestinal tract (with impaired digestion, sluggish bowels, constipation, incl. hemorrhoids) associated with impaired bile secretion, and genitourinary tract (cystitis, urethritis, etc.). It is also used as an antidyscratic (= blood purifier; tea, h. p.) for chronic skin diseases (incl. cases of syphilitic origin, atopic eczema = chronic eczema of internal origin) and chronic rheumatic complaints. To enhance the effects in problems of the genitourinary tract, the fluid intake (incl. herbal teas) should be more than 2 liters per day.

Caution: Stillingia should be used only as directed by an experienced practitioner. It should not be used during pregnancy and lactation, in cases of peptic ulcers and biliary and bowel obstructions. At higher doses than recommended it causes gastrointestinal irritations (with nausea, vomiting, diarrhea). Milky juice of the fresh root is a strong skin irritant.

References: (2) Vol. 3, p. 579; (3) Vol. 6b, p. 553; (15) p. 199; (20) p. 225; (29) p. 111; (35) p. 664; (41) Vols. 1-7; (44) p. 545; (47) p. 2622; (52) p. 757; (65) p. 180; (66) p. 471.

STONEROOT

Other Common Name(s): horse balm, richweed
Botanical Name(s): *Collinsonia canadensis* L. [Fam.: Lamiaceae (Labiatae)]

Root

Constituents: Volatile oil (with α- and β-pinene, limonene, caryophyllene, etc.), Lamiaceae tannins (rosmarinic acid and other caffeic acid derivatives), triterpenoid saponins, mucilaginous polysaccharides, etc. It possibly contains bitter principles (diterpenoid lactones).

Properties: Aromatic, bitter tonic, antispasmodic, astringent, diuretic.

Uses: Internally it is used (as a tea, h. p.) for inflammatory and spastic conditions of the gastrointestinal tract (loss of appetite, nonulcer dyspepsia with flatulence, cramps, diarrhea, ulcerative colitis, incl. hemorrhoids) and genitourinary tract (cystitis, gravel, nonobstructive urinary stones), and for primary dysmenorrhea. To enhance the effects in problems of the genitourinary tract, the fluid intake (incl. herbal teas) should be more than 2 liters per day. Externally it is used (as a poultice) for bruises, small cuts, and boils.

Caution: It should not be taken during pregnancy and lactation. At higher doses than recommended it may cause gastrointestinal irritations (with nausea, vomiting) and dizziness.

References: (1) Vol. 4, p. 956; (3) Vol. 4, p. 249; (15) p. 72; (18) p. 262; (20) p. 253; (36) pp. 48, 475; (44) p. 171; (45) p. 191; (47) p. 1056.

STORAX

Other Common Name(s): 1) Levant storax 2) American storax
Botanical Name(s): 1) *Liquidambar orientalis* Mill. 2) *Liquidambar styraciflua* L. [Fam.: Hamamelidaceae]
Balsam (storax; here: prepared storax; 1: Levant storax 2: American storax) Crude storax exuded from tappings made to the trunk is dissolved in benzene, filtered, then freed from the solvent to produce the prepared storax.
Constituents: Cinnamic acid (free cinnamic acid, cinnamyl-cinnamate, phenylpropyl-cinnamate), volatile oil, vanillin, etc. American storax is much richer in phenylpropyl-cinnamate and contains only traces of vanillin.
Properties: Antibacterial, antifungal, expectorant.
Uses: Externally it is used (as a paint: Compound Benzoin Tincture) chiefly for small cuts, and (as a paint, ointment) for eczema, fungal skin infections (= dermatomycosis) and itching. Internally it is used (as an inhalation) for inflammations of upper respiratory tract (bronchitis, etc.; coughs due to thickened bronchial secretion), genitourinary tract (cystitis, etc.), and gastrointestinal tract (diarrhea, etc.). To enhance the effects in problems of the genitourinary tract, the fluid intake (incl. herbal teas) should be more than 2 liters per day. American storax is chiefly used as a flavor ingredient in tobacco industry.
Caution: In rare cases it may cause skin allergic reactions.

References: (1) Vol. 5, p. 698; (3) Vol. 5, p. 528; (9) p. 480; (11) p. 104; (36) p. 184; (37) p. 834; (48) p. 258; (49) Vol. 2, p. 432; (55) p. 139; (65) p. 147; (66) p. 474.

STRAWBERRY

Botanical Name(s): *Fragaria vesca* L. [Fam.: Rosaceae]
Leaf
Constituents: Tannins (ellagitannins and oligomeric proanthocyanidins = OPCs), flavonoids (flavonols: rutin, etc.; flavan-3-ols = catechins; flavan-3, 4-ols = leucoanthocyanins), phenolic acids (caffeic and salicylic acids, etc.), volatile oil (traces), etc.
Properties: Astringent. Due to flavonoids and OPCs it can be considered a

valuable antioxidant.

Uses: Internally it is used (as a tea, h. p.) for minor inflammations of the gastrointestinal tract (diarrhea, ulcerative colitis, incl. hemorrhoids; also when minor hemorrhages are present, but on professional's advice). It is particularly recommended for children and the elderly. Externally it is used (as a mouthwash, gargle) for inflammations of the mouth and throat, (as a wash, wet compress) for minor skin inflammations, (as a poultice) for wounds, ulcers, hemorrhoids, and (as an enema) for hemorrhoids. Due to its safety and antioxidant effect, it is used as an ingredient in caffeine-free household teas.

Caution: There are no reports of contraindications or side effects when used properly except rare cases of allergic reactions, if allergic to strawberries.

References: (1) Vol. 5, p. 182; (3) Vol. 4, p. 1046; (8) p. 267; (17) p. 225; (24) p. 126; (27) p. 140; (37) p. 556; (51) p. 98.

STRAWBERRY TREE

Other Common Name(s): arbute, cane apple tree
Botanical Name(s): *Arbutus unedo* L. [Fam.: Ericaceae]
Leaf
Constituents: Phenol glycosides (arbutin = hydroquinone-glucoside, etc.; ca. 1/3 –1/2 of that contained in uva-ursi), some free hydroquinone, tannins (gallotannins, ellagitannins; almost as much as uva-ursi), flavonoids (flavonols: quercetin and kaempferol glycosides), triterpenes (ursolic acid, etc.), bitter principles (iridoids, ursolic acid), etc.
Properties: Antibacterial, astringent. See UVA-URSI.
Uses: Internally it is sometimes used (as a tea, h. p.) for inflammations of the genitourinary tract (cystitis, urethritis, etc.; as a substitute for uva-ursi; see UVA-URSI) and gastrointestinal tract (diarrhea, etc.). As with uva-ursi, arbutin is extractable by cold maceration from the powdered leaves. So, to avoid tannins in cases of genitourinary problems, the tea can be prepared by cold maceration.
Caution: See UVA-URSI.

References: (1) Vol. 4, p. 326; (3) Vol. 3, p. 172; (27) p. 100; (45) p. 168.

STROPHANTHUS

Botanical Name(s): *Strophanthus gratus* (Wall. et Hook.) Franchet; *Strophanthus kombé* Oliv. [Fam.: Apocynaceae]
Seed (ripe, deprived of the awn)
Constituents: Its major active constituents are cardiac glycosides. *S. gratus* contains chiefly G-strophanthin (= ouabain = g-strophanthidin-rhamnoside). *S. kombé* contains chiefly k-strophanthin that is a mixture of three glyco-

sides (k-strophanthin α = cymarin, k-strophanthin β, k-strophanthin γ = strophanthoside; their aglycone is k-strophanthidin). It also contains steroidal saponins, fixed oil, etc.

Properties: Strophanthus cardiac glycosides exert similar effect to digitalis glycosides, but with a very fast onset of action. Strophanthus cardiac glycosides are very poorly absorbed orally therefore they are administered perlingually or by I.V. injection. See DIGITALIS.

Uses: Internally it is used (perlingually, I.V. injection: only pure glycosides) for acute / severe heart failure, as an emergency start-up therapy, and then followed by digitalis.

Caution: Strophanthus and its cardiac glycosides are toxic and not for self-treatment. They are used only as directed by a health professional. Strophanthus products should be standardized to the cardiac glycosides content. See DIGITALIS.

References: (1) Vol. 6, pp. 798, 808; (3) Vol. 6b, p. 576; (8) p. 535; (11) p. 120; (12) p. 591; (13) p. 186; (36) p. 317; (37) p. 1316; (46) p. 1539; (48) p. 745.

SUMAC, SMOOTH

Other Common Name(s): scarlet sumac
Botanical Name(s): *Rhus glabra* L. [Fam.: Anacardiaceae]
Fruit (ripe berry)
Constituents: Tannins (gallotaninns), organic acids (chiefly malic acid), phenolic acids (gallic acid), minerals (potassium and calcium malates), flavonoids (anthocyanins), lipids (fixed oil, phytosterols), etc.
Properties: Acidulous, refrigerant, astringent, anti-inflammatory, diuretic.
Uses: Internally it is used (as a tea, refreshing drink, h. p.) chiefly for feverish states, also beneficial for inflammatory conditions of the gastrointestinal and genitourinary tracts. Externally it is used (as a gargle, mouthwash) for inflammations of the mouth and throat.
Caution: There are no reports of contraindications or side effects when used properly. Internally should be used only ripe berries and at the recommended doses.

References: (1) Vol. 6, p. 454; (3) Vol. 6b, p. 127; (10) p. 261; (25) p. 250; (29) p. 98; (35) p. 779; (44) p. 471; (52) p. 668; (66) p. 414.

SUMAC, STAGHORN

Other Common Name(s): velvet sumac
Botanical Name(s): *Rhus hirta* (L.) Sudworth = *Rhus typhina* L. [Fam.: Anacardiaceae]
Fruit (ripe berry)
Constituents, Properties, Uses, and Caution: Almost the same as smooth sumac. See SUMAC, SMOOTH.

References: (1) Vol. 6, p. 463; (3) Vol. 6b, p. 128; (25) p. 250; (44) p. 472; (52) p. 669.

SUMAC, SWEET

Other Common Name(s): fragrant sumac
Botanical Name(s): *Rhus aromatica* Aiton [Fam.: Anacardiaceae]
Root bark
Constituents: Tannins (gallotannins), volatile oil (with sesquiterpenes, etc.), a phenol glycoside (orcinol-glucoside), phenolic acids (gallic acid), phytosterols (5- and 7-sterols), flavonoids (flavonols), triterpenes (squalene, oleanan derivatives), fixed oil, etc.
Properties: Astringent, anti-inflammatory, antimicrobial, diuretic, hemostatic. The astringent and hemostatic effects are due in large part to tannins. The anti-inflammatory effect is due in large part to flavonoids, gallic acid and phytosterols. The antimicrobial effect is due in large part to phenolics (orcinol-glucoside, gallic acid) and partly the volatile oil. The diuretic effect is due at least in part to flavonoids and the volatile oil.
Uses: Internally it is used (as a tea, h. p.) for inflammations (also when minor hemorrhages are present) of the gastrointestinal tract (diarrhea, ulcerative colitis, incl. hemorrhoids) and genitourinary tract (urinary incontinence, childhood enuresis, cystitis, urethritis, minor pyelonephritis), and for menorrhagia / hypermenorrhea (= prolonged / heavy menstruation). Externally it is used (as a wash) for minor skin inflammations, and (as a poultice) for boils.
Caution: There are no reports of contraindications or side effects when used properly. For any kind of hemorrhage use it on professional's advice.

References: (1) Vol. 6, p. 450; (3) Vol. 6b, p. 125; (8) p. 486; (10) p. 261; (13) p. 421; (19) p. 91; (37) p. 1188; (41) Vols. 1-7; (44) p. 471; (46) p. 1358; (47) p. 2312; (66) p. 414.

SUMBUL

Botanical Name(s): *Ferula sumbul* (Kauffm.) Hook. f. = *Ferula moschata* (Reinsch) Koso-Pol.; *Ferula suaveolens* Aitch. et Hemsl. [Fam.: Apiaceae (Umbelliferae)]
Root (sumbul root, musk root)
Constituents: Volatile oil and resin (*F. sumbul*: musk-like aroma; *F. suaveolens*: angelica-like aroma), organic acids (angelic, butyric and valerianic acids, etc.), bitter principles, coumarins (umbelliferone, etc.), etc.
Properties: Aromatic, bitter tonic, antispasmodic, sedative, hypnotic.
Uses: It is used as a fixative in perfumery and flavor ingredient in liqueur industry. Internally it is used (as a tea, h. p.; at low doses) for inflammatory and spastic conditions of the gastrointestinal tract (diarrhea, vomiting, gastroenteritis, irritable bowel syndrome) and upper respiratory tract (spastic bronchitis, bronchial asthma), for primary dysmenorrhea (= painful men-

struation without pathology), and (usually combined with other herbs) for nervousness, insomnia and menopausal nervous disorders.

Caution: Sumbul should not be taken during pregnancy and lactation. At doses higher than recommended, it exerts narcotic effect. Alcoholic drinks may interact with sumbul. A possible combination of sumbul with sedative, hypnotic, and antidepressant drugs should be made only by a health professional. Otherwise, there are no reports of contraindications or side effects when used properly.

References: (2) Vol. 2, p. 709; (3) Vol. 4, p. 987; (5) Vol. 1, p. 499; (8) p. 262; (10) p. 262; (35) p. 781; (37) p. 523; (47) p. 2642; (65) p. 144; (66) p. 482.

SUNDEW

Botanical Name(s): *Drosera rotundifolia* L.; *Drosera ramentacea* Burch. ex Harv. et Sond.; *Drosera longifolia* L. p.p.; *Drosera intermedia* Hayne; etc. [Fam.: Droseraceae]
Aerial part
Constituents: Naphthoquinones (ramentaceone = 7-methyljuglone, plumbagin = 2-methyljuglone, droserone = 3-hydroxyplumbagin, etc.; free and glucosides), flavonoids (flavonols: quercetin, etc.), mucilage, etc.
Properties: Antispasmodic (bronchial active), antitussive (chiefly cough suppressant effect), antibacterial (against *Staphylococcus* spp., *Streptococcus* spp., etc.), antifungal, anti-inflammatory (by inhibiting the biosynthesis of prostaglandins). Most of the effects are attributed to naphthoquinones.
Uses: Internally it is used (as a tea, h. p.) for minor inflammatory and spastic conditions of the upper respiratory tract (bronchitis, laryngitis with hoarseness, bronchial asthma; coughs: irritating dry cough, whooping cough), also gastrointestinal tract (diarrhea, etc.). Externally it is used (as a poultice) for wounds, and (fresh plant) for freckles, warts (common w., plantar w.) and corns.
Caution: There are no reports of contraindications or side effects when used properly. Products should be prepared with extracts standardized to the naphthoquinones content.

References: (2) Vol. 2, p. 536; (3) Vol. 4, p. 723; (6) p. 106; (8) p. 229; (13) p. 407; (16) p. 78; (17) p. 188; (19) p. 214; (20) p. 100; (23) pp. 222, 403; (31) p. 505; (37) p. 439; (46) p. 486; (47) p. 1232; (48) p. 415; (49) Vol. 2, p. 226; (51) p. 92.

SUNFLOWER

Botanical Name(s): *Helianthus annuus* L. [Fam.: Asteraceae (Compositae)]
Sunflower oil
It is the fixed oil obtained by cold expression from the seeds.
Constituents: Chiefly glycerides (fatty acids component: chiefly linoleic acid = an omega-6 fatty acid and oleic acid), also phytosterols (5-sterols: β-

sitosterol, etc.; 7-sterols: stigmastenol, etc.) and α-tocopherol. The fatty acids component depends on genetic factors and climate.

Properties: Nutrient, demulcent, emollient.

Uses: Sunflower oil is chiefly used as nutrient and dietetic oil, alternative to corn and safflower oils. In cosmetic and food industries it is used as an ingredient in creams, ointments, soaps, and soft gelatin capsules, among others. Due to linoleic acid and β-sitosterol it is beneficial for high cholesterol.

Caution: As an oil rich in unsaturated fatty acids, sunflower oil should be stored in nonmetallic containers and protected from the air, light and heat.

Flower (ligulate flower)

Constituents: Flavonoids (flavonols, anthocyanins), triterpenoid saponins, diterpenes, carotenoids (lutein, etc.), a biogenic amine (choline), etc.

Properties and Uses: It is chiefly used as a coloring ingredient in herbal teas. Internally it is chiefly used in traditional medicine as an antipyretic for feverish states.

Caution: There are no reports of contraindications or side effects when used properly.

References: (1) Vol. 5, p. 410; (3) Vol. 5, p. 28; (8) p. 302; (11) p. 72; (24) p. 304; (27) p. 157; (37) p. 647; (46) p. 691; (47) p. 1518; (48) p. 151.

SYRIAN RUE

Botanical Name(s): *Peganum harmala* L. [Fam.: Zygophyllaceae]

Seed

Constituents: Indole alkaloids of β-carboline group (harman alkaloids: chiefly harmine = banisterine, etc.), quinazoline alkaloids (peganine = vasicine), fixed oil, etc.

Properties: Antispasmodic, analgesic, narcotic.

Uses: Syrian rue has been used in traditional medicine. Internally it has been used for colicky states of the gastrointestinal, biliary and genitourinary tracts. Externally it has been used (as a poultice) for wounds.

Caution: Syrian rue is a toxic hallucinogenic herb therefore is no longer used. Harmine, found also in Ayahuasca (q. v.), has shown CNS stimulant effect, and at high doses to be hallucinogenic. At high doses, Syrian rue causes cardiac depression and even respiratory paralysis.

References: (3) Vol. 6a, p. 490; (8) p. 412; (13) p. 287; (31) p. 176; (36) pp. 440, 504; (37) p. 1035; (48) p. 973; (65) p. 262; (81) p. 347.

TAMARIND

Botanical Name(s): *Tamarindus indica* L. [Fam.: Fabaceae (Caesalpiniaceae)]

Pod (crude pulp preserved with sugar)

368

Constituents: Organic acids (chiefly tartaric acid, etc.; very rich), minerals (tartrates: rich in potassium hydrogen tartrate), invert sugar (very rich), pectin, proteins, fat, fragrant constituents, etc.

Properties: Acidulous, refrigerant, mild laxative. Most of the effects are attributed to its organic acids and invert sugar.

Uses: Internally it is used (as a tea, h. p.) for feverish and thirsty states, and (as a tea, h. p.; usually combined with other herbs) for minor constipation and as an adjuvant for hepatobiliary disorders. As a mild laxative it is also recommended for infants.

Caution: There are no reports of contraindications or side effects when used properly.

References: (1) Vol. 6, p. 893; (3) Vol. 6c, p. 8; (8) p. 547; (9) p. 484; (12a) p. 147; (27) p. 322; (28) p. 112; (36) p. 182; (37) p. 1343; (48) p. 24; (49) Vol. 2, p. 392; (65) p. 172; (66) p. 484.

TANSY

Botanical Name(s): *Tanacetum vulgare* L. = *Chrysanthemum vulgare* (L.) Bernh. [Fam.: Asteraceae (Compositae)]

Aerial part, flower

Constituents: Volatile oil (chiefly with α-thujone / β-thujone / camphor, depending on chemotype; flowers are richer), bitter principles (sesquiterpene lactones: tanacetin, etc.), etc.

Properties: Aromatic, bitter tonic, stomachic, carminative, antispasmodic, anthelmintic (against pinworms = *Oxyuris* spp.), emmenagogue.

Uses: Internally it is used (as a tea, h. p.) for loss of appetite and nonulcer dyspepsia (with flatulence, minor cramps, minor constipation, etc.), and as enema for pinworm infestation. At low doses, it may also be used for primary dysmenorrhea (= painful menstruation without pathology) and secondary amenorrhea and oligomenorrhea (= ceased / infrequent / scanty menstruation without pathology). Externally it is used (as a poultice) for minor cuts and wounds, (as a liniment that contains tansy oil) for rheumatic pains, and (powdered flower) as an insect-repellent (against moths and fleas).

Caution: Tansy should not be taken during pregnancy and lactation. Before using it for gynecologic disorders, the problem should be judged by a health professional. Abuses to induce abortion, by taking the herb at high doses or by taking tansy oil, have resulted in intoxication due to β-thujone (neurotoxic!; cf. SAGE; THUJA; WORMWOOD). It may cause allergic contact dermatitis to persons hypersensitive to other Asteraceae plants (e. g. arnica, chamomile, feverfew, ragweed, yarrow) that contain sesquiterpene lactones. When used as a flavor ingredient in some alcoholic beverages (Chartreuse, etc.), the raw material or extract must be thujone-free or should contain it within limits.

References: (2) Vol. 3, p. 628; (3) Vol. 3, p. 902; (8) p. 155; (13a) p. 82; (15) p. 205; (20) p. 254; (27) p. 323; (36) p. 288; (37) p. 328; (46) p. 1586; (47) p. 2668; (51) p. 210; (66) p. 485.

TARRAGON

Other Common Name(s): estragon, French tarragon
Botanical Name(s): *Artemisia dracunculus* L. [Fam.: Asteraceae (Compositae)]

Aerial part

Constituents: Volatile oil (with estragole, etc.; some chemotypes with elemicin, eugenol, etc.), bitter principles (sesquiterpene lactones), coumarins, flavonoids, etc.

Properties: Aromatic, bitter tonic, antihyperglycemic.

Uses: Tarragon is chiefly used as a flavor ingredient much like mugwort (see MUGWORT), incorporated in herbal vinegars, seasonings and beverages, beneficial for loss of appetite and as an adjuvant for diabetes.

Caution: Tarragon should not be taken during pregnancy and lactation. Otherwise, there are no reports of contraindications or side effects when used properly.

References: (1) Vol. 4, p. 371; (3) Vol. 3, p. 269; (9) p. 487; (37) p. 135; (45) p. 171; (48) p. 525.

TEA

Other Common Name(s): Chinese tea
Botanical Name(s): *Camellia sinensis* (L.) Kuntze = *Thea sinensis* L. [Fam.: Theaceae]

Leaf and **leaf bud** (green / black / oolong)

Best qualities are obtained when plugged "two leaves and a bud".

Green tea: fresh material, before being dried, undergoes a short heating (with or without moisture). Black tea: fresh material before being dried, undergoes up to one hour fermentation. Oolong tea: fresh material before being dried, undergoes a partial fermentation. These are practices, in general.

Constituents: Purine alkaloids (chiefly caffeine, some theobromine and theophylline), polyphenols, phenolic acids, volatile oil. In green tea, as polyphenols are catechin derivatives (chiefly epigallocatechin gallate = EGCG; catechins are flavan-3-ols) and flavonols, etc. In black tea, as polyphenols are condensed tannins (thearubigenes, proanthocyanidins), etc.

Properties: CNS stimulant, mild diuretic, cardiac stimulant, antioxidant, cancer preventive (green tea is stronger). It exerts also "vitamin P"-like effect (= helps in normalizing an increased microvascular permeability and fragility), in which black tea is stronger.

Uses: Internally it is consumed mainly as a popular stimulant beverage for short-term fatigue, advisable due also to the other mentioned effects. Black tea decoction is taken for diarrhea, and can be applied externally (as a wash, wet compress) for minor skin inflammations, cuts, wounds, burns, (as a mouthwash) for minor inflammations of the mouth, and (as a wet cotton, drops, irrigation with the tea) for nosebleed.

370

Caution: For the side effects of caffeine see COFFEE. Ingestion of considerable amounts of black tea, particularly if it is prepared by decoction, may result in gastrointestinal irritations (with constipation, etc.).

References: (1) Vol. 4, p. 628; (3) Vol. 3, p. 626; (5) Vol. 1, p. 208; (7) p. 210; (8) p. 111; (9) p. 489; (11) p. 184; (13) p. 266; (16) p. 149; (22) pp. 137, 249; (37) p. 262; (48) p. 1075; (70) p. 176.

TEA TREE

Botanical Name(s): *Melaleuca alternifolia* Cheel. [Fam.: Myrtaceae]
Tea tree oil
It is the volatile oil obtained by steam distillation from the leaves and twigs.
Constituents: Monoterpenes (chiefly terpinen-4-ol, also α- and γ-terpinene, 1,8-cineole, etc., small amounts of 3-carene; depending on chemotype), etc.
Properties: Antibacterial (against *P. acnes*, *E. coli*, *S. aureus*, etc.), antifungal (against *C. albicans*, *Trichophyton* spp., *Tinea pedis*), antiprotozoal (against *Trichomonas vaginalis*).
Uses: Externally it is used (as a gel, lotion) for common acne (= acne vulgaris), skin infections, insect bites, etc., (as a paint) for fungal nail infections, (as a vaginal suppository / capsule, etc.) for vulvovaginitis and leukorrhea associated with fungal / protozoal / bacterial infections, and (as a gargle, mouthwash: diluted) for bacterial / fungal infections of the oral cavity.
Caution: It may cause skin irritations or allergic reactions. To minimize chances of side effects, the oil should be of high quality (standardized to the terpinen-4-ol content, contain 1,8-cineole and 3-carene within limits), and protected from air, light and heat.

References: (2) Vol. 3, p. 182; (3) Vol. 5, p. 750; (9) p. 110; (13) p. 418; (22) p. 222; (37) p. 874; (48) p. 559.

THUJA

Other Common Name(s): Eastern white cedar, eastern arborvitae, northern white cedar, swamp cedar
Botanical Name(s): *Thuja occidentalis* L. [Fam.: Cupressaceae]
Leaves and tops
Constituents: Volatile oil (with α- and β-thujone), lignans (desoxypodophyllotoxin), water-soluble polysaccharides, flavonoids, tannins (proanthocyanidins), etc.
Properties: Immunomodulant, antiviral, rubefacient, counterirritant. The immunomodulant effect (chiefly by increasing T-lymphocyte count) is due to water-soluble polysaccharides. The antiviral effect (incl. papillomaviruses) is due in large part to desoxypodophyllotoxin and thujones. It is rubefacient and counterirritant due in large part to the volatile oil.
Uses: Internally it is used (as an h. p.; usually combined with other immu

nomodulant herbs) to prevent, ease, and shorten the duration of microbial or viral infections of the upper respiratory and genitourinary tracts, and to reduce their relapse. Externally it is used (as an ointment) for rheumatic and neuralgic pains and (as a paint: tincture) for warts (common w., plantar w.).
Caution: Thuja should not be used internally during pregnancy and lactation, and in infants and children under 12 years of age. Doses higher than recommended, and especially when the oil is taken internally, cause gastrointestinal irritations (with gastroenteritis) and genitourinary tract (cystitis, nephritis), and intoxicating effect in the CNS (epileptiform seizures) due to β-thujone (cf. SAGE; TANSY). For further caution concerning immunomodulants see ECHINACEA; BETA GLUCANS.

References: (1) Vol. 6, p. 956; (3) Vol. 6c, p. 155; (6) p. 269; (8) p. 555; (13) p. 554; (16) p. 194; (19) p. 139; (36) p. 478; (37) p. 1373; (41) Vols. 1-7; (46) p. 1600; (51) p. 238; (66) p. 488.

THYME

Other Common Name(s): 1) common thyme, garden thyme, thyme 2) Spanish thyme
Botanical Name(s): 1) *Thymus vulgaris* L. 2) *Thymus zygis* L. [Fam.: Lamiaceae (Labiatae)]
Aerial part (rubbed)
Constituents: Volatile oil (see Thyme oil), Lamiaceae tannins (rosmarinic acid and other caffeic acid derivatives), flavonoids, triterpenoid saponins, bitter principles, etc. Volatile oil accounts for most of the effects. Rosmarinic acid and related caffeic acid derivatives have been shown to inhibit the biosynthesis of leukotrienes and prostaglandins, and to exert choleretic, antibacterial and antiviral effects.
Properties: Aromatic, expectorant (chiefly bronchial secretagogue effect, due to the volatile oil), antispasmodic (bronchial / gastrointestinal active), stomachic (due to bitter principles and phenolic acids), carminative, antiinflammatory (by inhibiting the biosynthesis of prostaglandins), and antibacterial, antifungal and anthelmintic (due to phenols of the volatile oil: thymol, carvacrol). Thyme exerts also diuretic effect.
Uses: In culinary practice thyme is used to flavor soup, meat and fish, and it is also beneficial due to its antioxidant effect. Internally it is used (as a tea, h. p.) for inflammatory and spastic conditions of the upper respiratory tract (spastic bronchitis, laryngitis, bronchial asthma, the common cold; coughs due to thickened bronchial secretion, whooping cough; also as a diaphoretic hot tea) and gastrointestinal tract (with impaired digestion, heartburn, flatulence, bloating, diarrhea). Externally it is used (as a mouthwash, gargle) for inflammations of the mouth and throat, (as a mouthwash, chewing) for bad breath, and (as a wash) for wounds.
Caution: Unless consumed in small amounts as a spice, thyme should not be taken during pregnancy and lactations. Otherwise, there are no reports of

contraindications or side effects when used properly.

Thyme oil

It is the volatile oil obtained by steam distillation from the fresh aerial parts.

Constituents: There are different chemotypes (thymol type, 1,8-cineole type, etc.). The preferred chemotype (thymol type) contains chiefly thymol, also p-cymene, carvacrol, etc.

Properties: Expectorant, antibacterial, antifungal, antispasmodic, anthelmintic. The effects are due in large part to thymol, a monoterpenoid phenol.

Uses: (Thyme oil, thymol): Internally it is used (as an inhalation, cough drop; in a combination product) for inflammations of the upper respiratory tract (common cold, bronchitis, laryngitis; coughs due to thickened bronchial secretion, spastic dry cough), and (as an enema) for intestinal worms (pinworms = *Oxyuris* spp.). Externally it is used (as a mouthwash, gargle) for inflammations of the mouth and throat, and (as an ointment) for inflammations of the upper respiratory tract and rheumatic pains.

Caution: Internally, thyme oil or thymol should be avoided during pregnancy and lactation. The undiluted oil causes skin irritations. Otherwise, there are no reports of contraindications or side effects when used properly.

References: (1) Vol. 6, p. 974; (3) Vol. 6c, p. 161; (6) p. 95; (8) p. 557; (9) p. 492; (12) pp. 727, 782; (13) p. 108; (16) p. 78; (17) p. 578; (19) p. 227; (20) p. 256; (22) p. 122; (23) p. 220; (27) p. 330; (36) p. 263; (46) p. 1618; (47) p. 2702; (48) p. 545; (59) p. 259.

THYME, LEMON

Botanical Name(s): *Thymus × citriodorus* (Pers.) Schreb. ex Schwiegg. et Körte [Fam.: Lamiaceae (Labiatae)]

Aerial part

Constituents: Volatile oil (with geraniol, citral, etc.), Lamiaceae tannins (rosmarinic acid and other caffeic acid derivatives), flavonoids, etc.

Properties: Aromatic, stomachic, mild antimicrobial.

Uses: Lemon thyme is used in culinary practice and food industry (in spice blends) to flavor salads. It exhibits beneficial effects on the gastrointestinal tract due also to the antimicrobial action of geraniol and citral.

Caution: There are no reports of contraindications or side effects when used properly.

References: (1) Vol. 6, p. 968; (5) Vol. 1, p. 1077; (9) p. 493; (31) pp. 560, 562.

THYME, WILD

Other Common Name(s): creeping thyme, mother-of-thyme

Botanical Name(s): *Thymus serpyllum* L. [Fam.: Lamiaceae (Labiatae)]

Aerial part (leaves and flowering tops)

Constituents: Volatile oil (with carvacrol, some thymol, etc.), Lamiaceae tannins (rosmarinic acid and other caffeic acid derivatives), bitter principles, flavonoids, triterpenoid saponins, etc.

Properties: Compared to garden thyme (see THYME) it is milder in action. Its aroma is somehow different, as the essential oil contains more carvacrol and less thymol.

Uses: Internally it is used (as a tea, h. p.) much like garden thyme but for minor disorders. See THYME.

Caution: There are no reports of contraindications or side effects when used properly.

References: (1) Vol. 6, p. 970; (3) Vol. 6c, p. 169; (8) p. 556; (9) p. 492; (17) p. 555; (19) p. 185; (37) p. 1374; (46) p. 1615; (47) p. 2544; (48) p. 545.

TICKSEED

Other Common Name(s): bur marigold, three-lobe beggar ticks, water agrimony

Botanical Name(s): *Bidens tripartita* L. [Fam.: Asteraceae (Compositae)]

Aerial part

Constituents: Tannins, bitter principles, flavonoids (chalcones, aurones, etc.), coumarins (umbelliferone, etc.), polysaccharides, volatile oil, polyacetylenes, thiophenes, carotenoids, etc.

Properties: Astringent, anti-inflammatory, antibacterial, hemostatic, diuretic, choleretic. The effects are mild.

Uses: Internally it is used (as a tea, h. p.) for inflammations (also when minor hemorrhages are present) of the genitourinary tract (cystitis, gravel, nonobstructive urinary stones) and gastrointestinal tract (diarrhea, ulcerative colitis, etc., incl. hemorrhoids), as an adjuvant for menorrhagia / hypermenorrhea (= prolonged / heavy menstruation), and as a diaphoretic hot tea for the common cold and feverish states. To enhance the effects in problems of the genitourinary tract, the fluid intake (incl. herbal teas) should be more than 2 liters per day. Externally it is used (as a mouthwash, gargle) for inflammations of the mouth and throat, (as a wash, wet compress, poultice) for eczema, ulcers and wounds, and (as a hair rinse) for hair loss.

Caution: Before using it for hemorrhages (uterine bleedings, etc.), the problem should be judged by a health professional. If bitter principles are sesquiterpene lactones, which is very possible (Heliantheae tribe!), it may cause allergic contact dermatitis to persons hypersensitive to other Asteraceae plants (e. g. arnica, chamomile, feverfew, ragweed, tansy, yarrow) that contain them. The toxic unsaturated pyrrolizidine alkaloids (= UPAs) are seldom found in the Heliantheae tribe (tickseed belongs here). Nevertheless, manufacturers should run tests for them. Otherwise, there are no reports of contraindications or side effects when used properly.

References: (2) Vol. 2, p. 236; (3) Vol. 3, p. 440; (10) p. 51; (15) p. 42; (18) p. 284; (36) p. 475; (41) Vols. 1-7; (42) Vol. 3, p. 495; (45) p. 177; (86) Vol. 1, p. 307; (87) Vol. 2, p. 229; (95) p. 254.

TOADFLAX

Other Common Name(s): butter and eggs, common toadflax, yellow toad-flax

Botanical Name(s): *Linaria vulgaris* Mill. [Fam.: Scrophulariaceae]

Aerial part

Constituents: Bitter principles (iridoids: aucubin, etc.), flavonoids (chiefly flavones: linarin; also aurones: aureusin, etc.), a quinazoline alkaloid (linarine), mucilaginous polysaccharides, and it is reported to contain cyanogenic glycosides, among others.

Properties: Diuretic, cholagogue, laxative, antimicrobial. The effects are mild.

Uses: Internally it is used (as a tea, h. p.) for inflammations of the genitourinary tract (cystitis, urinary incontinence, urethritis, prostatitis), as an adjuvant for early stages of benign prostatic hyperplasia (= BPH), minor cases of hepatobiliary disorders (with impaired bile flow) and minor constipation. To enhance the effects in problems of the genitourinary tract, the fluid intake (incl. herbal teas) should be more than 2 liters per day. Externally it is used (as a poultice) for minor wounds, ulcers, boils and hemorrhoids, and (as an ointment) for hemorrhoids.

Caution: Toadflax should not be taken during pregnancy and lactation. It should be used only as directed by an experienced practitioner. Manufacturers should evaluate cyanogenic glycosides and alkaloids.

References: (3) Vol. 5, p. 513; (24) p. 218; (27) p. 195; (31) p. 278; (35) p. 815; (36) p. 49; (37) p. 829; (41) Vols. 1-7; (47) p. 1760; (51) p. 183.

TOLU BALSAM TREE

Botanical Name(s): *Myroxylon balsamum* (L.) Harms var. *balsamum* = *Myroxylon toluiferum* Kunth [Fam.: Fabaceae (Leguminosae)]

Balsam (tolu balsam, tolu)

It is obtained by deep V-shaped incisions made to the trunk.

Constituents: Cinnamein (a mixture: esters of benzoic and cinnamic acids with benzyl alcohol), resin (esters of the same acids with toluresinotannol), free benzoic and cinnamic acids, and some vanillin, farnesol, etc.

Properties: Aromatic, antimicrobial, mild expectorant.

Uses: Internally it is used (as a syrup, lozenge, etc.) for minor inflammations of the upper respiratory tract (bronchitis, tracheitis, laryngitis, etc.; irritating dry coughs). It is widely used as a flavor ingredient in syrupy medicines and confectionery products, and as a fixative in perfumery. Externally it is used as an ingredient in Friar's Balsam, which is applied to wounds and ulcers.

Caution: In some hypersensitive individuals it may cause skin allergic reactions.

References: (1) Vol. 5, p. 898; (3) Vol. 5, p. 934; (9) p. 65; (10) p. 267; (11) p. 105; (13) p. 137; (36) p. 183; (37) p. 176; (46) p. 125; (48) p. 257.

TOMATO

Botanical Name(s): *Lycopersicon esculentum* Mill. = *Solanum lycopersicum* L. [Fam.: Solanaceae]
Fruit (ripe)
Constituents: Besides water, it contains invert sugar (very rich), carotenoids (rich in lycopene, lycoxanthin, etc.), minerals (rich in potassium, etc.), organic acids, etc. Only the unripe fruit contains tomatine and other toxic glycoalkaloids (glycosidic steroidal alkaloids), while ripe and processed fruit contains its aglycone, tomatidine (non-toxic).
Properties and Uses: Ripe tomato has values as a natural supplement of carotenoids (lycopene, etc.), which are strong antioxidants, valuable for the prevention of cancer and chronic diseases. Lycopene is soluble in fats and oils, so cooking tomato sauce with vegetable oils will be a valuable natural supplement of lycopene. Tomato is also considered a good supplement of potassium. Traditional medicine recommends the freshly prepared tomato juice, to be taken in the morning (on empty stomach) as a laxative for habitual constipation.
Caution: Ripe tomato should not be consumed in cases of diarrhea. The consumption of raw green tomato should be avoided as it contains tomatine (see: Constituents), which is toxic. Otherwise, there are no reports of contraindications or side effects with a normal consumption.

References: (1) Vol. 5, p. 726; (3) Vol. 5, p. 598; (12) p. 611; (27) p. 264; (48) p. 772; (75) p. 249.

TONKA

Other Common Name(s): Dutch tonka
Botanical Name(s): *Dipteryx odorata* (Aubl.) Willd. = *Coumarouna odorata* Aubl. [Fam.: Fabaceae (Leguminosae)]
Bean (seed)
Constituents: Coumarins (very rich in coumarin), fixed oil, phytosterols, volatile oil, starch, sugars, gum, etc.
Properties: Aromatic and bitter tonic, due in large part to coumarins (see Uses).
Uses: It is used as a flavor ingredient in tobacco and liqueur industries, and as a fragrance ingredient in perfumery. Coumarin has been shown to cause liver injuries, but only in animal tests. In some countries it is still allowed within standard limits in different products. There are new reports, which show the immunomodulating effect of coumarin, with hopes of treating certain tumors.
Caution: Tonka bean should not be taken for any kind of self-treatment.

376

References: (3) Vol. 4, p. 697; (9) p. 208; (11) p. 135; (12) p. 800; (13) p. 322; (36) p. 231; (37) pp. 371, 424; (48) p. 273.

TORMENTIL

Other Common Name(s): cinquefoil
Botanical Name(s): *Potentilla erecta* (L.) Räusch. = *Potentilla tormentilla* Stokes [Fam.: Rosaceae]
Root
Constituents: Tannins (chiefly proanthocyanidins, some ellagitannins), a triterpenoid pseudosaponin (tormentoside = diglucoside of tormentillic acid), flavonoids, phenolic acids, etc.
Properties: Astringent, hemostatic, antimicrobial. The effects are due in large part to tannins.
Uses: Internally it is used (as a tea, h. p.) for inflammations of the gastrointestinal tract (diarrhea, minor peptic ulcers, Crohn's disease, ulcerative colitis; also when minor hemorrhages are present, but on professional's advice). Externally it is used (as a mouthwash, gargle, paint) for inflammations of the mouth and throat, inflamed and bleeding gums, (as a vaginal irrigation / sitz bath / wash) for leukorrhea and vulvovaginitis, (as a wash, wet compress, poultice) for hemorrhoids, minor skin inflammations, eczema, cuts and wounds, (as a wet cotton, drops, irrigation with the tea) for nosebleed, and (as a partial bath, paint) for chilblains.
Caution: As with other herbs very rich in tannins, at higher doses than recommended it causes gastrointestinal irritations. Otherwise, there are no reports of contraindications or side effects when used properly.

References: (1) Vol. 6, p. 259; (3) Vol. 6a, p. 843; (7) p. 213; (8) p. 459; (10) p. 268; (13) p. 341; (16) pp. 87, 148; (19) p. 231; (23) p. 92; (24) p. 333; (27) p. 330; (35) p. 819; (37) p. 1113; (46) p. 1629; (47) p. 2716; (51) p. 96.

TRAGACANTH MILKVETCH

Botanical Name(s): *Astragalus gummifer* Labill.; *Astragalus microcephalus* Willd.; and some other *Astragalus* spp. [Fam.: Fabaceae (Papilionaceae)]
Gum tragacanth
It is a dried exudate (produced naturally, or after incisions) of the stem and branches.
Constituents: A mixture of polysaccharides (tragacanthin, water-soluble; bassorin, water insoluble), starch, but no enzymes.
Properties: Emulsifier, demulcent, bulk laxative, emollient.
Uses: Gum tragacanth is used in pharmaceutical and food industries mainly in the production of emulsions and suspensions, as a binding ingredient in tablets and lozenges, and more seldom as a thickening ingredient. It is still an ingredient in some laxative combination products.

Caution: Compound laxatives that contain gum tragacanth should be taken with sufficient liquids and avoided in bowel obstruction.

References: (1) Vol. 4, p. 411; (3) Vol. 3, p. 300; (8) p. 87; (9) p. 498; (11) p. 41; (12) p. 354; (13) p. 364; (36) p. 210; (37) p. 151; (48) p. 97.

TRAILING ARBUTUS

Other Common Name(s): gravel plant
Botanical Name(s): *Epigaea repens* L. [Fam.: Ericaceae]
Leaf
Constituents: A phenol glycoside (arbutin = hydroquinone-glucoside), triterpenes (ursolic acid, etc.), tannins (condensed and hydrolyzable t.), gallic acid, etc.
Properties: Urinary antiseptic, astringent. It acts much like uva-ursi, but milder. See UVA-URSI.
Uses: Internally it is used (as a tea, h. p.) chiefly for minor inflammations of the genitourinary tract (cystitis, urethritis, etc.). To enhance the effects, urine should be slightly alkaline (this can be done by consuming a diet rich in vegetables and / or taking about a teaspoonful / day of baking soda) and the fluid intake (incl. herbal teas) should be more than 2 liters per day. It is also used for inflammations of the gastrointestinal tract (diarrhea, etc.).
Caution: See UVA-URSI.

References: (3) Vol. 4, p. 786; (5) Vol. 1, p. 458; (35) p. 53; (44) p. 211.

TREE-OF-HEAVEN, CHINESE

Other Common Name(s): Chinese sumac, stinktree
Botanical Name(s): *Ailanthus altissima* (Mill.) Swingle = *Ailanthus glandulosa* Desf. [Fam.: Simaroubaceae]
Bark (root bark, stem inner bark)
Constituents: Bitter principles (nortriterpenes of quassinoid type: ailanthone, glaucarubinone, etc.), indole alkaloids (canthin-6-one, etc.), tannins, etc.
Properties: Plasmodicidal (against *Plasmodium falciparum*, causative for malignant tertian malaria), amebicidal (against *Entamoeba histolytica*, causative for amebic dysentery), antibacterial, bitter tonic, astringent. The antiprotozoal effect is due to nortriterpenes. Canthin-6-one has shown antibacterial effect.
Uses: Internally it is used (as a tea, h. p.) for malignant tertian malaria, chronic diarrhea and amebic dysentery, and may be beneficial for hepatic amebiasis. It is also used for loss of appetite and nonulcer dyspepsia (with fullness, flatulence, etc.).

Caution: There are no reports of contraindications or side effects when used properly. At higher doses than recommended it causes gastrointestinal irritations (with nausea, vomiting, diarrhea), headache, dizziness, etc.

References: (1) Vol. 4, p. 147; (3) Vol. 2, p. 1156; (12) p. 96; (31) p. 168; (37) p. 33; (41) Vols. 1-7; (66) p. 92.

TRICHOSANTHES

Other Common Name(s): Chinese cucumber, Mongolian snakegourd
Botanical Name(s): *Trichosanthes kirilowii* Maxim. [Fam.: Cucurbitaceae]
Root
Constituents: Triterpenes (karounidiol, karounidiol-3-benzoate), triterpenoid saponins, phytosterols (7-sterols, 5-sterols), trichosanthin (= compound Q: a linear polypeptide composed of more than 200 amino acids), etc.
Properties: Anti-inflammatory, antimicrobial, expectorant (bronchial secretagogue effect), laxative, demulcent, emollient. Trichosanthin has been shown to be abortifacient, antiviral (against HIV), and immunomodulant, with cytostatic effect against certain tumors (trophoblastic tumors).
Uses: Internally it is used (as a tea, h. p.) for inflammations of the upper respiratory tract (bronchitis, etc.; coughs due to thickened bronchial secretion), gastrointestinal tract (with minor constipation) and liver (chronic hepatitis). Trichosanthes is also used as an anti-inflammatory and antidyscratic (= blood purifier; tea, h. p.) for atopic eczema (= chronic eczema of internal origin) and chronic rheumatic complaints. In China, purified trichosanthin is used clinically to induce abortion. Externally it is used (as a poultice) for boils and carbuncles.
Caution: Unless advised by a health professional, trichosanthes should not be taken during pregnancy. It should not be used in diarrhea. At higher doses than recommended it causes gastrointestinal irritations (with nausea, vomiting, diarrhea). Trichosanthin is not for self-treatment. Only health professionals administer purified trichosanthin and are aware of its contraindications and side effects.

References: (3) Vol. 6c, p. 254; (31) p. 115; (36) p. 507; (37) p. 1400; (41) Vols. 1-7; (48) p. 220; (52) p. 814; (53) p. 39; (79) p. 128.

TURKEY CORN

Other Common Name(s): 1) Turkey corn, squirrel corn 2) Dutchman's breeches
Botanical Name(s): 1) *Dicentra canadensis* (Goldie) Walp. 2) *Dicentra cucullaria* (L.) Bernh. [Fam.: Papaveraceae]
Root (tuber)

Constituents: Isoquinoline alkaloids of various types (aporphine, cularine, phthalideisoquinoline, morphinan, benzylisoquinoline, protopine types), with some differences between two species.

Properties: Based on traditional use and result from animal tests with isolated alkaloids, it possibly exerts sedative, hypnotic, antispasmodic, and analgesic effects.

Uses: It is chiefly used in traditional medicine. Internally it is used (as a tea) to alleviate colicky states of genitourinary tract, Parkinson's disease (= a chronic neurologic disorder, with muscular weakness and tremor, sluggish movement and abnormal gait) and Ménière's disease (= a sudden attack, with violent dizziness, nausea and vomiting, ringing in the ear).

Caution: Root of Turkey corn or Dutchman's breeches is toxic. Unless advised by a health professional, it should not be used during pregnancy and lactation. Alcoholic drinks may interact with it. A possible combination of it with sedative, hypnotic, and antidepressant drugs should be made only by a health professional.

References: (1) Vol. 4, p. 1155; (3) Vol. 4, p. 525; (10) p. 270; (12a) p. 525; (35) p. 822; (41) Vols. 1-7; (52) p. 253.

TURMERIC

Other Common Name(s): common turmeric, curcuma, Indian saffron, yellow ginger

Botanical Name(s): *Curcuma longa* L. = *Curcuma domestica* Valeton [Fam.: Zingiberaceae]

Root

Constituents: Curcuminoid pigments (curcumin, desmethoxycurcumin, bisdesmethoxycurcumin, etc.; richer than Javanese t.), volatile oil (less than Javanese t.; with sesquiterpenes: ar-turmerone, etc., no xanthorhizol), polysaccharides (starch, ukonanes), etc.

Properties: Aromatic, bitter tonic, choleretic, cholagogue, antispasmodic, carminative, antioxidant, cholesterol reducing, liver protective, anti-inflammatory and analgesic (NSAID-like effect, by inhibiting biosynthesis of prostaglandins), antibacterial, antiviral, antifungal, immunomodulant, antitumoral. The effects are due in large part to curcuminoids and the volatile oil. The immunomodulant effect may be due at least in part to ukonanes.

Uses: It is chiefly used as a flavor and coloring ingredient in food industry (in curry powder, etc.) and culinary practice. Internally it is used (as a tea, h. p.) for nonulcer dyspepsia (with fullness, flatulence, etc.), which are mostly associated with hepatobiliary disorders (impaired bile secretion and flow, chronic cholecystitis and cholangitis, nonobstructive gallstones), for rheumatic complaints (incl. rheumatoid arthritis), and as a dietary aid to the prevention of cancer. Combined with celandine and peppermint it is used to alleviate complaints following a cholecystectomy. For primary dysmenorrhea

380

it can be used same as ginger (see: GINGER). Externally (as a poultice) may be helpful for eczema, psoriasis, and dermatomycosis.

Caution: Unless consumed in small amounts as a flavor, turmeric should not be taken in cases of obstructive gallstones and during pregnancy. In cases of nonobstructive gallstones it can be used but only on health professional's advice. Before using it for dysmenorrhea, the gynecologic problem should be judged by a health professional. At higher doses than recommended it may cause gastrointestinal irritations (with nausea, vomiting) and a consumption of excessive amounts for prolonged periods may cause fatty liver. Otherwise, there are no reports of contraindications or side effects when used properly.

References: (1) Vol. 4, p. 1088; (3) Vol. 4, p. 380; (6) p. 148; (8) p. 206; (9) p. 499; (12) p. 686; (13) p. 143; (16) p. 131; (17) p. 181; (19) p. 66; (22) p. 73; (26) p 235; (29) p. 39; (37) p. 373; (46) p. 421; (48) p. 296; (59) p. 115; (65) p. 182.

TURMERIC, JAVANESE

Other Common Name(s): Temu lawak
Botanical Name(s): *Curcuma xanthorrhiza* Roxb. [Fam.: Zingiberaceae]
Root
Constituents: Volatile oil (richer than turmeric; with sesquiterpenes: ar-curcumene, etc., incl. xanthorhizol; no ar-turmerone), curcuminoid pigments (less than turmeric; curcumin, etc.), polysaccharides (starch, no ukonanes), etc.
Properties: Aromatic, bitter tonic, choleretic, cholagogue, carminative, antioxidant, liver protective, anti-inflammatory, antitumoral, antibacterial, antiviral. Due to its higher volatile oil content (with xanthorhizol, a pungent principle), the aromatic pungent flavor is stronger than in turmeric. Due to its lower content in curcuminoids, the hepatobiliary and anti-inflammatory effects are somehow weaker than in turmeric. See also TURMERIC.
Uses: Javanese turmeric is used much like turmeric, with some differences in effects (see Constituents, Properties, for both). See TURMERIC.
Caution: See TURMERIC.

References: (1) Vol. 4, p. 1096; (3) Vol. 4, p. 384; (8) p. 204; (9) p. 499; (12) p. 299; (13) p. 143; (16) p. 130; (17) p. 185; (19) p. 88; (22) p. 73; (37) p. 373; (48) p. 298

UMCKALOABO

Botanical Name(s): *Pelargonium reniforme* Curtis; *Pelargonium sidoides* DC [Fam.: Geraniaceae]
Root bark
Constituents: Coumarins (chiefly umckalin = 5-methoxy-scopoletin, also scopoletin, scopolin = scopoletin-glucoside, etc.), tannins (hydrolyzable t.),

phenolic acids (gallic acid, etc.), flavonoids (flavan-3-ols = catechins), minerals (silicic acid, as soluble silicates), biogenic amines, etc.

Properties: Antibacterial (against *Staphylococcus aureus*, *Streptococcus haemolyticus*, *Escherichia coli*, etc.), antiviral, immunomodulant, anti-inflammatory, antioxidant. The antibacterial effect is due to phenolics (tannins, gallic acid). Coumarins and tannins may account at least in part for the immunomodulating effect. Scopoletin has shown anti-inflammatory, antispasmodic, antibacterial and antifungal effects.

Uses: Internally it is used (as a tea, h. p.) for inflammations chiefly of the upper respiratory tract (the common cold, bronchitis, sinusitis, pharyngitis, etc.), also gastrointestinal tract (diarrhea, etc.) and liver (chronic hepatitis).

Caution: Umckaloabo is best avoided during pregnancy and lactation. It should not be used in severe liver and kidney disorders. A concomitant use of umckaloabo with anticoagulants (warfarin, etc.) and / or platelet aggregation inhibitors (aspirin, etc.) should be avoided as it may potentiate their effect. Otherwise, there are no reports of contraindications or side effects when used properly.

References: (6) p. 325; (8) p. 413; (13) p. 419; (31) p. 364; (57) p. 595; (72) nr. 10001; (91) p. 508.

USNEA

Botanical Name(s): *Usnea florida* (L.) Fries; *Usnea aspera* (Eschw.) Waino; *Usnea barbata* (L.) Wigg.; *Usnea hirta* Hoffm.; etc. [Fam.: Usneaceae]

Usnea spp. are lichens (= symbiotic association of a fungi with algae) but commonly called mosses.

Thallus (= a complete plant body, which is not differentiated into root, stem and leaves)

Constituents: Dibenzofurans (rich in usnic acid, etc.), depsidones (lichenic acids: usnaric acid, etc.; bitter tasting), polysaccharides (D-glucans: the water-insoluble lichenin and water-soluble isolichenin), etc.

Properties: Antibacterial, demulcent, bitter tonic, mild immunomodulant. Usnic acid accounts in large part for the antibacterial effect (against *Staphylococcus* spp., *Streptococcus* spp., *Mycobacterium* spp., etc.). The immunomodulating effect may be due to water-soluble polysaccharides, enhanced by bitter principles (lichenic acids).

Uses: Topically it is used (as a lozenge) for inflammations of the mouth and throat, and (as an ointment, powder, spray) for minor skin infections. Internally it is used (as a tea, h. p.) for loss of appetite and inflammations of the gastrointestinal tract (gastroenteritis, diarrhea).

Caution: In rare cases, products applied to the skin may cause contact skin irritations especially when exposed to strong sunrays. This is due to usnic acid. Otherwise, there are no reports of contraindications or side effects when used properly.

References: (3) Vol. 6c, p. 363; (5) Vol. 2, p. 156; (13a) p. 301; (19) p. 38; (23) pp. 68, 213; (31) p. 342; (36) p. 217; (37) pp. 826, 1430; (41) Vols. 1-7; (42) Vol. 1, pp. 158, 163, 167; (72) nr. 62065.

UVA-URSI

Other Common Name(s): bearberry
Botanical Name(s): *Arctostaphylos uva-ursi* Spreng. [Fam.: Ericaceae]
Leaf
Constituents: Phenol glycosides (arbutin = hydroquinone-glucoside, etc.), some free hydroquinone, flavonoids (flavonols: hyperin, etc.), tannins (gallotannins, ellagitannins), triterpenes (ursolic acid, etc.), phenolic acids, bitter principles (iridoids, ursolic acid), etc.
Properties: Antibacterial (against *Staphylococcus* spp., *Escherichia coli*, *Pseudomonas* spp., *Proteus* spp., etc.), astringent. In the gastrointestinal tract hydroquinone is liberated from arbutin, then conjugated and as such reaches urinary pathways. Hydroquinone (= 1,4-dihydroxy-benzene), a phenolic compound, accounts for the antibacterial effect. Depending on the amount and the product used, uva-ursi exerts mild to strong astringent effect. Hyperin is a mild diuretic.
Uses: Internally it is used (as a tea, h. p.) for inflammations of the genitourinary tract (cystitis, urethritis, prostatitis, pyelonephritis). To enhance the effects, urine should be slightly alkaline (e. g. by consuming a diet rich in vegetables and / or taking about a teaspoonful / day of baking soda) and the fluid intake (incl. herbal teas) should be more than 2 liters per day.
Caution: Uva-ursi should not be taken during pregnancy and lactation. It should not be used in infants and children under 12 years of age. Due to the high tannin content uva-ursi may cause constipation and gastrointestinal irritations (with nausea, vomiting). Therefore, the tea should not be prepared by boiling but by infusing the crushed leaves or by macerating in room temperature the powdered leaves. It is best used as a standardized product to arbutin or hydroquinone content. A normal daily dose of uva-ursi leaf is about 10 grams. In view of this, capsules should contain a dried extract and not powdered leaf alone. Uva-ursi products should not be taken for more than one week and more than five times in one-year, because hydroquinone has shown hepatotoxic effect.

References: (1) Vol. 4, p. 329; (3) Vol. 3, p. 177; (6) pp. 187, 329; (7) p. 247; (12) p. 696; (13) p. 303; (14) p. 211; (17) p. 599; (19) p. 34; (22) p. 95; (23) p. 247; (46) p. 1640; (47) p. 2759; (48) p. 243.

UZARA

Other Common Name(s): Xysmalobium undulatum
Botanical Name(s): *Xysmalobium undulatum* (L.) R. Br. [Fam.: Asclepiadaceae]

383

Root
Constituents: Tannins (possibly gallotannins), cardiac glycosides (chiefly uzarin, uzaroside, etc.) and their free aglycones (uzarigenin, etc.), etc.
Properties: Antidiarrheal (chiefly by inhibiting the intestinal peristalsis), antispasmodic. Unless taken at very high doses, the cardioactivity of uzara glycosides is very mild. This is because the configuration of C / D ring junction in uzarigenin is different from that of digitoxigenin (in digitalis) and related aglycones (in lily-of-the-valley, spring adonis, strophanthus, etc.).
Uses: Internally it is used (as an h. p.) for acute diarrhea. With a rational treatment, uzara stops the diarrhea, pains, and vomiting.
Caution: Uzara products should be standardized to the cardiac glycosides content. Doses higher than recommended should be avoided as they will exert digitalis-like effects. Unless advised by a health professional, uzara should not be combined with cardioactive glycosides or herbs (digoxin, lily-of-the-valley, etc.). Otherwise, there are no reports of contraindications or side effects when used properly.

References: (2) Vol. 3, p. 794; (3) Vol. 6c, p. 543; (6) p. 154; (8) p. 597; (12) p. 597; (13) p. 194; (19) p. 235; (23) p. 95; (37) p. 1485.

VALERIAN

Other Common Name(s): officinal valerian
Botanical Name(s): *Valeriana officinalis* L. [Fam.: Valerianaceae]
Root (rhizome with roots)
Constituents: Dried root and alcoholic extracts contain volatile oil (with monoterpenes: bornyl esters, borneol, α- and β-pinene, etc.; sesquiterpenes: valerenic acid, valeranone, etc.), baldrinals (= degraded compounds of valepotriates), valepotriates (only small amounts; fresh root is much richer), phenolic acids, etc. Dried root and special extracts contains GABA (= gamma-aminobutyrric acid). Not all extracts contain it.
Properties: Sedative, hypnotic, antispasmodic, muscle relaxant, anticonvulsant, mild antiulcer (= prevents or helps in healing peptic ulcers). Depending on cases, at low doses, valerian has shown to be mild stimulant of the nervous and cardiovascular systems. Volatile oil and sesquiterpenes as a whole have shown sedative and antispasmodic effects. Baldrinals have shown sedative effect. Valerian has shown GABA-mimetic activity (increases levels and binding affinity of GABA to its receptors), which explains most of the mentioned effects. Valeranone has also shown antiulcerogenic effect.
Uses: Internally it is used (as an h. p., tea) for problems due to nervous tension and anxiety such as difficulties to concentrate, insomnia, nervous cardiovascular disorders (minor tachycardia = rapid heartbeat, hypertension), gastrointestinal complaints (flatulence, cramps, irritable bowel syndrome, diarrhea, etc.), uterine cramps (incl. dysmenorrhea = painful menstruation without pathology), mild withdrawal syndromes (after stopping a

384

prolonged use of alcohol or benzodiazepines), and as an adjuvant for peptic ulcers. As a sleeping aid it is taken ½-1 hour before bedtime.

Caution: Alcoholic drinks may interact with valerian (at higher doses). A possible combination of it with sedative, hypnotic and antidepressant drugs should be made only by a health professional. Before using it for uterine cramps, the gynecologic problem should be judged by a health professional. It should not be used in children under 3 years, and it should be avoided its use under 12 years as well as during pregnancy and lactation. Otherwise, there are no reports of contraindications or side effects when used properly.

References: (1) Vol. 6, p. 1079; (3) Vol. 6c, p. 375; (6) p. 210; (7) p. 80; (8) p. 576; (9) p. 507; (12) p. 457; (13) p. 131; (14) p. 214; (16) p. 177; (17) p. 603; (19) p. 35; (20) p. 260; (22) p. 154; (23) p. 290; (28) p. 210; (37) p. 1436; (46) p. 1649; (47) p. 2770; (48) p. 595; (59) p. 267; (66) p. 494; (67) p. 436.

VANILLA

Botanical Name(s): *Vanilla planifolia* Jacks. = *Vanilla fragrans* (Salisb.) Ames [Fam.: Orchidaceae]

Fruit (vanilla pod, vanilla bean)

It consists of the fully-grown but unripe capsule, which has undergone a curing process before drying.

Constituents: Vanillin (= 3-methoxy-4-hydroxy-benzaldehyde), traces of 4-hydroxy-benzaldehyde and other aromatic compounds. It also contains sugars, organic acids, tannins, mucilaginous polysaccharides, etc. Fresh pod contains vanilloside = vanillin-4-β-glucoside.

Properties: Aromatic, and it is claimed to be aphrodisiac.

Uses: Vanilla and vanilla tincture are used as flavor ingredients in food and pharmaceutical industries, and culinary practice.

Caution: In hypersensitive persons vanilla pods (not vanillin) may cause allergic reactions. Otherwise, there are no reports of contraindications or side effects when used and consumed properly.

References: (3) Vol. 6c, p. 391; (5) Vol. 1, p. 1116; (9) p. 510; (11) p. 61; (12) p. 664; (36) p. 222; (37) p. 1440; (46) p. 1673.

VERBENA, LEMON

Botanical Name(s): *Aloysia citriodora* Palau = *Aloysia triphylla* (L' Hér.) Britton = *Lippia citriodora* Kunth, nom. illeg. [Fam.: Verbenaceae]

Leaf

Constituents: Volatile oil (with citral a = geranial, citral b = neral, limonene, caryophyllene, etc.), iridoids, phenolic acids, flavonoids (6-hydroxy- and 6-methoxy-flavone), mucilaginous polysaccharides, tannins, minerals (potassium, etc.), etc.

Properties: Aromatic, bitter tonic, sedative, antispasmodic, antimicrobial. Lemon verbena oil has shown antispasmodic and antimicrobial effects.

385

Among 6-hydroxy- and 6-methoxy-flavones there are compounds that have shown antispasmodic, liver protective, antioxidant, and platelet aggregation inhibitory effects.

Uses: <u>Internally</u> it is used (as a tea, h. p.) for nonulcer dyspepsia (with irritable stomach and minor upper abdominal pains, flatulence and intestinal cramps), minor cases of anxiety, headache and insomnia, and as a diaphoretic hot tea for feverish states and the common cold.

Caution: There are no reports of contraindications or side effects for the herb when used properly.

References: (1) Vol. 5, p. 690; (3) Vol. 5, p. 526; (20) p. 179; (29) p. 8; (31) p. 388; (37) p. 51; (48) p. 569.

VERVAIN, BLUE

Other Common Name(s): American blue vervain, wild hyssop
Botanical Name(s): *Verbena hastata* L. [Fam.: Verbenaceae]
Aerial part
Constituents: Not well known. It is reported to contain iridoids (hastatoside, verbenalin). It possibly contains principles similar to European vervain (see VERVAIN, EUROPEAN).
Properties and Uses: Much like European vervain (see VERVAIN, EUROPEAN).
Caution: Until its constituents are better known, it should be used with the same caution as European vervain (see VERVAIN, EUROPEAN).

References: (3) Vol. 6c, p. 423; (25) p. 172; (35) p. 832; (44) p. 591; (52) p. 843.

VERVAIN, EUROPEAN

Botanical Name(s): *Verbena officinalis* L. [Fam.: Verbenaceae]
Aerial part
Constituents: Iridoids (verbenalin, hastatoside, etc.), phenylethanoid glycosides (acteoside = verbascoside, etc.), flavonoids (flavones: luteolin, etc.), tannins, mucilaginous polysaccharides, volatile oil (traces), etc.
Properties: Bitter tonic, diuretic, mild laxative, astringent, demulcent, emollient, antifungal (against *Tinea* spp.). Iridoids have shown bitter tonic, choleretic, liver protective, laxative, diuretic, anti-inflammatory, antibacterial, antiviral, antifungal and immunomodulant effects, among others. Verbenalin has shown parasympathomimetic activity and European vervain may affect organs that are innervated by parasympathetic nervous system (heart, bronchi, gastrointestinal tract, uterus, urinary bladder, etc.). A parasympathetic stimulation decreases the heart rate, increases gastrointestinal secretions and motility, and contracts smooth muscles of bronchi, uterus, and urinary bladder, among others. Acteoside has shown anti-inflammatory (by in-

hibiting the biosynthesis of leukotrienes) and liver protective effects.

Uses: <u>Internally</u> it is only incorporated in herbal teas or other products used for disorders of the gastrointestinal, hepatobiliary, upper respiratory and genitourinary tracts, and in antidyscratic (= blood purifying) teas used for atopic eczema (= chronic eczema of internal origin) and chronic rheumatic complaints. <u>Externally</u> it is used (as a wash, wet compress, poultice) for minor skin inflammations, wounds, ulcers, Tinea capitis (= fungal infection of the scalp) and other itching conditions.

Caution: Unless advised by a health professional, European vervain should not be taken during pregnancy and lactation. At higher doses than recommended it causes gastrointestinal irritations (with nausea, vomiting, diarrhea), among others. See also Properties.

References: (1) Vol. 6, p. 1108; (3) Vol. 6c, p. 422; (6) p. 102; (8) p. 583; (15) p. 227; (17) p. 611; (20) p. 263; (24) p. 120; (27) p. 336; (29) p. 121; (35) p. 831; (47) p. 2796; (48) p. 607; (51) p. 158.

VETIVER

Other Common Name(s): khus, khus-khus
Botanical Name(s): *Chrysopogon zizanioides* (L.) Roberty = *Vetiveria zizanioides* (L.) Nash. = *Andropogon muricatus* Retz. [Fam.: Poaceae (Gramineae)]
<u>Root</u>
Constituents: Volatile oil (with sesquiterpenes: vetivenols, vetivenones, vetivones, β-isokhusenic acid, etc.; depending on origin), bitter principles, sugars (rich), resin, etc.
Properties: Aromatic, bitter tonic, antimicrobial, antispasmodic, carminative, analgesic. It is also reported to be emmenagogic.
Uses: Vetiver root is chiefly used as a flavor ingredient in food industry. Its volatile oil has myrrh-like aroma and is used as a fragrance ingredient and fixative in cosmetics and perfumery. <u>Internally</u> it is used (as a tea, h. p.) for loss of appetite and nonulcer dyspepsia (with flatulence, minor cramps), and as a diaphoretic hot tea for feverish states and the common cold. In traditional practice it is also used as an insect-repellent for moths, fleas, etc.
Caution: Vetiver should not be taken during pregnancy and lactation. It is best used as directed by an experienced practitioner.

References: (3) Vol. 6c, p. 433; (5) Vol. 2, p. 1126; (36) p. 495; (37) p. 1449; (41) Vols. 1-7; (52) p. 847; (57) p. 875.

VIOLET, SWEET

Other Common Name(s): English violet, sweet blue violet
Botanical Name(s): *Viola odorata* L. [Fam.: Violaceae]
<u>Root</u> (rhizome)
Constituents: Volatile oil (with methyl salicylate, etc.), a phenol glycoside

(gaultherin = methylsalicylate glycoside), saponins, an emetine-like alkaloid, etc.

Properties: Mild expectorant (bronchial secretagogue effect).

Uses: <u>Internally</u> it is used (as a tea, h. p.; usually combined with other herbs) for inflammations of the upper respiratory (bronchitis, laryngitis, etc.; coughs due to thickened bronchial secretions). Due to its mild ipecac-like / cowslip-like expectorant effects it has been designated as German ipecac.

Caution: There are no reports of contraindications or side effects when used properly. At higher doses than recommended it may cause gastrointestinal irritations (with nausea, vomiting).

<u>Aerial part</u>

Constituents: Triterpenoids (saponins, friedelin, etc.), phytosterols, phenol glycosides, phenolic acids, flavonoids, an emetine-like alkaloid, volatile oil, etc.

Properties, Uses, and Caution: The same as root, but milder.

References: (1) Vol. 6, p. 1143; (3) Vol. 6c, p. 479; (8) p. 588; (15) p. 232; (23) p. 215; (24) p. 335; (27) p. 339; (35) p. 834; (37) p. 1453; (46) p. 1757; (47) p. 2821; (48) p. 113.

VIRGIN'S BOWER

Other Common Name(s): clematis

Botanical Name(s): *Clematis virginiana* L.; *Clematis recta* L.; *Clematis vitalba* L. [Fam.: Ranunculaceae]

<u>Aerial part</u>

Constituents: (Dried herb): Anemonin (= protoanemonin dimer); (fresh herb): protoanemonin (an unstable compound); and (fresh or dried): saponins, phytosterols, alkanes, etc.

Properties: (Dried herb): Diuretic, antimicrobial. (Fresh herb): Counterirritant / vesicant (depending on concentrations) and analgesic. Anemonin is non-toxic and has shown antimicrobial effect. Protoanemonin is toxic and a strong local irritant (cf. PULSATILLA).

Uses: Clematis is chiefly used in traditional medicine. <u>Internally</u> it is used (only dried herb; as a tea; combined with other herbs) for inflammatory and spastic conditions of the genitourinary tract, and as an antidyscratic (= blood purifier) for atopic eczema (= chronic eczema of internal origin) and chronic rheumatic complaints. To enhance the effects in problems of the genitourinary tract, the fluid intake (incl. herbal teas) should be more than 2 liters per day. <u>Externally</u> it is used (as a poultice: fresh herb) for rheumatic pains, and (as wash, wet compress: dried herb) for bacterial and fungal skin infections.

Caution: Internally should be used only dried herb and as directed by an experienced practitioner. Even dried, virgin's bower should not be taken during pregnancy as it may still contain protoanemonin (teratogenic, abortifacient!; cf. PULSATILLA). Fresh herb should be handled with care (see Properties), even when used externally. If taken internally, fresh herb (also dried herb at higher doses than recommended) causes strong gastrointestinal irritations (with vomiting, diarrhea), etc.

References: (3) Vol. 4, p. 148; (5) Vol. 2, p. 306; (25) p. 22; (27) p. 131; (36) p. 508; (35) p. 205; (37) p. 340; (47) pp. 1007, 1013; (48) p. 747; (51) p. 76.

WAHOO

Other Common Name(s): Eastern burningbush, euonymus
Botanical Name(s): *Euonymus atropurpurea* Jacq. [Fam.: Celastraceae]
Root bark
Constituents: A bitter principle (furan-3-carboxylic acid), a sugar alcohol (dulcitol), tannins, cardiac glycosides (with aglycone: digitoxigenin), etc.
Properties: (At low doses): Choleretic, cholagogue, diuretic. (At high doses): Laxative. Due to the cardiac glycosides it exerts also digitalis-like effects.
Uses: Internally it is used (at low doses; as an herbal combination product) for hepatobiliary disorders (impaired bile secretion and flow, chronic cholecystitis) and nonulcer dyspepsia (with sluggish bowels, minor constipation). In traditional medicine it is also used (at low doses, combined with other herbs) as an antidyscratic (= blood purifier) for atopic eczema (= chronic eczema of internal origin).
Caution: Wahoo should be used only as directed by an experienced practitioner. Doses higher than recommended should be avoided (cardiac glycosides!). It should not be taken in cases of biliary obstruction. In cases of nonobstructive gallstones, during pregnancy and lactation, and in minor cardiac edemas it can be used but only on health professional's advice. A possible combination with cardiac glycosides or herbs (digoxin, lily-of-the-valley, etc.) should be made only by a health professional.

References: (3) Vol. 4, p. 865; (5) Vol. 1, p. 481; (10) p. 277; (15) p. 85; (18) p. 221; (25) p. 275; (35) p. 762; (37) p. 499; (41) Vols. 1-7; (46) p. 570; (47) p. 1334.

WALNUT

Other Common Name(s): English walnut, Persian walnut
Botanical Name(s): *Juglans regia* L. [Fam.: Juglandaceae]
Leaf
Constituents: Tannins (ellagitannins), a naphthoquinone (juglone), a naphthohydroquinone (hydrojuglone and its glucoside), flavonoids (flavonols, etc.), phenolic acids (caffeic, chlorogenic, ferulic and gallic acids, etc.), volatile oil, etc.
Properties: Astringent, antibacterial, antifungal (against *Tinea* spp.), anti-inflammatory, "vitamin P"-like (= helps in normalizing an increased microvascular permeability and fragility).
Uses: Externally it is used (as a wash, wet compress, poultice) for minor

bacterial or fungal infections of the skin (incl. Tinea capitis = fungal infection of the scalp), eczema, milk crust, ulcers, sore nipples, wounds and sunburns, (as a partial bath) for tired and sweating feet, (as a mouthwash, gargle) for inflammations of the mouth and throat, and (as a vaginal irrigation / sitz bath / wash) for leukorrhea and vulvovaginitis. Internally it is used (as a tea, h. p.) for minor inflammations of the gastrointestinal tract (diarrhea, ulcerative colitis, etc.).

Caution: There are no reports of contraindications or side effects when used properly.

References: (3) Vol. 5, p. 328; (5) Vol. 1, p. 619; (8) p. 327; (13) p. 339; (16) p. 27; (17) p. 319; (19) p. 238; (22) p. 213; (23) p. 333; (27) p. 233; (37) p. 740; (46) p. 978; (47) p. 1663; (48) p. 419; (51) p. 242.

WATER MINT

Botanical Name(s): *Mentha aquatica* L. [Fam.: Lamiaceae (Labiatae)]
Leaf
Constituents: Volatile oil (with menthofuran, also linalool, menthol, etc.), Lamiaceae tannins (rosmarinic acid and other caffeic acid derivatives), etc.
Properties: Aromatic, antispasmodic, cholagogue, carminative, astringent. The effects are mild.
Uses: Water mint is used in traditional medicine. Internally it is used (as a tea) for minor gastrointestinal cramps, flatulence and diarrhea, and minor cases of primary dysmenorrhea (= painful menstruation without pathology).
Caution: There are no reports of contraindications or side effects when used properly. Nevertheless, as it contains menthofuran (the hepatotoxic metabolite of pulegone of pennyroyal), it should be used with caution.

References: (1) Vol. 5, p. 823; (3) Vol. 5, p. 775; (5) Vol. 1, p. 708; (35) p. 544; (37) p. 877; (48) p. 547.

WATER PEPPER

Other Common Name(s): smartweed
Botanical Name(s): *Polygonum hydropiper* L. [Fam.: Polygonaceae]
Aerial part
Constituents: Flavonoids (quercetin glycosides: rutin, etc.), tannins (chiefly hydrolyzable t.), minerals (potassium salts, etc.), volatile oil (with tadeonal; pungent), etc., but no vitamin K.
Properties: Hemostatic, astringent, diuretic.
Uses: Internally it is used (as a tea, h. p.) for minor internal hemorrhages such as menorrhagia / hypermenorrhea (= prolonged / heavy menstruation), postpartum hemorrhage (= h. following childbirth), as an adjuvant for metrorrhagia (= nonmenstrual uterine bleeding), for minor hemorrhages from intestinal tract (due to hemorrhoids, etc.), diarrhea, urinary tract (due to gravel or nonobstructive stones) and respiratory tract, and as a diaphoretic

hot tea for feverish states and the common cold. Externally it is used (as a wash, poultice, wet compress) for minor cuts and wounds, and hair loss.

Caution: There are no reports of contraindications or side effects when used properly. Nevertheless, before using it for internal bleedings, the problem should be judged by a health professional.

References: (3) Vol. 6a, p. 817; (6) p. 314; (10) p. 252; (12a) p. 169; (13) p. 148; (23) pp. 112, 374; (35) p. 743; (44) p. 423; (46) p. 1086; (47) p. 1573; (51) p. 66.

WATERLILY

Other Common Name(s): 1) white waterlily, European white waterlily 2) sweet-scented waterlily, American white waterlily
Botanical Name(s): 1) *Nymphaea alba* L. 2) *Nymphaea odorata* Aiton [Fam.: Nymphaeaceae]
Root (rhizome)
Constituents: Not well known. It is reported to contain tannins (gallotaninns, ellagitannins), starch (rich), sugars, phytosterols, alkanes (hexacosanol, etc.) and an alkaloid (in *N. alba*: nympheine?).
Properties: Astringent, antidiarrheal.
Uses: Externally it is used (as a mouthwash, gargle) for inflammations of the mouth and throat, (as a vaginal irrigation / sitz bath / wash) for vulvovaginitis and leukorrhea, and (as a poultice) for boils. Internally it is used (as a tea, h. p.) for diarrhea. In traditional medicine it is also used as mild sedative-hypnotic for insomnia and as an anaphrodisiac for hyperactive sexual desires.
Caution: There are no reports of contraindications or side effects when used properly.

References: (1) Vol. 5, p. 925; (3) Vol. 6a, p. 285; (15) p. 150; (25) p. 14; (35) p. 484; (41) Vols. 1-7; (47) p. 1997; (51) p. 71.

WILLOW

Other Common Name(s): 1) purple willow / osier 2) laurel / bay willow 3) brittle / crack willow 4) violet / daphne willow; etc.
Botanical Name(s): 1) *Salix purpurea* L. 2) *Salix pentandra* L. 3) *Salix fragilis* L. 4) *Salix daphnoides* Vill.; etc. [Fam.: Salicaceae]
Bark (from young branches)
Constituents: Phenol glycosides (salicin = glucoside of salicyl alcohol, salicortin, 2'-acetyl-salicortin, etc.), flavonoids (isosalipurposide, etc.), tannins (condensed t.), phenolic acids (caffeic, syringic and ferulic acids, etc.), etc. Concentrations of salicin and related compounds depend on species, clones, and harvesting period. White willow (S. alba L.) contains much less salicin.
Properties: Anti-inflammatory, analgesic, antipyretic, astringent. Salicin and related glycosides, in the intestinal tract liberate salicyl alcohol, which

is oxidized in the liver into salicylic acid. As with aspirin, salicylic acid is the active compound, which accounts for the NSAID-like effect (anti-inflammatory, analgesic, antipyretic) by inhibiting the biosynthesis of inflammatory prostaglandins. Salicin lacks the acetyl residue of aspirin, which binds to thromboxane synthetase of platelets, so it doesn't influence the biosynthesis of thrombocytes (= platelets). Due to tannins it also exerts astringent effect.

Uses: Internally it is used (as a standardized extract, often in a combination product) for minor cases of rheumatic complaints (incl. rheumatoid arthritis), headaches and feverish states. It is also used (as a tea) for inflammations of the gastrointestinal tract (diarrhea, etc.; also when minor hemorrhages are present, but on professional's advice). Externally it is used (as a wash, wet compress) for minor skin inflammations, wounds and ulcers, and (as a vaginal irrigation / sitz bath / wash) for leukorrhea.

Caution: As with aspirin, in persons hypersensitive to salicylates, it may cause allergic reactions. Willow bark products (capsules, dragées, tablets, liquid preparations) should contain extracts standardized to the phenol glycosides content (expressed as salicin) and not powdered herb, which contains negligible amounts of active constituents per capsule and the like. It should not be tried to substitute aspirin as a platelet aggregation inhibitor (see Properties). At higher doses than recommended, willow bark tea may cause gastrointestinal irritations (with nausea, constipation). Otherwise, there are no reports of contraindications or side effects when used properly.

References: (2) Vol. 3, p. 469; (3) Vol. 6b, p. 233; (6) p. 233; (7) p. 156; (8) p. 502; (13) p. 422; (14) p. 224; (17) p. 517; (20) p. 268; (22) p. 200; (27) p. 299; (46) p. 1397; (47) p. 2394; (48) p. 253; (51) p. 242.

WILLOW HERB

Other Common Name(s): 1) small-flower willow herb 2) great willow herb, fireweed; etc.
Botanical Name(s): 1) *Epilobium parviflorum* Schreb. 2) *Epilobium angustifolium* L. = *Chamaenerion angustifolium* (L.) Scop.; etc. [Fam.: Onagraceae (Oenotheraceae)]
Aerial part
Constituents: Flavonoids (flavonols: myricetin glycosides or quercetin glycosides, depending on species), phytosterols (5-sterols: β-sitosterol, β-sitosterolin = β-sitosterol-glucoside, β-sitosterol esters), tannins (gallotannins), etc.
Properties: Anti-inflammatory, antiedematous, antioxidant, mild antimicrobial, astringent. The anti-inflammatory, antiedematous and antioxidant effects are due to flavonols, phytosterols and tannins. The antimicrobial effect is due in large part to gallic acid (liberated from gallotannins). β-Sitosterol and β-sitosterolin exert anti-inflammatory effect by inhibiting the

392

biosynthesis of prostaglandins and leukotrienes.

Uses: <u>Internally</u> it is chiefly used (as a tea, h. p.) for micturition problems associated with early stages of benign prostatic hyperplasia (= BPH: stages I and II). It is also used for inflammations of the gastrointestinal tract (diarrhea, ulcerative colitis, etc., incl. hemorrhoids; also when minor hemorrhages are present, but on professional's advice) and may be beneficial for inflammations of the genitourinary tract (cystitis, urethritis, prostatitis, etc.). <u>Externally</u> it is used (as a wet compress, poultice) for minor wounds.

Caution: There are no reports of contraindications or side effects when used properly. Nevertheless, before using willow herb products for BPH, the prostate problem should be judged by a health professional. Willow herb is best used as a standardized product to flavonols and sterols.

References: (1) Vol. 5, pp. 57, 63; (3) Vol. 3, p. 832; (6) p. 198; (8) p. 244; (17) p. 199; (31) pp. 405, 457; (37) p. 478; (44) p. 212.

WINTER CHERRY

Other Common Name(s): strawberry tomato
Botanical Name(s): *Physalis alkekengi* L. [Fam.: Solanaceae]
Fruit (ripe)
Constituents: Carotenoids (zeaxanthin dipalmitate, cryptoxanthin), flavonoids (flavones: luteolin, etc.), vitamin C (rich), organic acids (citric acid, etc.), sugars, pectin, bitter principles (steroidal lactones: physalins A-C), etc.
Properties: Acidulous, stomachic, laxative, diuretic, antioxidant. The effects are mild.
Uses: It is mainly consumed fresh as an edible fruit and a natural supplement of vitamin C. It is recommended for digestive complaints (loss of appetite, impaired digestion, minor constipation) and genitourinary complaints in general (including gravel, nonobstructive urinary stones). To enhance the effects in problems of the genitourinary tract, the fluid intake (incl. herbal teas) should be more than 2 liters per day.
Caution: Other plant parts of winter cherry may contain solanaceous alkaloids. Therefore, before incorporating dried fruits in herbal teas, manufacturers should run tests accordingly. Otherwise, there are no reports of contraindications or side effects when used properly.
Note: The fruit of another related species, cherry tomato: *Physalis peruviana* L., contains similar constituents and is used much like winter cherry.

References: (3) Vol. 6a, p. 637; (5) Vol. 1, p. 828; (27) p. 86; (28) p. 184; (35) p. 191; (37) p. 1074; (47) p. 2110; (51) p. 178; (52) p. 591.

WINTER'S BARK

Botanical Name(s): *Drimys winteri* J. R. et G. Forst [Fam.: Winteraceae]

Bark
Constituents: Volatile oil (with eugenol, 1,8-cineole, pinenes, etc.), sesquiterpenes (drimenin, drimenol, confertifolin, polygodial, etc.; many of them are pungent), tannins, flavonoids (flavonols), resin, mannitol, etc.
Properties: Aromatic, stomachic, diuretic, antimicrobial, analgesic.
Uses: Winter's bark is chiefly used as a spice for its pungent flavor and in liqueur / liquor industry. Internally it is used (as a tea, h. p.) for loss of appetite and nonulcer dyspepsia (with flatulence, minor cramps, etc.) and for inflammations of the gastrointestinal tract (diarrhea, etc.). Externally it is used (as a wash) for minor skin inflammations, wounds and ulcers, (as a cotton swab or pasty mass applied to the tooth, or by chewing the herb) for toothache, and (as a partial bath) for rheumatic pains.
Caution: Winter's bark should not be taken during pregnancy and lactation. Otherwise, there are no reports of contraindications or side effects when used properly.

References: (1) Vol. 4, p. 1192; (3) Vol. 4, p. 720; (10) p. 284; (27) p. 108; (35) p. 850; (36) p. 37; (37) p. 438; (41) Vols. 1-7; (52) p. 264.

WINTERGREEN

Other Common Name(s): checkerberry
Botanical Name(s): *Gaultheria procumbens* L. [Fam.: Ericaceae]
Wintergreen oil
It is the volatile oil obtained by steam distillation from the fresh leaves of wintergreen (*Gaultheria procumbens* L.) or the fresh bark of sweet birch (*Betula lenta* L. [Fam.: Betulaceae]), after they have undergone fermentation. The intact fresh wintergreen leaves and sweet birch bark contain gaultherin (= monotropitoside = a methyl salicylate glycoside). With fermentation it liberates methyl salicylate, which is almost the exclusive constituent of natural wintergreen oil. With wintergreen oil is to be understood also the synthetic methyl salicylate. The three sorts have some differences in the aroma. This is due to other components present in natural oils.
Properties: Aromatic, antimicrobial, anti-inflammatory, rubefacient, counterirritant, analgesic.
Uses: Wintergreen oil is chiefly used as a flavor ingredient in mouthwashes, chewing gums, etc., to which it adds its antiseptic effect. Synthetic methyl salicylate is used (as a liniment, ointment combination product) for rheumatic pains (chiefly muscular) and neuralgic pains, among others.
Caution: Wintergreen oil may cause allergic reactions to persons hypersensitive to salicylates (e. g. aspirin). To be considered is also the fact that the skin absorbs it rapidly. Otherwise, there are no reports of contraindications or side effects when used properly.

References: (3) Vol. 3, p. 438; Vol. 4, p. 1104; (8) p. 277; (9) p. 512; (11) p. 94; (12) p. 745; (22) p. 206; (48) p. 252; (55) p. 142; (65) p. 539.

WITCH HAZEL

Botanical Name(s): *Hamamelis virginiana* L. [Fam.: Hamamelidaceae]
Leaf, bark
Constituents: (Leaf): Tannins (chiefly condensed t.: oligomeric proantho-cyanidins = OPCs, etc.; small amounts of a gallotannin: hamamelitannin), flavonoids (flavonols), phenolic acids (gallic and caffeic acids), volatile oil, etc. (Bark): Tannins (chiefly hamamelitannin; some condensed t.), phenolic acids (gallic acid), volatile oil, etc.
Properties: Astringent, anti-inflammatory, wound-healing, hemostatic (topical action). Hamamelis has also shown antioxidant, "vitamin P"-like (= helps in normalizing an increased microvascular permeability and fragility) and topical vasoconstrictor effects. The effects are attributed in large part to phenolics (tannins, flavonoids, gallic acid) and partly to the volatile oil.
Uses: Externally it is used (as a wash, ointment, cream, poultice, etc.) for skin inflammatory conditions (eczemas, diaper rash, etc.), wounds, burns, ulcers (incl. sore nipples), varicose veins in the legs, hemorrhoids, (as a cream with hamamelis water) for eczemas, diaper rash, sunburn and other skin inflammatory conditions, (as a vaginal irrigation / sitz bath / wash) for leukorrhea and vulvovaginitis, and (as a mouthwash, gargle) for inflammations of the mouth and throat. Internally it is used (as a tea, h. p.; at low doses) for inflammations of the gastrointestinal tract (diarrhea, ulcerative colitis, incl. hemorrhoids; also when minor hemorrhages are present).
Caution: There are no reports of contraindications or side effects when used properly. For intestinal bleedings it should be used on professional's advice.

References: (1) Vol. 5, p. 368; (3) Vol. 5, p. 9; (6) pp. 171, 340; (7) p. 285; (8) p. 295; (11) p. 141; (12) p. 880; (13) p. 339; (16) p. 24; (17) p. 270; (19) p. 249; (20) p. 270; (23) pp. 112, 348; (36) p. 228; (46) p. 715; (47) p. 1503; (48) p. 389; (66) p. 298.

WOODRUFF

Other Common Name(s): sweet woodruff
Botanical Name(s): *Galium odoratum* (L.) Scop. = *Asperula odorata* L. [Fam.: Rubiaceae]
Aerial part
Constituents: Coumarins (coumarin, etc.), bitter principles (iridoids: asper-uloside, etc.), phenolic acids (p-coumaric, gallic and caffeic acids, etc.), n-alkanes (n-heptacosane, etc.), anthranoids, etc.
Properties: Aromatic, mild sedative, antispasmodic, diuretic, bitter tonic.
Uses: Sweet woodruff is chiefly used as a fragrance ingredient in perfumery and as a flavor ingredient in food industry. Internally it is used (as a tea, h. p.; combined with other herbs) for insomnia, headaches, primary dysmenor-rhea (= painful menstruation without pathology), loss of appetite and non-ulcer dyspepsia (with minor cramps, etc.) associated with minor spasti conditions of the hepatobiliary tract, and for minor peripheral venous disorders

(varicose veins in the legs, hemorrhoids) and thrombophlebitis (= inflammation of a vein associated with an attached blood clot / thrombus). Externally
it is used (as a wash, wet compress) for minor skin inflammations, wounds
and ulcers.

Caution: There are no reports of contraindications or side effects when used
properly. Nevertheless, before using it for dysmenorrhea, the gynecologic
problem should be judged by a health professional.

References: (1) Vol. 5, p. 222; (3) Vol. 4, p. 1088; (8) p. 275; (9) p. 514; (24) p. 342; (27) p. 320; (28) p. 217; (31) p. 571; (37) pp. 371, 570; (48) p. 273; (51) p. 190.

WORMWOOD

Botanical Name(s): *Artemisia absinthium* L. [Fam.: Asteraceae (Compositae)]

Aerial part (leaves and flowering tops)

Constituents: Bitter principles (sesquiterpene lactones: absinthin, anab-
sinthin, etc.), volatile oil (with β-thujone, thujyl alcohol and thujyl acetate,
or other terpenes; depending on chemotype), phenolic acids (caffeic acid,
etc.), flavonoids (flavonols), etc.

Properties: Bitter tonic, aromatic, choleretic, mild cholagogue, antispasmodic, carminative, antipyretic, antibacterial (against *Staphylococcus* spp.,
Pseudomonas spp., *Klebsiella* spp.), antiprotozoal (against *Plasmodium*
spp.). It possibly exerts mild immunomodulant effect.

Uses: Internally it is used (as a tea, h. p.) for loss of appetite and nonulcer
dyspepsia (with fullness, flatulence, burping, heartburn, minor cramps,
sluggish bowels) associated with impaired bile secretion and flow, and for
feverish states, decreased immune response, convalescence and minor fatigue. In the production of alcoholic bitters, are often used extracts freed in a
selective way from most of thujone. Externally it is used (as a mouthwash)
for bad breath.

Caution: It should not be taken for prolonged period, particularly at higher
doses than recommended as it may lead to absinthism, a chronic intoxication
due to β-thujone, which has been shown to be neurotoxic (cf. SAGE; TAN-
SY; THUJA). At higher doses than recommended it may cause gastrointestinal irritations (with nausea, vomiting, diarrhea). In seldom cases it may
cause allergic contact dermatitis to persons hypersensitive to other Asteraceae plants (e. g. arnica, chamomile, feverfew, ragweed, tansy) that contain
sesquiterpene lactones. Otherwise, there are no reports of contraindication
or side effects when used properly.

References: (1) Vol. 4, p. 360; (3) Vol. 3, p. 254; (8) p. 77; (9) p. 1; (12) p. 486; (13) p. 164; (15) p. 32; (16) p. 139; (17) p. 35; (19) p. 245; (23) p. 129; (28) p. 96; (29) p. 15; (46) p. 118; (51) p. 212.

WORMWOOD, SWEET

Other Common Name(s): annual wormwood, sweet Annie
Botanical Name(s): *Artemisia annua* L. [Fam.: Asteraceae (Compositae)]
Aerial part (qing hao)
Constituents: Bitter principles (sesquiterpene lactones: artemisinin, arteannuin B, etc.), volatile oil (with artemisia ketone, etc.), flavonoids, etc.
Properties: Plasmodicidal. Artemisinin (= arteannuin = qinghaosu) has been shown to be effective against *Plasmodium falciparum*, causative for malignant tertian malaria, even its multi-resistant strains.
Uses: Artemisinin and its derivative, arteether, are used for the treatment of resistant forms of malaria.
Caution: Artemisinin and its derivatives are used only by prescription.

References: (1) Vol. 4, p. 364; (12) p. 672; (13) p. 527; (36) pp. 170, 428; (37) p. 134; (48) p. 623; (53) p. 322.

WORMWOOD, YIN-CHEN

Other Common Name(s): capillaris, capillary artemisia
Botanical Name(s): *Artemisia capillaris* Thunb. [Fam.: Asteraceae (Compositae)]
Aerial part
Constituents: Volatile oil (with pinenes, polyacetylenes, etc.), chromones (capillarisin, etc.), flavonoids (chiefly methoxy-flavones), polyacetylenes (capillin, capillene, etc.), coumarins (scoparone = 6,7-dimethyl-aesculin = 6,7-dimethoxy-coumarin, etc.), phenolic acids, etc.
Properties: Aromatic, bitter tonic, choleretic, antispasmodic, anti-inflammatory, diuretic. Capillarisin has shown choleretic effect, to which may contribute phenolic acids. Many methoxy-flavones have shown anti-inflammatory, antioxidant, antiviral, antibacterial, antifungal, and antispasmodic effects. Polyacetylenes have shown antifungal and antibacterial effects. Scoparone has shown liver protective effect.
Uses: Internally it is used (as a tea, h. p.) for loss of appetite and nonulcer dyspepsia (with flatulence, bloating, minor cramps, etc.), inflammations of the hepatobiliary tract (chronic hepatitis, chronic cholecystitis) and genitourinary tract (cystitis, etc.), and for feverish states.
Caution: Yin-chen wormwood should not be taken in cases of biliary obstruction. In cases of nonobstructive gallstones it can be used but only on health professional's advice. Otherwise, there are no reports of contraindications or side effects when used properly.

References: (1) Vol. 4, p. 367; (29) p. 15; (31) pp. 48, 344, 364, 394; (36) p. 508; (41) Vols. 1-7; (45) p. 170; (52) p. 74.

YAM

Botanical Name(s): *Dioscorea alata* L.; *Dioscorea batatas* Decne.; *Dioscorea esculenta* (Lour.) Burkill; etc. [Fam.: Dioscoreaceae]
Root (tuber)
Constituents: Starch (very rich), mucilaginous polysaccharides, sugars (fructose, galactose), etc. Compared to wild yam (see YAM, WILD) it is almost saponin-free.
Properties: Nutrient, demulcent.
Uses: Internally it is used as an adjuvant (tea, h. p.) for inflammations of the gastrointestinal tract (diarrhea, etc.) and hemorrhoids. From yam is produced starch (Dioscorea starch), which is used much like arrowroot starch (see ARROWROOT).
Caution: See ARROWROOT.

References: (3) Vol. 4, p. 675; (5) Vol. 1, p. 427; (12) p. 566.

YAM, WILD

Botanical Name(s): *Dioscorea villosa* L. [Fam.: Dioscoreaceae]
Root (rhizome)
Constituents: Steroidal saponins (dioscin, gracillarin, etc.; with aglycone: diosgenin), polysaccharides (very rich in starch; possibly some mucilaginous polysaccharides), tannins, minerals, etc.
Properties: Demulcent, emollient. The effects are due to the high starch content, small concentrations of saponins, and possibly mucilage.
Uses: Internally it is used (as a tea, h. p.) for inflammations of the gastrointestinal tract (gastritis, diarrhea, etc.). Due to the steroidal saponins it may be beneficial for high cholesterol (see FENUGREEK). Externally it is used (as a wet compress, poultice, cream) for minor skin inflammations.
Caution: There are no reports of contraindications or side effects when used properly. Creams that contain only wild yam extracts, with no progesterone incorporated, exert only emollient (= softening and soothing) effect.

References: (3) Vol. 4, p. 673; (12) p. 566; (15) p. 78; (22) p. 187; (25) p. 204; (35) p. 863; (36) pp. 295, 512; (37) p. 420; (42) Vol. 2, p. 145.

YARROW

Other Common Name(s): milfoil
Botanical Name(s): *Achillea millefolium* L. [F.: Asteraceae (Compositae)]
Aerial part
Constituents: Volatile oil (with an azulene: chamazulene; etc.), bitter principles (sesquiterpene lactones: achillicin, etc.), flavonoids (flavones: apigenin, luteolin, their glycosides, etc.), coumarins, proline-betaines (betonicine, stachydrine), polyacetylenes, phenolic acids, etc. Depending on

398

chemotype, the herb can be free of sesquiterpene lactones and the oil can be chamazulene-free accordingly.

Properties: Aromatic, bitter tonic, choleretic, cholagogue, anti-inflammatory, antispasmodic, emmenagogue, astringent, antimicrobial. The bitter tonic and hepatobiliary effects are due to the bitter sesquiterpene lactones, proline-betaines and phenolic acids. Yarrow volatile oil has shown anti-inflammatory and antimicrobial effects. Yarrow (flower, essential oil) acts and is used much like chamomile. Phenolic acids are also astringents.

Uses: Internally it is used (as a tea, h. p.) for loss of appetite and nonulcer dyspepsia (with flatulence, minor cramps, minor diarrhea) associated with impaired bile secretion and flow, for inflammatory and spastic conditions of the genitourinary tract (cystitis, etc.), primary dysmenorrhea (= painful menstruation without pathology), inflammations of the upper respiratory tract (the common cold and feverish states; also as a diaphoretic hot tea). Externally it is used (as a wash, wet compress, poultice) for minor skin inflammations, wounds and hemorrhoids, (as an enema) for hemorrhoids, (as an irrigation / sitz bath / wash; often combined with other herbs) for leukorrhea, vulvovaginitis, primary dysmenorrhea, and (as a mouthwash) for inflammations of the mouth.

Caution: Before using it for dysmenorrhea and other gynecologic disorders, the problem should be judged by a health professional. Yarrow may cause allergic contact dermatitis to persons hypersensitive to other Asteraceae plants (e. g. arnica, chamomile, feverfew, ragweed, tansy) that contain sesquiterpene lactones. Otherwise, there are no reports of contraindications or side effects when used properly.

References: (1) Vol. 4, p. 46; (3) Vol. 2, p. 890; (8) p. 18; (9) p. 518; (12) p. 483; (13) p. 122; (14) p. 227; (16) p. 129; (17) p. 395; (19) p. 200; (23) p. 125, (28) p. 101; (37) p. 13; (46) p. 1; (47) p. 1911; (48) p. 337; (51) p. 206.

YARROW, MUSK

Other Common Name(s): black milfoil, musk herb, iva herb
Botanical Name(s): *Achillea moschata* Wulfen in Jacq. [Fam.: Asteraceae (Compositae)]

Aerial part
Constituents: Volatile oil (with 1,8-cineole, camphor, valeraldehyde, etc.), bitter principles (sesquiterpene lactones), coumarins (scopoletin), flavonoids (apigenin), etc.

Properties: Aromatic, bitter tonic, antimicrobial, antispasmodic, diuretic. The effects are mild.

Uses: Internally it is used (as a tea, h. p.) for loss of appetite and nonulcer dyspepsia (with flatulence, minor cramps, etc.), and (usually combined with other herbs) for inflammations of the upper respiratory and genitourinary tracts. Externally it is used (as a wash, wet compress, poultice) for minor skin inflammations and wounds. It is also used as a flavor ingredient in some bitters (e. g. Iva Bitter).

Caution: At higher doses than recommended it may cause gastrointestinal irritations (with nausea, vomiting, diarrhea). Otherwise, there are no reports of side effects when used properly.

References: (1) Vol. 4, p. 52; (3) Vol. 2, p. 892; (5) Vol. 1, p. 13; (24) p. 455; (37) p. 13; (52) p. 8.

YELLOW CHASTE WEED

Other Common Name(s): yellow immortelle, everlasting flower, sandy everlasting
Botanical Name(s): *Helichrysum arenarium* Moench. [Fam.: Asteraceae (Compositae)]
Flower
Constituents: Flavonoids (isosalipurposide, helechrysins A and B, etc.), phenolic acids (caffeic acid derivatives), bitter principles (sesquiterpene lactones, etc.), phthalides, volatile oil, tannins, coumarins, triterpenes (ursolic acid), phytosterols (5-sterols: β-sitosterol, etc.), etc.
Properties: Choleretic, cholagogue, bitter tonic, antioxidant, liver protective, diuretic, anti-inflammatory, antiallergic, antispasmodic. The hepatobiliary effects (possibly mild artichoke-like) are due in large part to phenolic acids and flavonoids. The anti-inflammatory, antiallergic and antispasmodic effects (possibly by inhibiting the biosynthesis of prostaglandins and leukotrienes) may be due in large part to phytosterols, coumarins, phthalides, and sesquiterpene lactones.
Uses: Internally it is used (as a tea, h. p.; usually combined with other herbs) for nonulcer dyspepsia (with fullness, nausea, change of bowel habits) associated with minor inflammatory and spastic conditions of the hepatobiliary tract (impaired bile secretion and flow, chronic cholecystitis, nonobstructive gallstones). It has also been tried with good results for minor inflammatory and spastic conditions of the upper respiratory tract (spastic bronchitis, allergic rhinitis, bronchial asthma, whooping cough) and chronic skin disorders (eczema, psoriasis). Externally it is used (as a poultice, ointment) for skin inflammations, minor burns (incl. sunburn), varicose veins (incl. hemorrhoids), eczema and psoriasis. Due to its intensive yellow color, it is incorporated in herbal teas mainly to enhance their appearance.
Caution: Yellow chaste weed should not be taken in cases of biliary obstruction. In cases of nonobstructive gallstones it can be used but only on health professional's advice. It may cause allergic contact dermatitis to persons hypersensitive to other Asteraceae plants (e. g. arnica, chamomile, feverfew, ragweed, tansy, yarrow) that contain sesquiterpene lactones. Otherwise, there are no reports of side effects when used properly.

References: (3) Vol. 5, p. 34; (8) p. 303; (9) p. 315; (12) p. 821; (17) p. 287; (19) p. 195; (24) p. 192; (37) p. 648; (46) p. 533; (47) p. 1469; (51) p. 204.

YELLOW ROOT

Botanical Name(s): *Xanthorhiza simplicissima* Marshall [Fam.: Ranunculaceae]
Root
Constituents: According to old reports, it contains isoquinoline alkaloids chiefly of protoberberine type (berberine, jatrorrhizine), also aporphine type (magnoflorine). It is often found as an adulterant of goldenseal, but it doesn't contain hydrastine.
Properties: Based on reported constituents it possibly acts like barberry and coptis . See BARBERRY; COPTIS.
Uses: Internally it is used (as a tea, h. p.) chiefly for disorders of the gastrointestinal and hepatobiliary tracts, much like barberry and coptis, and partly like goldenseal. See BARBERRY; COPTIS.
Caution: See BARBERRY.

References: (3) Vol. 6c, p. 525; (25) p. 240; (37) p. 197; (44) p. 602.

YERBA MANSA

Other Common Name(s): apache beads
Botanical Name(s): *Anemopsis californica* (Nutt.) Hook et Arn. [Fam.: Saururaceae]
Root
Constituents: Volatile oil (with eugenol methyl ether, thymol, piperitone, estragole = methylchavicol, 1,8-cineole, etc.), lignans (asarinin = sesamin isomer, and possibly others), etc.
Properties: Antimicrobial, antispasmodic. Thymol is antimicrobial. Eugenol methyl ether (= methyleugenol = 4-allylveratrole) has shown antispasmodic effect. There are lignans that have shown anti-inflammatory, liver protective, immunomodulant and antimicrobial effects.
Uses: Internally it is used (as a tea, h. p.) for inflammatory and spastic conditions of the gastrointestinal tract (diarrhea, etc.), upper respiratory tract (the common cold, pharyngitis, bronchitis, etc.; spastic dry coughs) and genitourinary tract (cystitis, urethritis), and primary dysmenorrhea (= painful menstruation without pathology). Externally it is used (as a mouthwash, gargle) for inflammations of the mouth and throat, (as a wash, wet compress) for wounds, and (as a sitz bath) for anal and genital inflammations and primary dysmenorrhea.
Caution: At higher doses than recommended yerba mansa may cause gastrointestinal irritations (with nausea, vomiting). Otherwise, there are no reports of contraindications or side effects when used properly.

References: (3) Vol. 3, p. 84; (5) Vol. 1, p. 82; Vol. 3, p. 288; (29) p. 10; (31) p. 480; (42) p. 304; (44) p. 73; (52) p. 50.

401

YERBA SANTA

Other Common Name(s): California yerba santa
Botanical Name(s): *Eriodictyon californicum* (Hook. et Arn.) Torr. = *Eriodictyon glutinosum* Benth. [Fam.: Hydrophyllaceae]
Leaf (often with thin twigs)
Constituents: Flavonoids (rich in flavanones: homoeriodictyol, etc.), volatile oil (pungent taste), tannins (hydrolyzable t.), organic acids (formic acid and acetic acids, etc.), saponins (?), etc.
Properties: Taste suppressant (blocks the bitter taste, without influencing the sweet, acid or salt taste), anti-inflammatory, antioxidant, antimicrobial, expectorant, antispasmodic, diuretic. Possibly, the taste suppressant effect is due to homoeriodictyol and closely related flavanones.
Uses: Internally it is used as a flavor ingredient to mask or correct the bitter taste of some drugs, and (as a tea, h. p.) for inflammations of the upper respiratory tract (the common cold, laryngitis, bronchitis, bronchial asthma, etc.; irritating dry cough, whooping cough) and genitourinary tract (cystitis, urethritis, etc.). It is also used as an antidyscratic (= blood purifier) for chronic rheumatic complaints. To enhance the effects in problems of the genitourinary tract, the fluid intake (incl. herbal teas) should be more than 2 liters per day. Externally it is used (as a poultice) for wounds, rheumatic pains, insect bites, bruises and sprains.
Caution: There are no reports of contraindications or side effects when used properly.
Note: Other species used similarly are, narrow-leaf yerba santa: *Eriodictyon angustifolium* Nutt.; hairy yerba santa: *Eriodictyon trichocalyx* A. Heller.; wooly yerba santa: *Eriodictyon tomentosum* Benth.; and thick-leaf yerba santa: *Eriodictyon crassifolium* Benth.

References: (2) Vol. 2, p. 614; (3) Vol. 4, p. 799; (8) p. 247; (9) p. 520; (10) p. 291; (12a) p. 393; (29) p. 48; (31) pp. 375, 388; (35) p. 865; (36) p. 288; (37) p. 481; (44) p. 220; (47) p. 1288; (52) p. 285; (65) p. 23; (66) p. 275.

YLANG YLANG

Botanical Name(s): *Cananga odorata* J.D. Hook. et T. Thompson [Fam.: Annonaceae]
Ylang ylang oil
It is the volatile oil obtained by steam distillation from the fresh flowers.
Constituents: Monoterpenes (linalool, geraniol, geranyl acetate, methyl benzoate, pinenes, etc.), sesquiterpenes (farnesol, caryophyllene, etc.), phenylpropanoids (eugenol, isoeugenol, etc.), etc.
Properties: Aromatic.
Uses: It is widely used in perfumery, cosmetics, and aromatherapy.
Caution: Ylang ylang oil has not shown irritating or allergic effects.

402

References: (3) Vol. 3, p. 649; (5) Vol. 1, p. 211; (9) p. 521; (37) p. 264.

YOHIMBE

Other Common Name(s): johimbe
Botanical Name(s): *Pausinystalia yohimbe* (K. Schum.) Pierre ex Beille = *Corynanthe yohimbe* K. Schum. [Fam.: Rubiaceae]
Bark
Constituents: Indole alkaloids, chiefly yohimbine, also its stereoisomer α-yohimbine (= rauwolscine), and smaller amounts of other closely related alkaloids.
Properties: Aphrodisiac, due in large part to yohimbine. At low doses yohimbine increases blood pressure. At higher doses it dilates peripheral blood vessels and lowers blood pressure. Yohimbine exerts also local anesthetic effect. Due to the presence of other alkaloids the overall effect of the herb is different from pure yohimbine.
Uses: <u>Internally</u> it is used (chiefly as yohimbine, also as a standardized h. p.) for erectile dysfunction and urinary incontinence.
Caution: Yohimbe may cause tachycardia, anxiety, insomnia, headache, nausea and tremor, among others. It should not be combined with MAOI antidepressant drugs (e. g. phenelzine) or herbs (e. g. St. Joh's wort) as it may potentiate their effect. It should not be used in liver and kidney disorders. Yohimbe is best used on health professional's advice. Yohimbine is a prescription drug.

References: (2) Vol. 3, p. 317; (3) Vol. 6a, p. 482; (6) p. 292; (11) p. 169; (12) p. 1029; (13) p. 256; (46) p. 1783; (48) p. 1015; (67) p. 496.

YOHIMBE, FALSE

Other Common Name(s): pseudocinchona
Botanical Name(s): *Corynanthe pachyceras* K. Schum. = *Pausinystalia pachyceras* (K. Schum.) De Wild. [Fam.: Rubiaceae]
Bark
Constituents: Indole alkaloids, including corynanthine and a yohimbine stereoisomer (α-yohimbine = rauwolscine), among others. No yohimbine is found present.
Properties: Antipyretic, mild sedative, mild antihypertensive.
Uses: <u>Internally</u> it is used (as a tea, h. p.) for feverish states and the common cold, and as an adjuvant for minor hypertension. It is claimed to be aphrodisiac and recommended for erectile dysfunction.
Caution: False yohimbe should be used only as directed by an experienced practitioner as it contains potential alkaloids.

References: (1) Vol. 4, p. 1029; (52) p. 570.

YUCCA

Other Common Name(s): 1) aloe yucca, dagger plant, Spanish bayonet, yucca 2) Adam's needle, yucca 3) soapweed, soapwell, yucca 4) Mojave yucca; etc.

Botanical Name(s): 1) *Yucca aloifolia* L. 2) *Yucca filamentosa* L. 3) *Yucca glauca* Nutt 4) *Yucca schidigera* Roezl ex Ortgies; etc. [Fam.: Agavaceae]

Root

Constituents: Steroidal saponins, with aglycones depending on species and origin such as tigogenin and smilagenin in aloe yucca, and sarsasapogenin in Adam's needle; etc.

Properties and Uses: Internally may be beneficial for high cholesterol (due to steroidal saponins; see FENUGREEK). It is claimed to be anti-inflammatory and effective for rheumatic complaints (incl. rheumatoid arthritis). Externally it is used (as a wash, wet compress, poultice) for minor skin inflammations and (as a hair wash / rinse) for dandruff.

Caution: There are no reports of contraindications or side effects when used properly.

References: (2) Vol. 3, p. 804; (3) Vol. 6c, p. 547; (9) p. 524; (21) p. 397; (29) p. 124; (42) Vol. 2, p. 33; (44) pp. 603, 606; (52) p. 878.

ZEDOARY

Botanical Name(s): *Curcuma zedoaria* (Christm.) Roscoe [Fam.: Zingiberaceae]

Root (tuber) (zedoary root, Indian arrowroot)

Constituents: Volatile oil (with zingiberene, 1,8-cineole, α-pinene, camphene, camphor, borneol, etc.), curcuminoids (curcumin, demethoxycurcumin, etc.), ethyl ester of p-methoxy cinnamic acid, starch (rich), proteins, mucilaginous polysaccharides, etc.

Properties: Aromatic, stomachic, choleretic, carminative, antispasmodic, antimicrobial.

Uses: Zedoary is chiefly used as a spice, sometimes to replace turmeric in curry powder (cf. TURMERIC). Zedoary, especially zedoary oil, is used in liqueur / liquor industry. From fresh tubers is also prepared starch (arrowroot starch; see ARROWROOT). Internally it is used (as a tea, h. p.; usually combined with other herbs) for loss of appetite and nonulcer dyspepsia (with fullness, flatulence, minor cramps, etc.) associated with impaired bile secretion and flow, for inflammatory conditions of the upper respiratory tract (bronchitis, colds), and as a tonic.

Caution: There are no reports of contraindications or side effects when used properly and consumed as a spice in moderate amounts.

References: (1) Vol. 4, p. 1098; (3) Vol. 4, p. 387; (8) p. 208; (35) p. 866; (36) p. 504; (37) p. 372; (46) p. 1805.

GLOSSARY OF MEDICAL TERMS

Abortifacient: inducing abortion.

Acidulous: having a sour or acid taste.

Adaptogenic: increasing adaptation and resistance to physical, chemical and biologic (non-infectious) stressors.

Adjuvant: aiding or enhancing the effects of a medication.

Anabolic: promoting anabolism (= biosynthesis of macromolecular body substances such as proteins).

Analeptic: restoring or stimulating central nervous system.

Analgesic: relieving pain.

Anaphrodisiac: decreasing hyperactive sexual desires.

Anesthetic (here local anesthetic)**:** inducing a temporary loss of local sensation by blocking sensory nerves.

Anthelmintic: destroying or expelling intestinal parasitic worms.

Antiallergic: relieving allergy.

Antiarrhythmic: preventing or relieving cardiac arrhythmias.

Antibacterial: killing or inhibiting the growth of bacteria.

Anticoagulant: delaying or inhibiting blood clotting.

Anticonvulsant: relieving or inhibiting convulsions.

Antidepressive (= antidepressant)**:** relieving or preventing psychic depression.

Antidiarrheal: relieving or stopping diarrhea.

Antidyscratic (= blood purifier = depurative = blood cleanser)**:** an agent, which by enhancing the excretion of bodily wastes through hepatobiliary, urinary and gastrointestinal tracts, helps in correcting dyscrasia (= an imbalanced condition in general, esp. of blood). These agents are still recommended for chronic rheumatic complaints and atopic eczema (= chronic eczema of internal origin), among others.

Antiedematous: relieving or preventing edemas.

Antiemetic: preventing, relieving or stopping vomiting.

Antiexudative: relieving or preventing exudation (= oozing of fluids from blood vessels, usually associated with inflammation).

Antifungal: killing or inhibiting the growth of fungi.

Anti-gout: relieving or preventing gout (= inflamed and painful joints, associated with deposition of urates in and around the joints).

Antihidrotic: preventing or inhibiting sweat secretions.

Antihistaminic: tending to counteract the effects of histamine, a biogenic amine found normally in our body in certain levels. Histamine is a mediator of allergic reactions. It constricts bronchi, dilates capillaries, and increases gastric secretion, among other effects.

Antihyperglycemic: reducing hyperglycemia (= elevated blood sugar).

Antihypertensive: reducing hypertension (= high blood pressure).

Anti-inflammatory: relieving or preventing inflammation (= a local tissue reaction marked esp. by redness, heat, swelling and pain, due to injuries or infections).

Antimalarial: relieving or preventing malaria.

Antimicrobial: killing or inhibiting the growth of microbes (= microorganisms, esp. bacteria).

Antimitotic: inhibiting or disrupting mitosis (= a type of cell division).

Antineoplastic: inhibiting or preventing neoplasms (= abnormal growths).

Antioxidant: preventing oxidation and protecting from the formation of free radicals.

Antiprotozoal: killing or inhibiting the growth of protozoa (= single-celled organisms such as amebas).

Antipruritic: relieving or checking pruritus (= itching).

Antipyretic (= febrifuge): reducing fever.

Antirheumatic: relieving or preventing rheumatism (= painful inflammation esp. in the joints and muscles).

Antiseptic: preventing or controlling sepsis (= a widespread bacterial infection).

Antispasmodic: relieving or preventing spasms or cramps.

Antithyrotropic: preventing the iodination of precursors of thyroxine and triiodothyronine, both iodine-containing thyroid hormones.

Antitussive: relieving or checking cough.

Antiulcer: preventing or healing peptic ulcers.

Antiviral: killing or inhibiting the growth of viruses.

Anxiolytic (= antianxiety): relieving or checking anxiety.

Aphrodisiac: stimulating sexual desire.

Astringent: drawing together soft tissues (e. g. the skin).

Bitter tonic: stimulating appetite and improving digestion. Bitter botanicals, in moderate amounts, stimulate appetite, increase secretions of the mouth, stomach, liver, and pancreas, restore the normal tonus of the gastrointestinal smooth musculature (incl. biliary tract), aid the absorption of foods, and exert mild immunostimulant effect (by strengthening chiefly the first line / non-specific immune defense).

Blood purifier: see **Antidyscratic**.

Bronchodilatory: dilating the bronchi.

Carcinogenic: causing cancer.

Cardioactive: acting upon the heart.

Cardiotonic: increasing the contractility of the heart muscle.

Carminative: expelling gas from the gastrointestinal tract.

Cholagogue (= Cholagogic): promoting bile flow.

Choleretic: promoting bile secretion by the liver.

Counterirritant: producing a superficial inflammation and irritation (after external application). Counterirritants are stronger than rubefacients (q. v.).

Cytostatic: preventing or retarding the cell growth and multiplication.

Cytotoxic: having harmful or destroying effects upon cells.

Decoction: a liquid preparation made by putting an herb in water, bringing to a boil, simmering for a time, and then straining.

406

Demulcent: covering mucous membranes and soothing them when inflamed.

"Detoxify": diminish the effects of toxins or remove them through body excretions.

Diaphoretic: increasing or inducing perspiration.

Digestant: aiding the digestion, breaking down of foods.

Diuretic: increasing urine excretion and flow.

Drastic: strong purgative (q. v.)

Emetic: inducing vomit.

Emmenagogue (= Emmenagogic): promoting menstruation.

Emollient: covering, softening the skin and soothing it when inflamed or damaged superficially.

Estrogens: female sex hormones (e. g. estradiol), which are responsible for the estrus (= a state of female sexual excitability) and the development of female secondary sexual characteristics.

Estrogen-like: this term comprises pro-estrogenic and anti-estrogenic elements. Some herbs contain the so-called phytoestrogens (e. g. isoflavones), whose metabolites have been shown to inhibit binding of stronger estrogens (e. g. estradiol) to their receptors therefore they are considered antiestrogens. Depending on the hormone imbalance stage (when estrogens level is lower than expected) they may exert proestrogenic effects.

Euphoriant: inducing euphoria.

Expectorant: facilitating the expulsion of secretions from the respiratory tract.

Febrifuge: see **Antipyretic.**

Galactagogue: promoting the secretion of milk in nursing mothers.

Hemostatic: checking hemorrhage.

Hepatotoxic: having harmful or toxic effects upon liver.

Hypnotic: inducing sleep.

Immunomodulant: adjusting the immune response. Usually, at low doses they stimulate it (= immunostimulant effect), at high doses they decrease or suppress it (immunosuppressant effect).

Immunostimulant: stimulating the immune response.

Infusion: a liquid preparation made by pouring boiling water on an herb, letting the mixture to steep for a time, and then straining.

Insecticidal: killing insects.

Keratolytic: braking down the horny outer layer of the skin.

Laxative: facilitating defecation, relieving constipation.

Maceration: a liquid preparation made by putting an herb in a solvent (water, etc.), letting the mixture at room temperature to steep for a time, and then straining.

Narcotic: inducing mental numbness or unconsciousness.

Nootropic: increasing cognitive function.

NSAID-like: acting in a similar way to nonsteroidal anti-inflammatory drugs (e. g. aspirin, ibuprofen, etc.), i. e. relieving or preventing inflammation, and exerting analgesic and antipyretic effects.

Oxytocic: stimulating contractions of the uterine smooth musculature and promoting rapid childbirth.

Parasympatholytic: challenging the effects or blocking the action of parasympathetic nervous system (= a division of the autonomic nervous system).

Parasympathomimetic: stimulating or enhancing the effects of parasympathetic nervous system (= a division of the autonomic nervous system).

Pediculicide: destroying lice.

Phototoxic: causing toxic effects (esp. skin irritations) by exposure to strong sunrays. This may happen after handling herbs, spices or essential oils rich in furanocoumarins (esp. of linear type) or taking their teas or products.

Platelet aggregation inhibitory: inhibiting the aggregation or adhesion of blood platelets (= thrombocytes), preventing the formation of thrombi.

Prolactin (Lat. *lac* = milk): a hormone secreted by the anterior lobe of pituitary gland (= hypophysis). It stimulates and maintains the secretion of milk after childbirth and promotes the growth of breast tissue. Elevated levels of prolactin are associated with amenorrhea (= ceased, infrequent menstruation), among others.

Purgative (= cathartic): causing the evacuation of bowels. Purgatives are stronger than laxatives (q. v.).

Refrigerant: relieving fever and thirst; cooling.

Rubefacient: causing redness of the skin (after external application).

Secretagogue: digestive secretagogue (= increasing secretions of the mouth, stomach, liver, and pancreas); bronchial secretagogue (increasing secretions of the upper respiratory tract, incl. bronchi).

Sedative: calming an irritable state esp. of the central nervous system.

Sialagogue: increasing the flow of saliva.

Stomachic: stimulating the stomach function.

Sympatholytic: challenging the effects or blocking the action of sympathetic nervous system (= a division of the autonomic nervous system).

Sympathomimetic: stimulating or enhancing the effects of sympathetic nervous system (= a division of the autonomic nervous system).

Taeniafuge: expelling tapeworms.

Teratogenic: causing abnormal growth of fetus.

Tonic: invigorating, increasing the tonus.

Uterotonic: restoring or increasing the tonus of uterine musculature.

Vasoconstrictor: constricting or making narrower blood vessels.

Vasodilator: dilating or making wider blood vessels.

Vasotonic: restoring or increasing the tonus of blood vessels.

Venotonic: restoring or increasing the tonus of veins.

Vesicant: causing blisters.

"Vitamin P"-like: helps in normalizing an increased microvascular permeability and fragility.

Vulnerary: wound-healing.

GLOSSARY OF CHEMICAL TERMS

Acetophenones: derivatives of acetophenone (= methyl phenyl ketone).

Acetylenes: see **Polyacetylenes**.

Aglycone: non-sugar moiety of a glycoside (q. v.).

Alcohol Glycosides: glycosides (q. v.) that as an aglycone moiety have an alcohol, more exactly a phenol-alcohol.

Aldehyde Glycosides: glycosides (q. v.) that as an aglycone moiety have an aldehyde, more exactly a phenol-aldehyde.

Alkaloids: compounds (chiefly basic; alkaloid = alkali-like) mostly of plant origin, which contain one or more nitrogen atoms, normally in a heterocyclic ring. They exert a marked physiological action on human and animal organisms.

Anthranoids: anthracene derivatives, particularly those based on 1,8-dihydroxy-9,10-anthraquinone, commonly referred to as hydroxyanthraquinones or anthraquinones, which are chiefly found as glycosides (commonly referred to as anthraquinone glycosides) but also as free compounds.

Balsams: mixtures of a resin (q. v.) and "volatile oil". Their "volatile oil" is chiefly constituted of high-boiling compounds (benzoic acid, cinnamic acid, and their esters), but also low-boiling compounds (e. g. vanillin). Sometimes this name is incorrectly applied to oleoresins (q. v.).

Benzofurans: derivatives of benzofuran (= coumarone), which itself is formed by a combination of benzene and furan.

Benzoquinones: derivatives of p-benzoquinone.

Bioflavonoids: see **Flavonoids**.

Biogenic Amines: organic derivatives of ammonia (alkyl-substituted compounds: betaine, choline, etc.; aryl-substituted compounds: phenylethylamine, tyramine, histamine, etc.), which exert a marked physiological action. Norepinephrine and epinephrine are also biogenic amines, but they are not found in plants.

Bitter Principles: compounds of different groups such as iridoids (q. v.), etc., which have a marked bitter taste.

Carbohydrates: compounds which consist of carbon, hydrogen and oxygen, and in which hydrogen and oxygen are generally in the same proportions as in water.

Cardiac Glycosides: glycosides (q. v.) that as an aglycone moiety have a steroidal alcohol with a five-membered lactone ring (cardenolide type) or six-membered lactone ring (bufadienolide type). They exert a marked physiological action upon the cardiac muscle.

Carotenoids: tetraterpenoids, found in plants as red to yellow pigments.

Chromones: derivatives of chromone (= benzo-γ-pyrone), a compound formed by a combination of benzene and γ-pyrone.

Clovamides: amides of caffeic acid with dopa (= 3,4-dihydroxyphenylalanine).

Coumarins: derivatives of coumarin (benzo-α-pyrone = 1,2-benzopyrone) that on its part is considered formally a lactone of cis-o-hydroxycinnamic acid. They occur also as glycosides.

Coumestans (= coumarono-coumarins): compounds formed by a combination of coumarone (= benzofuran) and coumarin.

Cyanogenic Glycosides: glycosides (q. v.) that yield hydrocyanic acid as one of their products of hydrolysis.

Cyclitols: polyalcohols based on cyclohexane.

Depsides: ester-like derivatives of two or more phenolic acids.

Depsidones: depsides (q. v.) with one -O- linkage making a third ring.

Dibenzofurans: derivatives of dibenzofuran, which itself is formed by a combination of two benzene rings and one furan ring between them.

Essential Oils: see **Volatile Oils**.

Fats: substances constituted mainly of esters of glycerol (= glycerin) with fatty acids (q. v.). At ordinary temperatures they have a semisolid or solid consistency.

Fatty Acids: long-chain carboxylic acids, present in fats and fixed oils as esters of glycerol. They are saturated (without double bonds), monounsaturated (with one double bond), and polyunsaturated (with more than one double bond).

Fixed Oils: substances constituted mainly of esters of glycerol with fatty acids (mainly unsaturated fatty acids). At ordinary temperatures they usually have a liquid consistency.

Flavonoids (= bioflavonoids): derivatives of flavan (= 2-phenylbenzopyran = 2-phenylchromane) such as flavones, flavonols, flavanones and anthocyanidins, or isoflavan (= 3-phenylbenzopyran = 3-phenylchromane) such as isoflavones (q. v.), which contain free, methylated or glycosidically bound phenol groups. Generally, they are yellow (Lat. *flavus* = yellow), red or blue in color.

Furanochromones (= furochromones): phenolic compounds formed by a linear combination of furan with chromone (= benzo-γ-pyrone, q. v.).

Furanocoumarins (= furocoumarins): compounds formed by a linear or angular combination of furan with coumarin derivatives. Linear compounds (e. g. bergaptene) are phototoxic.

"Glucokinin": it is a coined name. It tells that among the known or unknown constituents of a botanical, there is a constituent with antihyperglycemic effect.

Glycone: sugar moiety of a glycoside (q. v.).

Glucosinolates (= isothiocyanate glucosides): glycosides that under the action of an enzyme (myrosinase) liberate volatile isothiocyanates (= mustard oils). The sugar moiety is glucose.

Glycosides: compounds made of two moieties, namely aglycone (= non-sugar component) and glycone (= sugar component). Aglycone can be an alcohol, an aldehyde (phenol-aldehyde), phenolic compounds (hydroquinone,

410

flavonoids, anthraquinones, etc.), etc. Glycone or sugar moiety can be one glucose and the resulting glycoside is a glucoside (e.g. arbutin = hydroquinone-glucoside), one rhamnose and the resulting glycoside is a rhamnoside (e. g. adonitoxol = adonitoxigenol-rhamnoside), etc.

Gum-oleoresins: natural mixtures of **oleoresins** (q. v.) and **gums** (q. v.).

Gums: mixtures of polysaccharides, which ooze as viscous solutions from plants after injuries and then harden after contact with air. They form viscous sticky solutions with water.

Inulin: a polysaccharide made of almost only fructose units.

Iridoids: bitter tasting monoterpenoid lactones.

Isoflavones: flavonoids (q. v.), which are derivatives of 3-phenylbenzopyran (= 3-phenylchromane), found (mostly) free or as glycosides. They are isomers of flavones (see **Flavonoids**).

Isothiocyanates: (= Mustard oils): volatile compounds liberated after the enzymatic hydrolysis of glucosinolates (q. v.).

Lectins (= phytohemagglutinins): proteins and glycoproteins that have the quality of combining with specific sugars such as those of glycoproteins and glycolipids located on the surface of the red blood cells, lymphocytes, etc., and agglutinate them.

Lignans: dimers of phenylpropanoid compounds, often found as constituents of resins.

Lignin: a polymer of phenylpropanoid compounds (e. g. coniferyl alcohol), which with cellulose is found in certain cell walls of woody plants.

Monosaccharides: carbohydrates, as simple sugars.

Mucilages: (= mucilaginous polysaccharides): mixtures of polysaccharides, which with water form non-sticky viscous solutions.

Mucilaginous polysaccharides: see **Mucilages**

Mustard oils (= isothiocyanates): see **Isothiocyanates**

Naphthodianthrones (= naphthoanthraquinones): dimers of anthraquinones (cf. **Anthranoids**).

Naphthoquinones: compounds based on 1,4-naphthoquinone (= quinone of naphthalene).

Oleo-gum-resins or **Gum-oleoresins** (q. v.)

Oleoresins: natural mixtures of resins (q. v.) and volatile oils (q. v.). They are sometimes incorrectly designated as balsams (q. v.).

Pectins: polysaccharides constituted of monosaccharides and uronic acids (esp. galacturonic acid).

Phenol Glycosides: glycosides (q. v.) that as an aglycone moiety have a phenol.

Phenolic Acids: phenol-carboxylic compounds derived either from benzoic acid (e. g. gallic acid) or cinnamic acid (e. g. caffeic acid).

Phlobaphenes: red insoluble polymers of condensed tannins.

Phospholipids (= phosphatides): complex lipids constituted of phosphoric acid, fatty acids, an alcohol (glycerol, sphingosin) and an N base (choline).

Phytoestrogens: plant constituents with estrogen-like effect, whose metabolites have been shown to inhibit binding of stronger estrogens to their receptors therefore regarded as antiestrogens. Depending on the hormone imbalance stage, when estrogens level is lower than expected, they may exert proestrogenic effects. Chemically they are a diverse group of natural compounds such as coumestans (e.g. coumestrol), isoflavones (e.g. genistein, daidzein, formononetin), flavanones (e.g. 8-prenyl-naringenin), stilbenes (e.g. resveratrol), lignans (enterodiol).

Phytosterols: plant sterols such as 5-sterols (β-sitosterol, etc., very seldom cholesterol), 7-sterols (α-spinasterol, etc.), and 5 & 7-sterols (ergosterol, etc.). Other plant sterols are phytoecdysteroids = phytoecdysones (ecdysterone, cyasterone, etc.) and withanolides (withaferin A, withanolide E, etc.).

Polyacetylenes: hydrocarbons that in their structure have more than one acetylenic group (triple bond). Often they are called acetylenes.

Prolin-betaines: compounds formed by a combination of pyrrolidine and betaine (a biogenic amine, q. v.).

Resins: amorphous, nonvolatile and complex mixtures of resin acids, resin alcohols, resin phenols, esters and inert resenes.

Saponins: glycosides (q. v.) that as their aglycone moiety (= sapogenin) have a steroidal or triterpenoid alcohol. Their water solutions foam upon shaking (Lat. *sapo* = soap).

Starch: a polysaccharide, namely a polymer of glucose.

Stilbenoids: (incl. stilbenes and phenanthrenes): phenolic compounds, derivatives of diphenyl ethene or diphenyl ethane.

Sugar Alcohols: polyalcohols, which occur in plants naturally or are obtained by reduction (hydrogenation) of aldehyde or keto groups of monosaccharides (q. v.).

Sugars: a common name for carbohydrates (q. v.) with sweet taste.

Tannins: complex nitrogen-free polyphenolic compounds, which can combine with animal proteins of the skin or other tissues and cause tightening, astringent or tanning effects. They are classified in two major groups, namely in hydrolyzable tannins (gallotannins, ellagitanins) and condensed tannins (proanthocyanidins).

Thiophenes: derivatives of thiophene (a sulfur containing heterocyclic compound). Many thiophenes have acetylenic substituents.

Volatile Oils (= essential oils = ethereal oils): steam-distilling liquids found mainly as such in plants. They contain a complex mixture of odoriferous compounds. At ordinary temperature they evaporate, compared to fixed oils, which do not.

Waxes: complex mixtures of esters of fatty acids (long and straight chain, mostly saturated fatty acids) with alcohols (mostly monovalent, straight chain alcohols).

Xanthones: derivatives of dibenzo-γ-pyrone, often found as glycosides. They are yellow to red-yellow in color.

412

THERAPEUTIC CHECKLIST

NERVOUS SYSTEM DISORDERS

Nervousness; Restlessness; Anxiety

• ASHWAGANDHA • BALM, LEMON • BUPLEURUM • CELERY • DEER'S TONGUE • DITTA-NY, WHITE • GELSEMIUM • DOGWOOD, JAMAICA • GOTU KOLA • HOPS • HOREHOUND, BLACK • INDIAN PIPE • KAVA • LADY'S SLIPPER • LAVENDER • LINDEN • PASSION-FLOWER • POPPY, CALIFORNIA • RAUWOLFIA • SKULLCAP • ST. JOHN'S WORT • SUMBUL • VALERIAN • VERBENA, LEMON

Anxiety; Insomnia

• ASHWAGANDHA • BALM, LEMON • DOGWOOD, JAMAICA • HAWTHORN • HOPS • HOREHOUND, BLACK • KAVA • LADY'S SLIPPER • LAVENDER • LEMONGRASS • LINDEN • OAT • PASSIONFLOWER • POPPY, CALIFORNIA • POPPY, FIELD • SKULLCAP • ST. JOHN'S WORT • SUMBUL • VALERIAN • VERBENA, LEMON • WATERLILY • WOODRUFF

Depressive Mood; Minor Depression

• DAMIANA • GINKGO • GINSENG, SIBERIAN • KAVA • LAVENDER • MARJORAM • NUT-MEG • RHODIOLA • SAFFRON • ST. JOHN'S WORT

Headache; Migraine

• AMBRETTE • BALM, LEMON • BETONY, WOOD • BLUE FLAG • BUTTERBUR, PURPLE • CATNIP • CLARY SAGE • DEVIL'S CLAW • DOGWOOD, JAMAICA • ERGOT • FEVERFEW • GELSEMIUM • GINKGO • LADY'S SLIPPER • LAVENDER • LOVAGE, CHINESE • MAGNOLIA • MARJORAM • PATCHOULY • PEONY, CHINESE • RADISH, BLACK • RHODIOLA • VERBE-NA, LEMON • WILLOW • WOODRUFF

Impaired Cognitive Function

• BACOPA • GINKGO • GINSENG • GOTU KOLA • PEONY, CHINESE

Epilepsy (= a chronic CNS disorder, with sudden convulsive seizures, associated with abnormal electrical activity of the brain)

• DITTANY, WHITE • GOTU KOLA • HORSE NETTLE • INDIAN PIPE • LADY'S SLIPPER • MISTLETOE, AMERICAN • MUDAR • PASSIONFLOWER • SKUNK CABBAGE

Parkinson's Disease (= a chronic neurologic disorder, with muscular weakness and tremor, sluggish movement and abnormal gait)

• CORYDALIS • SCOPOLIA • TURKEY CORN

Alcoholism

• EPIMEDIUM • KUDZU • PASSIONFLOWER • SAGE, CHINESE

Neuralgic Pains (= Neuralgias; incl. Sciatica); Headache
[external applications]

• ACONITE • AMMONIAC • BITTER CANDYTUFT • CAJUPUT • CALAMUS • CAMPHOR • CAPSICUM • CEDAR, EASTERN RED • CROTON • DONG QUAI • FIR • GARLIC • HEMLOCK, POISON • HENBANE • HORSERADISH • HORSERADISH TREE • LAVENDER • NETTLE • PELLITORY, SPANISH • PEPPER • PEPPER TREE, PERUVIAN • PEPPERMINT • PINE •

413

PRICKLY ASH, SOUTHERN • PULSATILLA • RUE • SAVIN • ST. JOHN'S WORT • STAVESA-CRE • THUJA • WINTERGREEN

AUDITORY DISORDERS

Tinnitus (= subjective perception of noise in the ears); **Impaired Hearing**

• BUPLEURUM • GINKGO • LYCIUM

Vertigo (= a type of dizziness, like that after spinning); **Ménière's Disease** (= a disorder characterized by chronic attacks of violent dizziness, nausea, vomiting, ringing in the ear, and hearing loss)

• BUPLEURUM • CORYDALIS • GINKGO • LYCIUM • PEONY, CHINESE • PERIWINKLE, LESSER • TURKEY CORN

OPHTHALMOLOGIC DISORDERS

Age-related Macular Degeneration (= AMD = degeneration of the yellowish spot in the central part of the retina); **Vascular Retinopathy** (= pathologic condition of the retina, chiefly associated with diabetes, hypertension, arteriosclerosis)

• BILBERRY • BUCKWHEAT • GINKGO • GRAPE • LYCIUM • PERIWINKLE, LESSER
See also **VARIOUS EFFECTS AND USES (Antioxidants)**

CARDIOVASCULAR DISORDERS

Heart Failure (= Congestive Heart Failure = Cardiac Insufficiency / Failure = a clinical condition associated with insufficient cardiac output)

• ADONIS, SPRING • ARJUNA • CANADIAN HEMP • CERBERA • CEREUS, NIGHT-BLOOMING • DIGITALIS • ERYSIMUM • FORSKOHLII • HAWTHORN • LILY-OF-THE-VALLEY • MILKWEED • MILKWEED, BUTTERFLY • OLEANDER • SQUILL • SCOTCH BROOM • STROPHANTHUS

Arrhythmias (= cardiac arrhythmias = altered rhythm of the heartbeat, here chiefly as tachycardia = rapid heartbeat)

• BALM, LEMON • DIGITALIS • EPIMEDIUM • HAWTHORN • KAVA • MOTHERWORT • KUDZU • MOUNTAIN LAUREL • PASSIONFLOWER • POPPY, FIELD • RAUWOLFIA • RHO-DODENDRON • SCOTCH BROOM • VALERIAN

Hypertension (= Arterial Hypertension = high blood pressure)

• ARJUNA • BEAR'S GARLIC • BUTTERBUR, PURPLE • CUDWEED, MARSH • DONG QUAI • EPIMEDIUM • EUCOMMIA • FEVER BARK TREE, AUSTRALIAN • GALANGAL, GREATER • GARLIC • GOTU KOLA • HAWTHORN • HELLEBORE, WHITE • HIBISCUS • KUDZU • LESPEDEZA • MISTLETOE, EUROPEAN • MOSSY STONECROP • MOTHERWORT • OLIVE • ONION • PEONY, TREE • PERIWINKLE, LESSER • RAUWOLFIA • RHODODENDRON • VA-LERIANA • YOHIMBE, FALSE

Hypotension (= Arterial Hypotension = low blood pressure)

414

• CALAMUS • CEREUS, NIGHT-BLOOMING • HORSERADISH TREE • HYSSOP • MILK THIS-TLE • MUIRA PUAMA • RHODIOLA • ROSEMARY • SCOTCH BROOM

Arteriosclerosis (= a complex condition associated with changes in the arterial walls as they become thicker and less elastic, chiefly due to atherosclerosis = deposition of fatty materials under the inner layer of the wall of arteries)
See **METABOLIC DISORDERS (High Cholesterol; High Triglycerides; Diabetes Mellitus; Overweight), Hypertension** (= Arterial Hypertension = high blood pressure), and **VARIOUS EFFECTS AND USES (Antioxidants)**

Coronary Heart Disease (= a condition associated with insufficient blood supply to the heart, chiefly due to atherosclerosis = deposition of fatty materials under the inner layer of the wall of arteries); **Angina Pectoris** (= chest pain associated with insufficient blood supply to the heart)

• DONG QUAI • EPIMEDIUM • GARLIC • HAWTHORN • KHELLA • KUDZU • LOVAGE, SICHUAN • SAGE, CHINESE • SCOTCH BROOM
See also **Arteriosclerosis**

Cerebrovascular Disease (= a complex condition associated with changes in the brain blood flow)

• GINKGO • HOLY BASIL • LOVAGE, SICHUAN • PEONY, CHINESE • PERIWINKLE, LESSER • SAGE, CHINESE
See also **Arteriosclerosis**

Intermittent Claudication (= pain / cramp / weakness in the legs on walking associated with deficient blood supply); **Raynaud's Disease** (= pale or red-blue patchy fingers / toes associated with spasms of small arteries)

• DONG QUAI • EPIMEDIUM • GARLIC • GINKGO • KUDZU • LOVAGE, SICHUAN • PRICKLY ASH, SOUTHERN • SAGE, CHINESE

Postthrombotic Syndrome (= symptoms associated with the presence of a blood clot / thrombus in a blood vessel or heart chamber); **Thrombophlebitis** (= inflammation of a vein associated with an attached blood clot / thrombus)

• Bromelain (see PINEAPPLE) • BUTCHER'S BROOM • HORSE CHESTNUT • MELILOT, YELLOW • Papain (see PAPAYA) • WOODRUFF

Varicose Veins in the Legs (= swollen and tortuous veins in the superficial tissue of the legs); **Hemorrhoids** (= varicose veins in the wall of rectum)

• BUTCHER'S BROOM • GOTU KOLA • GRAPE • HORSE CHESTNUT • MELILOT, YELLOW • WITCH HAZEL • WOODRUFF • YELLOW CHASTE WEED

RESPIRATORY DISORDERS

Inflammations of the Upper Respiratory Tract (The Common Cold = Acute Rhinitis; Sinusitis; Pharyngitis; Laryngitis; Tracheitis; Bronchitis)

• AERVA • AGARWOOD, CHINESE • AKEBIA • ALLSPICE • AMMONIAC • ANDROGRAPHIS • ANEMARRHENA • ANGELICA • ANISE • ANISE, STAR • ARNICA, FALSE • ASAFETIDA • ASARABACCA • BACOPA • BAILAHUÉN • BALLOON VINE • BASIL • BAY • BAYRUM-TREE

• BEAR'S BREECH • BEAR'S GARLIC • BEEBALM • BENZOIN TREE • BETONY, WOOD • BIT-
TER CANDYTUFT • BITTERSWEET • BLACK CHERRY • BONESET • BROOKLIME • BU-
PLEURUM • BUTTERBUR, PURPLE • BUTTERWORT • CABBAGE • CAJUPUT • CALAMUS •
CAMPHOR • CAPER, THREE-LEAF • CARAWAY • CARDAMOM • CARDAMOM, AMOMUM •
CAREX, SAND • CARLINE THISTLE • CATALPA, SOUTHERN • CEDAR, EASTERN RED •
CHAMOMILE, GERMAN • CHAPARRAL • CHEQUÉN • CHESTNUT, SPANISH • CHICKWEED •
CLOVE • COCILLANA • CODONOPSIS • COLTSFOOT • COPAIBA • COSTUS • COW PARSNIP,
AMERICAN • COWSLIP • CRESS, GARDEN • CRESS, INDIAN • CRESS, WATER • CUBEB •
CUDWEED, FRAGRANT • CUDWEED, MARSH • DAISY, GARDEN • DEER'S TONGUE • DEV-
IL'S BIT • DILL • DONG QUAI • DUCKWEED • EASTERN HEMLOCK • ELDER, DWARF • EL-
DER, EUROPEAN • ELECAMPANE • ELECAMPANE, BRITISH / JAPANESE • EPHEDRA •
EPIMEDIUM • ERYNGO • EUCALYPTUS • EYEBRIGHT • FENNEL • FENUGREEK • FIR • FLY
TRAP • FRANKINCENSE TREE • GALANGAL, GREATER • GALANGAL, LESSER • GALBA-
NUM • GAYFEATHER • GINGER • GINGER, CANADIAN WILD • GINGER, CREPE • GOLDEN-
ROD • GRINDELIA • GROUND IVY • GUAIACUM • HART'S TONGUE • HEARTSEASE • HEMP
NETTLE • HOLY BASIL • HOREHOUND • HORSERADISH • HYSSOP • IPECAC • IVY, ENG-
LISH • JUBA'S BUSH • JUNIPER • KHAT • LABRADOR TEA, MARSH • LICORICE • LINDEN •
LIPPIA, MEXICAN • LOUSEWORT, CANADIAN • LOVAGE • LOVAGE, CHINESE • LUNG-
WORT • LYSIMACHIA • MAGNOLIA • MAIDENHAIR FERN • MALABAR NUT TREE • MAL-
LOW • MAPLE, SUGAR • MARCELA • MARJORAM • MARSHMALLOW • MEADOWSWEET •
MOSS, ICELAND • MOSS, LUNGWORT • MOSS, OAK • MOUSE-EAR • MULLEIN • MUSTARD
• MUSTARD, GARLIC • MUSTARD, HEDGE • MUSTARD, WHITE • MYRRH • MYRTLE •
NETTLE, WHITE • NEW JERSEY TEA • NUTMEG • ONION • OREGANO • ORRIS • OSHA •
PATCHOULY • PAU D'ARCO • PEONY, TREE • PEPPER • PEPPER TREE, PERUVIAN • PEP-
PERMINT • PERUVIAN BALSAM TREE • PICRORHIZA • PINE • PIPSISSEWA • PLANTAIN •
PLATYCODON • POLYPODY • POPLAR • POPPY, FIELD • PRICKLY ASH, SOUTHERN • PUL-
SATILLA • PULSATILLA, CHINESE • QUILLAJA • RADISH, BLACK • RED CLOVER • RUD-
BECKIA • RUPTUREWORT • SAFFLOWER • SAGE • SAGE, GREEK • SANDALWOOD • SANI-
CLE, EUROPEAN • SAVORY • SAXIFRAGE, BURNET • SCHISANDRA • SENEGA • SKULL-
CAP, BAIKAL • SKUNK CABBAGE • SLIPPERY ELM • SLOE • SOAPWORT, RED • SOAP-
WORT, WHITE • SOLOMON'S SEAL, AROMATIC • SOUTHERNWOOD • SPEEDWELL •
SPIKENARD • SPURGE, PILL- THYME • THYME, WILD • TOLU BALSAM TREE • TRICHO-
SANTHES • BEARING • ST. JOHN'S WORT • STILLINGIA • STORAX • SUMBUL • SUNDEW •
UMCKALOABO • VIOLET, SWEET • YARROW • YARROW, MUSK • YELLOW CHASTE WEED
• YERBA MANSA • YERBA SANTA • ZEDOARY

Spastic Conditions of the Upper Respiratory Tract (Spastic Bronchitis, etc.); Bronchial Asthma

• AGARWOOD, CHINESE • AMMONIAC • ANEMARRHENA • ANISE • ASAFETIDA • ASARA-
BACCA • ASHWAGANDHA • BELLADONNA • BITTERSWEET • BLACK CHERRY • BONDUC
• BORAGE • BUTTERBUR, PURPLE • BUTTERWORT • CALAMUS • CATALPA, SOUTHERN •
CODONOPSIS • COLTSFOOT • COSTUS • COW PARSNIP, AMERICAN • COWSLIP • DOG-
WOOD, JAMAICA • DONG QUAI • EPHEDRA • EVENING PRIMROSE • FLY TRAP • FOR-
SKOHLII • FRANKINCENSE TREE • GALBANUM • GELSEMIUM • GINKGO • GRINDELIA •
HOP TREE • HOREHOUND • HYSSOP • IVY, ENGLISH • JASMINE • JIMSON WEED • JUJUBE
• KHAT • KHELLA • LABRADOR TEA, MARSH • LICORICE • LIPPIA, MEXICAN • LIVER-
WORT • LOBELIA • LOVAGE, SICHUAN • MALABAR NUT TREE • MANDRAKE • MARCELA
• MARJORAM • MUSTARD, HEDGE • NEW JERSEY TEA • ONION • OREGANO • OSHA •
PICRORHIZA • PLATYCODON • POPPY, CALIFORNIA • QUEBRACHO, WHITE • SAXIFRAGE,
BURNET • SENEGA • SKULLCAP, BAIKAL • SKUNK CABBAGE • SPIKENARD • SPURGE,
PILL-BEARING • SUMBUL • SUNDEW • THYME • YELLOW CHASTE WEED • YERBA SANTA

Allergic Conditions of the Upper Respiratory Tract (Allergic Rhinitis, etc.)

• BUTTERBUR, PURPLE • CAT'S CLAW • DUCKWEED • MAGNOLIA • PEONY, TREE • SKULL-
CAP, BAIKAL • SPURGE, PILL-BEARING • YELLOW CHASTE WEED

416

Coughs

• AERVA • AMMONIAC • ANEMARRHENA • ANISE • ARNICA, FALSE • ASARABACCA • BACOPA • BAY • BEEBALM • BETHROOT • BITTERSWEET • BLACK CHERRY • BUTTER-BUR, PURPLE • BUTTERWORT • CAJUPUT • CALAMUS • CAMPHOR • CARDAMOM • CARDAMOM, AMOMUM • CAREX, SAND • CARRAGEEN ALGAE • CEDAR, EASTERN RED • CHEQUÉN • CHERRY LAUREL • CHESTNUT, SPANISH • CHICKWEED • COCILLANA • COLTSFOOT • COPAIBA • COSTUS • COW PARSNIP, AMERICAN • COWSLIP • CUBEB • CUDWEED, FRAGRANT • CUDWEED, MARSH • DEVIL'S BIT • DILL • EASTERN HEMLOCK • ELDER, DWARF • ELDER, EUROPEAN • ELECAMPANE • ELECAMPANE, BRITISH / JAPA-NESE • EPIMEDIUM • ERYNGO • EUCALYPTUS • FENNEL • FENUGREEK • FIR • FLY TRAP • GALANGAL, GREATER • GALANGAL, LESSER • GALBANUM • GAYFEATHER • GINGER • GINGER, CANADIAN WILD • GINGER, CREPE • GRINDELIA • GUAIACUM • HART'S TONGUE • HEARTSEASE • HOLY BASIL • HOREHOUND • HORSERADISH • HYSSOP • IPE-CAC • IVY, ENGLISH • JUNIPER • LABRADOR TEA, MARSH • LICORICE • LINDEN • LIPPIA, MEXICAN • LOUSEWORT, CANADIAN • LOVAGE • LUNGWORT • LYSIMACHIA • MAIDEN-HAIR FERN • MALABAR NUT TREE • MALLOW • MAPLE, SUGAR • MARSHMALLOW • MOSS, ICELAND • MULLEIN • MYRTLE • NETTLE, WHITE • ONION • OREGANO • ORRIS • OSHA • PATCHOULY • PEACH • PEPPER • PEPPER TREE, PERUVIAN • PEPPERMINT • PINE • PLANTAIN • PLATYCODON • POLYPODY • POPLAR • POPPY, FIELD • POPPY, OPIUM • PRICKLY ASH, SOUTHERN • QUEBRACHO, WHITE • QUILLAJA • RADISH, BLACK • RUP-TUREWORT • SAFFLOWER • SAGE • SAGE, GREEK • SANICLE, EUROPEAN • SAVORY • SAXIFRAGE, BURNET • SCHISANDRA • SENEGA • SKUNK CABBAGE • SLIPPERY ELM • SOAPWORT, RED • SOAPWORT, WHITE • SPEEDWELL • SPIKENARD • SPURGE, PILL-BEARING • STILLINGIA • STORAX • SUNDEW • THYME • THYME, WILD • TOLU BALSAM TREE • TRICHOSANTHES • VIOLET, SWEET • YERBA MANSA • YERBA SANTA

Whooping Cough

• BUTTERWORT • CATALPA, SOUTHERN • CHESTNUT, SPANISH • COWSLIP • DOGWOOD, JAMAICA • EASTERN HEMLOCK • ERYNGO • FIR • FLY TRAP • GRINDELIA • HORE-HOUND, BLACK • IVY, ENGLISH • LABRADOR TEA, MARSH • LIPPIA, MEXICAN • MAID-ENHAIR FERN • MULLEIN • NEW JERSEY TEA • SUNDEW • THYME • YELLOW CHASTE WEED • YERBA SANTA

Feverish States; The Common Cold

1) Diaphoretic (= increasing / inducing perspiration) hot teas prepared with
• AKEBIA • ARNICA, FALSE • BAILAHUÉN • BALM, LEMON • BEEBALM • BETONY, WOOD • BONESET • CALAMINT • CAREX, SAND • CATNIP • CINNAMON • CINNAMON, WHITE • CORNFLOWER • CUDWEED, FRAGRANT • ELDER, EUROPEAN • GINGER • HEARTSEASE • HEATHER • HEMIDESMUS • HOLLY • HOLY BASIL • HYSSOP • JUBA'S BUSH • LEMONGRASS • LINDEN • LOCUST, BLACK • MARCELA • MEADOWSWEET • MULLEIN • OREGANO • OSWEGO TEA • PENNYROYAL, AMERICAN • PENNYROYAL, EUROPEAN • PINE • PRICKLY ASH, SOUTHERN • RUDBECKIA • SKULLCAP • SLOE • TICKSEED • VER-BENA, LEMON • VETIVER • WATER PEPPER

2) Antipyretics (= botanicals that reduce fever); Bitter Tonics
• ANDROGRAPHIS • ANEMARRHENA • ANGOSTURA • ASH, EUROPEAN • BACCHARIS TRIMERA • BAILAHUÉN • BLESSED THISTLE • BOG BEAN • BONDUC • BONESET • CALA-MUS • CANCHALAGUA • CARLINE THISTLE • CASCARA AMARGA • CASCARILLA • CEDRON • CENTAURY • CHANG SHAN • CHAPARRO • CHIRATA • CINCHONA • COPALCHI • DEER'S TONGUE • DEVIL'S CLAW • DOGWOOD, FLOWERING • FEVER BARK TREE, AUS-TRALIAN • GARDENIA • HEMP AGRIMONY • HONEYSUCKLE • HOP TREE • INDIAN PIPE • JUBA'S BUSH • MEADOWSWEET • MELIA • MOUNTAIN ASH, AMERICAN • MYROBALAN, BELLERIC • NEEM • NUT GRASS • OLIVE • PAU D'ARCO • REHMANNIA • SANDARAC TREE • SANICLE, MARYLAND • SIMARUBA • SPIGELIA • SUNFLOWER • WILLOW • WORM-WOOD • WORMWOOD, YIN-CHEN • YARROW • YOHIMBE, FALSE

3) Refrigerants (here: botanicals that relieve fever and thirst)

• ACEROLA • BARBERRY • CRANBERRY • CURRANT, BLACK • ELDER, EUROPEAN • HIBISCUS • JUJUBE • MULBERRY • PINEAPPLE • RASPBERRY • ROSE • SEA BUCKTHORN • SUMAC, SMOOTH • SUMAC, STAGHORN • TAMARIND • WINTER CHERRY
See also VARIOUS EFFECTS AND USES (**Vitamin C Supplements**)

Nosebleed

• NETTLE • OAK • SHEPHERD'S PURSE • TEA • TORMENTIL

Pulmonary Tuberculosis
[herbs rich in silicic acid, used as adjuvants]

• HORSETAIL • LUNGWORT • KNOTWEED

ORAL CAVITY AND THROAT DISORDERS

Inflammation of the Mouth (= Stomatitis = inflammations of the mouth in general); **Inflammation of the Gums** (= Gingivitis); **Canker Sore; Denture Sore; Inflammation of the Throat** (= Sore Throat = Pharyngitis; incl. Tonsillitis and Laryngitis)

• ACEROLA • ACHYRANTHES • AGRIMONY • AJUGA • ALDER • ANGELICA • ARNICA • AVENS • BALM, LEMON • BARBERRY • BASIL • BAYBERRY • BEAR'S BREECH • BEE-BALM • BENZOIN TREE • BETONY, WOOD • BILBERRY • BISTORT • BLACKBERRY • BLOODROOT • BURNET • BURNET, THORN • CALAMUS • CALENDULA • CAMPHOR • CAPSICUM • CARLINE THISTLE • CASCARILLA • CATECHU • CHAMOMILE, GERMAN • CHESTNUT, SPANISH • CINNAMON, WHITE • CLARY SAGE • CLOVE • COLTSFOOT • CRANESBILL • CRESS, GARDEN • CRESS, SCURVY • CRESS, WATER • CUDWEED, FRAGRANT • CUDWEED, MARSH • DAISY, GARDEN • DILL • EASTERN HEMLOCK • ECHINACEA • ELDER, EUROPEAN • EUCALYPTUS • FLEABANE, CANADA • FROSTWEED • GALANGAL, LESSER • GAYFEATHER • GINGER • GOLDENROD • GOLDENSEAL • GUAIACUM • HART'S TONGUE FERN • HAZEL, EUROPEAN • HEAL ALL • HOLLYHOCK • HOP TREE • HORSERADISH TREE • HORSETAIL • HYSSOP • JAMBOLAN • JUJUBE • KINO, EUCALYPTUS • KINO TREE, INDIAN • KNOTWEED • LADY'S MANTLE • LOOSESTRIFE, PURPLE • LYSIMACHIA • MALLOW • MARJORAM • MARSHMALLOW • MASTIC TREE • MELILOT, YELLOW • MOSSY STONECROP • MOUNTAIN ASH, EUROPEAN • MOUNTAIN AVENS • MOUSE-EAR • MULBERRY • MYROBALAN, BELLERIC • MYROBALAN, CHEBULIC • MYRRH • NEEM • NETTLE, WHITE • NEW JERSEY TEA • OAK • OAK, GALL • OREGANO • OSHA • PATCHOULY • PELLITORY, SPANISH • PEPPER TREE, PERUVIAN • PERIWINKLE, LESSER • PLANTAIN • POPLAR • PRICKLY ASH, SOUTHERN • QUINCE • RASPBERRY • RESTHARROW • RHATANY • RHODIOLA • RHUBARB, CHINESE • ROSE • SAGE • SAGE, GREEK • SANICLE, EUROPEAN • SANTOLINA • SAXIFRAGE, BURNET • SEA LAVENDER • SHEPHERD'S PURSE • SILVERWEED • SLIPPERY ELM • SLOE • SNAKEROOT, VIRGINIA • SPEEDWELL • SPILANTHES • STRAWBERRY • SUMAC, SMOOTH • SUMAC, STAGHORN • TEA • TEA TREE • THYME • THYME, WILD • TICKSEED • TORMENTIL • USNEA • WALNUT • WATERLILY • WITCH HAZEL • YARROW • YELLOW ROOT • YERBA MANSA

Canker Sore (= aphthous stomatitis = painful ulcer of the mouth); **Denture Sore**

• AVENS • BARBERRY • BISTORT • CHAMOMILE, GERMAN • COPTIS • CRANESBILL • ECHINACEA • GOLDENSEAL • KINO, EUCALYPTUS • KINO TREE, INDIAN • MYRRH • RHATANY • SAGE • SILVERWEED • YELLOW ROOT

418

Thrush (= oral candidiasis = a fungal infection of the oral cavity, namely with Candida albicans)

• COWSLIP • GARLIC • SAVORY • SOAPWORT, RED • TEA TREE

Toothache

• CAJUPUT • CALAMUS • CLOVE • ECHINACEA • PELLITORY, SPANISH • PEPPER • PRICKLY ASH, SOUTHERN • SPILANTHES

Bad Breath (= Halitosis); **Ingredients for the Oral Hygiene**

• BASIL • BAY • CAMPHOR • CLOVE • CORIANDER • DILL • JUNIPER • MYRTLE • ORRIS • PARSLEY • PAPAYA • PATCHOULY • PENNYROYAL, EUROPEAN • PEPPERMINT • ROSEMARY • SAGE • SAGE, GREEK • THYME • WINTERGREEN • WORMWOOD

GASTROINTESTINAL DISORDERS

Loss of Appetite; Nonulcer Dyspepsia (= Indigestion: Fullness, Flatulence, Bloating, Burping, Minor Heartburn, Minor Upper Abdominal Pain, Nausea)

• AJUGA • ALETRIS • ALLSPICE • AMBRETTE • ANDROGRAPHIS • ANGELICA • ANGOSTURA • ANGURATÉ • ANISE • ANISE, STAR • ARTICHOKE • ATRACTYLODES, BAIZHU • BACCHARIS TRIMERA • BAILAHUÉN • BALM, LEMON • BALMONY • BARBERRY • BASIL • BAY • BEAR'S FOOT • BEAR'S GARLIC • BETONY, MARSH • BETONY, WOOD • BITTER CANDYTUFT • BLESSED THISTLE • BOG BEAN • BOLDO • BONESET • BROOKLIME • BUTTERNUT • CALAMINT • CALAMUS • CALUMBA • CAPSICUM • CHAMOMILE, ROMAN • CANCHALAGUA • CAPER BUSH • CARAWAY • CARAWAY, BLACK • CARDAMOM • CARDAMOM, AMOMUM • CARLINE THISTLE • CASCARA AMARGA • CASCARILLA • CEDRON • CELERY • CENTAURY • CHAPARRO • CHERVIL • CHICORY • CHIRATA • CINCHONA • CINNAMON • CLARY SAGE • CODONOPSIS • COLUMBO, AMERICAN • COMBRETUM MICRANTHUM • CONDURANGO • COPALCHI • COPTIS • CORIANDER • CORNFLOWER • COSTUS • CRESS, GARDEN • CRESS, SCURVY • CRESS, WATER • CULVER'S ROOT • CURRY, INDIAN • DAMIANA • DANDELION • DEVIL'S CLAW • DILL • DOGWOOD, ASIATIC • DOGWOOD, FLOWERING • DONG QUAI • ECLIPTA • ELECAMPANE • ELECAMPANE, BRITISH / JAPANESE • EUCOMMIA • FIGWORT • GALANGAL , GREATER • GALANGAL, LESSER • GARDENIA • GENTIAN • GINGER • GINGER, CANADIAN WILD • GOLDENSEAL • GRAINS-OF-PARADISE • HARONGA • HEAL ALL • HEMP AGRIMONY • HOP TREE • HOPS • HOREHOUND • HOREHOUND, BLACK • HORSERADISH • JUNIPER • LAVENDER • LOVAGE • LOUSEWORT, CANADIAN • MASTIC TREE • MATICO • MOSS, ICELAND • MUGWORT • MUSTARD, WHITE • MYROBALAN, BELLERIC • NEEM • NUT GRASS • NUTMEG • NUXVOMICA • OAT • ONION • ORANGE, BITTER • OSHA • OSWEGO TEA • PAPAYA • PELLITORY, SPANISH • PENNYROYAL, AMERICAN • PENNYROYAL, EUROPEAN • PEPPER • PEPPER TREE, PERUVIAN • PEPPERMINT • PICRORHIZA • PINEAPPLE • PIPSISSEWA • QUASSIA • QUINCE, FLOWERING • RADISH, BLACK • REHMANNIA • RHUBARB, CHINESE • ROSE • ROSEMARY • RUDBECKIA • SANTOLINA • SAXIFRAGE, BURNET • SIMARUBA • SKULLCAP • SKULLCAP, BAIKAL • SOUTHERNWOOD • SPEARMINT • SPEEDWELL • SPINACH • STONEROOT • SUMAC, SMOOTH • SUMAC, STAGHORN • TANSY • THYME • TRAILING ARBUTUS • TREE-OF-HEAVEN, CHINESE • TURMERIC • TURMERIC, JAVANESE • USNEA • VERBENA, LEMON • VETIVER • WAHOO • WINTER CHERRY • WINTER'S BARK • WORMWOOD, YIN-CHEN • YARROW • YARROW, MUSK • ZEDOARY • YELLOW ROOT

Gastritis (= inflammation of the stomach)

• AGRIMONY • AVENS • BACOPA • BARLEY • BITTER CANDYTUFT • CALAMUS • CAREX, SAND • CAT'S CLAW • CHAMOMILE, GERMAN • CODONOPSIS • CORIANDER • COSTUS •

CUDWEED, MARSH • DAISY, GARDEN • EYEBRIGHT • FENUGREEK • FLAX • GROUND IVY • LICORICE • LINDEN • LOCUST, BLACK • MALLOW • MARSHMALLOW • MOUNTAIN AVENS • NETTLE, WHITE • OAT • OKRA • PAU D'ARCO • PLATYCODON • POTATO • SLIPPERY ELM • ST. JOHN'S WORT • YAM, WILD

Peptic Ulcers (= sore erosions of the duodenal / gastric / esophageal lining)

• ANGURATÉ • BELLADONNA • BUTTERBUR, PURPLE • CABBAGE • CAT'S CLAW • CHAMOMILE, GERMAN • CLOVE • CUDWEED, MARSH • FLAX • GOTU KOLA • HENBANE • HOLY BASIL • HOLY THORN • LICORICE • MANDRAKE • MARSHMALLOW • MASTIC TREE • OAT • OKRA • Pectin (see APPLE) • PLATYCODON • SAUNDERS, RED • SEA BUCKTHORN • SLIPPERY ELM • TORMENTIL • VALERIAN

Thirsty States (without pathology)

• ACEROLA • BARBERRY • CURRANT, BLACK • HIBISCUS • JUJUBE • MULBERRY • PINEAPPLE • RASPBERRY • ROSE • SEA BUCKTHORN • SUMAC, SMOOTH • SUMAC, STAGHORN • TAMARIND • WINTER CHERRY

Motion Sickness (= Kinetosis = a sickness with dizziness and nausea, due to motion)

• GINGER • HENBANE

Intestinal Cramps; Spastic Conditions of the Gastrointestinal Tract (incl. Nausea; Vomiting)

• ACHYRANTHES • AGARIC • AGARWOOD, CHINESE • ASAFETIDA • ASHWAGANDHA • BEEBALM • BELLADONNA • BETONY, MARSH • BITTER CANDYTUFT • BLACK CHERRY • BONDUC • BUTTERBUR, PURPLE • CALAMUS • CARAWAY • CARAWAY, BLACK • CATNIP • CELANDINE • CHAMOMILE, GERMAN • CLOVE • COMBRETUM MICRANTHUM • CONDURANGO • CORIANDER • COSTUS • COW PARSNIP, AMERICAN • DITTANY, WHITE • DONG QUAI • FLY TRAP • FRANKINCENSE TREE • GALBANUM • GINGER • HENBANE • HOLY BASIL • HOP TREE • HYSSOP • JASMINE • JIMSON WEED • JUJUBE • KHELLA • LAVENDER • LEMONGRASS • LIPPIA, MEXICAN • LOCUST, BLACK • LOVAGE, CHINESE • MANDRAKE • MARCELA • MARJORAM • NEW JERSEY TEA • OREGANO • OSHA • PARSLEY • PATCHOULY • PEONY, CHINESE • PEONY, TREE • PEPPERMINT • POPPY, CALIFORNIA • POTATO • PULSATILLA • RUE • SAVORY • SCOPOLIA • SKULLCAP, BAIKAL • SPURGE, PILL-BEARING • SUMBUL • SUNDEW • TEA • THYME • UZARA • VALERIAN • VERBENA, LEMON • WOODRUFF • YERBA MANSA

Diarrhea; Enteritis (= inflammation of the intestine); Gastroenteritis (= inflammation of the stomach and intestine)

• ACEROLA • AERVA • AGRIMONY • ALDER • ALLSPICE • ANDROGRAPHIS • ANGOSTURA • APPLE • ARJUNA • ARROWROOT • ATRACTYLODES, BAI-ZHU • AVENS • BALLOON VINE • BARBERRY • BARLEY • BASIL • BAYBERRY • BEAR'S BREECH • BEAR'S GARLIC • BEDSTRAW • BEEBALM • BERGENIA • BILBERRY • BISTORT • BITTER CANDYTUFT • BLACK CHERRY • BLACKBERRY • BURNET • BUTTERNUT • CALAMUS • CALUMBA • CAROB • CARROT • CASCARILLA • CAT'S CLAW • CATECHU • CATNIP • CHAPARRAL • CHEQUÉN • CHESTNUT, SPANISH • CLOVE • CODONOPSIS • COFFEE • COMBRETUM MICRANTHUM • COPTIS • CORIANDER • COSTUS • COW PARSNIP, AMERICAN • CRANESBILL • CUBEB • CUDWEED, FRAGRANT • CUMIN • CURRANT, BLACK • CURRY, INDIAN • EVIL'S BIT • DILL • DOGWOOD, FLOWERING • EASTERN HEMLOCK • EUCALYPTUS • FEVER BARK TREE, AUSTRALIAN • FLEABANE, CANADA • FLY TRAP • FRANKINCENSE TREE • FROSTWEED • GALANGAL, GREATER • GALANGAL, LESSER • GALE, SWEET • GARLIC • GAYFEATHER • GINGER • GOLDENROD • GOLDENSEAL • GROUND IVY • GUARANÁ • HART'S TONGUE FERN • HAZEL, EUROPEAN • HEATHER • HENNA • HERB-ROBERT •

420

HOLY BASIL • HONEYSUCKLE • HYSSOP • JAMBOLAN • KINO, EUCALYPTUS • KINO TREE, INDIAN • KNOTWEED • LADY'S MANTLE • LOGWOOD • LOOSESTRIFE, PURPLE • LOUSEWORT, CANADIAN • LUNGWORT • LYSIMACHIA • MAPLE, SUGAR • MARCELA • MARJORAM • MASTIC TREE • MATICO • MEADOWSWEET • MOSS, ICELAND • MOSS, OAK • MOUNTAIN ASH, EUROPEAN • MOUNTAIN AVENS • MOUSE-EAR • MUIRA PUAMA • MYROBALAN, BELLERIC • MYROBALAN, CHEBULIC • MYRRH • MYRTLE • NETTLE • NETTLE, WHITE • NEW JERSEY TEA • NUT GRASS • NUTMEG • OAK • OAT • OREGANO • ORRIS • PARSLEY PIERT • PARTRIDGE BERRY • PATCHOULY • PAU D'ARCO • PEONY, TREE • PLANTAIN • PLATYCODON • POPPY, OPIUM • PRICKLY ASH, SOUTHERN • PSYL-LIUM • PULSATILLA, CHINESE • QUINCE • RASPBERRY • RHATANY • SAGE • SALEP • SANDALWOOD • SANDARAC TREE • SANICLE, EUROPEAN • SAUNDERS, RED • SAVORY • SCHISANDRA • SEA LAVENDER • SHEPHERD'S PURSE • SILVERWEED • SIMARUBA • SKULLCAP, BAIKAL • SLIPPERY ELM • SOLOMON'S SEAL, AROMATIC • SOUTHERNWOOD • SPEARMINT • SPEEDWELL • SPIKENARD • SPURGE, PILL-BEARING • ST. JOHN'S WORT • STERCULIA • STRAWBERRY • STRAWBERRY TREE • SUMAC, SMOOTH • SUMAC, STAG-HORN • SUMAC, SWEET • SUMBUL • SUNDEW • TEA • THYME • TICKSEED • TORMENTIL • UMCKALOABO • USNEA • UZARA • WALNUT • WATER MINT • WATER PEPPER • WATER-LILY • WILLOW • WILLOW HERB • WINTER'S BARK • WITCH HAZEL • YAM • YAM, WILD • YARROW • YERBA MANSA • YELLOW ROOT

Amebic Dysentery (= severe diarrhea due to amebiasis)
• BARBERRY • CALUMBA • CEDRON • CHAPARRO • COPTIS • CUBEB • GOLDENSEAL • IPECAC • PULSATILLA, CHINESE • SIMARUBA • SPURGE, PILL-BEARING • TREE-OF-HEAVEN, CHINESE • YELLOW ROOT

Sluggish Bowels; Minor Constipation

• AJUGA • AKEBIA • ALMOND • ANEMARRHENA • ARTICHOKE • ARTICHOKE, JERUSA-LEM • ASH, EUROPEAN • BACOPA • BALMONY • BARBERRY • BLUE FLAG • BOG BEAN • BONESET • BROOKLIME • BUTTERNUT • CANCHALAGUA • CAPER, THREE-LEAF • CAPSI-CUM • CAREX, SAND • CARLINE THISTLE • CENTAURY • CHAMOMILE, ROMAN • CHICO-RY • CINNAMON • COPAIBA • CORNFLOWER • COUCH GRASS • CRESS, GARDEN • CRESS, SCURVY • CRESS, WATER • CUBEB • CULVER'S ROOT • DAISY, GARDEN • DAMIANA • DANDELION • DODDER • DULSE • DYER'S BROOM • DYER'S BROOM • ELDER, EUROPEAN • FIG • FIGWORT • FUMITORY • GARDENIA • GENTIAN • GINGER • GRAPE • HEARTSEASE • HELLEBORE, BLACK • HEMP AGRIMONY • HORSERADISH • LICORICE • MELIA • MEZE-REON • MILK THISTLE • MOUNTAIN ASH, EUROPEAN • MULBERRY • MYROBALAN, BEL-LERIC • NUX-VOMICA • OLIVE • PEACH • PELLITORY, SPANISH • PEPPER TREE, PERUVI-AN • PICRORHIZA • PINEAPPLE • POLYPODY • QUINCE, FLOWERING • RADISH, BLACK • REHMANNIA • ROSE • SANICLE, MARYLAND • SLOE • STERCULIA • STILLINGIA • TAMA-RIND • TOADFLAX • TOMATO • TRICHOSANTHES • WAHOO • WINTER CHERRY • WORM-WOOD

Constipation

• AGAR • ALOE • BRYONY • BUCKTHORN • CARRAGEEN ALGAE • CASCARA SAGRADA • CASTOR • COLOCYNTH • DOCK, YELLOW • FLAX • FO-TI • FRANGULA • GUAR • JALAP • JALAP, INDIAN • MANNA • MAYAPPLE • PSYLLIUM • RHUBARB, CHINESE • SCAMMONY, MEXICAN • SENNA

Irritable Bowel Syndrome (= Mucous Colitis = Spastic Colon)

• AGARWOOD, CHINESE • ANISE • ASAFETIDA • ASHWAGANDHA • BELLADONNA • BIT-TER CANDYTUFT • BUTTERBUR, PURPLE • CARAWAY • CHAMOMILE, GERMAN • FENNEL • FENUGREEK • FLAX • GINGER • HENBANE • MARSHMALLOW • PEPPERMINT • PLATYCODON • PSYLLIUM • SLIPPERY ELM • STERCULIA • SUMBUL • VALERIAN

Inflammatory Bowel Disease (= Ulcerative Colitis and / or Crohn's Disease) (Ulcerative Colitis = inflammatory and ulcerative condition of the colon and adjacent portions of the large bowel) (Crohn's Disease = inflammatory condition of the lower portion of the small bowel, and partly colon)

• AVENS • BAYBERRY • BILBERRY • BISTORT • BURNET • CATECHU • CRANESBILL • EASTERN HEMLOCK • FRANKINCENSE TREE • FROSTWEED • HAZEL, EUROPEAN • HERB-ROBERT • JAMBOLAN • KNOTWEED • LADY'S MANTLE • LOGWOOD • LOOSESTRIFE, PURPLE • MALLOW • MARSHMALLOW • MATICO • MOUSE-EAR • NETTLE • OAK • PARSLEY PIERT • PLANTAIN • PSYLLIUM • SANICLE, EUROPEAN • SHEPHERD'S PURSE • SILVERWEED • SLIPPERY ELM • ST. JOHN'S WORT • STONEROOT • STRAWBERRY • SUMAC, SWEET • TICKSEED • TORMENTIL • WALNUT • WILLOW HERB • WITCH HAZEL

Intestinal Worms

1) Roundworms (= Ascaris spp.)
• ECLIPTA • EPAZOTE • MELIA • MELON • PUMPKIN • RUDBECKIA • SPIGELIA
2) Pinworms (= Oxyuris spp.)
• CARROT • ECLIPTA • GARLIC • QUASSIA • RUDBECKIA • TANSY • THYME
3) Hookworms (= Ancylostoma spp.; Necator spp.)
• ECLIPTA • EPAZOTE • MALE FERN • SPURGE, PILL-BEARING
4) Tapeworms (= Taenia spp.)
• KOUSSO • MALE FERN • MELON • PUMPKIN
5) Other botanicals with anthelmintic effects
• BEAR'S GARLIC • BETELNUT PALM • BUTTERNUT • CAJUPUT • CHIVE • CUCUMBER • DITTANY, WHITE • ELECAMPANE • GAMBOGE • JALAP, INDIAN • MEZEREON • MOUNTAIN ASH, AMERICAN • NEEM • SANTOLINA

Hemorrhoids (= piles = varicose veins in the wall of rectum)

• ALDER • AVENS • BALLOON VINE • BAYBERRY • BILBERRY • BISTORT • BLACKBERRY • BURNET • BUTCHER'S BROOM • BUTTERNUT • CALENDULA • CAT'S CLAW • CHAMOMILE, GERMAN • CRANESBILL • DANDELION • DOCK, YELLOW • EASTERN HEMLOCK • ELECAMPANE • EUCALYPTUS • FIGWORT • FLEABANE, CANADA • FRANKINCENSE TREE • GOLDENROD • GOLDENSEAL • GOTU KOLA • GRAPE • GROUND IVY • HART'S TONGUE FERN • HAZEL, EUROPEAN • HEAL ALL • HERB-ROBERT • HORSE CHESTNUT • KNOTWEED • LADY'S MANTEL • LOOSESTRIFE, PURPLE • LUNGWORT • MATICO • MELILOT, YELLOW • MILK THISTLE • MOUNTAIN AVENS • MULLEIN • MYRTLE • NETTLE • NETTLE, WHITE • OAK • OAK, GALL • PARSLEY PIERT • PARTRIDGE BERRY • PELLITORY-OF-THE-WALL • PEONY, EUROPEAN • PERUVIAN BALSAM TREE • PILEWORT • PLANTAIN • POPLAR • PSYLLIUM • RASPBERRY • RHATANY • RHODIOLA • SANICLE, EUROPEAN • SEA LAVENDER • SHEPHERD'S PURSE • SILVERWEED • SOLOMON'S SEAL, AROMATIC • ST. JOHN'S WORT • STILLINGIA • STONEROOT • STRAWBERRY • SUMAC, SWEET • TICKSEED • TOADFLAX • TORMENTIL • WATER PEPPER • WILLOW HERB • WITCH HAZEL • WOODRUFF • YAM • YARROW • YELLOW CHASTE WEED
See also **CARDIOVASCULAR DISORDERS (Varicose Veins)**

HEPATOBILIARY DISORDERS

Chronic Liver Inflammation (= Chronic Hepatitis); **Fatty Liver; Liver Damage; Cirrhosis** [adjuvants for Liver Cirrhosis]

• ANDROGRAPHIS • ASTRAGALUS • ATRACTYLODES, BAI-ZHU • BAILAHUÉN • BEET, RED • BEET, SUGAR • BUPLEURUM • DONG QUAI • ECLIPTA • EPIMEDIUM • EUCOMMIA • FRINGE TREE • GARDENIA • JASMINE • KUDZU • MILK THISTLE • PEONY, CHINESE

• PICRORHIZA • REHMANNIA • SAGE, CHINESE • SCHISANDRA • SCHISANDRA, JAPANESE • SOY • TRICHOSANTHES • UMCKALOABO • WORMWOOD, YIN-CHEN

Biliary Tract Inflammatory / Spastic Conditions (Cholecystitis = inflammation of the gallbladder; Cholangitis = inflammation of the bile duct; Nonobstructive Gallstones)

• ACHYRANTHES • AGRIMONY • AJUGA • ARTICHOKE • BAILAHUÉN • BARBERRY • BELLADONNA • BIRCH • BLUE FLAG • BOLDO • BUTTERBUR, PURPLE • BUTTERNUT • CELANDINE • COMBRETUM MICRANTHUM • COPTIS • DANDELION • ELECAMPANE • FRINGE TREE • FUMITORY • GOLDENSEAL • HEMP AGRIMONY • HOP TREE • HORSERADISH • JASMINE • KHELLA • LIVERWORT • LOCUST, BLACK • MILK THISTLE • OLIVE • PARSLEY • PEONY, CHINESE • PEPPERMINT • POLYPODY • POPPY, CALIFORNIA • PULSATILLA • ROSEMARY • TOADFLAX • TURMERIC • TURMERIC, JAVANESE • WAHOO • WOODRUFF • WORMWOOD, YIN-CHEN • YELLOW CHASTE WEED • YELLOW ROOT

Postcholecystectomy Syndrome (= complaints following a cholecystectomy)

• CELANDINE • PEPPERMINT • TURMERIC

GENITOURINARY DISORDERS

Inflammations of the Genitourinary Tract (Urethritis; Prostatitis; Cystitis; Ureteritis; Pyelonephritis; Nephritis)

• ACHYRANTHES • AERVA • AGRIMONY • AKEBIA • ANDROGRAPHIS • ARJUNA • ASPARAGUS • ASTRAGALUS • ATRACTYLODES, BAI-ZHU • BACOPA • BAILAHUÉN • BALLOON VINE • BASIL • BAY • BEAN, COMMON • BEAR'S BREECH • BEDSTRAW • BEET, RED • BERGENIA • BILBERRY • BIRCH • BROOKLIME • BUCHU • BUPLEURUM • BUTCHER'S BROOM • CAPER, THREE-LEAF • CARLINE THISTLE • CARROT • CEDAR, EASTERN RED • CELERY • CHAPARRAL • CHEQUÉN • CLUBMOSS • CODONOPSIS • COPAIBA • CORN • COUCH GRASS • CRANBERRY • CRESS, GARDEN • CRESS, INDIAN • CRESS, WATER • CUBEB • CUCUMBER • CUDWEED, FRAGRANT • CUDWEED, MARSH • CURRANT, BLACK • DAISY, GARDEN • DAMIANA • DANDELION • DEVIL'S BIT • DOGWOOD, ASIATIC • DYER'S GREEN • ELDER, DWARF • ELDER, EUROPEAN • ELECAMPANE • ELECAMPANE, BRITISH / JAPANESE • ERYNGO • EUCALYPTUS • EUCOMMIA • FLEABANE, CANADA • FRANKINCENSE TREE • FRINGE TREE • FROSTWEED • GALBANUM • GALE, SWEET • GARDENIA • GARLIC • GAYFEATHER • GOAT'S RUE • GOLDENROD • GRINDELIA • GROUND IVY • GUAIACUM • HART'S TONGUE FERN • HEATHER • HELLEBORE, BLACK • HOLLYHOCK • HORSERADISH • HORSETAIL • HYDRANGEA • JAVA TEA • JOE PYE • JUNIPER • KNOTWEED • LABRADOR TEA, MARSH • LINDEN • LINGONBERRY • LIVERWORT • LOCUST, BLACK • LOVAGE • LUNGWORT • MALLOW • MAPLE, SUGAR • MARCELA • MARJORAM • MARSHMALLOW • MASTIC TREE • MATICO • MEADOWSWEET • MOUSE-EAR • MYRTLE • NETTLE • NUT GRASS • OAT • OKRA • OREGANO • OSWEGO TEA • PARSLEY • PARSLEY PIERT • PARTRIDGE BERRY • PAU D'ARCO • PELLITORY-OF-THE-WALL • PEPPER TREE, PERUVIAN • PICHI • PIPSISSEWA • PLANTAIN • POPLAR • PRICKLY ASH, SOUTHERN • PULSATILLA • PULSATILLA, CHINESE • REHMANNIA • RESTHARROW • RUDBECKIA • RUPTUREWORT • SANDALWOOD • SANICLE, EUROPEAN • SANICLE, MARYLAND • SAVORY • SAXIFRAGE, BURNET • SCHISANDRA • SEA LAVENDER • SHEPHERD'S PURSE • SKULLCAP, BAIKAL • SLIPPERY ELM • SOAPWORT, RED • SOLOMON'S SEAL, AROMATIC • SOUTHERNWOOD • SPEEDWELL • SPIKENARD • SPILANTHES • SPURGE, PILL-BEARING • ST. JOHN'S WORT • STILLINGIA • STONEROOT • STORAX • STRAWBERRY TREE • SUMAC, SMOOTH • SUMAC, STAGHORN • SUMAC, SWEET • TICKSEED • TOADFLAX • TRAILING ARBUTUS • UVA-URSI • VIRGIN'S BOWER • WILLOW HERB • WORMWOOD, YIN-CHEN • YARROW • YARROW, MUSK • YERBA MANSA • YERBA SANTA

Gravel; Urinary Stones (= Urinary Calculi = Urolithiasis; here: nonobstructive stones); **Minor Spastic Conditions of the Genitourinary Tract**

• ACHYRANTHES • AERVA • AGARWOOD, CHINESE • AKEBIA • ASHWAGANDHA • AS-PARAGUS • ATRACTYLODES, BAI-ZHU • BACOPA • BEAN, COMMON • BEDSTRAW • BEL-LADONNA • BIRCH • BUTTERBUR, PURPLE • CAPER, THREE-LEAF • CARROT • CELERY • CLUBMOSS • CORN • COUCH GRASS • CURRANT, BLACK • DITTANY, WHITE • DYER'S BROOM • ELDER, DWARF • ERYNGO • FLEABANE, CANADA • GALBANUM • GOLDENROD • HART'S TONGUE FERN • HELLEBORE, BLACK • HORSETAIL • HYDRANGEA • JAVA TEA • JOE PYE • JUNIPER • KAVA • KHELLA • KNOTWEED • LOCUST, BLACK • LOVAGE • MAN-DRAKE • MARSHMALLOW • MOUSE-EAR • NETTLE • NETTLE, WHITE • NUT GRASS • PARSLEY • PARSLEY PIERT • PELLITORY-OF-THE-WALL • PICHI • POPPY, CALIFORNIA • RESTHARROW • RUPTUREWORT • SAXIFRAGE, BURNET • SCOPOLIA • SHEPHERD'S PURSE • SLIPPERY ELM • TICKSEED • TURKEY CORN • WINTER CHERRY • YARROW

Erectile Dysfunction (= impotence); **Low Sexual Drive** (= loss of libido)

• AGARWOOD, CHINESE • DOGWOOD, ASIATIC • ASHWAGANDHA • BONDUC • CARDA-MOM • CINNAMON • CNIDIUM • COSTUS • CRANESBILL • CUBEB • DAMIANA • EPIMEDI-UM • EUCOMMIA • GALANGAL, GREATER • GINSENG • GOTU KOLA • HORSERADISH TREE • JASMINE • LYCIUM • MATICO • MUIRA PUAMA • PATCHOULY • QUEBRACHO, WHITE • SCHISANDRA • SCHISANDRA, JAPANESE • VANILLA • YOHIMBE • YOHIMBE, FALSE

Benign Prostatic Hyperplasia (= BPH); **Prostate Cancer** (adjuvants for the prevention)

• BLACK COHOSH • CODONOPSIS • HYPOXIS ROOPERI • KUDZU • MELON • NETTLE • PLATYCODON • POPLAR • PUMPKIN • PYGEUM • RED CLOVER • SAW PALMETTO • SOY • TOADFLAX • WILLOW HERB

Childhood Enuresis (= bed-wetting)

• KAVA • PUMPKIN • ST. JOHN'S WORT • SUMAC, SWEET

Irritable Bladder; Urinary Incontinence

• AGRIMONY • BELLADONNA • DAMIANA • DOGWOOD, ASIATIC • GELSEMIUM • HOPS • KAVA • PICHI • POPLAR • PUMPKIN • SCHISANDRA • SCHISANDRA, JAPANESE • SUMAC, SWEET • TOADFLAX • YOHIMBE

GYNECOLOGIC DISORDERS

Premenstrual Syndrome = PMS (= symptoms that occur in the 7-10 days before menstruation: breast pain = mastodynia = mastalgia, nervousness, irritability, insomnia, emotional instability, depressive mood, fatigue, headache, pelvic discomfort, nausea, loss of appetite, dyspepsia, constipation, edema, etc.)

• BORAGE • BLACK COHOSH • BUPLEURUM • CHASTE TREE •• EVENING PRIMROSE
See also specific complaints (e. g. insomnia, nausea, loss of appetite, etc.)

Amenorrhea (here: secondary amenorrhea = absence of menstruation without pathology); **Oligomenorrhea** (here: secondary oligomenorrhea = infrequent / scanty menstruation without pathology)

• ACHYRANTHES • BUPLEURUM • CEDAR, EASTERN RED • CARROT • CHASTE TREE • CLARY SAGE • CUMIN • DEVIL'S COTTON • FALSE UNICORN • GINSENG • LIPPIA, MEXI-

424

CAN • PARSLEY • PARTRIDGE BERRY • PENNYROYAL, AMERICAN • PENNYROYAL, EU-
ROPEAN • PEONY, CHINESE • RUE • SAFFLOWER • SAGE, CHINESE • TANSY

Dysmenorrhea (here: primary dysmenorrhea = painful menstruation without pathology)

• ALETRIS • BALM, LEMON • BETONY, MARSH • BLACK COHOSH • BLACK HAW • BU-
PLEURUM • BUTTERBUR, PURPLE • CATNIP • CEDAR, EASTERN RED • CELERY • CHAM-
OMILE, GERMAN • CHAMOMILE, ROMAN • CLARY SAGE • CLOVE • CLUBMOSS • CRAMP
BARK • CUDWEED, FRAGRANT • DEVIL'S COTTON • DITTANY, WHITE • DOGWOOD, JA-
MAICA • DONG QUAI • GALANGAL, LESSER • GALBANUM • GELSEMIUM • GINGER •
GUAIACUM • HOPS • KAVA • LADY'S MANTLE • LOVAGE • LOVAGE, CHINESE •
MARCELA • OSHA • PARSLEY • PASSIONFLOWER • PENNYROYAL, AMERICAN • PENNY-
ROYAL, EUROPEAN • PEONY, CHINESE • PEONY, TREE • RASPBERRY • RUE • SAFFLOW-
ER • SAFFRON • SAGE, CHINESE • SANTOLINA • SAXIFRAGE, BURNET • SKULLCAP • SIL-
VERWEED • STONEROOT • SUMBUL • TANSY • TURMERIC • VALERIAN • WATER MINT •
WOODRUFF • YARROW • YERBA MANSA

Menopausal Syndrome (= symptoms associated with menopause: hot flashes,
sweating, tachycardia, insomnia, emotional instability, depressive mood, fatigue,
decreased vaginal lubrication, etc.)

• BLACK COHOSH • DONG QUAI • KUDZU • RED CLOVER • SOY
See also **Oligomenorrhea** and specific complaints (e. g. insomnia, depressive
mood, etc.)

Menorrhagia (= prolonged menstruation); **Hypermenorrhea** (= heavy menstruation); **Postpartum Hemorrhage** (= hemorrhage following childbirth)

• BETHROOT • BLUE COHOSH • CEREUS, NIGHT-BLOOMING • CRANESBILL • DOGWOOD,
ASIATIC • ERGOT • GINGER, CREPE • GOLDENSEAL • LADY'S MANTLE • MILKWEED •
MISTLETOE, AMERICAN • PARSLEY PIERT • PARTRIDGE BERRY • SHEPHERD'S PURSE •
SUMAC, SWEET • TICKSEED • WATER PEPPER

Metrorrhagia (= nonmenstrual uterine bleeding)

• BETHROOT • CHASTE TREE • LADY'S MANTLE • PARTRIDGE BERRY • SHEPHERD'S
PURSE • WATER PEPPER
See also **Menorrhagia, Hypermenorrhea, Postpartum Hemorrhage** for other bo-
tanicals used as adjuvants for metrorrhagia.

Leukorrhea (= Fluor albus = whitish / yellowish discharge from the vagina and / or
uterine cavity); **Vulvovaginitis** (= inflammation of the female external genitalia
and vagina chiefly due to fungal, protozoal, or bacterial infections)

• ALDER • BARBERRY • BASIL • BAY • BAYBERRY • BEDSTRAW • BETHROOT • BISTORT
• BLACKBERRY • CELERY • CHAMOMILE, GERMAN • CNIDIUM • COPAIBA • COPTIS •
CRANESBILL • CUBEB • CUDWEED, FRAGRANT • DOGWOOD, ASIATIC • EASTERN HEM-
LOCK • ECLIPTA • FIGWORT • GARLIC • GOLDENSEAL • HEARTSEASE • HORSERADISH •
INDIGO, WILD • LADY'S MANTLE • LOGWOOD • LOOSESTRIFE, PURPLE • MASTIC TREE •
MATICO • MYRTLE • NEEM • NETTLE, WHITE • NEW JERSEY TEA • OAK • OREGON
GRAPE • PAU D'ARCO • PEPPER TREE, PERUVIAN • PULSATILLA, CHINESE • SANDAL-
WOOD • SANTOLINA • SEA LAVENDER • TEA TREE • TORMENTIL • WALNUT • WATER-
LILY • WILLOW • WITCH HAZEL • YARROW • YELLOW ROOT

Endometriosis (= abnormal growth of the uterine lining outside the uterus)

• BORAGE • EVENING PRIMROSE

Morning Sickness (= Emesis gravidarum = vomiting in pregnancy)
• CAROB • GINGER • MOSS, ICELAND • QUINCE, FLOWERING

Milk Secretion

1) Botanicals used for deficient secretion
• ANISE • CARAWAY • DILL • FENNEL • GOAT'S RUE • SPURGE, PILL-BEARING
2) Botanicals used to stop it
• CHERVIL • PARSLEY • SAGE

Sore Nipples

• BISTORT • CHAMOMILE, GERMAN • OAK • PELLITORY-OF-THE-WALL • QUINCE • RHATANY • WALNUT • WITCH HAZEL

DERMATOLOGIC DISORDERS

Minor Skin Inflammations
[external applications]

• AERVA • AGRIMONY • ALDER • ALOE • ARJUNA • ARNICA • AVENS • BACCHARIS TRI-MERA • BAILAHUÉN • BALLOON-VINE • BAYBERRY • BEAR'S BREECH • BEAR'S FOOT • BEAR'S GARLIC • BEDSTRAW • BETHROOT • BILBERRY • BLACK CHERRY • BLACKBER-RY • BLUE FLAG • BORAGE • BURNET • BUTTERNUT • CAJUPUT • CALENDULA • CAREX, SAND • CARLINE THISTLE • CEDAR, EASTERN RED • CHAPARRAL • CHEQUÉN • CHERVIL • CHICKWEED • COLTSFOOT • COMFREY • COPAIBA • COSTUS • CRANESBILL • CUD-WEED, FRAGRANT • DAISY, GARDEN • DEVIL'S BIT • DITTANY, WHITE • EASTERN HEM-LOCK • ELDER, EUROPEAN • EYEBRIGHT • FENUGREEK • FIGWORT • FROSTWEED • GALE, SWEET • GARDENIA • GINGER, CREPE • GOLDENROD • GOLDENSEAL • GROUND IVY • HEMP AGRIMONY • HOLLYHOCK • HONEYSUCKLE • HYSSOP • JAMBOLAN • LOUSEWORT, CANADIAN • LYSIMACHIA • MALLOW • MARSHMALLOW • MEADOW-SWEET • MELIA • MOSS, ICELAND • MOSS, LUNGWORT • MOUNTAIN AVENS • MOUSE-EAR • MULLEIN • MYROBALAN, BELLERIC • MYROBALAN, CHEBULIC • NETTLE, WHITE • OAK, GALL • OAT • OKRA • PARSLEY PIERT • PAU D'ARCO • PELLITORY-OF-THE-WALL • PEONY, CHINESE • PEONY, EUROPEAN • PEONY, TREE • PERIWINKLE, LESSER • PIPSIS-SEWA • PLANTAIN • POPLAR • PRICKLY ASH, SOUTHERN • PSYLLIUM • QUINCE • RASP-BERRY • REHMANNIA • RUDBECKIA • SANDALWOOD • SANICLE, EUROPEAN • SANICLE, MARYLAND • SANTOLINA • SILVERWEED • SOLOMON'S SEAL, AROMATIC • SPURGE, PILL-BEARING • STRAWBERRY • SUMAC, SWEET • TEA • TORMENTIL • VERVAIN, EURO-PEAN • WINTER'S BARK • WITCH HAZEL • WOODRUFF • YAM, WILD • YARROW • YAR-ROW, MUSK • YELLOW CHASTE WEED • YUCCA

Eczema (= Dermatitis = eczema of external origin); **Atopic Eczema** (= Atopic Dermatitis = eczema of internal origin; incl. Milk Crust = Infantile Eczema)
[external applications]

• AGRIMONY • BALLOON VINE • BENZOIN TREE • BILBERRY • BIRCH • BITTERSWEET • BLUE FLAG • BURDOCK • BURNET • BUTTERNUT • CADE JUNIPER • CALENDULA • CHERVIL • CHICKWEED • COLTSFOOT • ECHINACEA • EVENING PRIMROSE • FENU-GREEK • FIGWORT • FLAX • GOTU KOLA • HEARTSEASE • HENNA • HOLY THORN • LOOSESTRIFE, PURPLE • LYSIMACHIA • MAGNOLIA • MALLOW • MELIA • MYROBALAN, BELLERIC • MYROBALAN, CHEBULIC • OAK • OAK, GALL • OLIVE • PAU D'ARCO • PEA-NUT • PERIWINKLE, LESSER • PINE • POKE • RED CLOVER • ROSEMARY • SANICLE, EU-ROPEAN • SAUNDERS, RED • SILVERWEED • SPEEDWELL • STORAX • TICKSEED • TOR-MENTIL • TURMERIC • WALNUT • WITCH HAZEL • YELLOW CHASTE WEED

426

Poison Ivy Dermatitis
[external applications]

• BEDSTRAW • GRINDELIA • Jewelweed (see POISON IVY) • PLANTAIN

Atopic Eczema (= Atopic Dermatitis = eczema of internal origin)
[internal applications]

• ASTRAGALUS • BEAN, COMMON • BITTERSWEET • DOCK, YELLOW • DUCKWEED • ECLIPTA • GINGER, CREPE • GUAIACUM • HEARTSEASE • NETTLE • NETTLE, WHITE • PEONY, CHINESE • PEONY, EUROPEAN • PEONY, TREE • RESTHARROW • SARSAPARILLA • TRICHOSANTHES • YELLOW CHASTE WEED
See also VARIOUS EFFECTS AND USES (**Antidyscratics** = blood purifiers = depuratives = blood cleansers)

Wounds; Cuts; Ulcers; Burns; Bacterial Skin Infections
[minor cases; expernal applications]

• ACHYRANTHES • AGRIMONY • AJUGA • ALDER • ALOE • AMMONIAC • ARJUNA • AR-NICA, FALSE • AVENS • BACCHARIS TRIMERA • BAILAHUÉN • BASIL • BAY • BAYBERRY • BEAR'S BREECH • BEDSTRAW • BENZOIN TREE • BETHROOT • BETONY, MARSH • BET-ONY, WOOD • BILBERRY • BISTORT • BLACK CHERRY • BLESSED THISTLE • BLOODROOT • BLUE FLAG • BURNET • BUTTERBUR, PURPLE • BUTTERNUT • CABBAGE • CALENDULA • CARLINE THISTLE • CEDRON • CHAMOMILE, GERMAN • CHAPARRAL • CHEQUÉN • CHERVIL • CHICKWEED • CLARY SAGE • COPAIBA • COSTUS • COW PARSNIP, AMERICAN • CRANESBILL • CRESS, GARDEN • CRESS, INDIAN • CRESS, SCURVY • CUDWEED, FRA-GRANT • CURRY, INDIAN • DAISY, GARDEN • DEVIL'S BIT • DOCK, YELLOW • DOGWOOD, FLOWERING • EASTERN HEMLOCK • ECHINACEA • ECLIPTA • EUCALYPTUS • FENU-GREEK • FIGWORT • FLEABANE, CANADA • FLY TRAP • FRANKINCENSE TREE • FRINGE TREE • FROSTWEED • GALBANUM • GALE, SWEET • GARDENIA • GAYFEATHER • GOLD-ENROD • GOTU KOLA • GROUND IVY • HART'S TONGUE FERN • HAZEL, EUROPEAN • HEAL ALL • HEARTSEASE • HEMP AGRIMONY • HENNA • HERB-ROBERT • HOLLYHOCK • HOLY THORN • HONEYSUCKLE • HOP TREE • HORSERADISH TREE • HORSETAIL • HYS-SOP • INDIGO, WILD • IVY, ENGLISH • JAMBOLAN • KNOTWEED • LADY'S MANTLE • LAVENDER • LIVERWORT • LOOSESTRIFE, PURPLE • LUNGWORT • LYSIMACHIA • MAR-JORAM • MASTIC TREE • MATICO • MELIA • MOSS, ICELAND • MOSS, LUNGWORT • MOSS, OAK • MOSSY STONECROP • MOUNTAIN AVENS • MOUSE-EAR • MULLEIN • MUS-TARD, GARLIC • MYROBALAN, BELLERIC • MYROBALAN, CHEBULIC • MYRRH • NEEM • NETTLE, WHITE • OAK • OREGANO • PARSLEY PIERT • PARTRIDGE BERRY • PAU D'ARCO • PELLITORY-OF-THE-WALL • PEONY, CHINESE • PEONY, EUROPEAN • PEPPER TREE, BRAZILIAN • PEPPER TREE, PERUVIAN • PERIWINKLE, LESSER • PERUVIAN BALSAM TREE • PIPSISSEWA • PLANTAIN • POPLAR • PULSATILLA • PULSATILLA, CHINESE • QUINCE • RASPBERRY • RHATANY • ROSEMARY • RUDBECKIA • SAFFLOWER • SANICLE, EUROPEAN • SANICLE, MARYLAND • SAUNDERS, RED • SAXIFRAGE, BURNET • SEA BUCKTHORN • SEA LAVENDER • SHEPHERD'S PURSE • SILVERWEED • SLIPPERY ELM • SNAKEROOT, VIRGINIA • SOUTHERNWOOD • SPEEDWELL • SPIKENARD • SPILANTHES • SPURGE, PILL-BEARING • ST. JOHN'S WORT • STONEROOT • STORAX • STRAWBERRY • SUNDEW • SYRIAN RUE • TANSY • TEA • TEA TREE • THYME • TICKSEED • TOADFLAX • TOLU BALSAM TREE • TORMENTIL • VERVAIN, EUROPEAN • VIRGIN'S BOWER • WALNUT • WATER PEPPER • WILLOW • WILLOW HERB • WINTER'S BARK • WITCH HAZEL • WOODRUFF • YARROW • YARROW, MUSK • YELLOW CHASTE WEED • YERBA MANSA • YERBA SANTA

Varicose Ulcers (= Ulcus Cruris = ulcers due to varicose veins)

• CABBAGE • CALENDULA • CHAMOMILE, GERMAN • DAISY, GARDEN • ECHINACEA • GOTU KOLA • HORSE CHESTNUT • LOOSESTRIFE, PURPLE • MILK THISTLE • PERUVIAN BALSAM TREE • ST. JOHN'S WORT

Boil (= furuncle = a suppurative swelling of the skin due to bacterial infection); **Carbuncle** (= a cluster of boils)

• AMMONIAC • ARNICA • ASHWAGANDHA • BIRCH • BURDOCK • CABBAGE • CEDRON • COMFREY • COW PARSNIP, AMERICAN • DAISY, GARDEN • DODDER • DONG QUAI • DUCKWEED • FENUGREEK • FLAX • HONEYSUCKLE • IVY, ENGLISH • MARSHMALLOW • MELILOT, YELLOW • MOSS, OAK • MUDAR • ONION • PAU D'ARCO • PLANTAIN • PSYLLIUM • SAGE, CHINESE • SLIPPERY ELM • SPIKENARD • STONEROOT • SUMAC, SWEET • TOADFLAX • TRICHOSANTHES • WATERLILY

Cold Sore (= fever sore / blister = infection caused by Herpes simplex virus)

• BALM, LEMON • ECHINACEA • MARJORAM • SAGE

Chilblain

• OAK • OAK, GALL • TORMENTIL

Fungal Skin Infections (= Dermatomycosis = fungal skin infections in general); **Athlete's Foot** (= ringworm of the feet = Tinea pedis); **Ringworm of the Nails** (= Tinea unguium); **Ringworm of the Scalp** (= Tinea capitis)

• ARNICA • BENZOIN TREE • BIRCH • CASHEW • CLOVE • CNIDIUM • COUCH GRASS • CRESS, INDIAN • ECLIPTA • GARLIC • GOA TREE • HENNA • LIVERWORT • LOVAGE, CHINESE • MOUNTAIN LAUREL • NEEM • POKE • PULSATILLA • PULSATILLA, CHINESE • QUILLAJA • SAUNDERS, RED • STORAX • TEA TREE • TURMERIC • USNEA • VERVAIN, EUROPEAN • VIRGIN'S BOWER • WALNUT

Scabies (= the itch)

• CADE JUNIPER • CARAWAY • CEDAR, EASTERN RED • GALE, SWEET • HORSE NETTLE • PERUVIAN BALSAM TREE • PINE

Pediculosis (= infestation with lice)

• NEEM • QUASSIA

Pruritus (= itching in general, incl. Lichen Planus = a skin itching condition); **Insect Bites**

• ARNICA • BALLOON VINE • CADE JUNIPER • CAJUPUT • DEVIL'S BIT • DITTANY, WHITE • FO-TI • LABRADOR TEA, MARSH • MOSSY STONECROP • NETTLE, WHITE • ONION • PARSLEY • PEPPERMINT • PINE • PLANTAIN • POPLAR • SNAKEROOT, VIRGINIA • SPILANTHES • STORAX • TEA TREE • VERVAIN, EUROPEAN • YERBA SANTA

Psoriasis (= a chronic skin disorder, with scaly red patches)

• BARBERRY • BLUE FLAG • BURDOCK • CASHEW • CHAULMOOGRA • CHICKWEED • COPTIS • GOA TREE • GOTU KOLA • JOJOBA • MOUNTAIN LAUREL • OLIVE • OREGON GRAPE • PINE • RED CLOVER • RUPTUREWORT • SARSAPARILLA • TURMERIC • YELLOW CHASTE WEED • YELLOW ROOT

Dandruff; Hair Loss

• BASIL • BEAR'S FOOT • BIRCH • BURDOCK • COUCH GRASS • COW PARSNIP, AMERICAN • CRESS, INDIAN • HEARTSEASE • NETTLE • ONION • QUILLAJA • ROSEMARY • SAFFLOWER • SAVIN • TICKSEED • WATER PEPPER • YUCCA

Common Acne (= Acne vulgaris = an inflammatory skin disorder in adolescents, with pimples in the face, chest or shoulders)

• ALOE • BARBERRY • CABBAGE • CAJUPUT • COPTIS • DAISY, GARDEN • HEARTSEASE • JOJOBA • OREGON GRAPE • PEONY, CHINESE • TEA TREE • YELLOW ROOT

Warts (Common Wart = Verruca vulgaris; Plantar Wart = Verruca plantaris); **Corns**

• BLOODROOT • CASHEW • CELANDINE • FIG • FLY TRAP • GARLIC • MAYAPPLE • MILKWEED • MOSSY STONECROP • MUDAR • SAVIN • SPURGE, PILL-BEARING • SUNDEW • THUJA

Genital Wart (= Venereal Wart = Condylomata acuminata = Verruca acuminata)

• CEDAR, EASTERN RED • MAYAPPLE • SAVIN

Excessive Sweating (= Hyperhidrosis)

• AGARIC • SAGE

Sweating Feet / Hands

• BAY • BIRCH • BLACKBERRY • MYRTLE • NEW JERSEY TEA • OAK • WALNUT

METABOLIC DISORDERS

High Cholesterol; High Triglycerides
[adjuvants; dietetic aids]

• ALOE • APPLE • ARTICHOKE • BEAR'S GARLIC • CARROT • CHIVE • EVENING PRIMROSE • FENUGREEK • FLAX • FO-TI • FRANKINCENSE TREE • GARLIC • GINGER • GINGER, CREPE • GINSENG • GINSENG, SIBERIAN • GUAR • GUGGUL • HIBISCUS • HYPOXIS ROOPERI • LESPEDEZA • OAT • OKRA • OLIVE • ONION • PLATYCODON • PSYLLIUM • PUMPKIN • SAFFLOWER • SALEP • SARSAPARILLA • SOAPWORT, RED • SOLOMON'S SEAL, AROMATIC • SOY • SUNFLOWER • YAM, WILD • YUCCA

Diabetes Mellitus
[adjuvants; dietetic aids]

• AERVA • ARTICHOKE, JERUSALEM • BEAN, COMMON • BILBERRY • BONDUC • BURNET, THORN • CASCARA AMARGA • COPALCHI • COUCH GRASS • DOGWOOD, ASIATIC • FEN-UGREEK • GALANGAL, GREATER • GINSENG • GINSENG, SIBERIAN • GOAT'S RUE • GUAR • GYMNEMA • HOLY BASIL • JAMBOLAN • KINO TREE, INDIAN • LYCIUM • MAIDENHAIR FERN • MULBERRY • OKRA • OLIVE • ONION • QUINCE, FLOWERING • SAUNDERS, RED • SOLOMON'S SEAL, AROMATIC • STEVIA • TARRAGON

Overweight
[adjuvants; aids to weight-loss diets]

• BLADDERWRACK • CAROB • CARRAGEEN ALGAE • DULSE • FRANKINCENSE TREE • GUAR • GUGGUL • GYMNEMA • SAMPHIRE • STERCULIA

Underweight (in convalescence)
[adjuvants]

• GINSENG, SIBERIAN

ENDOCRINE DISORDERS

Hyperthyroidism (= Basedow's Disease)

• BUGLEWEED

Endemic Goiter (= enlargement of thyroid gland due to iodine deficiency)

• BLADDERWRACK • NORI

Imbalance of Female Sex Hormones (disorders associated with)

See GYNECOLOGIC DISORDERS (**Premenstrual Syndrome = PMS; Amenorrhea; Oligomenorrhea; Menopausal Syndrome**)
See also • ALFALFA • RED CLOVER • SOY

ARTICULAR AND MUSCULOSKELETAL DISORDERS

Rheumatic Pains (articular, periarticular / nonarticular); **Muscular Pains** (= Myalgias)
[external applications]

• ACONITE • AMMONIAC • ANGELICA • ARNICA • ASH WEED • BACOPA • BALLOON VINE • BEEBALM • BITTER CANDYTUFT • BLUE FLAG • BRYONY • BUTTERNUT • CABBAGE • CAJUPUT • CALAMUS • CAMPHOR • CAPER, THREE-LEAF • CAPSICUM • CEDAR, EASTERN RED • CHAPARRAL • CINNAMON, WHITE • COW PARSNIP, AMERICAN • CRESS, GARDEN • CRESS, INDIAN • CRESS, SCURVY • CRESS, WATER • CROTON • DONG QUAI • DUCKWEED • ECHINACEA • EUCALYPTUS • FIR • GALBANUM • GARLIC • GINGER • GUAIACUM • HORSERADISH • HORSERADISH TREE • JASMINE • LABRADOR TEA, MARSH • LAVENDER • LEMONGRASS • LIVERWORT • MEZEREON • MOUNTAIN LAUREL • MUDAR • MUSTARD • MUSTARD, GARLIC • MUSTARD , WHITE • NEEM • NETTLE • NUTMEG • OAT • OREGANO • PELLITORY, SPANISH • PEPPER • PEPPER TREE, PERUVIAN • PEPPERMINT • PINE • PIPSISSEWA • POPLAR • PRICKLY ASH, SOUTHERN • PULSATILLA • ROSEMARY • RUE • SANDARAC TREE • SAVIN • SKUNK CABBAGE • SPILANTHES • ST. JOHN'S WORT • STAVESACRE • STEPHANIA • TANSY • THUJA • THYME • VIRGIN'S BOWER • WINTER'S BARK • WINTERGREEN • YERBA SANTA

Rheumatic Complaints (chiefly Rheumatoid Arthritis)
[internal applications]

• ACHYRANTHES • AGARWOOD, CHINESE • AKEBIA • ASH, EUROPEAN • ASHWAGANDHA • BALLOON VINE • BORAGE • Bromelain (see PINEAPPLE) • CAT'S CLAW • COWSLIP • DEVIL'S CLAW • DONG QUAI • ECLIPTA • EUCOMMIA • EVENING PRIMROSE • FEVERFEW • FRANKINCENSE TREE • GELSEMIUM • GINGER • GUAIACUM • GUGGUL • HEARTSEASE • HYPOXIS ROOPERI • INDIAN PIPE • LICORICE • LOVAGE, CHINESE • MEADOWSWEET • NETTLE • OLIVE • PEONY, CHINESE • PEONY, TREE • POKE • POPLAR • PRICKLY ASH, SOUTHERN • SPILANTHES • STEPHANIA • TURMERIC • WILLOW • YUCCA
See also VARIOUS EFFECTS AND USES (**Antidyscratics** = blood purifiers = depuratives = blood cleansers)

Gout (= crystal-induced arthritis = Arthritis urica)

• AUTUMN CROCUS

430

Osteoporosis

[adjuvants for the prevention of postmenopausal osteoporosis]

See GYNECOLOGIC DISORDERS (**Menopausal Syndrome**)

Sprains; Bruises (= Contusions)

• ANGELICA • ARNICA • ARNICA, FALSE • BEAR'S FOOT • BEDSTRAW • BLUE FLAG • Bromelain (see PINEAPPLE) • BRYONY • BUTTERNUT • CALENDULA • COMFREY • COW PARSNIP, AMERICAN • DEER'S TONGUE • FRINGE TREE • GALBANUM • HEMLOCK, POISON • HORSE CHESTNUT • HYSSOP • LABRADOR TEA, MARSH • MELILOT, YELLOW • MILKWEED, BUTTERFLY • MULLEIN • ONION • PEPPERMINT • PERUVIAN BALSAM TREE • POKE • QUILLAJA • RUE • SAFFLOWER • SOLOMON'S SEAL, AROMATIC • SPILANTHES • ST. JOHN'S WORT • STONEROOT • YERBA SANTA

FATIGUE; FEELING OF WEAKNESS; DECREASED MENTAL AND PHYSICAL PERFORMANCE; CONVALESCENCE

Adaptogens

• ASHWAGANDHA • ASTRAGALUS • CODONOPSIS • GINSENG • GINSENG, SIBERIAN • HOLY BASIL • Medicinal Mushrooms (Artist's Conk, Kawaratake, Maitake, Poria, Reishi, Shiitake, Suehirotake; see BETA GLUCANS) • SCHISANDRA • SCHISANDRA, JAPANESE

Minor Tonics (Bitter Tonics, Minor Immunomodulants, Minor Performance Enhancers, etc.)

• AGARWOOD, CHINESE • AJUGA • AMBRETTE • ANDROGRAPHIS • ANGOSTURA • ANGURATÉ • ARTICHOKE • BACCHARIS TRIMERA • BEAR'S FOOT • BEET, RED • BETONY, WOOD • BLESSED THISTLE • BOG BEAN • BONESET • BUPLEURUM • CALAMUS • CANCHALAGUA • CASCARILLA • CEDRON • CENTAURY • CHIRATA • CHLORELLA • CINCHONA • CINNAMON • CINNAMON, WHITE • COLUMBO, AMERICAN • COSTUS • CURRY, INDIAN • DAMIANA • DOGWOOD, ASIATIC • DOGWOOD, FLOWERING • EUCOMMIA • FENUGREEK • GALANGAL, GREATER • GALANGAL, LESSER • GENTIAN • GINGER • GRAINS-OF-PARADISE • HEMIDESMUS • HEMP AGRIMONY • HOLY BASIL • HONEYSUCKLE • HYSSOP • LICORICE • LYCIUM • MARCELA • MARJORAM • MATICO • MOSS, ICELAND • MOUNTAIN ASH, AMERICAN • NORI • NUX-VOMICA • OAT • OLIVE • PAU D'ARCO • PEONY, CHINESE • PEONY, EUROPEAN • PEPPER • QUASSIA • REHMANNIA • ROSEMARY • RUDBECKIA • SKULLCAP • SOY • TURMERIC • TURMERIC, JAVANESE • WORMWOOD

Tonics / Stimulants

• CACAO • CEREUS, NIGHT-BLOOMING • COFFEE • COLA • EPHEDRA • GUARANÁ • HORSERADISH TREE • JUJUBE • KHAT • MATÉ • MUIRA PUAMA • NUTMEG • RHODIOLA • TEA

VARIOUS EFFECTS AND USES

Immunomodulants

1) For common and relapsing infections especially in the upper respiratory and genitourinary tracts

• ASTRAGALUS • BETA GLUCANS • BUPLEURUM • CAT'S CLAW • CHAMOMILE, GERMAN • CODONOPSIS • ECHINACEA • ELDER, EUROPEAN • GINSENG, SIBERIAN • HEMP AGRIMONY • HONEYSUCKLE • INDIGO, WILD • MARCELA • Medicinal Mushrooms (Artist's Conk, Kawaratake, Maitake, Poria, Reishi, Shiitake, Suehirotake; see BETA GLUCANS) • OLIVE • QUILLAJA • RUDBECKIA • SCHISANDRA • SCHISANDRA, JAPANESE • THUJA • UMCKALOABO

2) For cancer
[mainly to enhance the effects of a therapy]

• ASTRAGALUS • BETA GLUCANS • CAT'S CLAW • Medicinal Mushrooms (Artist's Conk, Kawaratake, Maitake, Poria, Reishi, Shiitake, Suehirotake; see BETA GLUCANS) • MISTLETOE, EUROPEAN

Antitumorals
[botanicals with constituents that counteract or prevent the formation of malignant tumors]

• AERVA • ASHWAGANDHA • BIRCH • BUPLEURUM • CHAPARRAL • CINNAMON • DEER'S TONGUE • FLAX • GALANGAL, LESSER • GAYFEATHER • HENNA • HOLY THORN • JASMINE • Medicinal Mushrooms (Artist's Conk, Kawaratake, Maitake, Poria, Reishi, Shiitake, Suehirotake; see BETA GLUCANS) • MEZEREON • MISTLETOE, EUROPEAN • MUDAR • OLIVE • PAU D'ARCO • PEPPER TREE, BRAZILIAN • PERIWINKLE, MADAGASCAR • PLANTAIN • RHODIOLA • SEA BUCKTHORN • SOY • TONKA • TRICHOSANTHES • TURMERIC • TURMERIC, JAVANESE
See also **Immunomodulants** (for cancer)

Antioxidants
[here: botanicals with constituents that protect from the formation of free radicals]

• ACEROLA • ALFALFA • ALLSPICE • ARTICHOKE • ASHWAGANDHA • ATRACTYLODES, BAI-ZHU • BARBERRY • BEARSFOOT • BILBERRY • BOLDO • BUCKWHEAT • CABBAGE • CACAO • CAPER BUSH • CAPER, THREE-LEAF • CLOVE • CRESS, GARDEN • CRESS, INDIAN • CRESS, SCURVY • CRESS, WATER • CUDWEED, FRAGRANT • CURRANT, BLACK • DOGWOOD, ASIATIC • EASTERN HEMLOCK • EPIMEDIUM • FO-TI • GINKGO • GINSENG • GRAINS-OF-PARADISE • GRAPE • GUARANÁ • HAWTHORN • HONEYSUCKLE • HORSERADISH • JUJUBE • KUDZU • LEMON • LEMONGRASS • LESPEDEZA • LYCIUM • MARJORAM • MATICO • MILK THISTLE • MUSTARD, GARLIC • MUSTARD, WHITE • OLIVE • OREGANO • OSWEGO TEA • Paprika (see CAPSICUM) • PEPPER • LOOSESTRIFE, PURPLE • RADISH, BLACK • REHMANNIA • ROOIBOS • ROSE • ROSEMARY • SAFFRON • SAGE • SAGE, GREEK • SAGE, RED-ROOT • SAMPHIRE • SAVORY • SEA BUCKTHORN • SPRUCE • STRAWBERRY • TEA • THYME • TOMATO • TURMERIC • TURMERIC, JAVANESE • VERBENA, LEMON • WINTER CHERRY • YERBA SANTA

Antidyscratics (= blood purifiers = depuratives = blood cleansers)
[botanicals used for atopic eczema = chronic eczema of internal origin, and chronic rheumatic complaints]

• AJUGA • AKEBIA • ALETRIS • ASH WEED • ASPARAGUS • ASTRAGALUS • BALMONY • BEAN, COMMON • BEDSTRAW • BIRCH • BITTERSWEET • BLUE FLAG • BROOKLIME • BRYONY • BURDOCK • CAPER, THREE-LEAF • CAREX, SAND • CEDAR, EASTERN RED • CELERY • CHERVIL • CHICKWEED • COMBRETUM MICRANTHUM • COUCH GRASS • CRESS, WATER • CURRANT, BLACK • DAISY, GARDEN • DANDELION • DEVIL'S BIT • DODDER • DUCKWEED • DYER'S BROOM • ECLIPTA • ELDER, EUROPEAN • ELECAMPANE • FIGWORT • FO-TI • FUMITORY • GALE, SWEET • GARDENIA • GINGER, CREPE • GOLDENROD • GUAIACUM • HEARTSEASE • HEMIDESMUS • HOLLY • HORSERADISH • JAVA TEA • JOE PYE • LABRADOR TEA, MARSH • LICORICE • MANACÁ • MEZEREON • MUS-

TARD, GARLIC • NETTLE • NETTLE, WHITE • PARSLEY • PELLITORY-OF-THE-WALL • PILEWORT • QUINCE, FLOWERING • RED CLOVER • REHMANNIA • RESTHARROW • RUP-TUREWORT • SALSIFY, SPANISH • SARSAPARILLA • SAUNDERS, RED • SAXIFRAGE, BUR-NET • SLOE • SOAPWORT, RED • SORREL • SPEEDWELL • SPIKENARD • STILLINGIA • TRICHOSANTHES • VIRGIN'S BOWER • WAHOO • YELLOW CHASTE WEED • YERBA SAN-TA

Antimalarials

• CEDRON • CHANG SHAN • CINCHONA • COPALCHI • DOGWOOD, FLOWERING • NEEM • TREE-OF-HEAVEN, CHINESE • WORMWOOD, SWEET

Insecticides; Insect-repellents

• AMBRETTE • BASIL • BAY-RUM-TREE • CAJUPUT • CEDAR, EASTERN RED • GALE, SWEET • LEMONGRASS • NEEM • PATCHOULY • PENNYROYAL, AMERICAN • PENNY-ROYAL, EUROPEAN • PYRETHRUM • QUASSIA • SANTOLINA • SPILANTHES • TANSY • VETIVER

Potassium Supplements

• ARTICHOKE, JERUSALEM • ASPARAGUS • AVOCADO • BACOPA • CHERVIL • CRESS, GARDEN • DANDELION • GRAPE • JAVA TEA • POTATO • TAMARIND • TOMATO

Vitamin C Supplements

• ACEROLA • BARBERRY • CRESS, GARDEN • CRESS, INDIAN • CRESS, SCURVY • CUR-RANT, BLACK • HORSERADISH • JUJUBE • MOUNTAIN ASH, EUROPEAN • Paprika (see CAPSICUM) • ROSE • SEA BUCKTHORN • WINTER CHERRY

Skin Care and Cosmetic Ingredients (excluding fragrance ingredients)

• ALMOND • ALOE • AVOCADO • CACAO • CALENDULA • CARNAUBA WAX PALM • CAS-TOR • CLUBMOSS • CUCUMBER • JOJOBA • KELP • NARAS • OLIVE • PEACH • PEANUT • QUINCE • SAFFLOWER • SEA BUCKTHORN • STERCULIA • SUNFLOWER

Suspending, Emulsifying, Gelling, Thickening, and Binding Ingredients

• AGAR • CAROB • CARRAGEEN ALGAE • GUAR • GUM ARABIC TREE • KELP • SALEP • STERCULIA • TRAGACANTH MILKVETCH

Flavor Ingredients

• AGARIC • ALLSPICE • AMBRETTE • ANGELICA • ANGOSTURA • ANISE • ANISE, STAR • ASAFETIDA • BASIL • BACCHARIS TRIMERA • BAILAHUÉN • BAY • BAY-RUM-TREE • BEAR'S GARLIC • BETONY, MARSH • BETONY, WOOD • BLACK CHERRY • BLESSED THIS-TLE • CALAMINT • CALAMUS • CAPER BUSH • CARAWAY • CARAWAY, BLACK • CAR-DAMOM • CARDAMOM, AMOMUM • CARLINE THISTLE • CASCARILLA • CELERY • CHER-RY LAUREL • CHERVIL • CHIVE • CINNAMON • CINNAMON, WHITE • CLARY SAGE • CLOVE • COFFEE • CORIANDER • COSTUS • CRESS, GARDEN • CRESS, INDIAN • CRESS, SCURVY • CRESS, WATER • CUBEB • CUMIN • CURRY, INDIAN • DEER'S TONGUE • DILL • EUCALYPTUS • FENNEL • FIG • GALANGAL, GREATER • GALANGAL, LESSER • GALBA-NUM • GALE, SWEET • GENTIAN • GINGER • GINGER, CANADIAN WILD • GRAINS-OF-PARADISE • GUARANÁ • HORSERADISH • HORSERADISH TREE • HYSSOP • JASMINE • JUNIPER • LEMON • LEMONGRASS • LICORICE • LIME • LIPPIA, MEXICAN • LOCUST, BLACK • LOVAGE • MAIDENHAIR FERN • MARJORAM • MATICO • MUGWORT • MOSS, ICELAND • MULBERRY • MUSTARD • MUSTARD, GARLIC • MUSTARD, WHITE • NUTMEG • ORANGE, BITTER • OREGANO • OREGANO, MEXICAN • ORRIS • PEPPER • PEPPER TREE, PERUVIAN • PEPPERMINT • PIPSISSEWA • QUASSIA • QUINCE • RADISH, BLACK • RASP-BERRY • ROSE • ROSEMARY • SAFFRON • SAGE • SAGE, GREEK • SAGE, SPANISH • SAR-

SAPARILLA • SAVORY • SAXIFRAGE, BURNET • SOUTHERNWOOD • SPEARMINT • STEVIA • STORAX • SUMBUL • TANSY • TARRAGON • THYME • THYME, LEMON • TOLU BALSAM TREE • TONKA • TURMERIC • TURMERIC, JAVANESE • VANILLA • VETIVER • WINTERGREEN • WINTER'S BARK • WOODRUFF • WORMWOOD • YARROW, MUSK • YERBA SANTA • ZEDOARY

Fragrance Ingredients

• AMBRETTE • BASIL • BAY • BENZOIN TREE • CARAWAY • CARAWAY, BLACK • CASCARILLA • CEDAR, EASTERN RED • CLARY SAGE • COPAIBA • CORIANDER • COSTUS • DEER'S TONG • EASTERN HEMLOCK • EUCALYPTUS • FIR • FRANKINCENSE TREE • GALBANUM • GINGER, CANADIAN WILD • HYSSOP • JASMINE • LAVENDER • LEMONGRASS • LIME • MASTIC TREE • MOSS, OAK • ORRIS • PATCHOULY • PENNYROYAL, AMERICAN • PENNYROYAL, EUROPEAN • PERUVIAN BALSAM TREE • PINE • ROSE • ROSEMARY • SAGE • SAGE, SPANISH • SANDALWOOD • SANDARAC TREE • SUMBUL • TOLU BALSAM TREE • TONKA • VETIVER • WOODRUFF • YLANG YLANG

Coloring Ingredients; Appearance Enhancers

• ALKANET • ANNATTO • CORNFLOWER • ELDER, EUROPEAN • GARDENIA • HOLLYHOCK • LARKSPUR, FORKING • MULBERRY • PEONY, EUROPEAN • POPPY, FIELD • SAFFLOWER • SAFFRON • SAUNDERS, RED • SUNFLOWER • TURMERIC • YELLOW CHASTE WEED

REFERENCES

(1) Hänsel, R., Keller, K., Rimpler, H., Schneider, G. (Eds.): *Hagers Handbuch der Pharmazeutischen Praxis*, 5th Ed., Springer-Verlag, Berlin, Vol. 4 (1992), Vol. 5 (1993), Vol. 6 (1994).

(2) Blaschek, W., Hänsel, R., Keller, K., Reichlig, J., Rimpler, H., Schneider, G. (Eds.): *Hagers Handbuch der Pharmazeutischen Praxis*, 5th Ed., Springer-Verlag, Berlin, subsequent Vol. 2 (1998), subsequent Vol. 3 (1998).

(3) List, P. H., Hörhammer, L. (Eds.): *Hagers Handbuch der Pharmazeutischen Praxis*, 4th Ed., Springer-Verlag, Berlin, Vol. 2 (1969), Vol. 3 (1972), Vol. 4 (1973), Vol. 5 (1976), Vol. 6a (1977), Vol. 6b (1979), Vol. 6c (1979).

(4) Frerichs, G., Arends, G., Zörnig, H. (Eds.): *Hagers Handbuch der Pharmazeutischen Praxis*, 2nd Ed. (rev.), Verlag von Julius Springer, 2 Vols., 1938.

(5) Hoppe, H. A.: *Drogenkunde*, 8th Ed., Walter de Gruyter, Berlin, Vol. 1 (1975), Vol. 2 (1977), Vol. 3 (1987).

(6) Wagner, H., Wiesenauer, M.: *Phytotherapie*, Gustav Fischer Verlag, Stuttgart, 1995.

(7) Schulz, V., Hänsel, R.: *Rationale Phytotherapie*, 3rd Ed., Springer-Verlag, Berlin, 1996.

(8) Braun, H., Frohne, D.: *Heilpflanzenlexikon*, 6th Ed., Gustav Fischer Verlag, Stuttgart, 1994.

(9) Leung, A. Y., Foster, S.: *Encyclopedia of Common Natural Ingredients*, 2nd Ed., John Wiley & Sons, New York, 1996.

(10) Wren, R. C., revised by Williamson, E. M. and Evans, F. J.: *Potter's New Cyclopaedia of Botanical Drugs and Preparations*, C. W. Daniel Co., Saffron Walden, 1988.

(11) Robbers, J. E., Speedie, M. K., Tyler, V. E.: *Pharmacognosy and Pharmacobiotechnology*, Williams & Wilkins, Baltimore, 1996.

(11a) Tyler, V. E., Brady, L. R., Robbers, J. E.: *Pharmacognosy*, 9th Ed., Lea & Fabiger, Philadelphia, 1988.

(12) Hänsel, R., Sticher, O., Steinegger, E.: *Pharmakognosie-Phytopharmazie*, 6th Ed., Springer-Verlag, Berlin, 1999.

(12a) Steinegger, E., Hänsel, R.: *Pharmakognosie*, 5th Ed., Springer-Verlag, Berlin, 1992.

(12b) Steinegger, E., Hänsel, R.: *Pharmakognosie*, 3rd Ed., Springer-Verlag, Berlin, 1972.

(13) Wagner, H.: *Arzneidrogen und Ihre Inhaltsstoffe* (*Pharmazeutische Biologie*, Bd. 2), 6th Ed., Wissenschaftliche Verlagsgesellschaft mbH, Stuttgart, 1999.

(13a) Wagner, H.: *Pharmazeutische Biologie*, Bd. 2 (*Drogen und Ihre Inhaltsstoffe*), 5th Ed., Gustav Fischer Verlag, Stuttgart, 1993.

(13b) Wagner, H.: *Pharmazeutische Biologie*, Bd. 2 (*Drogen und Ihre Inhaltsstoffe*), 2nd Ed., Gustav Fischer Verlag, Stuttgart, 1980.

(14) Bradley, P. R. (Ed.): *British Herbal Compendium,* BHMA, Bournemouth, 1992.

(15) *British Herbal Pharmacopoeia*, 2nd Ed., BHMA, Bournemouth, 1983.

(16) Reuter, H. D.: *Therapie mit Phytopharmaka*, Gustav Fischer Verlag, Ulm, 1997.

(17) Wichtl, M. (Ed.): *Teedrogen und Phytopharmaka*, 3rd Ed., Wissenschaftliche Verlagsgesellschaft mbH, Stuttgart, 1997.

(18) Frohne, D., Jensen, U.: *Systematik des Pflanzenreichs*, 5th Ed., Wissenschaftliche Verlagsgesellschaft mbH, Stuttgart, 1998.

(19) Schilcher, H., Kammerer, S.: *Leitfaden Phytotherapie*, Urban & Fischer Verlag, München, 2000.

(20) Newall, C. A., Anderson, L. A., Phillipson, J. D.: *Herbal Medicines*, The Pharmaceutical Press, 1996.

(21) Foster, S., Tyler, V. E.: *Tyler's Honest Herbal*, 4th Ed., The Haworth Herbal Press, New York, 1999.

(22) Robbers, J. E., Tyler, V. E.: *Tyler's Herbs of Choice,* The Haworth Herbal Press, New York, 1999.

(23) Weiss, R. F., Fintelmann, V.: *Lehrbuch der Phytotherapie*, 9th Ed., Hippokrates Verlag, Stuttgart, 1999.

(24) Pahlow, M.: *Das Grosse Buch der Heilpflanzen*, Gräfe und Unzer, München, 1979.

(25) Foster, S., Duke, J.: *A Field Guide to Medicinal Plants,* Houghton Mifflin Co., Boston, 1990.

(26) Duke, J.: *Dr. Duke's Essential Herbs*, Rodale Inc., Emmaus, 1999.

(27) Cecchini, T.: *Enciclopedia delle Erbe Medicinali*, De Vecchi Editore, Milano, 1992.

(28) Penso, G.: *Piante Medicinali nella Terapia Medica*, 2nd Ed., Organizzazione Editoriale Medico Farmaceutica, Milano, 1987.

(29) McGuffin, M., Hobbs, C., Upton, R., Goldberg, A. (Eds.): *American Herbal Products Association's Botanical Safety Handbook*, CRC Press, Boca Raton, 1997.

(30) Duke, J.: *Handbook of Medicinal Herbs*, CRC Press, Boca Raton, 1995.

(31) Harborne, J. B., Baxter, H.: *Phytochemical Dictionary*, Taylor & Francis, London, 1993.

(32) Gibbs, R. D.: *Chemotaxonomy of Flowering Plants*, McGill-Queen's University Press, Montreal, 4 Vols., 1974.

(33) Steinmetz, E. F.: *Codex Vegetabilis*, E. F. Steinmetz, Amsterdam, Netherlands, 1957.

(34) McGuffin, M., Kartesz, J. T., Leung A. Y, Tucker, A. O.: *Herbs of Commerce*, 2nd Ed., American Herbal Products Association, Silver Spring, 2000.

(35) Grieve, M.: *A Modern Herbal*, Harcourt, Brace & Company, 1931, 2 Vols. (reprint Dover Publications, New York, 1971).

(36) Evans, W. C.: *Trease and Evans' Pharmacognosy*, WB Saunders Company Ltd., London, 1996.

(37) Burger, A., Wachter, H.: *Hunnius Pharmazeutisches Wörterbuch*, 8th Ed., Walter de Gruyter, Berlin, 1998.

(38) Blumenthal, M. et al. (Eds.): *The Complete Commission E Monographs*, American Botanical Council, Austin, 1998.

(39) Skenderi, G.: *Chemical and Pharmacological Bases of Phytotherapy* (Pharmacy Postgraduate Lectures, in Albanian), Tirana, 1975-1985

(40) Moore, M.: *Medicinal Plants of the Mountain West*, 2nd Ed., Museum of New Mexico Press, 2003.

(41) Buckingham, J. (Ed.): *Dictionary of Natural Products*, 7 Vols., Chapman & Hall, London, 1994.

(42) Hegnauer, R.: *Chemotaxonomie der Pflanzen*, Birkhäuser Verlag, Basel: Vol. 1 (1962), Vol. 2 (1963), Vol. 3 (1964), Vol. 4 (1966), Vol. 5 (1969), Vol. 6 (1973).

(43) Kartesz, T.: *A Synonymized Checklist of the Vascular Flora of the United States, Canada, and Greenland*, 2nd ed., Timber Press, Portland, 2 Vols., 1994.

(44) Moerman, D. E.: *Native American Ethnobotany*, Timber Press, Portland, 1998.

(45) Chevallier, A.: *The Encyclopedia of Medicinal Plants*, DK Publishing Inc., New York, 1996.

(46) Benigni, R., Capra, C., Cattorini, P. E.: *Piante Medicinali* (Chimica, Farmacologia e Terapia), Inverni & Della Beffa, Milano, Vol. 1 (1962), Vol. 2 (1964).

(47) Madaus, G.: *Lehrbuch der Biologischen Heilmittel*, Georg Thieme Verlag, Leipzig, 1938, 3 Vols. (reprint Georg Olms Verlag, Hildesheim, 1976).

(48) Bruneton, J.: *Pharmacognosy*, 2nd Ed. (translated by Hatton, C. K.), Intercept Ltd., London, 1999.

(49) Paris, R. R., Moyse, H.: *Précis de Matière Médicale*, Masson & Co., Paris, Vol. 1 (1965), Vol. 2 (1967), Vol. 3 (1971).

(50) Jacob, L. S.: *Pharmacology*, 3rd Ed., Williams & Wilkins, Baltimore, 1992.

(51) Bäsler, F.: *Heilpflanzen*, Neumann Verlag, Radebeul, 1956.

(52) Hocking, G. M.: *A Dictionary of Natural Products*, Plexus Publishing, Inc., Medford, 1997.

(53) Foster, S., Chongxi, Y.: *Herbal Emissaries*, Healing Arts Press, Rochester, 1992.

(54) Huang, K. C.: *The Pharmacology of Chinese Herbs*, 2nd Ed., CRC Press, Boca Raton, 1999.

(55) Pratt, R., Youngken, H. W.: *Pharmacognosy*, 2nd Ed., J. B. Lippincott Co., Philadelphia, 1956.

(56) Janson, M.: Dr. *Janson's New Vitamin Revolution*, Avery, New York, 2000.

(57) Johnson, T.: *CRC Ethnobotany Desk Reference*, CRC Press, Boca Raton, 1999.

(58) Tyler, V. E.: *Hoosier Home Remedies*, Purdue University Press, West Lafayette, 1985.

(59) *WHO monographs on selected medicinal plants*, Vol. 1, WHO Geneva, 1999.

(59a) *WHO monographs on selected medicinal plants*, Vol. 2, WHO Geneva, 2002.

(60) Shetler, G. S., Skog, L. E.: *A Provisional Checklist of Species for Flora North America*, Missouri Botanical Garden, St. Louis, 1978.

(61) Schultes, R. E., Raffauf, R. F.: *The Healing Forest*, Dioscorides Press, Portland, 1990.

(62) Balick, M. J., Cox, P. A.: *Plants, People, and Cultures,* Scientific American Library, New York, 1996.

(63) Craker, L. E., Simon, J. E. (Eds.): *Herbs, Spices, and Medicinal Plants*, Haworth Press, Inc., New York, Vol. 1 (1992), Vol. 2 (1991), Vol. 3 (1996), Vol. 4 (1995).

(64) Fernald, M. L.: *Gray's Manual of Botany*, 8th Ed., American Book Company, New York, 1950.

(65) Sollmann, T.: *A Manual of Pharmacology*, 7th Ed., W. B. Saundres Company, Philadelphia, 1948.

(66) Potter, S. O. L.: *Therapeutics, Materia Medica and Pharmacy*, 12th Ed., P. Blakiston's Son & Co., Philadelphia, 1912.

(67) Delgado, J.M., Remers, W. A. (Eds.): *Wilson and Gisvold's Textbook of Organic Medicinal and Pharmaceutical Chemistry*, 10th Ed., Lippincott-Raven, Philadelphia, 1998.

(68) DerMarderosian, A. (Ed.): *Guide to Popular Natural Products*, Facts and Comparisons, St. Louis, 1999.

(69) Balch, J. F., Balch, P. A.: *Prescription for Nutritional Healing*, 2nd Ed., Avery Publishing Group, Garden City Park, 1997.

(70) Weil, A.: *Spontaneous Healing*, Fawcett Columbine, New York, 1995.

(71) Hudson, T.: *Women's Encyclopedia of Natural Medicine*, Keats Publishing, Los Angeles, 1999.

(72) *Rote Liste 1994*, BPI (Ed.), Editio Cantor Verlag, Aulendorf

(73) *Codex Galenica 1992*, Galenica AG, Bern.

(74) *Dictionnaire Vidal 1993*, French & European Publications, Paris.

(75) Bratman, S., Kroll, D. (Eds.): *Natural Health Bible*, Prima Publishing, 1999.

(76) Kuhn, M. A., Winston, D.: Winston & Kuhn's Herbal Therapy & Supplements, 2nd. Ed., Wolters Kluwer, LWW, Philadelphia, etc., 2008

(77) Harvey, A.: *Drugs from Natural Products*, Ellis Horwood, New York, 1993.

(78) Reis, S. von, Lipp, F. J.: *New Plant Sources for Drugs and Foods from The New York Botanical Garden Herbarium*, Harvard University Press, Cambridge, 1982.

(79) Balick, M. J. et al. (Eds.): *Medicinal Resources of the Tropical Forest*, Columbia University Press, New York, 1996.

(80) Burger, A. (Ed.): *Medicinal Chemistry*, 2nd Ed., Interscience Publishers, New York, 1960.

(81) Schultes, R. E., Reis, S. von (Eds.): *Ethnobotany, Evolution of a Discipline*, Dioscorides Press, Portland, 1995.

(82) Brinker, F.: *Herb Contraindications and Drug Interactions*, Eclectic Medical Publications, Sandy, 1998.

(83) Berkow, R. et al. (Eds.): *The Merck Manual of Medical Information, Home Edition*, Pocket Books, New York, 1997.

(84) Tierney, Jr., et al. (Eds.): *Current Medical Diagnosis & Treatment*, 41st Ed., Lange Medical Books / McGraw-Hill, New York, 2002.

(85) Defacqz, Ed.: *L' Officine*, 16th Ed., Vigot Frères Editeurs, Paris, 1923.

(86) Mashkovskij, M. D.: *Lekarstvenie Sredstva*, 13th Ed., Torsing, Harkov, 2 Vols., 1997.

(87) Craciun, F., Bojor, O., Mircea, A.: *Farmacia naturii*, Editura Ceres, Bucuresti, Vol. 1 (1976), Vol. 2 (1977).

(88) Mowrey, D. B.: *Herbal Tonic Therapies*, Keats Publishing, New Canaan, 1993.

(89) Murray, M. T.: *The Healing Power of Herbs*, 2nd Ed., Prima Publishing, Rocklin, 1995.

(90) Hoffmann, D.: *Medical Herbalism*, Healing Arts Press / Inner Traditions, Rochester, 2003.

(91) *Die Präparate-Liste 2000*, Urban & Fischer Verlag, München, 2000.

(92) Tierra, M.: *The Way of Chinese Herbs*, Pocket Books / Simon & Schuster, New York, 1998.

(93) Germano, C., Ramazanov, Z.: *Arctic Root* (Rhodiola rosea), Kensington Publishing Corp., New York, 1999.

(94) *Remington: The Science and Practice of Pharmacy*, 21st Ed., Lippincott Williams & Wilkins, Philadelphia, 2006.

(95) Kovaleva, N. G.: Lecenie Rastenijami, Izdatelstvo "Medicina", Moskva, 1971

(96) Winston, D., Maimes, S.: *Adaptogens*, Healing Arts Press, Rochester, 2007.

438

INDEX

Monographs (in capitals), Common Names (in regular types), Latin Botanical Names (in italics), Disorders and Various Effects and Uses (in bold types). In the THERAPEUTIC CHECKLIST (pp. 413-434), disorders are classified according to the organ systems. Ds = disorders

439

440

442

444

445

446

447

449

454

456

457

458

460

461

462

463

464

465

466

468

470

474

476

478